NEUROLOGY AND NEUROSURGERY ILLUSTRATED

NEUROLOGY AND NEUROSURGERY ILLUSTRATED

KENNETH W. LINDSAY PhD FRCS

Consultant Neurosurgeon, Institute of Neurological Sciences;
Honorary Clinical Senior Lecturer, University of Glasgow, UK
Formerly Consultant Neurosurgeon, Royal Free Hospital;
Honorary Senior Lecturer, Royal Free Hospital School of Medicine,
University of London, UK

IAN BONE FRCP (L and G)

Consultant Neurologist, Institute of Neurological Sciences;
Honorary Clinical Senior Lecturer, University of Glasgow,
UK

ROBIN CALLANDER FFPh FMAA AIMI

Medical Illustrator
Formerly Director of Medical Illustration, University of Glasgow

SECOND
EDITION

CHURCHILL LIVINGSTONE
EDINBURGH LONDON MELBOURNE AND NEW YORK 1991

CHURCHILL LIVINGSTONE
Medical Division of Pearson Professional Ltd

Distributed in the United States of America by
Churchill Livingstone Inc., 650 Avenue of the Americas,
New York, 10011, and by associated companies, branches
and representatives throughout the world.

First Edition 1986
Second edition 1991
    Reprinted 1992 (twice)
    Reprinted 1993 (twice)
    Reprinted 1994
    Reprinted 1995 (twice)

ISBN 0-443-04345-0

British Library Cataloguing in Publication Data.
A catalogue record for this book is available from the British Library.

The
publisher's
policy is to use
paper manufactured
from sustainable forests

Printed in Hong Kong
LYP/08

FOREWORD

Ideally, medical students should learn even the first principles of neurology from patients, not from books. One reason is that in real life patients present with symptoms, not with a diagnosis. Another reason is that the 'human interest' helps to retain factual information — after all, emotions and memory are processed in adjoining parts of the brain.

Textbooks should serve only as a frame of reference for the non-specialist. The design of the book by Lindsay, Bone and Callander makes it stand out against its competitors in several respects. The most conspicuous feature is the wealth of figures and diagrams, which make any other text look like a barren desert of words. Neurosurgery has been fully integrated as it should be. Yet the urge to achieve completeness has been firmly resisted. The subjects that interest only experts have been left out, with some sections in small print as a compromise. The chapters about the differential diagnosis of common symptoms will enhance the usefulness of the book in everyday practice. Finally, the authors have kept clear of many tenacious myths that perpetuate themselves through generations of textbooks (to name but a few: that enophthalmos is part of Horner's syndrome, that the Hoffmann reflex or finger jerk is a pathological sign, or that a slow pulse rate and a high blood pressure are useful signs of impending transtentorial herniation).

One can always quibble about details, and particularly about classifications. The only solution is for every teacher to write his or her personal text book. In my case I was so impressed with the general organisation of the book, that it was a pleasure to read through the first edition and submit my own views about a number of sections. I am sure that many students and general practitioners will use and cherish this book.

1991

J. van Gijn
Professor and Chairman
University Department of Neurology
Utrecht, The Netherlands.

PREFACE TO SECOND EDITION

This new edition updates the whole text and takes into account recent advances in imaging such as magnetic resonance scanning. The section on infection has been expanded in view of the neurological importance of disorders such as AIDS. In addition, there is further information on new developments in brain protection and tumour management.

As before, we thank our numerous friends and colleagues who have proffered suggestions and advice. In particular, we are most grateful to Professor van Gijn who has provided detailed comments throughout the book. Again we thank our families for their continual support.

1990

K.W. Lindsay
I. Bone
R. Callander

CONTENTS

GENERAL APPROACH TO HISTORY AND EXAMINATION

NERVOUS SYSTEM — HISTORY

An accurate description of the patient's neurological symptoms is an important aid in establishing the diagnosis; but this must be taken in conjunction with information from other systems, previous medical history, family and social history and current medication. Often the patient's history requires confirmation from a relative or friend.

The following outline indicates the relevant information to obtain for each symptom, although some may require further clarification.

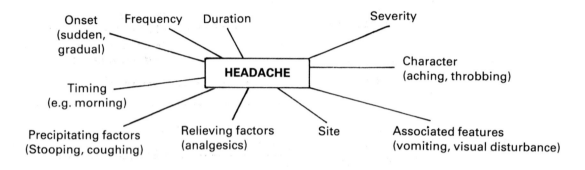

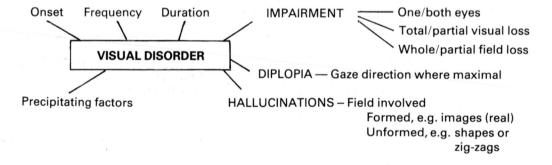

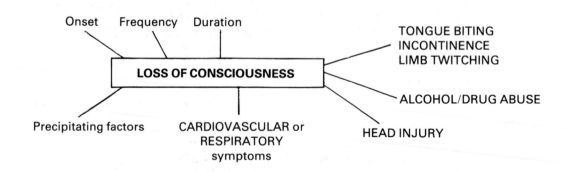

NERVOUS SYSTEM — HISTORY

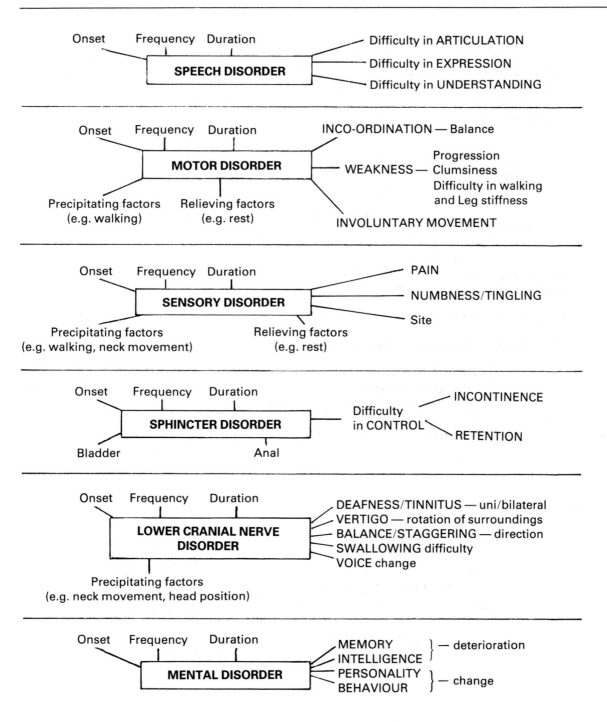

Onset Frequency Duration

SPEECH DISORDER
— Difficulty in ARTICULATION
— Difficulty in EXPRESSION
— Difficulty in UNDERSTANDING

Onset Frequency Duration

MOTOR DISORDER

Precipitating factors
(e.g. walking)

Relieving factors
(e.g. rest)

INCO-ORDINATION — Balance

WEAKNESS — Progression
Clumsiness
Difficulty in walking
and Leg stiffness

INVOLUNTARY MOVEMENT

Onset Frequency Duration

SENSORY DISORDER

Precipitating factors
(e.g. walking, neck movement)

Relieving factors
(e.g. rest)

— PAIN
— NUMBNESS/TINGLING
— Site

Onset Frequency Duration

SPHINCTER DISORDER

Bladder   Anal

Difficulty
in CONTROL
— INCONTINENCE
— RETENTION

Onset Frequency Duration

**LOWER CRANIAL NERVE
DISORDER**

Precipitating factors
(e.g. neck movement, head position)

DEAFNESS/TINNITUS — uni/bilateral
VERTIGO — rotation of surroundings
BALANCE/STAGGERING — direction
SWALLOWING difficulty
VOICE change

Onset Frequency Duration

MENTAL DISORDER

MEMORY
INTELLIGENCE } — deterioration
PERSONALITY
BEHAVIOUR } — change

3

NERVOUS SYSTEM — EXAMINATION

Neurological disease may produce systemic signs and systemic disease may affect the nervous system. A complete general examination must therefore accompany that of the central nervous system. In particular, note the following:

Temperature	Evidence of weight loss	Septic source, e.g. teeth, ears,
Blood pressure	Breast lumps	Skin marks, e.g. rashes
Neck stiffness	Lymphadenopathy	cafe-au-lait spots
Pulse irregularity	Hepatic and splenic	angiomata
Carotid bruit	enlargement	Anterior fontanelle } in baby
Cardiac murmurs	Prostatic irregularity	Head circumference
Cyanosis/respiratory insufficiency		

CNS examination is described systematically from the head downwards and includes:

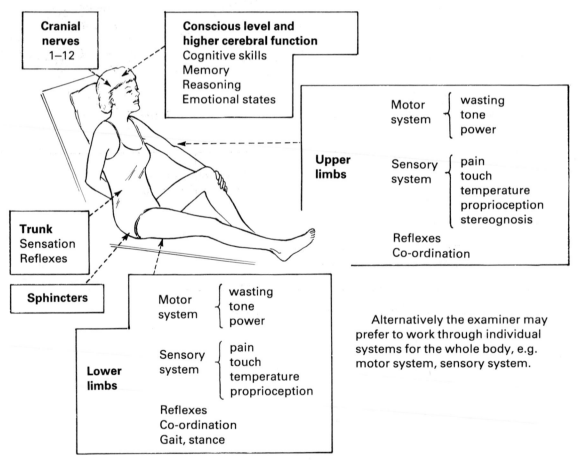

Cranial nerves 1–12

Conscious level and higher cerebral function
Cognitive skills
Memory
Reasoning
Emotional states

Upper limbs
Motor system { wasting / tone / power
Sensory system { pain / touch / temperature / proprioception / stereognosis
Reflexes
Co-ordination

Trunk
Sensation
Reflexes

Sphincters

Lower limbs
Motor system { wasting / tone / power
Sensory system { pain / touch / temperature / proprioception
Reflexes
Co-ordination
Gait, stance

Alternatively the examiner may prefer to work through individual systems for the whole body, e.g. motor system, sensory system.

EXAMINATION — CONSCIOUS LEVEL ASSESSMENT

A wide variety of systemic and intracranial problems produce depression of conscious level. Accurate assessment and recording are essential to determine deterioration or improvement in a patient's condition. In 1974 Teasdale and Jennett, in Glasgow, developed a system for conscious level assessment. They discarded vague terms such as stupor, semicoma and deep coma, and described conscious level in terms of EYE opening,
VERBAL response and
MOTOR response.
The Glasgow coma scale is now used widely in Britain and in many centres throughout the world. Recording is consistent irrespective of the status of the observer and can be carried out just as reliably by nurse as by neurosurgeon.

EYE OPENING

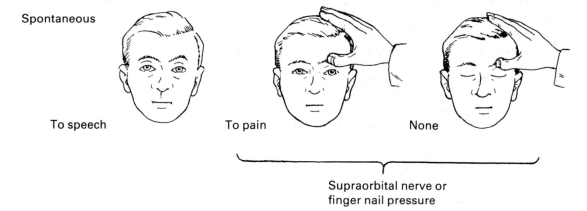

Spontaneous

To speech   To pain   None

Supraorbital nerve or
finger nail pressure

VERBAL RESPONSE

Orientated — Knows place, e.g. Royal Free Hospital
and time, e.g. day, month and year

Confused — Talking in sentences but disorientated in time and place

Words — Utters occasional words rather than sentences

Sounds — Groans or grunts, but no words

None

EXAMINATION — CONSCIOUS LEVEL ASSESSMENT

MOTOR RESPONSE

Obeys commands

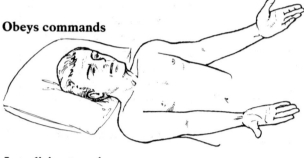

'Hold up your arms'

Localising to pain

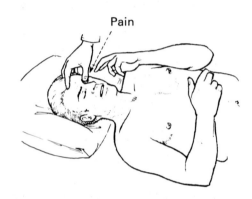

Pain

Apply a painful stimulus to the supraorbital nerve, e.g. rub thumb nail in the supraorbital groove, increasing pressure until a response is obtained. If the patient responds by bringing the hand up beyond the chin = 'localising to pain'. (Pressure to nail beds or sternum at this stage may not differentiate 'localising' from 'flexing'.)

Flexing to pain

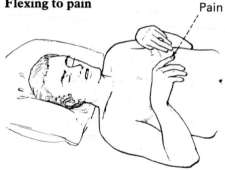

Pain

If the patient does not localise to supraorbital pressure, apply pressure with a pen or hard object to the nail bed. Record elbow flexion as 'flexing to pain'. Spastic wrist flexion may or may not accompany this response.

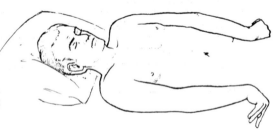

Extending to pain

If in response to the same stimulus elbow extension occurs, record as 'extending to pain'. This is always accompanied by spastic flexion of the wrist.

None

Before recording a patient at this level, ensure that the painful stimulus is adequate.

During examination the motor response may vary. Supraorbital pain may produce an extension response, whereas finger nail pressure produces flexion. Alternatively one arm may localise to pain; the other may flex. When this occurs record the *best* response during the period of examination (this correlates best with final outcome). For the purpose of conscious level assessment use only the *arm* response. Leg response to pain gives less consistent results, often producing movements arising from spinal rather than cerebral origin.

EXAMINATION — HIGHER CEREBRAL FUNCTION

COGNITIVE SKILL

	Dominant hemisphere disorders
Listen to language pattern — hesitant — fluent	Expressive dysphasia Receptive dysphasia
Does the patient understand simple/complex spoken commands? e.g. 'Hold up both arms, touch the right ear with the left fifth finger.'	Receptive dysphasia
Ask the patient to name objects.	Nominal dysphasia
Does the patient read correctly?	Dyslexia
Does the patient write correctly?	Dysgraphia
Ask the patient to perform a numerical calculation, e.g. serial 7 test, where 7 is subtracted serially from 100.	Dyscalculia
Can the patient recognise objects? e.g. ask patient to select an object from a group.	Agnosia
	Non-dominant hemisphere disorders
Note patient's ability to find his way around the ward or his home.	Geographical agnosia
Can the patient dress himself?	Dressing apraxia
Note the patient's ability to copy a geometric pattern, e.g. ask patient to form a star with matches or copy a drawing of a cube.	Constructional apraxia

7

EXAMINATION — HIGHER CEREBRAL FUNCTION

MEMORY test

Testing requires alertness and is not possible in a confused or dysphasic patient.

IMMEDIATE memory — Digit span — ask patient to repeat a sequence of 5, 6 or 7 random numbers.

RECENT memory — Ask patient to describe present illness, duration of hospital stay or recent events in the news.

REMOTE memory — Ask about events and circumstances occurring more than 5 years previously.

VERBAL memory — Ask patient to remember a sentence or a short story and test after 15 minutes.

VISUAL memory — Ask patient to remember objects on a tray and test after 15 minutes.

Note: Retrograde amnesia — loss of memory of events leading up to a brain injury or insult.

Post-traumatic amnesia — permanent loss of memory of events for a period following a head injury.

REASONING AND PROBLEM SOLVING

Test patient with two-step calculations, e.g. 'I wish to buy 12 articles at 7 pence each. How much change will I receive from £1?'

Ask patient to reverse 3 or 4 random numbers.

Ask patient to explain proverbs.

The examiner must compare patient's present reasoning ability with expected abilities based on job history and/or school work.

EMOTIONAL STATE

Note: Anxiety or excitement

Depression or apathy

Emotional behaviour

Uninhibited behaviour

Slowness of movement or responses.

CRANIAL NERVE EXAMINATION

OLFACTORY NERVE (I)

Test using aromatic non-irritant materials, e.g. soap, tobacco.

One nostril is closed while the patient sniffs with the other.

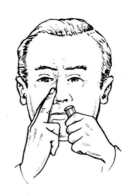

OPTIC NERVE (II)

Visual acuity

severe deficit — Can patient see light? movement?
Can patient count fingers?

mild deficit — Record reading acuity with wall or hand chart.

N.B. *Refractory error* (i.e. inadequate focussing on the retina, e.g. hypermetropia, myopia) can be overcome by testing reading acuity through a pinhole. This concentrates a thin beam of vision on the macula.

Jaeger type card for near vision, labelled according to size [N5 (smallest print) – N48 (largest print)].

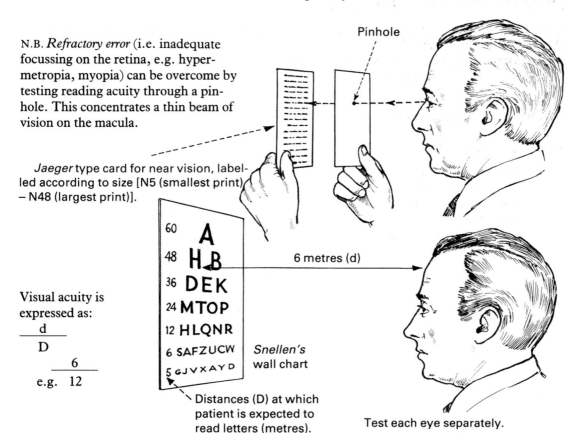

Pinhole

Visual acuity is expressed as:

$$\frac{d}{D}$$

e.g. $\frac{6}{12}$

6 metres (d)

60 A
48 H B
36 DEK
24 MTOP
12 HLQNR
6 SAFZUCW
5 GJVXAYD

Snellen's wall chart

Distances (D) at which patient is expected to read letters (metres).

Test each eye separately.

9

CRANIAL NERVE EXAMINATION

Visual fields

1. Gross testing by CONFRONTATION.
Compare the patient's fields of vision by advancing a moving finger or, more accurately, a red 5 mm pin from the extreme periphery towards the fixation point. This maps out 'cone' vision. A 2 mm pin will define central field defects which may only manifest as a loss of colour perception.

In the temporal portion of the visual field the physiological blind spot may be detected. A 3 mm object should disappear here.

The patient must fixate on the examiner's pupil.

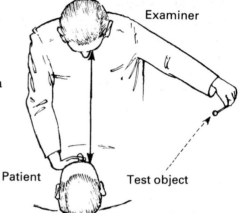

2. Peripheral visual fields are more sensitive to a *moving* target and are tested with a GOLDMANN PERIMETER.

The patient fixes on a central point. A point of light is moved centrally from the extreme periphery. The position at which the patient observes the target is marked on a chart. Repeated testing from multiple directions provides an accurate record of visual fields.

Central fields are charted in a similar manner using a smaller light source of lesser intensity.

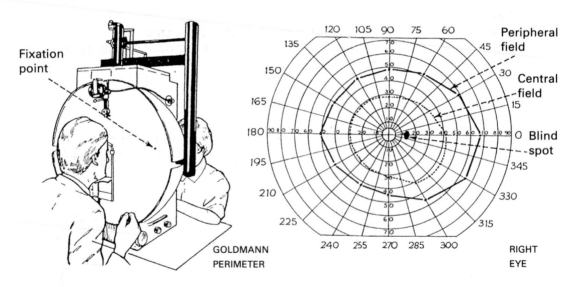

The HUMPHREY FIELD ANALYSER records the threshold at which the patient observes a static light source of increasing intensity. This is particularly valuable for central field testing.

CRANIAL NERVE EXAMINATION

Optic fundus (*Ophthalmoscopy*)

Ask the patient to fixate on a distant object away from any bright light. Use the right eye to examine the patient's right eye and the left eye to examine the patient's left eye.

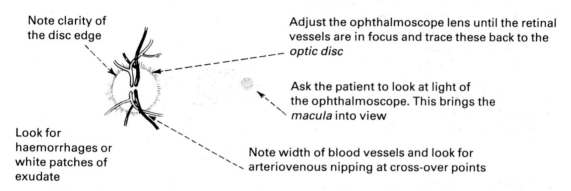

Note clarity of the disc edge

Adjust the ophthalmoscope lens until the retinal vessels are in focus and trace these back to the *optic disc*

Ask the patient to look at light of the ophthalmoscope. This brings the *macula* into view

Look for haemorrhages or white patches of exudate

Note width of blood vessels and look for arteriovenous nipping at cross-over points

If small pupil size prevents fundal examination, then dilate pupil with homatropine. This is contraindicated if either an acute expanding lesion or glaucoma is suspected.

Pupils

Note: Size

Shape

Equality

Reaction to light: both pupils constrict when light is shone in either eye

Reaction to accommodation and convergence: pupil constriction occurs when gaze is transferred to a near point object.

A lesion of the *optic nerve* will abolish pupillary response to light on the same side as well as in the contra-lateral eye.

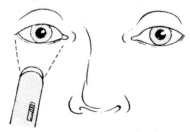

When light is shone in the *normal* eye, it and the contralateral pupil will constrict.

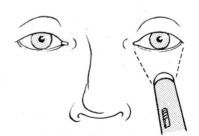

11

CRANIAL NERVE EXAMINATION

OCULOMOTOR (III), TROCHLEAR (IV) AND ABDUCENS (VI) NERVES

A lesion of the III nerve produces impairment of eye and lid movement as well as disturbance of pupillary response.

Pupil: The pupil dilates and becomes 'fixed' to light.

Shine torch in *affected* eye — contralateral pupil constricts (its III nerve intact). Absent or impaired response in illuminated eye

When light is shone into the *normal* eye, only the pupil on that side constricts

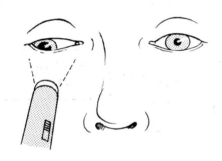

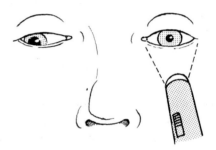

Ptosis: Ptosis is present if the eyelid droops over the pupil when the eyes are fully open.

Since the levator palpebrae muscle contains both skeletal and smooth muscle, ptosis signifies either a III nerve palsy or a sympathetic lesion.

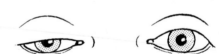

Ocular movement

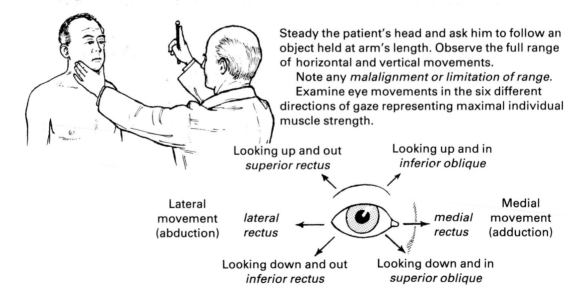

Steady the patient's head and ask him to follow an object held at arm's length. Observe the full range of horizontal and vertical movements.

Note any *malalignment or limitation of range.*

Examine eye movements in the six different directions of gaze representing maximal individual muscle strength.

Looking up and out
superior rectus

Looking up and in
inferior oblique

Lateral movement (abduction)
lateral rectus

medial rectus
Medial movement (adduction)

Looking down and out
inferior rectus

Looking down and in
superior oblique

CRANIAL NERVE EXAMINATION

Question patient about *diplopia;* the patient is more likely to notice this before the examiner can detect impairment of eye movement. If present:

– note the *direction of maximum displacement* of the images and determine the pair of muscles involved
– identify the source of the *outer image* (from the defective eye) using a transparent coloured lens.

e.g.

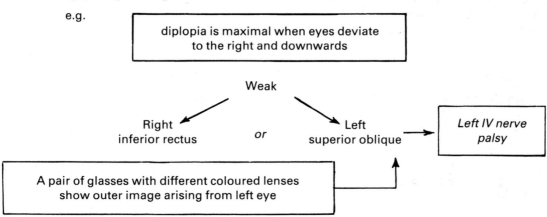

Conjugate movement: Note the ability of the eyes to move together (conjugately) in horizontal or vertical direction or tendency for gaze to fix in one particular direction.

Nystagmus: This is an upset in the normal balance of eye control. A slow drift in one direction is followed by a fast corrective movement. Nystagmus is maximal when the eyes are turned in the direction of the fast phase. Nystagmus 'direction' is usually described in terms of the fast phase and may be horizontal or vertical. Test as for other eye movements, but remember that 'physiological' nystagmus can occur when the eyes deviate more than 30° from central gaze.

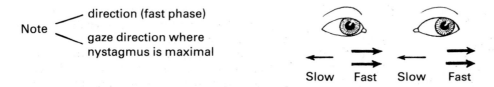

e.g. Nystagmus to the left maximal on left lateral gaze.

13

CRANIAL NERVE EXAMINATION

TRIGEMINAL NERVE (V)

Test *pain* (pin prick) sensation   } over
       temperature (cold object or   } whole
             hot/cold tubes) } face
     light touch

Compare each side.
Map out the sensory deficit,
testing from the abnormal
to the normal region.

Does distribution involve
     – a *root* pattern?
     – or a *brain stem* 'onion skin' pattern?

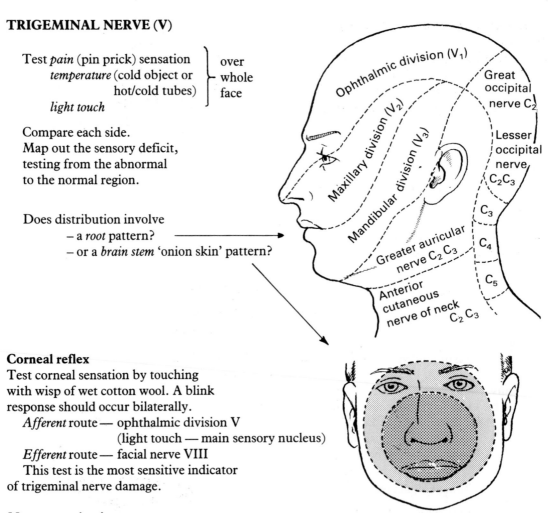

Corneal reflex
Test corneal sensation by touching
with wisp of wet cotton wool. A blink
response should occur bilaterally.
     Afferent route — ophthalmic division V
                   (light touch — main sensory nucleus)
     Efferent route — facial nerve VIII
     This test is the most sensitive indicator
of trigeminal nerve damage.

Motor examination
Observe for wasting and thinning of temporalis muscle — 'hollowing out' the temporalis fossa.
     Ask the patient to clamp jaws together. Feel temporalis and masseter muscles. Attempt to open patient's jaws by applying pressure to chin. Ask patient to open mouth. If pterygoid muscles are weak the jaw will deviate to the weak side, being pushed over by the unopposed pterygoid muscles of the good side.

CRANIAL NERVE EXAMINATION

TRIGEMINAL NERVE (V) *(contd)*
Jaw jerk
Ask patient to relax jaw. Place finger
on the chin and tap with hammer:
Slight or absent jerk — normal
Increased jerk — upper motor neuron lesion.

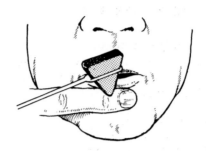

FACIAL NERVE (VII)
Observe patient as he talks and smiles, watching for:
  – eye closure
  – asymmetrical elevation of one corner of mouth
  – flattening of nasolabial fold.
Patient is then instructed to:

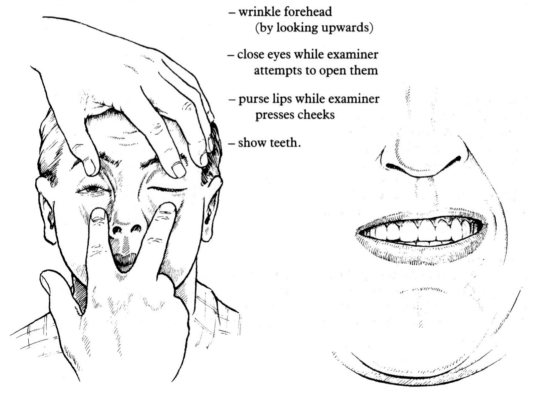

  – wrinkle forehead
     (by looking upwards)

  – close eyes while examiner
     attempts to open them

  – purse lips while examiner
     presses cheeks

  – show teeth.

Taste may be tested by using sugar, tartaric acid or sodium chloride. A small quantity of each substance is placed on the appropriate side of the protruded tongue.

CRANIAL NERVE EXAMINATION

AUDITORY NERVE (VIII)
Cochlear component

Test by whispering numbers into one ear while masking hearing in the other ear by occluding and rubbing the external meatus. If hearing is impaired, examine external meatus and the tympanic membrane with auroscope to exclude wax or infection.

Differentiate conductive (middle ear) deafness from perceptive (nerve) deafness by:

1. *Weber's test:* Hold base of tuning fork against the vertex. Ask patient if sound is heard more loudly in one ear.

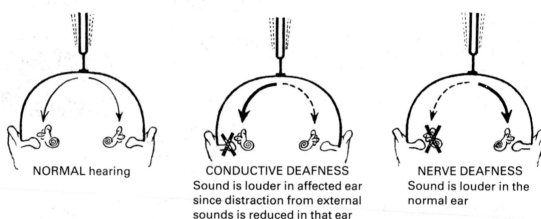

NORMAL hearing

CONDUCTIVE DEAFNESS
Sound is louder in affected ear since distraction from external sounds is reduced in that ear

NERVE DEAFNESS
Sound is louder in the normal ear

2. *Rinne's test:* Hold the base of a vibrating tuning fork against the mastoid bone. Ask the patient if note is heard. When note disappears — hold tuning fork near the external meatus. Patient should hear sound again since air conduction via the ossicles is better than bone conduction.

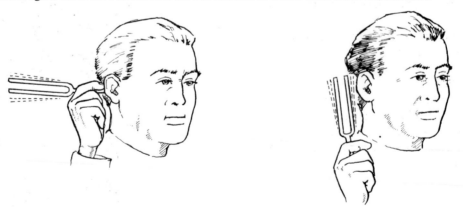

In *conductive deafness*, bone conduction is better than air conduction.
In *nerve deafness*, both bone and air conduction are impaired.

Further auditory testing and examination of the **vestibular component** requires specialised investigation (see pages 60 – 62).

16

CRANIAL NERVE EXAMINATION

GLOSSOPHARYNGEAL NERVE (IX): VAGUS NERVE (X)

These nerves are considered jointly since they are examined together and their actions are seldom individually impaired.

Note patient's *voice* — if there is vocal cord paresis (X), voice may be high pitched. (Vocal cord examination is best left to an ENT specialist.)

Note any *swallowing* difficulty or nasal regurgitation of fluids.

Ask patient to open mouth and say '*Ah*'. Note any *asymmetry* of palatal movements (X nerve palsy).

Gag reflex

Depress patient's tongue and touch palate, pharynx or tonsil on one side until the patient 'gags'. Compare sensitivity on each side (*afferent* route — IX nerve) and observe symmetry of palatal contraction (*efferent* route — X nerve).

Absent gag reflex = loss of sensation and/or loss of motor power.
(Taste in the posterior third of the tongue (IX) is impractical to test.)

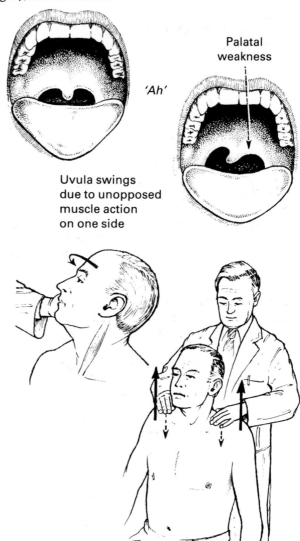

'Ah'

Palatal weakness

Uvula swings due to unopposed muscle action on one side

ACCESSORY NERVE (XI)
Sternomastoid

Ask patient to rotate head against resistance. Compare power and muscle bulk on each side. Also compare each side with the patient pulling head forward against resistance.
N.B. The left sternomastoid turns the head to the right and *vice versa*.

Trapezius

Ask patient to 'shrug' shoulders and to hold them in this position against resistance. Compare power on each side. Patient should manage to resist any effort to depress shoulders.

17

CRANIAL NERVE EXAMINATION

HYPOGLOSSAL NERVE (XII)

Ask patient to open mouth; inspect tongue.

Look for – evidence of atrophy (increased folds, wasting)

            – fasciculation (small wriggling movements).

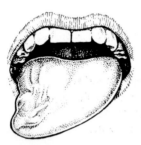

Ask patient to protrude tongue. Note any difficulty or deviation. (N.B. apparent deviation may occur with facial weakness – if present, assess tongue in relation to teeth.)

Tongue deviates towards side of weakness.

Note any disturbance in patient's speech.

EXAMINATION — UPPER LIMBS

MOTOR SYSTEM

Appearance

Note: – any *asymmetry* or *deformity*

– muscle *wasting*⎫ If in doubt, measure circumference at fixed distance above/below
– muscle *hypertrophy*⎭ joint. Note muscle group involved.

– muscle *fasciculation* – irregular, non-rhythmical contraction of groups of motor units, increased after exercise and on smacking muscle surface.
N.B. Fasciculation may occur in normal individuals, particularly in the orbicularis oculi. Distinguish from 'fibrillation', which is excessive activity of a single motor unit and is only detectable with electromyography.

Tone

Ensure that the patient is relaxed, and assess tone by alternately flexing and extending the elbow or wrist.

Note: – decrease in tone

– increase in tone ⎰ *'Clasp-knife':* the initial resistance to the movement is suddenly overcome (upper motor neuron lesion).
'Lead-pipe': a steady increase in resistance throughout the movement (extrapyramidal lesion).
'Cog-wheel': ratchet-like increase in resistance (extrapyramidal lesion).

Power

If a pyramidal weakness is suspect (i.e. a weakness arising from damage to the motor cortex or descending motor tracts (see pages 189 – 193) the following test is simple, quick, yet sensitive.

Ask the patient to hold arms outstretched with the hands supinated for up to one minute. The eyes are closed (otherwise visual compensation occurs). The weak arm gradually pronates and drifts downwards.

With possible involvement at the spinal root or nerve level (lower motor neuron), it is essential to test individual muscle groups to help localise the lesion.

When testing muscle groups, think of *root* supply and *nerve* supply.

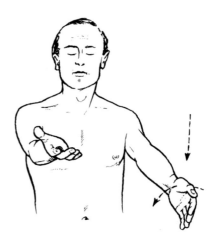

EXAMINATION — UPPER LIMBS

Test for *Serratus anterior:*

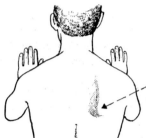

C5, C6, C7 roots
Long thoracic nerve

Patient presses
arms against wall

Look for winging
of scapula

Shoulder abduction

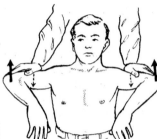

Deltoid:
C5, C6 roots
Axillary nerve

Arm (at more
than 15° from
the vertical)
abducts against
resistance

Elbow flexion

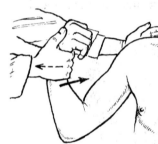

Biceps: **C5, C6** roots
Musculocutaneous
nerve

Arm flexed against
resistance with
the hand fully
supinated

Elbow extension

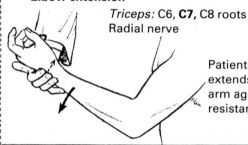

Triceps: C6, **C7,** C8 roots
Radial nerve

Patients
extends
arm against
resistance

Brachioradialis: C5, **C6** roots.
Radial nerve

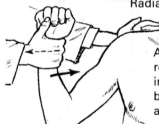

Arm flexed against
resistance with hand
in mid-position
between pronation
and supination

Finger extension

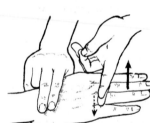

Extensor digitorum:
C7, C8 roots
Posterior inter-
osseous nerve

Patient extends
fingers against
resistance

Thumb extension — terminal phalanx

Extensor pollicis longus and brevis: **C7,** C8 roots
Posterior interosseous nerve

Thumb is extended against resistance

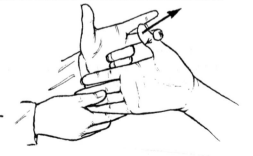

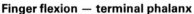

Finger flexion — terminal phalanx

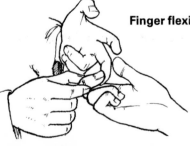

Flexor digitorum profundus I and II: C7, **C8** roots
Median nerve
Flexor digitorum profundus III and IV: C7, **C8** roots
Ulnar nerve

Examiner tries to extend patient's flexed terminal phalanges

EXAMINATION — UPPER LIMBS

Thumb opposition

Opponens pollicis: C8, **T1** roots. Median nerve

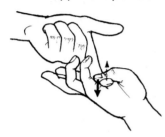

Patient tries to touch
the base of the
5th finger with
thumb against
resistance

Finger abduction

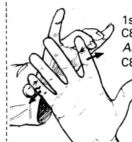

1st *dorsal interosseus:*
C8, **T1** roots. Ulnar nerve
Abductor digiti minimi:
C8, **T1** roots. Ulnar nerve

Fingers abducted
against resistance

[Note: not all muscle groups are included in the foregoing, but only those required to identify and differentiate nerve and root lesions.]

SENSATION
Pain
Pin prick with a sterile pin provides a simple method of testing this important modality. Firstly, check that the patient detects the pin as 'sharp', i.e. painful, then rapidly test each dermatome in turn.

Memorising the dermatome distribution is simplified by noting that 'C7' extends down the middle finger.

If pin prick is impaired, then more carefully map out the extent of the abnormality, moving from the abnormal to the normal area.

Light touch
This is tested in a similar manner, using a wisp of cotton wool.

Temperature
Temperature testing seldom provides any additional information. If required, use a cold object or hot and cold test tubes.

21

EXAMINATION — UPPER LIMBS

Joint position sense

Hold the sides of the patient's finger or thumb and demonstrate 'up and down' movements.

Repeat with the patient's eyes closed. Ask patient to specify the direction of movement.

Ask the patient, with eyes closed, to touch his nose with his forefinger or to bring forefingers together with the arms outstretched.

Vibration

Place a vibrating tuning fork (usually 128 c/s) on a bony prominence, e.g. radius. Ask the patient to indicate when the vibration, if felt, ceases. If impaired, move more proximally and repeat. Vibration testing is of value in the early detection of demyelinating disease and peripheral neuropathy, but otherwise is of limited benefit.

If the above sensory functions are normal and a cortical lesion is suspected, it is useful to test for the following:

Two point discrimination: the ability to discriminate two blunt points when simultaneously applied to the finger, 5 mm apart (cf, 4 cm in the legs).

Blunt ends

5mm

Sensory inattention (perceptual rivalry): the ability to detect stimuli (pin prick or touch) in both limbs, when applied to both limbs simultaneously.

Stereognosis: the ability to recognise objects placed in the hand.

Graphaesthesia: the ability to recognise numbers or letters traced out on the palm.

REFLEXES

Biceps jerk C5, C6 roots. Musculocutaneous nerve

Supinator jerk C6, C7 roots. Radial nerve

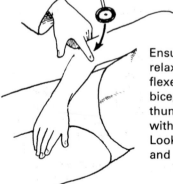

Ensure patient's arm is relaxed and slightly flexed. Palpate the biceps tendon with the thumb and strike with tendon hammer. Look for elbow flexion and biceps contraction.

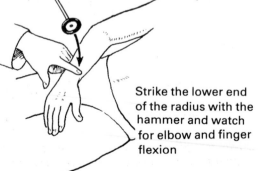

Strike the lower end of the radius with the hammer and watch for elbow and finger flexion

EXAMINATION — UPPER LIMBS

Triceps jerk

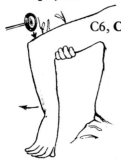

C6, **C7,** C8 roots. Radial nerve. Strike the patient's elbow a few inches above the olecranon process. Look for elbow extension and triceps contraction.

Hoffman reflex C7, C8

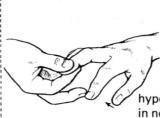

Flick the patient's terminal phalanx, suddenly stretching the flexor tendon on release. Thumb flexion indicates hyperreflexia. (May be present in normal subjects with brisk tendon reflexes.)

Reflex enhancement
When reflexes are difficult to elicit, enhancement occurs if the patient is asked to 'clench the teeth'.

CO-ORDINATION
Inco-ordination (ataxia) is often a prominent feature of cerebellar disease (see page 178). Prior to testing, ensure that power and proprioception are normal.

Inco-ordination
Finger – nose testing

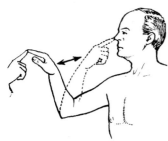

Ask patient to touch his nose with finger (eyes open). Look for jerky movements — DYSMETRIA or an INTENTION TREMOR (tremor only occurring on voluntary movement).
Ask patient to alternately touch his own nose then the examiner's finger as fast as he can. This may exaggerate the intention tremor and may demonstrate DYSDIADOCHOKINESIA — an inability to perform rapidly alternating movements.

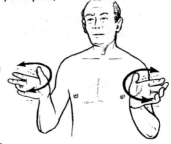

This may also be shown by asking the patient to rapidly supinate and pronate the forearms or to perform rapid and repeated tapping movements.

Arm bounce

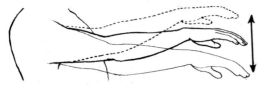

Downward pressure and sudden release of the patient's outstretched arm causes excessive swinging

Rebound phenomenon

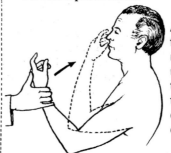

Ask the patient to flex elbow against resistance. Sudden release may cause the hand to strike the face due to delay in triceps contraction

23

EXAMINATION — TRUNK

SENSATION Test pin prick and light touch in dermatome distribution as for the upper limbs.
Levels to remember: T5 — at *nipple*
T10 — at *umbilicus*
T12 — at *inguinal ligament*.

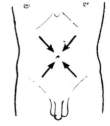

Abdominal reflexes: T7 – T12 roots. Stroke or lightly scratch the skin towards the umbilicus in each quadrant in turn. Look for abdominal muscle contraction and note if absent or impaired. (N.B. Reflexes may be absent in obesity, after pregnancy, or after abdominal operations.)

Cremasteric reflex: L1 root. Scratch inner thigh. Observe contraction of cremasteric muscle causing testicular elevation.

SPHINCTERS

Examine abdomen for distended bladder.

Note evidence of urinary or faecal incontinence.

Note tone of anal sphincter during rectal examination.

Anal reflex: S4, S5 roots. A scratch on the skin beside the anus causes a reflex contraction of the anal sphincter.

EXAMINATION — LOWER LIMBS

MOTOR SYSTEM

Appearance: Note: – *asymmetry* or *deformity*
– muscle *wasting*
– muscle *hypertrophy*
– muscle *fasciculation*
} as in the upper limbs.

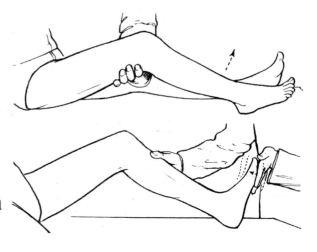

Tone

Try to relax the patient and alternately flex and extend the knee joint. Note the resistance.

Roll the patient's legs from side to side. Suddenly lift the thigh and note the response in the lower leg. With increased tone the leg kicks upwards.

Clonus

Ensure that the patient is relaxed. Apply sudden and sustained flexion to the ankle. A few oscillatory beats may occur in the normal subject, but when this persists it indicates increased tone.

EXAMINATION — LOWER LIMBS

Power

When testing each muscle group, think of *root* and *nerve* supply.

Hip flexion

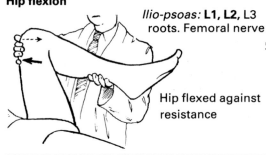

Ilio-psoas: **L1, L2,** L3 roots. Femoral nerve

Hip flexed against resistance

Hip extension

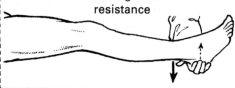

Gluteus maximus: **L5, S1,** S2 roots. Inferior gluteal nerve

Patient attempts to keep heel on bed against resistance

Hip abduction

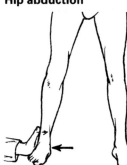

Gluteus medius and minimus and tensor fasciae latae: **L4, L5,** S1 roots. Superior gluteal nerve

Patient lying on back tries to abduct the leg against resistance

Hip adduction

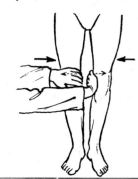

Adductors: **L2, L3,** L4 roots. Obturator nerve

Patient lying on back tries to pull knees together against resistance

Knee flexion

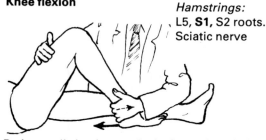

Hamstrings: L5, **S1,** S2 roots. Sciatic nerve

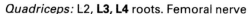

Patient pulls heel towards the buttock and tries to maintain this position against resistance.

Knee extension

Quadriceps: L2, **L3,** L4 roots. Femoral nerve

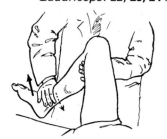

Patient tries to extend knee against resistance

Dorsiflexion

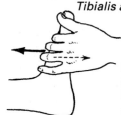

Tibialis anterior: **L4,** L5 roots. Deep peroneal nerve

Patient dorsiflexes the ankle against resistance. May have difficulty in walking on heels

Plantarflexion

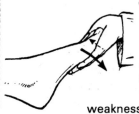

Gastrocnemius, soleus: **S1, S2,** roots. Tibial nerve.

Patient plantarflexes the ankle against resistance. May have difficulty in walking on toes before weakness can be directly detected

25

EXAMINATION — LOWER LIMBS

Toe extension

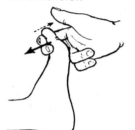

Extensor hallucis longus, extensor digitorum longus: **L5,** S1 roots. Deep peroneal nerve

Patient dorsiflexes the toes against resistance

Inversion

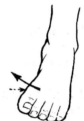

Tibialis posterior: **L4, L5** root. Tibial nerve

Patient inverts foot against resistance

Eversion

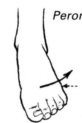

Peroneus longus and brevis: **L5, S1** roots. Superficial peroneal nerve

Patient everts foot against resistance

SENSATION

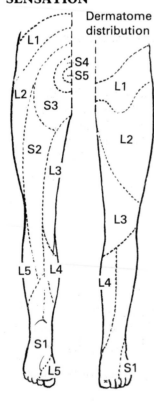

Dermatome distribution

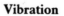

Test:
Pain   ⎤ follow the dermatome
Light touch   ⎬ distribution as in
(Temperature)   ⎦ the upper limb.

Joint position sense
Firstly, demonstrate flexion and extension movements of the big toe. Then ask patient to specify the direction with the eyes closed.
   If deficient, test ankle joint sense in the same way.

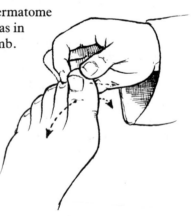

Vibration
Test vibration perception by placing a tuning fork on the malleolus. If deficient, move up to the head of the fibula or to the anterior superior iliac spine.

EXAMINATION — LOWER LIMBS

REFLEXES

Knee jerk: L2, L3, **L4** roots.

Ensure that the patient's leg is relaxed by resting it over examiner's arm or by hanging it over the edge of the bed. Tap the patellar tendon with the hammer and observe quadriceps contraction. Note impairment or exaggeration.

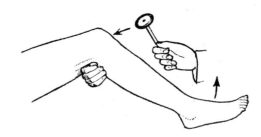

Ankle jerk: S1, S2 roots.

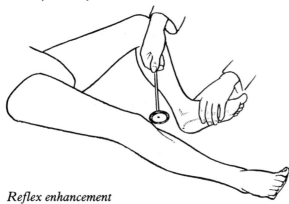

Externally rotate the patient's leg. Hold the foot in slight dorsiflexion. Ensure the foot is relaxed by palpating the tendon of tibialis anterior. If this is taut, then no ankle jerk will be elicited.

Tap the Achilles tendon and watch for calf muscle contraction and plantarflexion.

Reflex enhancement

When reflexes are difficult to elicit, they may be enhanced by asking the patient to clench the teeth or to try to pull clasped hands apart (Jendressik's manoeuvre).

Plantar response

Check that the big toe is relaxed. Stroke the lateral aspect of the sole and across the ball of the foot. Note the first movement of the big toe. Flexion should occur. Extension due to contraction of extensor hallucis longus (a 'Babinski' reflex) indicates an upper motor neuron lesion. This is usually accompanied by synchronous contraction of the knee flexors and tensor fasciae latae.

To avoid ambiguity do not touch the innermost aspect of the sole or the toes themselves.

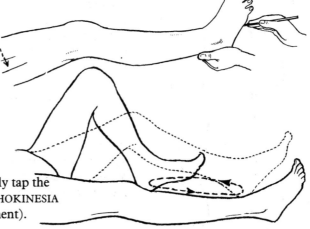

CO-ORDINATION

Ask patient to repeatedly run the heel from the opposite knee down the shin to the big toe. Look for ATAXIA (inco-ordination). Ask patient to repeatedly tap the floor with the foot. Note any DYSDIADOCHOKINESIA (difficulty with rapidly alternating movement).

EXAMINATION — POSTURE AND GAIT

Romberg's test

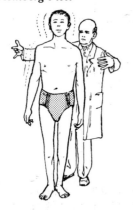

Ask patient to stand with the heels together, first with the eyes open, then with the eyes closed.

Note any excessive postural swaying or loss of balance

Present when eyes open or closed = cerebellar deficit (cerebellar ataxia)

Present only when eyes are closed = proprioceptive deficit (sensory ataxia)

GAIT

Note:
- Length of step and width of base
- Abnormal leg movements (e.g. excessively high step)
- Instability (gait ataxia)
- Associated postural movements (e.g. pelvic swinging)

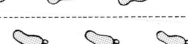

Normal

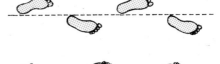

Abnormal

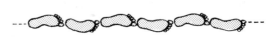

If normal, repeat with *tandem* walking, i.e. heel to toe. This will exaggerate any instability.

EXAMINATION OF THE UNCONSCIOUS PATIENT

HISTORY

Questioning relatives, friends or the ambulance team is an essential part of the assessment of the unconscious or the unco-operative patient.

> Has the patient sustained a head injury — leading to admission, or in the preceding weeks?
> Did the patient collapse suddenly?
> Did limb twitching occur?
> Have symptoms occurred in the preceding weeks?
> Has the patient suffered a previous illness?
> Does the patient take medication?

GENERAL EXAMINATION

Lack of patient co-operation does not limit general examination and this may reveal important diagnostic signs. In addition to those features described on page 4, also look for signs of head injury, needle marks on the arm and evidence of tongue biting. Also note the smell of alcohol, but beware of attributing the patient's clinical state solely to alcohol excess.

NEUROLOGICAL EXAMINATION

Conscious level: This assessment is of major importance. It not only serves as an immediate prognostic guide, but also provides a baseline with which future examinations may be compared. Assess conscious level as described previously (page 5) in terms of:

Eye opening		Verbal response		Motor response	
Spontaneous	4	Orientated	5	Obeying commands	5
To speech	3	Confused	4	Localising	4
To pain	2	Words	3	Flexing	3
None	1	Sounds	2	Extending	2
		None	1	None	1

A score may be applied to each category of the grading system and the total summed to give an overall value ranging from 3 – 4, e.g. no eye opening, no verbal response and extending to pain = 4.

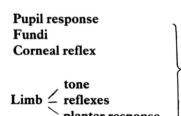

Pupil response
Fundi
Corneal reflex

Limb — tone / reflexes / plantar response

Lack of patient co-operation does not prevent objective assessment of these features described before, but other neurological features require a different approach

EXAMINATION OF THE UNCONSCIOUS PATIENT

Eye movements

Observe any **spontaneous** eye movements. 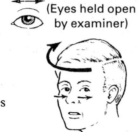 (Eyes held open by examiner)

Note whether the movements, if present, are *conjugate* (i.e. the eyes move in parallel) or *dysconjugate* (i.e. the eyes do not move in parallel).

Elicit the **oculocephalic (doll's eye) reflex.**
Rotation or flexion/extension of the head in a comatose patient produces transient eye movements in a direction opposite to the direction of movement.

These ocular movements assess midbrain and pontine function.

Elicit the **oculovestibular reflex** (caloric testing, see page 62).

Visual fields
In the unco-operative patient, the examiner may detect a hemianopic field defect when 'menacing' from one side fails to produce a 'blink'.

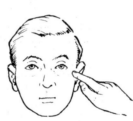

Facial weakness
Failure to 'grimace' on one side in response to bilateral supraorbital pain indicates a facial weakness.

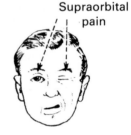
Supraorbital pain

Limb weakness
Detect by comparing the response in the limbs to painful stimuli. If pain produces an *asymmetric* response, then limb weakness is present.
(If the patient 'localises' with one arm, hold this down and retest to ensure that a similar response cannot be elicited from the other limb).

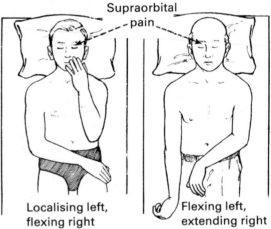
Supraorbital pain

e.g.

Localising left, flexing right

Flexing left, extending right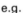

Both patients are in coma; both have an asymmetric response to pain indicating a right arm weakness and focal brain damage.

Pain stimulus applied to the toe nails or Achilles tendon similarly tests power in the lower limbs. Variation in tone, reflexes or plantar responses between each side also indicates a focal deficit. In practice, if the examiner fails to detect a difference in response to painful stimuli, these additional features seldom provide convincing evidence.

THE NEUROLOGICAL OBSERVATION CHART

Despite major advances in intracranial investigative techniques, none has replaced clinical assessment for monitoring the patient's neurological state. The neurological observation chart produced by Jennett and Teasdale incorporates the most relevant clinical features, i.e. *coma scale (eye opening, verbal and motor response), pupil size* and *reaction to light, limb responses* and *vital signs.* The frequency of observation (normally 2-hourly) depends on the individual patient's needs. The chart enables immediate evaluation of the trend in the patient's clinical state.

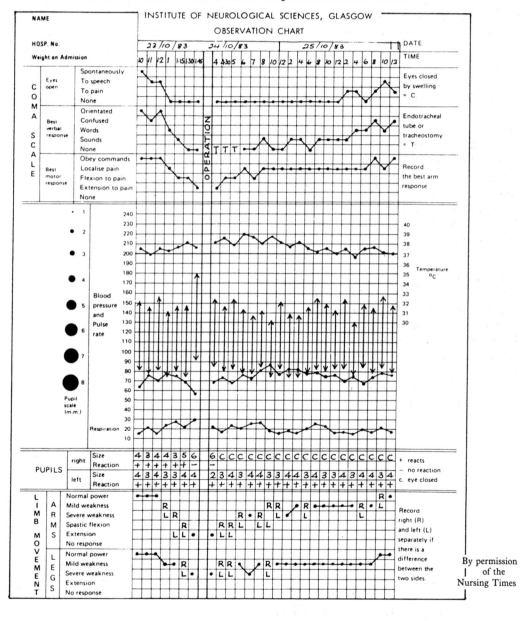

By permission
of the
Nursing Times

INVESTIGATIONS OF THE CENTRAL AND PERIPHERAL NERVOUS SYSTEMS

SKULL X-RAY

Despite the development of advanced radiological techniques, skull X-ray is still a useful preliminary investigation especially in head injured patients.

Standard views:
Lateral
Postero-anterior
Towne's (fronto-occipital)

Learn to distinguish normal skull markings and sites of calcification (pineal and choroid plexus).

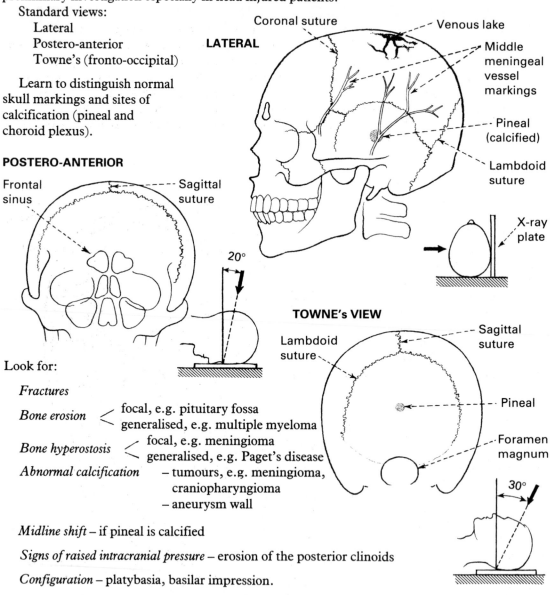

Look for:

Fractures

Bone erosion ⟨ focal, e.g. pituitary fossa
generalised, e.g. multiple myeloma

Bone hyperostosis ⟨ focal, e.g. meningioma
generalised, e.g. Paget's disease

Abnormal calcification – tumours, e.g. meningioma, craniopharyngioma
– aneurysm wall

Midline shift – if pineal is calcified

Signs of raised intracranial pressure – erosion of the posterior clinoids

Configuration – platybasia, basilar impression.

More specific views depend on clinical indications and the availability of other imaging techniques, e.g.

Base of skull (submentovertical) – cranial nerve palsies
Optic foramina – progressive blindness
Sella turcica – visual field defects
Petrous/internal auditory meatus – sensorineural deafness.

COMPUTERISED TOMOGRAPHY (CT) SCANNING

The development of this non-invasive technique in the 1970s revolutionised the investigative approach to intracranial pathology and its use has now been extended to the 'body' and spine.

A pencil beam of X-ray traverses the patient's head and a diametrically opposed detector measures the extent of its absorption. Computer processing, multiple rotating beams and detectors arranged in a complete circle around the patient's head enable determination of absorption values for multiple small blocks of tissue (voxels). Reconstruction of these areas on a two-dimensional display (pixels) provides the characteristic CT scan appearance. For routine scanning, slices are 5–10 mm wide. Slices of 2 mm width provide even greater detail but these 'high definition' views take longer to acquire and process and this technique is usually reserved for examination of the orbit, the pituitary region and the posterior fossa.

An *intravenous iodinated water-soluble contrast medium* is administered when the plain scan reveals an abnormality or if specific clinical indications exist, e.g. suspected arteriovenous malformation, acoustic neurilemmoma or intracerebral abscess — with these lesions the plain scan may appear normal. Intravenous contrast shows areas with increased vascularity or with impairment of the blood-brain barrier.

Intrathecal water-soluble contrast medium combined with CT scanning outlines the basal cisterns, the spinal cord and the lumbosacral nerve roots.

Intrathecal air, run up to the cerebellopontine angle more clearly outlines small acoustic neurilemmomas.

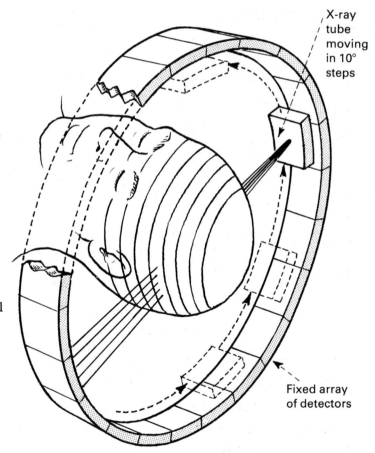

X-ray tube moving in 10° steps

Fixed array of detectors

35

COMPUTERISED TOMOGRAPHY (CT) SCANNING

NORMAL SCAN

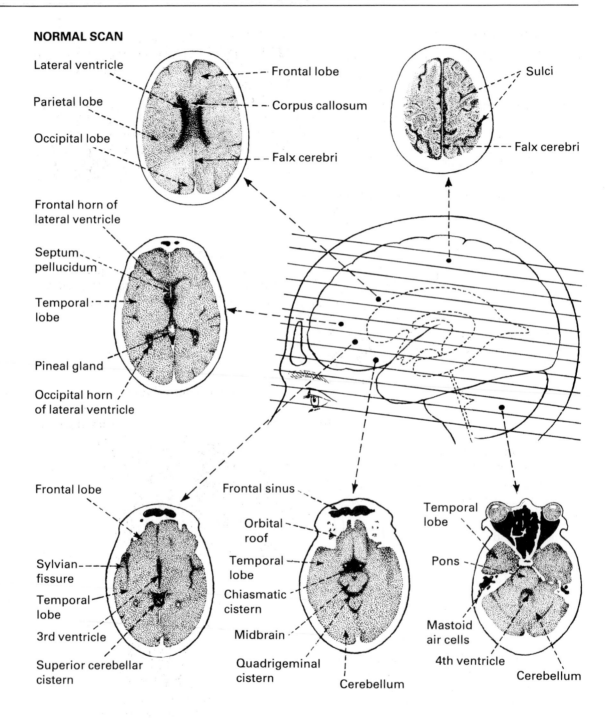

COMPUTERISED TOMOGRAPHY (CT) SCANNING

Coronal and sagittal reconstruction

Computer reconstruction of images in the sagittal or coronal planes may occasionally provide more information, but requires CT slices of narrow width, i.e. 2 mm. These are of particular value in demonstrating sellar and pineal region tumours and in lesions extending upwards from the skull base.

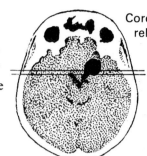
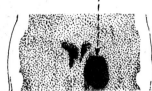

Coronal reconstruction showing relationships of an epidermoid cyst to the lateral ventricle.

Coronal CT scanning

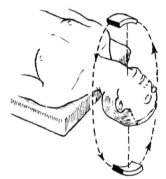

Coronal scan showing pneumocele arising from fracture in the orbital roof.

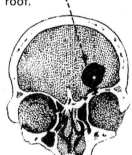

Full neck extension combined with maximal angulation of the CT gantry permits direct coronal scanning and may give greater definition than reconstructed views.

Orbital CT scanning

CT scanning clearly defines both normal and abnormal intraorbital contents and demonstrates any intracranial extension or bone destruction.

Normal orbit

Cavernous haemangioma

Optic nerve

Lateral rectus

Proptosis

Medial rectus

Spinal CT scanning

Plain CT of the spine provides useful information of disc disease, particularly at the lumbosacral level.

CT scanning after instilling intrathecal contrast (e.g. following myelography) more clearly demonstrates lesions compressing the spinal cord or the cervicomedullary junction. Sagittal or coronal reconstruction may also help.

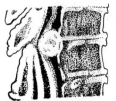

Sagittal reconstruction at T6/7 level showing cord compression from a large disc protrusion.

37

COMPUTERISED TOMOGRAPHY (CT) SCANNING

Interpretation of the cranial CT scan

Before contrast enhancement note:

VENTRICULAR SYSTEM

Size
Position
Compression of
one or more horns,
i.e. frontal, temporal
or occipital

WIDTH OF CORTICAL SULCI AND THE SYLVIAN FISSURES

SKULL BASE AND VAULT

Hyperostosis
Osteolytic lesion
Remodelling
Depressed fracture

MULTIPLE LESIONS may result from:

Tumour – metastases
         – lymphoma
Abscesses
Granuloma
Infarction
Trauma

ABNORMAL TISSUE DENSITY

Identify the site, and whether the lesion lies within or without the brain substance.
Note the 'MASS EFFECT':
– midline shift
– ventricular compression
– obliteration of the basal cisterns

High density
  Blood
  Calcification – tumour
              – arteriovenous
                 malformation/aneurysm
              – hamartoma
  (Calcification of the pineal gland, choroid plexus, basal ganglia and falx may occur in normal scans.)

Low density
  Infarction (arterial/venous)
  Tumour
  Abscess
  Oedema
  Encephalitis
  Resolving haematoma

Mixed density
  Tumour
  Abscess
  Arteriovenous malformation
  Contusion
  Haemorrhagic infarct

After contrast enhancement:
Look at the extent and pattern of contrast uptake in any abnormal region. Some lesions may only appear after contrast enhancement.

MAGNETIC RESONANCE IMAGING (MRI)

For many years, magnetic resonance techniques have aided chemical analysis in the food and petrochemical industries. The development of large-bore homogeneous magnets and computer assisted imaging (as in CT scanning) has extended its use to the mapping of hydrogen nuclei (i.e. water) densities and their effect on surrounding molecules in vivo. Since these vary from tissue to tissue, MRI can provide a detailed image of both head and body structures.

Physical basis

When a substance is placed in a magnetic field, spinning protons within the nuclei act like small magnets and align themselves within the field.

A superimposed electromagnetic pulse (radiowave) at a specific frequency displaces the hydrogen protons.

The transverse component of the magnetisation vector generates the MRI signal.

The T1 component (or spin-lattice relaxation) depends on the time taken for the protons to realign themselves with the magnetic field and reflects the way the protons interact with the 'lattice' of surrounding molecules and their return to thermal equilibrium.

Consider the effect on:
(a) *individual* protons

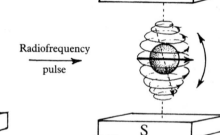

Radiofrequency pulse

(b) for *all* protons in the field

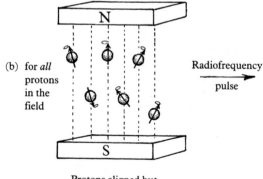

Radiofrequency pulse

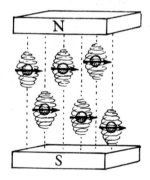

The T2 compound (spin-spin relaxation) is the time taken for the protons to return to their original 'out of phase' state and depends on the locally 'energised' protons and their return to electromagnetic equilibrium.

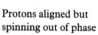

Protons aligned but spinning out of phase

Protons spin in phase (i.e. 'resonate')

A variety of different radiofrequency pulse sequences (saturation recovery (SR), inversion recovery (IR) and spin echo (SE)) combined with computerised imaging produce an image of either proton density or of T1 or T2 weighting depending on the sequence employed.

Rapidly flowing protons often give a reduced or absent MRI signal and the resultant flow 'void' can demonstrate vessels, aneurysms and arteriovenous malformations.

MAGNETIC RESONANCE IMAGING

Normal MRI images (T1/T2 weighting in relation to normal grey/white matter)

Axial views — head

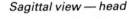
Sagittal view — head

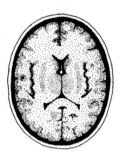

T1 weighted

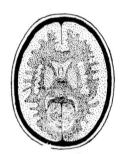

T2 weighted

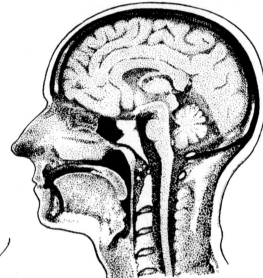

T1 weighted

*Cervicodorsal spine
(sagittal view)*

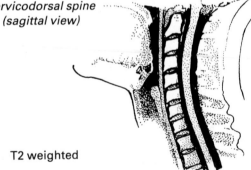

T2 weighted

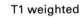
T2 weighted

Advantages (compared to CT scanning)
Can select any plane, e.g. coronal,
sagittal, oblique.
No ionising radiation.
More sensitive to tissue changes, e.g. demyelination plaques
(but not specific for each pathology,
i.e. does not distinguish demyelination
from ischaemia).
No bone artifacts, e.g. intracanalicular acoustic neuroma. ‒ ‒ ‒ ‒

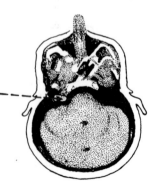

Disadvantages
Limited slice thickness — 3 mm (cf. CT — 1 mm).
Bone imaging limited to display of marrow.
Claustrophobia.
Cannot use with pacemaker or ferromagnetic implant.

T1 weighted

MAGNETIC RESONANCE IMAGING (MRI)

Interpretation of abnormal MRI image

Look for structural abnormalities and abnormal intensities indicating a change in tissue T1 or T2 weighting *in relation to normal grey and white matter.*

T1 relaxation time		T2 relaxation time		Lesion
Very prolonged (hypo-intense)	—	Prolonged (hyper-intense)	=	*Cyst, hygroma,* *cerebromalacia*
Prolonged (hypo-intense)	—	Prolonged (hyper-intense)	=	*Ischaemia, oedema,* *demyelination, most malignant tumours*
Short (hyper-intense)	—	Moderately prolonged (hyper-intense)	=	*Subacute/chronic haemorrhage* *Fat, e.g. dermoid tumour,* *lipoma,* *some metastases,* *atheroma*
Same (iso-intense)	—	Short (hypo-intense)	=	*Acute haemorrhage*
Same (iso-intense)	—	Same (iso-intense)	=	*Meningioma* (usually identified from structural change or from surrounding oedema

Paramagnetic enhancement

Some substances, e.g. gadolinium, induce strong local magnetic fields — particularly shortening the T1 component. After intravenous administration, leakage of gadolinium through regions of damaged blood-brain barrier produces marked enhancement of the MRI signal, e.g. in ischaemia, infection, tumours and demyelination. Gadolinium may also help to differentiate tumour tissue from surrounding oedema.

ULTRASOUND

When the probe (i.e. a transducer) — frequency 5–10 MHz, is applied to the skin surface, a proportion of the ultrasonic waves emitted are reflected back from structures of varying acoustic impedence and are detected by the same probe. These reflected waves are reconverted into electrical energy and displayed as a two-dimensional image (ß-mode).

When the probe is directed at moving structures, such as red blood cells within a blood vessel lumen, frequency shift of the reflected waves occurs (the Doppler effect) proportional to the velocity of flowing blood. Doppler ultrasound uses *continuous wave* (CW) or *pulsed wave* (PW). The former measures frequency shift anywhere along the path of the probe. Pulsed ultrasound records frequency shift at a specific depth.

Duplex scanning combines ß-mode with doppler, simultaneously providing images from the vessels from which the velocity is recorded.

These techniques permit assessment of both extracranial and intracranial vessels.

Extracranial

Normal vessels exhibit laminar flow and the probe detects a constant velocity.

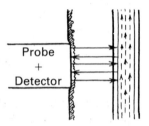

With stenosis the probe detects a wide spectrum of velocity

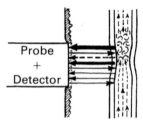

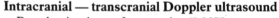

ß-mode (real time) scanning images the arterial wall rather than the passage of red blood cells — producing a 'map' of the lumen.

Intracranial — transcranial Doppler ultrasound

By selecting lower frequencies (2 MHz), ultrasound is able to penetrate the thinner parts of the skull bone. By combining this with a pulsed system, reliable measurements of flow velocity in the anterior, middle and posterior cerebral and basilar arteries are obtained.

Applications:

Assessment of intracranial haemodynamics in extracranial occlusive/stenotic vascular disease.

Detection of vasospasm in subarachnoid haemorrhage.

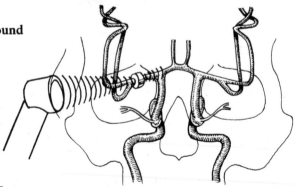

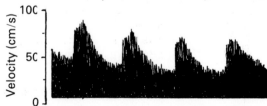

ANGIOGRAPHY

Many neurological and neurosurgical conditions require accurate delineation of both intra- and extracranial vessels. Angiography remains the standard technique, although digital subtraction angiography (DSA) may be of value in some conditions, e.g. carotid stenosis, sagittal sinus thrombosis.

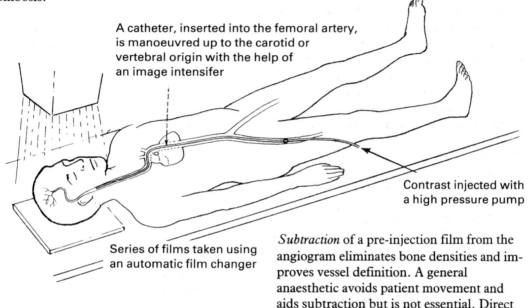

A catheter, inserted into the femoral artery, is manoeuvred up to the carotid or vertebral origin with the help of an image intensifer

Contrast injected with a high pressure pump

Series of films taken using an automatic film changer

Subtraction of a pre-injection film from the angiogram eliminates bone densities and improves vessel definition. A general anaesthetic avoids patient movement and aids subtraction but is not essential. Direct vessel puncture is rarely required.

Phase – arterial
– capillary   } Most information is now derived from the arterial phase.
– venous   Prior to the CT scan, the position of the cerebral veins helped localise intracranial structures.

CAROTID ANGIOGRAPHY

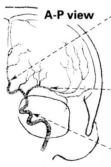

A-P view

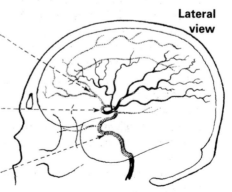

Lateral view

The *anterior cerebral arteries* run over the corpus callosum, supplying the medial aspects of the frontal lobes. Both anterior cerebral arteries may fill from each carotid injection.
The *middle cerebral artery* runs in the depth of the Sylvian fissure. Branches supply the frontal and temporal lobes.
The *internal carotid artery* bifurcates into the anterior and middle cerebral arteries.

Oblique views may aid identification of some lesions, e.g. aneurysms.

ANGIOGRAPHY

VERTEBRAL ANGIOGRAPHY

Towne's view

Lateral view

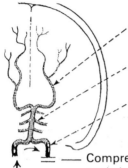

Posterior cerebral arteries supply the occipital lobes and parts of the parietal and temporal lobes
Basilar artery: branches supply the brain stem and cerebellum
Vertebral arteries: branches supply the spinal cord, brain stem and cerebellum

Contrast medium

Compression of the contralateral vertebral artery in the neck during contrast injection produces retrograde flow and demonstrates both vessels with one injection

Look for:
 Vessel *occlusion, stenosis* or *plaque formation*
 Aneurysms
 Arterio-venous malformations
 Abnormal *tumour circulation*
 Vessel *displacement* or *compression.*

Although superseded by the CT scan in tumour detection, angiography may give useful information about feeding vessels and the extent of vessel involvement with the tumour.

Complications

The development of non-ionic contrast mediums, e.g. iohexol, iopamidol, has considerably reduced the risk of complications during or following angiography; these seldom occur in the hands of experienced radiologists.

 Cerebral ischaemia: caused by emboli from an arteriosclerotic plaque broken off by the catheter tip, hypotension or vessel spasm following contrast injection.

 Contrast sensitivity: mild sensitivity to the contrast occasionally develops, but this rarely causes severe problems.

EMBOLISATION

Angiography combined with embolisation of specific vessels can be used as a precurser to operation to help minimise operative haemorrhage or as a treatment itself.

 Particles (e.g. Ivalon sponge) injected through the arterial catheter will occlude small vessels, e.g. those feeding meningioma, glomus jugulare tumours or spinal angioma.

 Small *balloons,* inflated then detached from the catheter tip will occlude high-flow systems with larger vessels, e.g. arteriovenous malformations, carotid-cavernous fistula. In some centres, radiologists inject rapidly setting 'glue' (isobutyl-2-cyanoacrylate) into arteriovenous malformations.

 These techniques carry some risk of cerebral (or spinal) infarct from inadvertent distal embolisation when used in the internal carotid or spinal systems.

44

DIGITAL SUBTRACTION ANGIOGRAPHY (DSA)

Digital subtraction angiography depends upon high-speed digital computing. Exposures taken before and after the administration of contrast agents are instantly subtracted 'pixel by pixel'. Data manipulation allows enhancement of small differences of shading as well as magnification of specific areas of study.

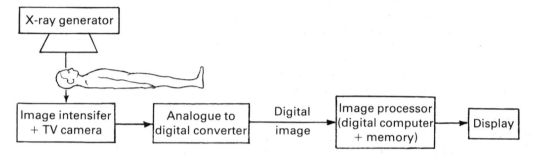

DSA results in improved contrast sensitivity, permitting the use of much lower concentrations of contrast material.

Intravenous contrast administration provides good definition of extracranial vessels, e.g. for investigation of transient ischaemic attacks.
Intra-arterial contrast injection is required for intracranial vessel display, e.g. for investigation of subarachnoid haemorrhage.

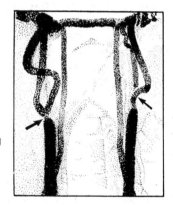

Computer enhancement of contrast showing moderate stenosis of both common carotid arteries with normal vertebral arteries.

Advantages of DSA over standard angiography
Fast, less costly technique
Less contrast required, therefore less risk (dose comparable to intravenous pyelogram).
Avoids intra-arterial injection for extracranial vessels.

Problems with DSA
Superimposition of vessels may mask pathology.
Limited spatial resolution may prevent visualisation of small intracranial vessels — even with intra-arterial injection.
Movement artefact (e.g. swallowing) may create image blurring.

RADIONUCLIDE IMAGING

There are two components to imaging with radioactive tracers — the detecting system and the labelled chemical. Each of these has become increasingly sophisticated in recent years.

Conventional gamma camera scanning

Following a blocking dose of potassium perchlorate (to prevent uptake in the choroid plexus and salivary glands), sodium pertechnetate, labelled with technetium^{99m}, is injected intravenously and its distribution within the brain detected with a gamma camera placed in the lateral, anterior or posterior positions.

Lateral   **Antero-posterior**

Abnormalities of isotope distribution result from:
– Increased vascularity, e.g. meningioma - - - - - - - - - →

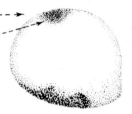

Increased radioisotope
uptake over the
hemispheric convexity

– Abnormal presence of blood, e.g. chronic subdural haematoma

– Breakdown of the blood-brain barrier, e.g. herpes simplex encephalitis.

Although still widely used in screening for large intracerebral lesions this technique has no role where X-ray CT scanning is available.

Single photon emission computed tomography (SPECT)

The technique also uses emitting tracers but, unlike conventional scanning, acquires data from multiple sites around the head. Similar computing to X-ray CT scanning provides a two-dimensional image depicting the radioactivity emitted from each 'pixel'. This gives improved definition and localisation. New radiochemicals produce images of cerebral blood flow.

Gamma-emitting radiopharmaceuticals are used. The ideal tracer properties for examining cerebral blood flow are:
    Passive diffusion across the blood-brain barrier
    'Trapping' within cells
    Slow clearance from brain
    Safety.

A ^{99}Tc^m-labelled derivative of propylamine oxime (HM PAO) fulfils these criteria and is the most promising pharmaceutical available. Of the total injected dose, 5% is taken up by the brain and 86% of this activity remains in the brain at 24 hours.

RADIONUCLIDE IMAGING

Single photon emission computed tomography (SPECT) *(contd)*
A rotating gamma camera is often used for detection, although new multidetector systems will produce higher quality images. Data is normally reconstructed to give axial images but coronal and sagittal sections can also be produced.

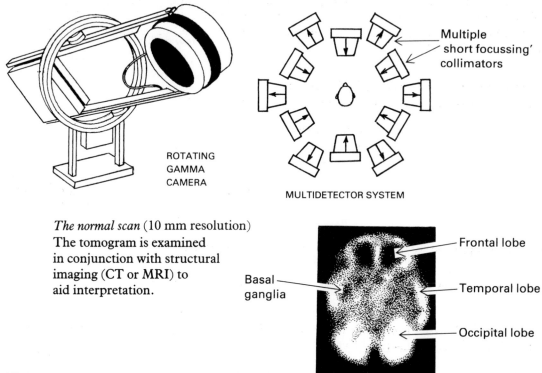

ROTATING
GAMMA
CAMERA

Multiple
short focussing'
collimators

MULTIDETECTOR SYSTEM

The normal scan (10 mm resolution)
The tomogram is examined
in conjunction with structural
imaging (CT or MRI) to
aid interpretation.

Basal ganglia

Frontal lobe

Temporal lobe

Occipital lobe

Clinical application
– Assessment of blood flow changes in DEMENTIA.
– Detection of early ischaemia in OCCLUSIVE and HAEMORRHAGIC CEREBROVASCULAR DISEASE and evaluation of EPILEPSY.

In focal epilepsy
an *ictal* scan will
often show a focal
increase in blood
flow...

...and an *interictal*
scan a larger focal
decrease in blood
flow.

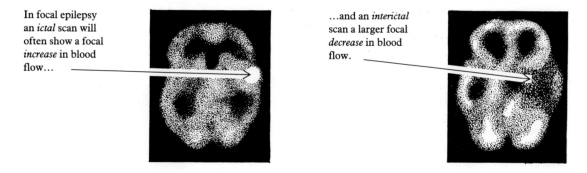

Such findings aid selection of patients for surgical treatment (see page 99).

RADIONUCLIDE IMAGING

Positron emission tomography (PET)

This new technique utilises positron-emitting isotopes (radionuclides) bound to compounds of biological interest to study specific physiological processes quantitatively. Positron-emitting isotopes depend on a cyclotron for production and their half-life is short, thus PET scanners only exist on adjacent sites. This limits availability for routine clinical use but PET scanners provide invaluable research information.

Each decaying positron results in the release of two photons in diametric opposition; these activate two coincidental detectors. Multiple pairs of detectors and computer processing techniques enable quantitative determination of local radio-activity (and density of the labelled compound) for each 'voxel'(a cube of tissue) within the imaged field. Reconstruction using similar imaging techniques to CT scanning produces the positron emission scan.

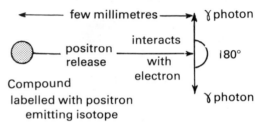

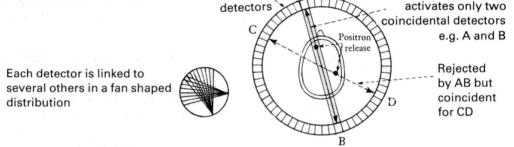

Each detector is linked to several others in a fan shaped distribution

Isotope	Binding compound		Measurement under study
^{15}Oxygen	Carbon monoxide	– inhalation	*Cerebral blood volume (CBV)*
^{15}Oxygen	Water	– i.v. bolus	*Cerebral blood flow (CBF)*
^{18}Fluorine	Fluorodeoxyglucose	– i.v. bolus	*Cerebral glucose metabolism (CMRgl)*
^{15}Oxygen	Oxygen	– inhalation	*Cerebral oxygen utilisation ($CMRO_2$)*
			Oxygen extraction factor (OEF)
^{11}Carbon	Drug, e.g. phenytoin	– i.v. bolus	*Drug receptor site*
^{11}Carbon	Methyl spiperone	– i.v. bolus	*Dopamine binding site*

Clinical and research uses

PET scanning is of particular value in elucidating the relationships between cerebral blood flow, oxygen utilisation and extraction in focal areas of ischaemia or infarction (page 237) and has been used to study patients with dementia, epilepsy and brain tumours. Identification of neurotransmitter and drug receptor sites has aided the understanding and management of psychiatric (schizophrenia) and movement disorders.

PET scan several days after a left middle cerebral infarct showing a reduction in blood flow

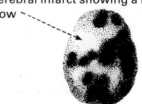

Oxygen utilisation is also reduced with a slight increase in oxygen extraction

48

ELECTROENCEPHALOGRAPHY (EEG)

Electroencephalography examines by means of scalp electrodes the spontaneous electrical activity of the brain. Tiny electrical potentials, which measure millionths of volts, are recorded, amplified and displayed on either 8 or 16 channels of a pen recorder. Low and high frequency filters remove unwanted signals such as muscle artefact and mains interference.

The system of electrode placement is referred to as the 10/20 system because the distance between bony points, i.e. inion to nasion, is divided into lengths of either 10% or 20% of the total, and the electrodes placed at each distance.

A switch changes recording from A (parasagittal) to B (transverse). Other electrode arrangements are also 'preset'. The numbering indicates the write out from top to bottom on an 8-channel record.

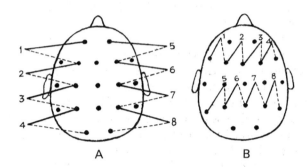

A   B

Normal rhythms

Alpha rhythm (8–13 Hz — cycles/second). Symmetrical and present posteriorly with the eyes closed—will disappear or 'block' with eye opening

Beta rhythm (>13 Hz). Symmetrical and present frontally. Not affected by eye opening

Theta rhythm (4-8 Hz) ⎰ Seen in children and young adults with
Delta rhythm <4 Hz) ⎱ frontal and temporal predominance

50uV | 1 sec

These 'immature' features should disappear in adult life as the EEG shows 'maturation'

As well as recording a resting EEG using various 'preset' electrode arrangements, stressing the patient by hyperventilation and photic stimulation (a flashing strobe light) may result in an electrical discharge supporting a diagnosis of epilepsy.

More advanced methods of telemetry and foramen ovale recording may be necessary

- to establish the diagnosis of 'epilepsy' if doubt remains
- to determine the exact frequency and site of the attacks
- to aid classification of seizure type.

Telemetry: utilises a continuous 24–48 hour recording of EEG, often combined with a videotape recording of the patient.

Foramen ovale recording: a needle electrode is passed percutaneously through the foramen ovale to record activity from the adjacent temporal lobe.

Magnetoencephalography

A new technique which measures changes in the magnetic field generated by the brain's electrical activity. It allows detection of the depth and location of current changes with better temporal and spatial resolution than the EEG.

INTRACRANIAL PRESSURE MONITORING

Although CSF pressure may be measured during lumbar puncture, this method is of limited value in intracranial pressure measurement:

An isolated pressure reading does not indicate the trend in intracranial pressure and pressure waves cannot be monitored.

Lumbar puncture is contraindicated in the presence of an intracranial mass.

Pressure gradients exist between different intracranial and spinal compartments, especially in the presence of brain shift.

Intracranial pressure is measured directly via a catheter inserted into the lateral ventricle. Alternatively, various devices are available to measure pressure on the hemisphere surface, either extradurally or through an opened dura. With these latter techniques, however, damping and pressure gradients may result in inaccuracies.

Technique

A ventricular catheter is inserted into the frontal horn of the lateral ventricle through a frontal burr hole situated two finger breadths from the midline, behind the hairline and anterior to the coronal suture.

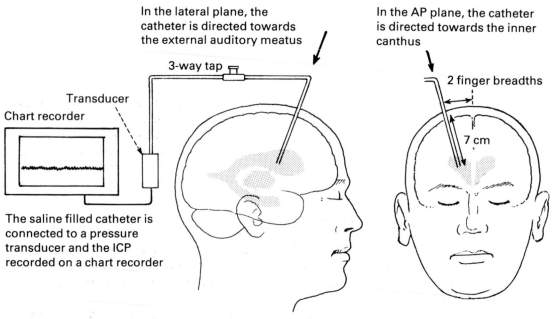

In the lateral plane, the catheter is directed towards the external auditory meatus

In the AP plane, the catheter is directed towards the inner canthus

3-way tap

2 finger breadths

Transducer

Chart recorder

7 cm

The saline filled catheter is connected to a pressure transducer and the ICP recorded on a chart recorder

Complications

Intracerebral haemorrhage following catheter insertion rarely occurs.

Ventriculitis seldom occurs provided monitoring does not continue for more than three days.

INTRACRANIAL PRESSURE MONITORING

NORMAL PRESSURE TRACE

Note waves caused by
pulse pressure and respiration

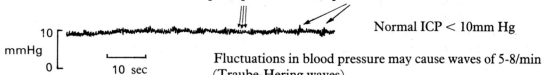

Normal ICP < 10mm Hg

Fluctuations in blood pressure may cause waves of 5-8/min
(Traube-Hering waves).

ABNORMAL PRESSURE TRACE

Look for: *Increase in the mean pressure* — >20 mmHg — moderate elevation
>40 mmHg — severe increase in pressure

N.B. As ICP increases, the amplitude of the pulse pressure wave increases.

β-waves

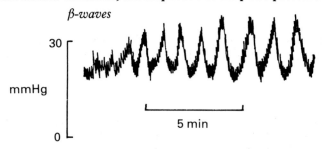

Frequency ½–2/min
Of variable amplitude
Often related to respiration

Plateau waves

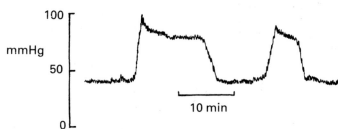

Elevation of ICP over 50 mmHg
lasting 5–20 minutes
Precede a severe continuous
rise in ICP and precursors of
further clinical deterioration

CLINICAL USES OF ICP MONITORING

1. Investigation of normal pressure hydrocephalus — the presence of ß waves for >5% of a 24-hour period suggests impaired CSF absorption and the need for a drainage operation.
2. Postoperative monitoring — a rise in ICP may precede clinical evidence of haematoma formation or cerebral swelling.
3. Small traumatic haematomas — ICP monitoring may guide management and indicate the need for operative removal.
4. ICP monitoring is required during treatment aimed at reducing a raised ICP.

EVOKED POTENTIALS – VISUAL, AUDITORY AND SOMATOSENSORY

RECORDING METHODS

Stimulation of any sensory receptor evokes a minute electrical signal (i.e. microvolts) in the appropriate region of the cerebral cortex. Averaging techniques permit recording and analysis of this signal normally lost within the background electrical activity. When sensitive apparatus is triggered to record cortical activity at a specific time after the stimulus, the background electrical 'noise' averages out, i.e. random positive activity subtracts from random negative activity, leaving the signal evoked from the specific stimulus.

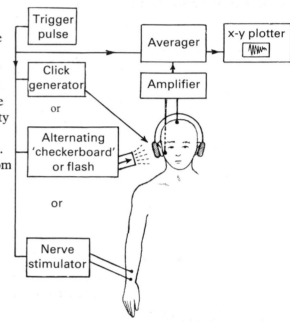

Visual evoked potential (VEP)

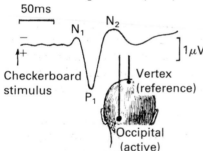

A stroboscopic flash diffusely stimulates the retina; alternatively an alternating checkerboard pattern stimulates the macula and produces more consistent results. The evoked visual signal is recorded over the occipital cortex. The first large positive wave (P_1) provides a useful point for measuring conduction through the visual pathways.

Uses: *Multiple sclerosis detection* — P_1 delayed in 90% of those with established disease.

Peroperative monitoring — pituitary surgery.

Brain stem auditory evoked potential (BAEP)

Electrical activity evoked in the first 10 milliseconds after a 'click' stimulus provides a wave pattern related to conduction through the auditory pathways in the VIII nerve and nucleus (waves I and II) and in the pons and midbrain (waves III – V). Longer latency potentials (up to 500 ms), recorded from the auditory cortex in response to a 'tone' stimulus, are of less clinical value.

Uses: *Hearing assessment* — especially in children.

Detection of intrinsic and extrinsic brain stem and cerebellopontine angle lesions, e.g. acoustic tumours.

Peroperative recording during acoustic tumour operations.

Assessment of brain stem function in coma.

EVOKED POTENTIALS – SOMATOSENSORY

Somatosensory evoked potentials (SEP)

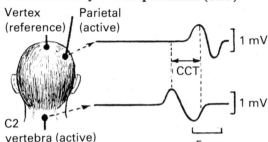

Vertex (reference)

Parietal (active)

1 mV

CCT

1 mV

C2 vertebra (active)

5 ms

The sensory evoked potential is recorded over the parietal cortex in response to stimulation of a peripheral nerve (e.g. median nerve). Other electrodes sited at different points along the sensory pathway record the ascending activity. Subtraction of the latencies between peaks provides conduction time between these sites.

Central conduction time (CCT)
Conduction time from the dorsal columns (or nuclei) to the parietal cortex.

Uses: *Detection of lesions in the sensory pathways* — brachial plexus injury
— spinal cord and brainstem tumours or demyelination.

Peroperative recording — straightening of scoliosis
— removal of spinal tumours/AVM } — spinal conduction
— aneurysm operation with temporary vessel occlusion — CCT.

MYELOGRAPHY

CT scanning and MRI are gradually replacing the need for myelography, but this still remains a useful (although invasive) method of screening the whole spinal cord and cauda equina for compressive or expanding lesions (e.g. disc disease or spondylosis, tumours, abscesses or cysts). Myelography may also clearly demonstrate lumbosacral or cervical root compression (although a normal study does not exclude the possibility of a laterally situated disc causing pressure on the distal root).

A water-soluble contrast medium is injected into the subarachnoid space via lumbar puncture (occasionally through a cervical puncture). Under direct screening with an image intensifier, the radiologist controls contrast flow up the spinal canal by varying the degree of patient tilt. X-rays provide a permanent record at the relevant levels.

Oblique view

Contrast should be screened up to the level of the conus medullaris (L1), i.e. RADICULOGRAPHY, for suspected root compression, e.g. disc disease. For suspected cord compression, the contrast is run up the whole length of the cord to the foramen magnum (page 379).

Note contrast filling the nerve roots

Problems

Arachnoiditis — previously a major complication with oil based contrast MYODIL, but rarely occurs with water soluble contrast.

Subdural injection (accidental) — prevents correct interpretation.

Haematoma — occurs rarely at the injection site.

Impaction of spinal tumour — may follow CSF escape and aggravate the effects of cord compression, leading to clinical deterioration.

53

LUMBAR PUNCTURE

Lumbar puncture permits: – acquisition of cerebrospinal fluid for analysis.
– CSF drainage and pressure reduction, e.g. in communicating hydrocephalus/CSF fistula.

TECHNIQUE

1. *Correct positioning of the patient is essential.* Open the vertebral laminae by drawing the knees up to the chest and flexing the neck. Ensure the back is perpendicular to the bed to avoid rotation of the spinal column.

2. Identify the site. The L3/L4 space lies level with the iliac crests and this is most often used, but since the spinal cord ends at L1 any space from L2/L3 to L5/S1 provides a safe approach.

3. Clean the area and insert a few millilitres of local anaesthetic.

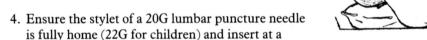

4. Ensure the stylet of a 20G lumbar puncture needle is fully home (22G for children) and insert at a slight angle towards the head, so that it parallels the spinous processes. Some resistance is felt as the needle passes through the ligamentum flavum, the dura and arachnoid layers.

L1
L2 – – Dura
L3 – – – Extradural fat
L4 – – – Ligamentum flavum
L5

5. Withdraw the stylet and collect the CSF. If bone is encountered, withdraw the needle and reinsert at a different angle. If the position appears correct yet no CSF appears, rotate the needle to free obstructive nerve roots.

A similar technique employing a TUOHY needle allows insertion of intra- or epidural cannula (for CSF drainage or drug instillation) or stimulating electrodes (for pain management).

Note: Do not perform lumbar puncture if raised intracranial pressure is suspect. Even a fine needle leaves a hole through which CSF will leak. In the presence of a space-occupying lesion, especially in the posterior fossa, CSF withdrawal creates a pressure gradient which may precipitate tentorial herniation.

CEREBROSPINAL FLUID

CSF COLLECTION
Subarachnoid haemorrhage (SAH), or puncture of a blood vessel by the needle, may account for blood stained CSF. To differentiate, collect CSF in three bottles.

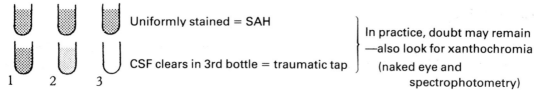

Uniformly stained = SAH

CSF clears in 3rd bottle = traumatic tap

In practice, doubt may remain
—also look for xanthochromia
(naked eye and
    spectrophotometry)

CSF PRESSURE MEASUREMENT
Check that the patient's head (foramen of Munro) is level with the lumbar puncture needle. Connect a manometer via a 3-way tap to the needle and allow CSF to run up the column. Read off the height.
Normal value: 100–150 mm CSF

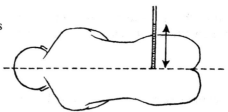

CSF ANALYSIS

Standard tests
1. Bacteriological – RBC and differential WBC (normal = < 5 WBCs per mm^3)
               – Gram stain and culture
               – appearance of supernatant. Xanthochromia (yellow staining) results from subarachnoid haemorrhage with RBC breakdown, high CSF protein or jaundice.
2. Biochemical   – protein (normal = 0.15–0.45 g/l)
                   – glucose (normal = 0.45–0.70 g/l)

Special tests
Suspected:
(i)   Malignant tumour   – cytology
(ii)   Tubercle   – Ziehl-Neelson stain, Lowenstein-Jensen culture
(iii) Non-bacterial infection – virology, fungal and parasitic studies
(iv) Demyelinating disease – γ globulin (normal = <12% of total protein) ⎱ not
                        oligoclonal bands   ⎰ pathognomonic

(v)   Neurosyphilis   – Wasserman test (WR),
                        Venereal Disease Research Lab. (VDRL),
                        Treponema pallidum immobilisation test (TPI)
(vi) Cryptococcus   – culture and antigen detection
(vii) HIV   – culture, antigen detection and
                      antiviral antibodies (anti-HIV-IgG).

ELECTROMYOGRAPHY/NERVE CONDUCTION STUDIES

Needle electromyography records the electrical activity occurring within a particular muscle.

Nerve conduction studies measure conduction in nerves in response to an electrical stimulus.

Both are essential in the investigation of diseases of nerve (neuropathy) and muscle (myopathy).

Repetitive nerve stimulation tests are important in the evaluation of disorders of neuromuscular transmission, e.g. myasthenia gravis.

ELECTROMYOGRAPHY

A concentric needle electrode is inserted into muscle. The central wire is the active electrode and the outer casing the reference electrode.

The potential difference between the two electrodes is amplified and displayed on an oscilloscope. An audio monitor enables the investigator to 'hear' the pattern of electrical activity.

Normal muscle at rest is electrically 'silent'; as the muscle gradually contracts, *motor unit potentials* appear...followed by the development of an *interference pattern*.

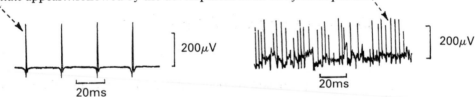

The recruitment of more and more motor units prevents identification of individual potentials

Abnormalities take the form of:
1. Spontaneous activity in muscle when at rest.
2. Abnormalities of the motor unit potential.
3. Abnormalities of the interference pattern.
4. Special phenomena, e.g. myotonia.

1. Spontaneous activity at rest

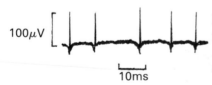

Fibrillation potentials are due to single muscle fibre contraction and indicate active denervation. They usually occur in neurogenic disorders, e.g. neuropathy, motor neuron disease, but can be seen in myopathies.

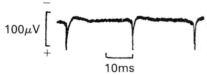

Positive sharp waves

Slow negative waves preceded by sharp positive spikes. Seen in chronically denervated muscle, e.g. motor neuron disease, but also in acute myopathy, e.g. polymyositis. These waves probably represent injury potentials.

ELECTROMYOGRAPHY/NERVE CONDUCTION STUDIES

Abnormalities (*contd*)

2. Motor unit potential

In myopathies and muscular dystrophies, potentials are polyphasic and of small amplitude and short duration.

In neuropathy, the surviving motor unit potentials are also polyphasic but of large amplitude and long duration.

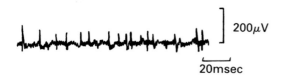 200μV

20msec

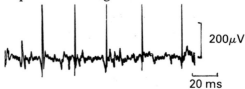 200μV

20 ms

The enlarged potentials result from collateral reinnervation.

3. Interference pattern

In myopathy, recruitment of motor units and the interference pattern remain normal. The interference pattern may even appear to increase due to fragmentation of motor units.

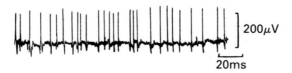 200μV

20ms

In neuropathy, there is a reduction in interference due to a loss of motor units under voluntary control.

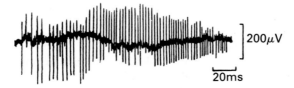 200μV

20ms

4. Myotonia

High frequency repetitive discharge may occur after voluntary movement. The amplitude and frequency of the potentials wax and wane giving rise to the typical 'dive bomber' sound on the audio monitor.

200μV

20ms

An abnormal myotonic discharge provoked by moving the needle electrode.

57

ELECTROMYOGRAPHY/NERVE CONDUCTION STUDIES

NERVE CONDUCTION STUDIES

Distal latency (latency from stimulus to recording electrodes), *amplitude* of the evoked response and *conduction velocity* all provide information on motor and sensory nerve function.

Conduction velocity: measurement made by stimulating or recording from two different sites along the course of a peripheral nerve.

$$\frac{\text{Distance between two sites}}{\substack{\text{Difference in conduction times} \\ \text{between two sites}}} = \text{Conduction velocity}$$

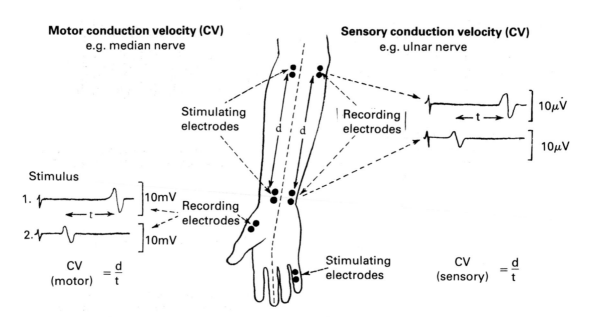

Normal values (motor)

Ulnar and median nerves – 50–60 m/s
Common peroneal nerve – 45–55 m/s

Normal values (sensory)

Ulnar and median nerves – 60–70 m/s
Common peroneal nerve – 50–70 m/s

Motor conduction velocities slow with age.
Body temperature is important; a fall of 1°C slows conduction in motor nerves by approximately 2 metres per second.

ELECTROMYOGRAPHY/NERVE CONDUCTION STUDIES

REPETITIVE STIMULATION

In the normal subject, repetitive stimulation of a motor nerve at a frequency of <30/second produces a muscle potential of constant form and amplitude. Increasing the stimulus frequency to >30/second results in fatigue manifest by a decline or 'decrement' in the amplitude. In patients with disorders of neuromuscular transmission, repetitive stimulation aids diagnosis:

Myasthenia gravis
A decrementing response occurs with a stimulus rate of 3–5/second.

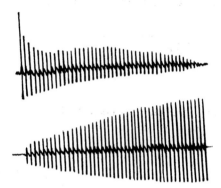

Myasthenic (Eaton Lambert) syndrome
With a stimulation rate of 20–50/second (i.e. rapid) a small amplitude response increases to normal amplitude — incrementing response.

SINGLE FIBRE ELECTROMYOGRAPHY

A standard concentric needle within muscle will record electrical activity 0.5–1 mm from its tip—sampling from up to 20 motor units. A 'single fibre' electromyography needle with a smaller recording surface detects electrical activity within 300 μm of its tip—sampling 1–3 muscle fibres from a single motor unit.

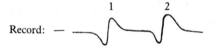

Parent axon from single anterior horn cell

Branch axons

Recording needle

Muscle fibres

Record: —

Action potentials recorded from two muscle fibres are not synchronous. The gap between each is variable and can be measured if the first recorded potential is 'locked' on the oscilloscope.

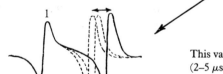

This variability is referred to as JITTER — normally 20–25 μs (2–5 μs due to transmission in the branch axon — 15–20 μs to variation in neuromuscular transmission).

Single fibre electromyography is valuable in the investigation of disorders of neuromuscular transmission as well as studying reinnervation in neuropathies.

NEURO-OTOLOGICAL TESTS

AUDITORY SYSTEM

Neuro-otological tests help differentiate conductive, cochlear and retrocochlear causes of impaired hearing. They supplement Weber's and Rinne's test (page 16).

PURE TONE AUDIOMETRY Thresholds for air and bone conduction are measured at different frequencies from 250 Hz to 8k Hz.

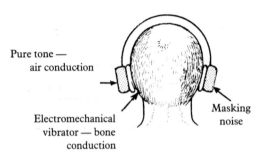

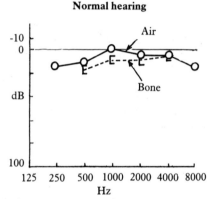

Normal hearing

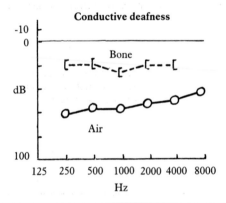

Conductive deafness

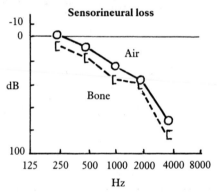

Sensorineural loss

TONE DECAY

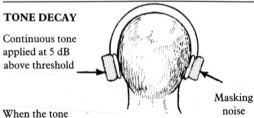

Continuous tone applied at 5 dB above threshold

When the tone disappears, the intensity is increased by 5 dB steps until the sound is heard for a 60 second period.

Tone decay is the inability to hear *continuous* sound at an intensity above the auditory threshold. It is of most value in detecting retrocochlear lesions.

Conduction deficit	– +5 dB required
Cochlear deficit	– +20 dB required

Retrocochlear deficit – >25 dB required

LOUDNESS DISCOMFORT

Tones of 100–120 dB produce discomfort in normal subjects and in patients with cochlear deafness. This contrasts to patients with conductive or retrocochlear deafness who experience little or no discomfort at high intensity.

NEURO-OTOLOGICAL TESTS

SPEECH AUDIOMETRY

This tests (i) sound intensity level at which the maximum percentage of words is perceived.

       (ii) the percentage score of words perceived when presented at 90 dB above the hearing threshold.

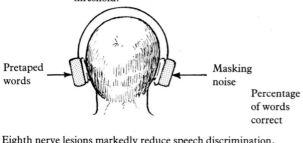

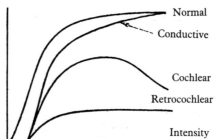

Eighth nerve lesions markedly reduce speech discrimination, but conductive and cochlear problems have some effect.

ACOUSTIC IMPEDENCE

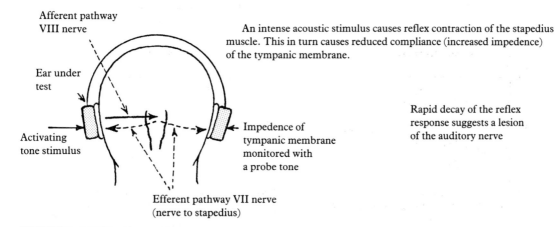

An intense acoustic stimulus causes reflex contraction of the stapedius muscle. This in turn causes reduced compliance (increased impedence) of the tympanic membrane.

Rapid decay of the reflex response suggests a lesion of the auditory nerve

AUDITORY BRAINSTEM EVOKED POTENTIAL

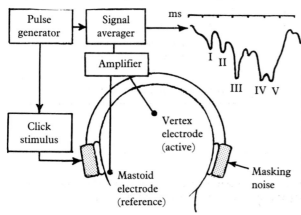

Averaging techniques (page 52) permit the recording and analysis of small electrical potentials evoked in response to auditory stimuli. Activity in the first 10 ms provides information about the VIII nerve and nucleus (waves I and II) and the pons and midbrain (waves III – V). Lesions of the VIII nerve diminish the amplitude and/or the latency of wave I or II and increase the wave I to V interpeak latency. In comparison, cochlear lesions seldom affect either wave pattern or latency.

61

NEURO-OTOLOGICAL TESTS

VESTIBULAR SYSTEM
Caloric testing (vestibulo-ocular reflex)
Compensatory mechanisms may mask clinical evidence of vestibular damage — spontaneous and positional nystagmus. Caloric testing provides useful supplementary information and may reveal undetected vestibular dysfunction.

Method: Water at 30°C is injected into the external auditory meatus. Nystagmus usually develops after a 20 second delay and lasts for more than a minute. The test is repeated after 5 minutes with water at 44°C.

    Cold water effectively reduces the vestibular output from one side, creating an imbalance and producing eye drift towards the irrigated ear. Rapid corrective movements result in 'nystagmus'. Hot water (44°C) reverses the convection current, increases the vestibular output and changes the direction of the nystagmus.

N.B. Ice water ensures a maximal stimulus when caloric testing for brain death or head injury prognostication.

Stimulus is maximal with the head supported 30° from the horizontal (with the lateral semicircular canal in a vertical plane).

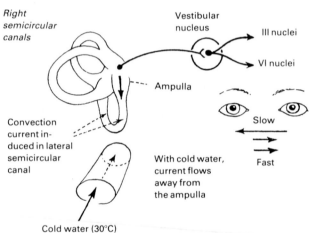

Time from onset of irrigation to the cessation of nystagmus is plotted for each ear, at each temperature.

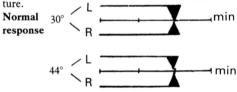

    Damage to the labyrinth, vestibular nerve or nucleus results in one of two abnormal patterns, or a combination of both.

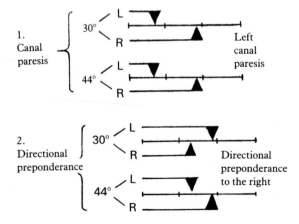

Electronystagmography: The potential difference across the eye (the corneoretinal potential) permits recording of eye movements with laterally placed electrodes and enables detection of spontaneous or reflex induced nystagmus in darkness or with the eyes closed. This eliminates optical fixation which may reduce or even abolish nystagmus.

Canal paresis implies reduced duration of nystagmus on one side. It may result from either a peripheral or central (brain stem or cerebellum) lesion on that side.

Directional preponderance implies a more prolonged duration of nystagmus in one direction than the other. It may result from a central lesion on the side of the preponderance or from a peripheral lesion on the other side.

These tests combined with audiometry should differentiate a peripheral from a central lesion.

CLINICAL PRESENTATION, ANATOMICAL CONCEPTS AND DIAGNOSTIC APPROACH

HEADACHE — GENERAL PRINCIPLES

Headache is a common symptom arising from psychological, otological, ophthalmological, neurological or systemic disease. In clinical practice psychological 'tension' headache is encountered most frequently.

Definition
Pain or discomfort between the orbits and occiput, arising from pain-sensitive structures.

Intracranial pain-sensitive structures are:
venous sinuses, cortical veins, basal arteries, dura of anterior, middle and posterior fossae.

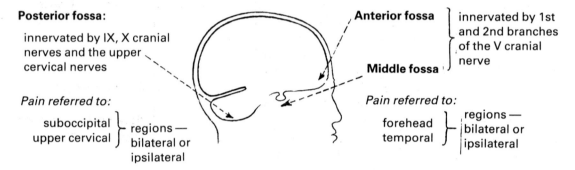

Posterior fossa:

innervated by IX, X cranial nerves and the upper cervical nerves

Pain referred to:

suboccipital ⎫
upper cervical ⎭ regions —
bilateral or
ipsilateral

Anterior fossa ⎫ innervated by 1st
  ⎬ and 2nd branches
  ⎰ of the V cranial
Middle fossa ⎭ nerve

Pain referred to:

forehead ⎫ regions —
temporal ⎭ bilateral or
ipsilateral

Extracranial pain-sensitive structures are:
Scalp vessels and muscles, orbital contents, mucous membranes of nasal and paranasal spaces, external and middle ear, teeth and gums.

In view of the many causes of head pain an accurate history and examination are essential to direct appropriate investigation and treatment.

Points from the history
1. *Character* of headache — sharp, dull, stabbing, throbbing.
2. *Site* — unilateral, bilateral, frontal, temporal, occipital.
3. *Mode of onset* — sudden, gradual.
4. *Frequency/duration* — one acute attack, recurrent attacks, chronic.
5. *Timing* — morning, night.
6. *Accompanying symptoms* — vomiting, double vision, watering eye, etc.
7. *Precipitating factors* — posture, exercise, food, hunger, noise, stress, coughing, menstruation, etc.

Examination
Full general examination, including:
  Ocular — acuity, tenderness, strabismus
  Teeth and scalp
  Percussion over frontal and maxillary sinuses.
Full neurological examination.

HEADACHE — DIAGNOSTIC APPROACH

The above clinical features all provide important diagnostic clues. Most information is derived from determining: – whether or not this is the first attack
– whether onset is acute or gradual (days or weeks)
– whether previous attacks have occurred
– whether attacks have recurred for many years (chronic).
The following table classifies causes in these categories:

ACUTE Cause	Associated features which (if present) aid diagnosis	RECURRENT ATTACKS	Further investigations (if required)
Sinusitis	preceding 'cold' nasal discharge	+	X-ray nasal sinuses
Migraine	visual/neurological aura, nausea, vomiting	+	
Cluster headache	lacrimation, rhinorrhoea	+	
Glaucoma	'misting' of vision 'haloes' around objects	+	Ophthalmological referral
Retrobulbar neuritis	loss of vision (unilateral)	–	Visual evoked response
Post-traumatic	preceding head injury		Skull X-ray, CT scan
Drugs/toxins	on vasodilator drugs		
Haemorrhage	instantaneous onset vomiting, neck stiffness impaired conscious level		CT scan, lumbar puncture (see page 54)
Infection (meningitis, encephalitis)	as above but more gradual onset with pyrexia	+ (if CSF fistula)	
Hydrocephalus	impaired conscious level, leg weakness, impaired upward gaze	+	CT scan
SUBACUTE			
Infection (subacute, chronic meningitis, e.g. TB cerebral abscess.)	impaired conscious level, pyrexia, neck stiffness, focal neurological signs	–	CT scan lumbar puncture
Intracranial tumour Chronic subdural haema- Hydrocephalus toma	vomiting, papilloedema, impaired conscious level ± focal neurological signs	+	CT scan
Benign intracranial hypertension	vomiting, papilloedema	+	CT scan, CSF pressure monitoring
Temporal arteritis	thickened, tender, scalp arteries	–	ESR, temporal artery biopsy
CHRONIC			
Tension headache	anxiety, depression	+	
Ocular 'eye strain'	impaired visual acuity	+	Refractive errors
Drugs/toxins	on vasodilator drugs		
Cervical spondylosis	neck, shoulder, arm pain	+	X-ray cervical spine

HEADACHE — DIAGNOSTIC APPROACH

Headache in children

All causes of adult headache (except retrobulbar neuritis, glaucoma, temporal arteritis and cervical spondylosis) may cause headache in children. In this age group, the commonest type of headache is that accompanying any *febrile illness* or *infection of the nasal passages or sinuses*.

The clinician, however, must not take a complaint of headache lightly; the younger the child, the more likely the presence of an underlying organic disease. Pyrexia may not only represent a mild 'constitutional' upset, but may result from *meningitis, encephalitis* or *cerebral abscess*. The presence of neck stiffness and/or impaired conscious level indicates the need for urgent investigation.

Although *intracranial tumours* are uncommon in childhood, when they occur they tend to lie in the *midline* (e.g. medulloblastoma, pineal region tumours.) As a result, obstructive hydrocephalus often develops acutely with headache as a prominent initial symptom.

In a child with 'unexplained' headache, *skull X-ray* and preferably *CT scan* should be performed:

- if the presentation is acute
- if the severity progressively increases
- if school performance declines, or other symptoms, e.g. personality change, develop
- if the head circumference increases
- if the child is under 5 years.

HEADACHE — SPECIFIC CAUSES

TENSION HEADACHE

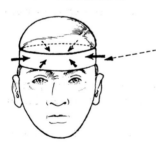

This is a common form of headache experienced by most people at some time of their lives.

Characteristics: Diffuse, dull, aching, 'band-like' headache, worse on touching the scalp and aggravated by noise; associated with 'tension' but not with other physical symptoms.
Duration: Many hours — days.
Frequency: Infrequent or daily; worse towards the end of the day.
May persist over many years.

Mechanism: 'Muscular' due to persistent contraction, e.g. clenching teeth, head posture, furrowing of brow.

Treatment: Reassurance
Benzodiazepines, e.g. diazepam (short course)
Antidepressants.

HEADACHE — SPECIFIC CAUSES

MIGRAINE
Migraine is a common, often familial disorder characterised by *unilateral throbbing headache*.

Onset: Childhood or early adult life.

Incidence: Affects 5-10% of the population.

Female: male ratio: 2:1.

Family history: Obtained in 70% of all sufferers.

Two recognisable forms exist:

CLASSIC MIGRAINE
An *aura* or warning of visual, sensory or motor type followed by headache – throbbing, unilateral, worsened by bright light, relieved by sleep, associated with nausea and, occasionally, vomiting.

COMMON MIGRAINE
The *aura* is absent. The headache has similar features, but it is often poorly localised and its description may merge with that of 'tension' headache.

The aura of classic migraine may take many forms. The visual forms comprise: flashing lights, zig-zags (fortifications), scintillating scotoma (central vision) and may precede visual field defects. Such auras are of retinal or visual (occipital) cortex origin.

The headache is paroxysmal, lasting from 2 to 48 hours and rarely occurring more frequently than twice weekly.

Mechanism
Whether migraine is primarily a VASCULAR or NEURONAL disorder remains controversial. Studies of regional cerebral blood flow and metabolism support the neuronal hypothesis and suggest a defect in neurotransmitter release (serotonin).

TYPES OF 'CLASSIC' MIGRAINE (COMPLICATED MIGRAINE)
Basilar: Characterised by bilateral visual symptoms, unsteadiness, dysarthria, vertigo, limb parasthesia, even tetraparesis. Loss of consciousness may ensue and precede the onset of headache. This form of migraine frequently affects young women.

Hemiplegic: Characterised by an aura of unilateral paralysis (hemiplegia) which can persist for some days after the headache has settled. Often misdiagnosed as a 'stroke'. When familial, mendelian dominant inheritance is noted. Recovery is the rule.

Ophthalmoplegic: Characterised by extraocular nerve palsies, usually the IIIrd, rarely the VIth. These may result from dilatation of the internal carotid artery with stretching of the III or VI cranial nerve within the cavernous sinus.

Dysphasia, memory disturbance, vertigo or a hemisensory disturbance may also occur.

Focal neurological disturbance without headache may result from a *migraine equivalent*.

HEADACHE — SPECIFIC CAUSES

Precipitating factors in Migraine

The migraine sufferer can often identify exogenous factors which induce attacks. Dietary factors include alcohol, chocolate and cheese (high tyramine content). Attacks in women are often more common premenstrually and when on the oral contraceptive. They may disappear in pregnancy. Stress, physical fatigue, exercise, sleep deprivation and minor head trauma may all precipitate attacks.

Diagnosis

From clinical history, supported by:

- a positive family history
- the presence of travel sickness or migraine variants (abdominal pains) in childhood
- age of onset — childhood, adolescence, early adult life, menopause.

Distinguish from:

- partial (focal) epilepsy (in hemiplegic or hemisensory migraine)
- aneurysmal dilatation compressing III cranial nerve (in ophthalmoplegic migraine)
- transient ischaemic attack (in hemiplegic or hemisensory migraine)
- arteriovenous malformation — gives well localised but chronic headache
- hypoglycaemia.

Management

1. Identification and avoidance of precipitatory factors.
2. Prophylaxis:

    Justification – frequent and severe attacks.

    Commonly used drugs – Pizotifen (powerful antiserotonin)

    Propranolol (beta adrenergic receptor blocker)

    Methysergide (powerful antiserotonin — use with caution in view of the side effects, e.g. retroperitoneal fibrosis).

3. Treatment of an attack:

    Poor gastrointestinal absorption of drugs during attack.

    Metoclopramide will enhance absorption of soluble aspirin, etc.

    Ergotamine tartrate may be used in severe attacks. In a severely prolonged episode (status migrainosus), hydrocortisone i.v. will halt the attack. $5HT_1$ agonists.

CLUSTER HEADACHES (Histamine cephalgia)

Cluster headaches occur less frequently than migraine, and more often in men than women, with onset in early middle age.

Characteristics: Severe unilateral pain around the eye, *associated with* conjunctival injection, lacrimation, rhinorrhoea and, occasionally, a transient Horner's syndrome.

Duration: 10 minutes to 2 hours.

Frequency: Once to many times per day, often wakening from sleep at night. 'Clusters' of attacks separated by weeks or even many months. Alcohol may precipitate the attacks.

Mechanism: Serum histamine levels rise during the attacks, hence the alternative name 'histamine cephalgia'.

Treatment: Antihistamines give disappointing results. Ergotamine and methysergide are useful prophylactics. Lithium administration may benefit. Use prednisolone 30 mg daily for 10 days in refractory cases.

HEADACHE — SPECIFIC CAUSES

POST-TRAUMATIC HEADACHE
A 'common migraine' or 'tension-like' headache may arise after head injury and accompany other symptoms including light-headedness, irritability, difficulty in concentration and in coping with work. Although once thought to have a purely 'psychological' origin, especially with impending litigation, it is now recognised that injuries severe enough to cause loss of consciousness or a period of post-traumatic amnesia result in some neuronal damage, requiring several weeks to recover.

Treatment: As for tension headache.

GIANT CELL (TEMPORAL) ARTERITIS
Giant cell arteritis causes headache in the elderly. This is severe and throbbing in nature and overlies the involved vessel — usually the superficial temporal artery, although the condition may affect any extra- or intracranial vessels. *Palpation* reveals a thickened, tender, but nonpulsatile artery.

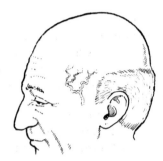

Jaw claudication: pain when chewing or talking due to ischaemia of the masseter muscles is pathognomonic and occurs in a high proportion of patients.
Visual symptoms are common with blindness or diplopia.
Associated systemic symptoms — weight loss, lassitude and generalised muscle aches — polymyalgia rheumatica in one-fifth of cases.
Duration: the headache is intractable, lasting until treatment commences.

Mechanism:
Large and medium-sized arteries undergo intense 'giant cell' infiltration, with fragmentation of the lamina and narrowing of the lumen, resulting in distal ischaemia as well as stimulating pain sensitive fibres. Occlusion of important end arteries, e.g. the ophthalmic artery, may result in blindness; occlusion of the basilar artery may cause brain stem or bilateral occipital infarction.

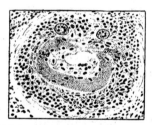

Thickened wall with giant cell infiltrate

Diagnosis: ESR usually high. C-reactive protein and hepatic alkaline phosphatase elevated. Biopsy of 1 cm length of temporal artery is often diagnostic.

Treatment: Urgent treatment, prednisolone 60 mg daily, prevents visual loss or brain-stem stroke, as well as relieving the headache. Monitoring the ESR allows gradual reduction in steroid dosage over several weeks to a maintenance level, e.g. 5 mg daily. Most patients eventually come off steroids; 25% require long-term treatment.

HEADACHE — SPECIFIC CAUSES

HEADACHE FROM RAISED INTRACRANIAL PRESSURE

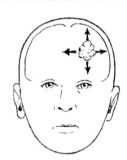

Characteristics:
– generalised.
– aggravated by bending or coughing.
– worse in the morning on awakening; may awaken patient from sleep.
– the severity of the headache gradually progresses.
Associated features:
– vomiting in later stages.
– transient loss of vision (obscuration) with sudden change
   in posture.
– eventual impairment of conscious level.
Management: further investigations are essential — CT scan.

HEADACHE DUE TO INTRACRANIAL HAEMORRHAGE

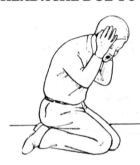

Characteristics:
– instantaneous onset.
– severe pain, spreading over the vertex to the occiput, or
   described as a 'sudden blow to the back of the head'.
– patient may drop to knees or lose consciousness.
Associated features:
– usually accompanied by vomiting.
– focal neurological signs suggest a haematoma.
Management: further investigation — CT scan/lumbar puncture
   (see Meningism, page 71).

NON-NEUROLOGICAL CAUSES OF HEADACHE

Local causes:
Sinuses: Well localised. Worse in morning. Affected by posture, e.g. bending.
   X-ray — sinus opacified. Treatment — decongestants or drainage.
Ocular: Refraction errors may result in 'muscle contraction' headaches — resolves when
   corrected with glasses.
   Glaucoma does not produce headache without other symptoms, e.g. misting of vision,
   'haloes'. Cupping seen on fundoscopy.
Dental disease: Discomfort localised to teeth. Check for malocclusion.
   Check temporomandibular joints.

Systemic causes:
Headache may accompany any febrile illness or may be the presenting feature of accelerated
hypertension or metabolic disease, e.g. hypoglycaemia, hypercalcaemia.
   Many drugs, e.g. dipyridamole and toxins, e.g. caffeine may also cause headache.

70

MENINGISM

Evidence of meningeal irritation caused by infection or subarachnoid haemorrhage results in characteristic clinical features:

SYMPTOMS

1. Headache
2. Vomiting
3. Photophobia

SIGNS

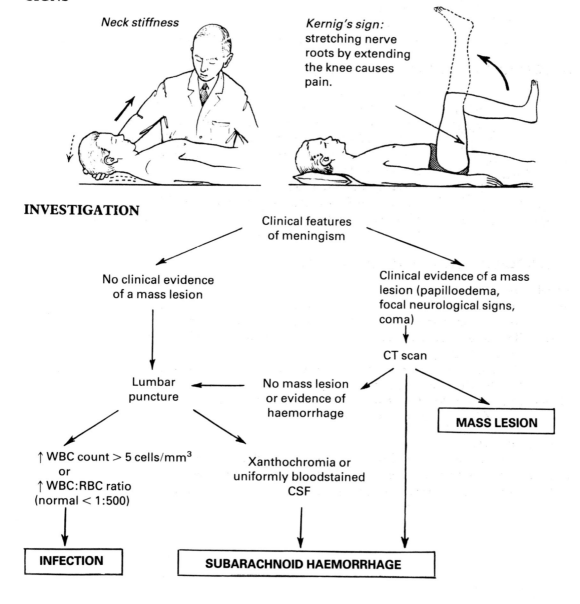

Neck stiffness

Kernig's sign: stretching nerve roots by extending the knee causes pain.

INVESTIGATION

Clinical features of meningism

No clinical evidence of a mass lesion

Clinical evidence of a mass lesion (papilloedema, focal neurological signs, coma)

CT scan

Lumbar puncture ← No mass lesion or evidence of haemorrhage

MASS LESION

↑ WBC count > 5 cells/mm³
or
↑ WBC:RBC ratio
(normal < 1:500)

Xanthochromia or uniformly bloodstained CSF

INFECTION

SUBARACHNOID HAEMORRHAGE

71

RAISED INTRACRANIAL PRESSURE

The skull is basically a rigid structure. Since its contents – brain, blood and cerebrospinal fluid (CSF) – are incompressible, an increase in one constituent or an expanding mass within the skull results in an increase in intracranial pressure (ICP) – the 'Monro Kellie doctrine'.

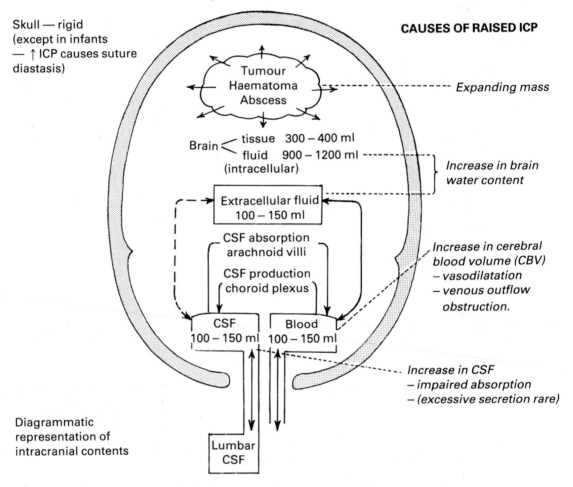

Skull — rigid
(except in infants
— ↑ ICP causes suture
diastasis)

CAUSES OF RAISED ICP

Tumour
Haematoma
Abscess

----------- Expanding mass

Brain ⟨ tissue 300 – 400 ml
       ⟨ fluid   900 – 1200 ml ------
       (intracellular)

⎫ Increase in brain
⎬ water content

Extracellular fluid
100 – 150 ml

CSF absorption
arachnoid villi

Increase in cerebral
blood volume (CBV)
– vasodilatation
– venous outflow
  obstruction.

CSF production
choroid plexus

CSF   Blood
100 – 150 ml   100 – 150 ml

Increase in CSF
– impaired absorption
– (excessive secretion rare)

Diagrammatic
representation of
intracranial contents

Lumbar
CSF

Compensatory mechanisms for an expanding intracranial mass lesion:

Immediate ⎰ 1. ↓ CSF volume — CSF outflow to the lumbar theca
          ⎱ 2. ↓ Cerebral blood volume
Delayed —   3. ↓ Extracellular fluid

RAISED INTRACRANIAL PRESSURE

CEREBROSPINAL FLUID (CSF)

Secreted at a rate of 500 ml per day from the choroid plexus, CSF flows through the ventricular system and enters the subarachnoid space via the 4th ventricular foramina of Magendie and Luschka.

Under normal conditions, CSF flows freely through the subarachnoid space and is absorbed into the venous system through the arachnoid villi. If flow is obstructed at any point in the pathway, *hydrocephalus* with an associated rise in intracranial pressure develops, as a result of continued CSF production. With an expanding intracranial mass lesion, normal pressure is initially maintained by CSF expulsion to the expandable lumbar theca. Further expansion and subsequent brain shift may obstruct the free flow of CSF not only to the lumbar theca but also to the arachnoid villi, causing an acute rise in intracranial pressure.

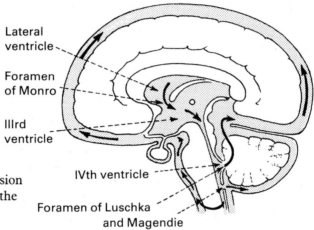

Lateral ventricle

Foramen of Monro

IIIrd ventricle

IVth ventricle

Foramen of Luschka and Magendie

BRAIN WATER/OEDEMA

Cerebral oedema — an excess of brain water — may develop around an intrinsic lesion within the brain tissue, e.g. tumour or abscess or in relation to traumatic or ischaemic brain damage, and contribute to the space-occupying effect.

Different forms of cerebral oedema exist:

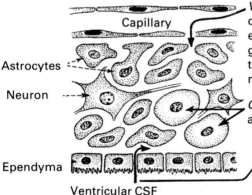

Capillary

Astrocytes

Neuron

Ependyma

Ventricular CSF

Vasogenic: excess fluid (protein rich) passes through defective vessel walls to the extracellular space — especially in the white matter. The extracellular fluid gradually infiltrates throughout normal brain tissue towards the ventricular CSF and this drainage route may aid clearance.

Cytotoxic: fluid accumulates within cells — neurons and glia i.e. intracellular.

Interstitial: when obstructive hydrocephalus develops CSF is forced through to the extracellular space especially in the periventricular white matter.

With *ischaemic* damage, as cell metabolism fails, intracellular Na^+ and Ca^{2+} increases and the cells swell i.e. cytotoxic oedema. Capillary damage follows and vasogenic oedema supervenes.

RAISED INTRACRANIAL PRESSURE

CEREBRAL BLOOD FLOW (CBF)/CEREBRAL BLOOD VOLUME (CBV)
Blood flow is dependent on blood pressure and the vascular resistance:

$$\text{Flow} = \frac{\text{Pressure}}{\text{Resistance}}$$

Inside the skull, intracranial pressure must be taken into account:

$$\text{Cerebral blood flow (CBF)} = \frac{\text{Cerebral perfusion pressure (CPP)}}{\text{Cerebral vascular resistance (CVR)}} \text{ (i.e. systemic BP — intracranial pressure)}$$

Under normal conditions the cerebral blood flow is coupled to the energy requirements of brain tissue. Various regulatory mechanisms acting on the arterioles maintain a cerebral blood flow sufficient to meet the metabolic demands.

FACTORS AFFECTING THE CEREBRAL VASCULATURE
Chemoregulation
– Change in extracellular pH or an accumulation of metabolic by-products directly affect the vessel calibre.
– Any change in arteriolar PCO_2 has a direct effect on cerebral vessels, but only a reduction of PO_2 to < 50 mmHg has a significant effect.
Autoregulation
– A change in the cerebral perfusion pressure results in a compensatory change in vessel calibre.

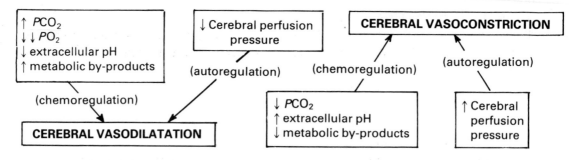

Any change in blood vessel diameter results in considerable variation in cerebral blood volume and this, in turn, directly affects intracranial pressure.

Energy requirements differ in different parts of the brain. In the white matter, flow is 20 ml/100 g/min, whereas in the grey matter flow is as high as 100 ml/100 g/min.

RAISED INTRACRANIAL PRESSURE

CEREBRAL BLOOD FLOW *(contd)*

Autoregulation is a compensatory mechanism which permits fluctuation in the cerebral perfusion pressure within certain limits without significantly altering cerebral blood flow.

A drop in cerebral perfusion pressure produces vasodilatation (probably due to a direct 'myogenic' effect on the vascular smooth muscle) thereby maintaining flow; a rise in the cerebral perfusion pressure causes vasoconstriction.

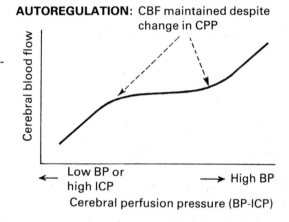

Neurogenic influences appear to have little direct effect on the cerebral vessels but they may alter the range of pressure changes over which autoregulation acts.

Autoregulation fails when the cerebral perfusion pressure falls below 60 mmHg or rises above 160 mmHg. At these extremes, cerebral blood flow is more directly related to the perfusion pressure.

In damaged brain (e.g. after head injury or subarachnoid haemorrhage), autoregulation is impaired; a drop in cerebral perfusion pressure is more likely to reduce cerebral blood flow and cause ischaemia. Conversely, a high cerebral perfusion may increase the cerebral blood flow, break down the blood-brain barrier and produce cerebral oedema as in hypertensive encephalopathy.

INTRACRANIAL PRESSURE (ICP)

Intracranial pressure, measured relative to the foramen of Monro, under normal conditions ranges from 0–135 mm CSF (0–10 mmHg) although very high pressures, e.g, 1000 mm CSF may occur transiently during coughing or straining.

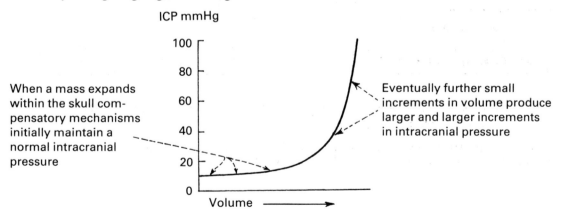

RAISED INTRACRANIAL PRESSURE

ICP (*contd*)

When intracranial pressure is monitored with a ventricular catheter, regular waves due to pulse and respiratory effects are recorded (page 51). As an intracranial mass expands and as the compensatory reserves diminish, transient pressure elevations (pressure waves) are superimposed. These become more frequent and more prominent as the mean pressure rises.

Eventually the rise in intracranial pressure and resultant fall in cerebral perfusion pressure reach a critical level and a significant reduction in cerebral blood flow occurs. Electrical activity in the cortex fails at flow rates about 20 ml/100 g/min. If autoregulation is already impaired these effects develop even earlier. When intracranial pressure reaches the mean arterial blood pressure, cerebral blood flow ceases.

INTERRELATIONSHIPS

Many factors affect intracranial pressure and these should not be considered in isolation. Inter-relationships are complex and feedback pathways may merely serve to compound the brain damage.

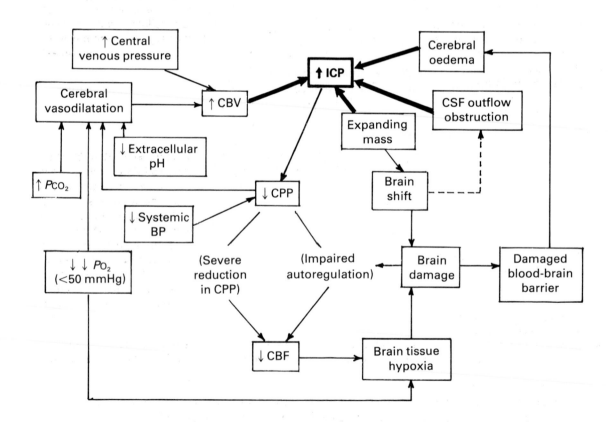

RAISED INTRACRANIAL PRESSURE

CLINICAL EFFECTS OF RAISED INTRACRANIAL PRESSURE

A raised ICP will produce symptoms and signs but does not cause neuronal damage provided cerebral blood flow is maintained. Damage does, however, result from brain shift — tentorial or tonsillar herniation.

Clinical features due to ↑ ICP:

1. *Headache* — worse in the mornings, aggravated by stooping and bending.
2. *Vomiting* — occurs with an acute rise in ICP.
3. *Papilloedema* — occurs in a proportion of patients with ↑ ICP. It is related to CSF obstruction and does not necessarily occur with brain shift alone. Increased CSF pressure in the optic nerve sheath impedes venous drainage and axoplasmic flow in optic neurons. Swelling of the optic disc and retinal and disc haemorrhages result. Vision is only at risk when papilloedema is both severe and prolonged.

BRAIN SHIFT — TYPES

TENTORIAL HERNIATION (lateral): a unilateral expanding mass causes tentorial (uncal) herniation as the medial edge of the temporal lobe herniates through the tentorial hiatus. As the intracranial pressure continues to rise, 'central' herniation follows.

SUBFALCINE 'MIDLINE' SHIFT: occurs early with unilateral space-occupying lesions. Seldom produces any clinical effect, although ipsilateral anterior cerebral artery occlusion has been recorded.

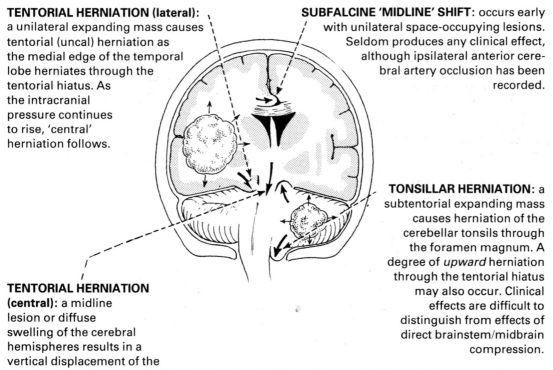

TONSILLAR HERNIATION: a subtentorial expanding mass causes herniation of the cerebellar tonsils through the foramen magnum. A degree of *upward* herniation through the tentorial hiatus may also occur. Clinical effects are difficult to distinguish from effects of direct brainstem/midbrain compression.

TENTORIAL HERNIATION (central): a midline lesion or diffuse swelling of the cerebral hemispheres results in a vertical displacement of the midbrain and diencephalon through the tentorial hiatus. Damage to these structures occurs either from mechanical distortion or from ischaemia secondary to stretching of the perforating vessels.

Unchecked lateral tentorial herniation leads to central tentorial and tonsillar herniation, associated with progressive brain stem dysfunction from midbrain to medulla.

RAISED INTRACRANIAL PRESSURE

CLINICAL EFFECTS OF BRAIN SHIFT

TENTORIAL HERNIATION — Lateral

The posterior cerebral artery is sometimes occluded but the resultant *homonymous hemianopia* is rarely detected in the acute stage

The rate of symptom progression is related to the rate of lesion expansion.

Pressure against the reticular formation in the midbrain causes *deterioration of conscious level*

Basilar artery

Anterior cerebral artery

Pressure from the edge of the tentorium cerebelli on the opposite cerebral peduncle (Kernohan's notch) may produce *limb weakness on the same side* as the lesion i.e. 'false localising sign'

Pons

III nerve

Internal carotid artery

Compression of the III nerve and oculomotor nucleus in the midbrain causes *pupil dilatation and failure to react to light.* [*Ptosis* and *impaired eye movements* are less easy to detect due to the associated depression of conscious level.]

(Optic nerves and chiasma are not illustrated)

TENTORIAL HERNIATION — Central

Diencephalon and midbrain damage from buckling and distortion and stretching of perforating vessels causes: *deterioration of conscious level. Pupils initially small, become moderately dilated and fixed to light*

Pressure on dorsal aspect (pretectum and superior colliculi) *impairs eye movements* – upward gaze is initially lost

Central tentorial herniation may progress to tonsillar herniation- - - -

Downward traction on pituitary stalk and hypothalamus may cause *diabetes insipidus*

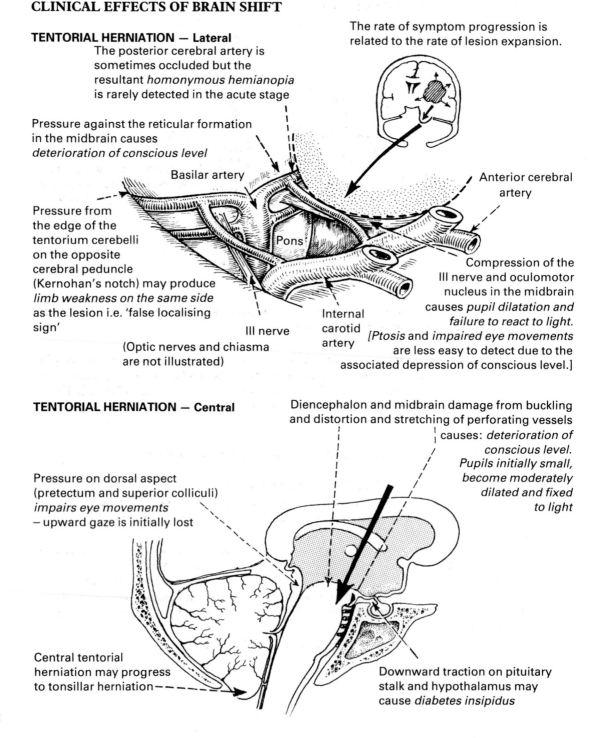

HEFFERS BOOKSELLERS
20 TRINITY STREET
CAMBRIDGE CB2 3NG
TEL: 01223 568568
FAX: 01223 568591
VAT: GB 213 4152 13

Neurology and neurosurgery ill		
0443043450	1	33.0
Neuroanatomy		
0443044791	1	17.5
Cognitive assessment for clin		
019262394X	1	17.5

==============================

TOTAL £ 68.0
DELTA 68.0

DATE: 8/ 6/96 TIME: 17:1
TILL 5 . OP 5 . BRANCH 1
RECEIPT NO. 79180

THANK YOU

RAISED INTRACRANIAL PRESSURE

CLINICAL EFFECTS OF BRAIN SHIFT (*contd*)

TONSILLAR HERNIATION

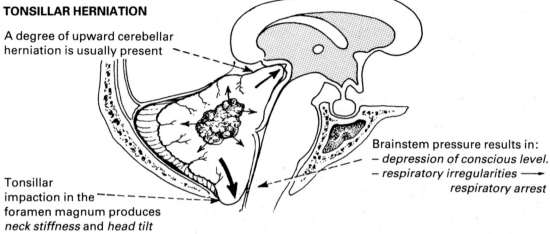

A degree of upward cerebellar herniation is usually present

Brainstem pressure results in:
– *depression of conscious level.*
– *respiratory irregularities* →
    respiratory arrest

Tonsillar impaction in the foramen magnum produces *neck stiffness* and *head tilt*

An injudicious lumbar puncture in the presence of a subtentorial mass may create a pressure gradient sufficient to induce tonsillar herniation.

N.B. Harvey Cushing described cardiovascular changes — an increase in blood pressure and a fall in pulse rate, associated with an expanding intracranial mass, and probably resulting from direct medullary compression. The clinical value of these observations is often overemphasised. They are often absent; when present they are invariably preceded by a deterioration in conscious level.

INVESTIGATIONS
Patients with suspected raised intracranial pressure require an urgent CT scan.

TREATMENT OF RAISED INTRACRANIAL PRESSURE
When a rising intracranial pressure is caused by an expanding mass, or is compounded by respiratory problems, treatment is clear-cut; the mass must be removed and blood gases restored to normal levels — by ventilation if necessary.

In some patients, despite the above measures, cerebral swelling may produce a marked increase in intracranial pressure. This may follow removal of a tumour or haematoma or may complicate a diffuse head injury. Artificial methods of lowering intracranial pressure may prevent brain damage and death from brain shift, although their use in some instances is controversial (see page 227).

Intracranial pressure is monitored with a ventricular catheter or surface pressure recording device (see page 50).

Treatment may be instituted when the mean ICP is >30 mmHg.

RAISED INTRACRANIAL PRESSURE

TREATMENT *(contd)*
Methods of reducing intracranial pressure

Mannitol infusion: An i.v. bolus of 100 ml of 20% mannitol infused over 15 minutes reduces intracranial pressure by establishing an osmotic gradient between the plasma and brain tissue. *This method 'buys' time prior to craniotomy in a patient deteriorating from a mass lesion.* Mannitol is also used 6 hourly for a 24–48 hour period in an attempt to reduce raised ICP. Repeated infusions, however, lead to equilibration and a high intracellular osmotic pressure, thus counteracting further treatment. In addition, repeated doses may precipitate lethal rises in arterial blood pressure and acute tubular necrosis. Its use is therefore best restricted for emergency situations.

Hyperventilation: If the patient is paralysed and hyperventilated — bringing the $P\text{CO}_2$ down to 3.5 kPa, the resultant vasoconstriction and reduction in cerebral blood volume lowers intracranial pressure. (A further drop in $P\text{CO}_2$ risks ischaemic damage due to severe vasoconstriction.) In many patients, however, adaptation to the new $P\text{CO}_2$ level occurs and after several hours the intracranial pressure gradually rises to previous levels.

CSF withdrawal: Removal of a few millilitres of CSF from the ventricle will immediately reduce the intracranial pressure. Within minutes, however, the pressure will rise and further CSF withdrawal will be required. In practice, this method is of limited value, since CSF outflow to the lumbar theca results in a diminished intracranial CSF volume and the lateral ventricles are often collapsed. Continuous CSF drainage may make most advantage of this method.

Barbiturate therapy: Some workers have advocated barbiturate therapy in the treatment of raised intracranial pressure following brain damage. This reduces neuronal activity and depresses cerebral metabolism; a fall in energy requirements may protect ischaemic areas and subsequent vasoconstriction may reduce cerebral blood volume and intracranial pressure. Although some experimental studies have shown encouraging results, clinical trials have yet to show convincing benefit. (See 'Brain protection', page 238.)

Steroids: There is no doubt that steroids play an important rôle in treating patients with intracranial tumours and surrounding oedema. Cell membranes are stabilised, but it is not certain that their beneficial effect in tumour management is a result of reducing ICP. Steroids appear to be of no value in the treatment of traumatic or ischaemic damage. Experimental evidence suggests that they may help if administered before the damage occurs, but clearly this is seldom of practical value.

COMA AND IMPAIRED CONSCIOUS LEVEL

Many pathological processes may impair conscious level and numerous terms have been employed to describe the various clinical states which result, including obtundation, stupor, semicoma and deep-coma. These terms result in ambiguity and inconsistency when used by different observers. Recording conscious level with the *Glasgow coma scale* (page 5) avoids these difficulties and clearly describes the level of consciousness. With this scale:

COMA = NO SPEECH, NO EYE OPENING, NO MOTOR RESPONSE

In this section we describe conditions which may present with, or lead to, coma. Patients experiencing 'transient disturbance of conscious level' require a different approach.

Pathophysiology of coma

A 'conscious' state depends on intact cerebral hemispheres, interacting with the ascending reticular activating system in the brain stem, midbrain, hypothalamus and thalamus. Lesions diffusely affecting the cerebral hemispheres, or directly affecting the reticular activating system cause impairment of conscious level:

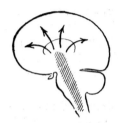

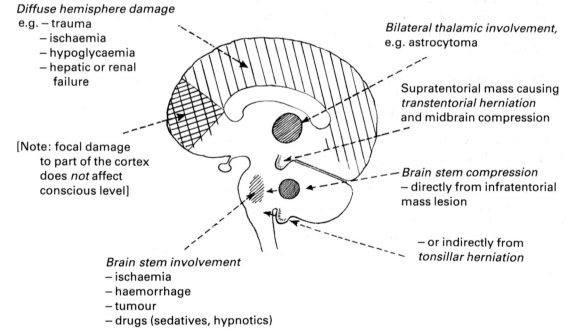

Diffuse hemisphere damage
e.g. – trauma
    – ischaemia
    – hypoglycaemia
    – hepatic or renal
      failure

[Note: focal damage
    to part of the cortex
    does *not* affect
    conscious level]

Bilateral thalamic involvement,
e.g. astrocytoma

Supratentorial mass causing
transtentorial herniation
and midbrain compression

Brain stem compression
– directly from infratentorial
mass lesion

– or indirectly from
tonsillar herniation

Brain stem involvement
  – ischaemia
  – haemorrhage
  – tumour
  – drugs (sedatives, hypnotics)

COMA AND IMPAIRED CONSCIOUS LEVEL

CAUSES

INTRACRANIAL

Trauma
Diffuse white matter injury
Haematoma – extradural
            – subdural
            – 'burst' lobe

Neoplastic
Tumour with oedema

Other
Epilepsy
Hydrocephalus

Vascular
Subarachnoid haemorrhage
'Spontaneous' intracerebral haematoma
Cerebral infarct with oedema and 'shift'
Vertebrobasilar infarct

Infective
Meningitis
Abscess
Encephalitis

EXTRACRANIAL

Metabolic
Hypo/hypernatraemia
Hypo/hyperkalaemia
Hypo/hypercalcaemia
Hypo/hyperglycaemia
Acidosis/alkalosis
Hypo/hyperthermia
Uraemia
Hepatic failure
Porphyria

Hypercapnia
Hypoxia

Endocrine
Diabetes
Hypopituitarism
Adrenal crisis (Addison's disease)
Hypo/hyperparathyroidism
Hypothyroidism

Respiratory insufficiency
Hypoventilation
Diffusion deficiency
Perfusion deficiency
Anaemia

Arterial occlusion
Reduced cerebral blood flow
Vertebral artery disease
Bilateral carotid disease

Decreased cardiac output
Vasovagal attack
Blood loss
Valvular disease
Myocardial infarction
Cardiac arrhythmias
Hypotensive drugs

Drugs
Sedatives
Opiates
Antidepressants
Anticonvulsants
Anaesthetic agents

Toxins
Alcohol
Carbon monoxide
Heavy metals

Psychiatric disease
Hysteria
Catatonia
Fugue states

COMA AND IMPAIRED CONSCIOUS LEVEL

Examination of the unconscious patient *(see pages 29,30)*

DIAGNOSTIC APPROACH
Questioning friends, relatives or the ambulance team, followed by general and neurological examination all provide important diagnostic information.

History

POSSIBLE CAUSE OF COMA/IMPAIRED CONSCIOUS LEVEL

Head injury leading to admission ⟶ *Diffuse shearing injury and/or intracranial haematoma*

Previous head injury (e.g. 6 weeks) ⟶ *Chronic subdural haematoma*

Sudden collapse ⟶ *Intracerebral haemorrhage*
Subarachnoid haemorrhage

Limb twitching, incontinence ⟶ *Epilepsy/postictal state*

Gradual development of symptoms ⟶ *Mass lesion, metabolic or infective cause*

Previous illness – diabetes ⟶ *Hypo- or (less likely) hyperglycaemia*

    – epilepsy ⟶ *Postictal state*

    – psychiatric illness ⟶ *Drug overdose*

    – alcoholism ⟶ *Drug toxicity*
      or drug abuse

    – viral infection ⟶ *Encephalitis*

    – malignancy ⟶ *Intracranial metastasis*

General examination

Note the presence of:

    Laceration, bruising, CSF leak ⟶ *Head injury*
    Internal auditory meatus – bleeding
            pus ⟶ *Cerebral abscess/meningitis*

    Enlarged head }
    Tense anterior fontanelle } In infant ⟶ *Raised intracranial pressure*

    Neck stiffness, retraction ⟶ *Tonsillar herniation*
    Positive Kernig's sign ⟶ *Meningitis*
    Tongue biting ⟶ *Epilepsy/postictal state*
    Emaciation, hepatomegaly, ⟶ *Intracranial metastasis*
      lymphadenopathy
    Infection source (ears, sinus, ⟶ *Cerebral abscess, meningitis*
      lungs, valvular disease — SBE)
    Pyrexia ⟶ *Subarachnoid, intracerebral, pontine haemorrhage*

COMA AND IMPAIRED CONSCIOUS LEVEL

DIAGNOSTIC APPROACH *(contd)*
General examination *(contd)*

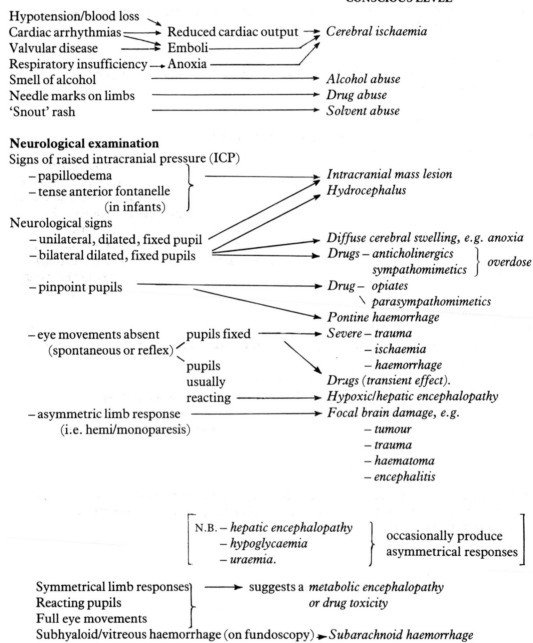

POSSIBLE CAUSE OF COMA/IMPAIRED
CONSCIOUS LEVEL

Hypotension/blood loss
Cardiac arrhythmias ⟶ Reduced cardiac output ⟶ *Cerebral ischaemia*
Valvular disease ⟶ Emboli
Respiratory insufficiency ⟶ Anoxia
Smell of alcohol ⟶ *Alcohol abuse*
Needle marks on limbs ⟶ *Drug abuse*
'Snout' rash ⟶ *Solvent abuse*

Neurological examination
Signs of raised intracranial pressure (ICP)
   – papilloedema ⟶ *Intracranial mass lesion*
   – tense anterior fontanelle *Hydrocephalus*
       (in infants)
Neurological signs
   – unilateral, dilated, fixed pupil ⟶ *Diffuse cerebral swelling, e.g. anoxia*
   – bilateral dilated, fixed pupils ⟶ *Drugs – anticholinergics*
                                        sympathomimetics } *overdose*
   – pinpoint pupils ⟶ *Drug – opiates*
                         \ *parasympathomimetics*
                       Pontine haemorrhage

   – eye movements absent   pupils fixed ⟶ *Severe – trauma*
       (spontaneous or reflex)   *– ischaemia*
                            pupils   *– haemorrhage*
                            usually   *Drugs (transient effect).*
                            reacting ⟶ *Hypoxic/hepatic encephalopathy*
   – asymmetric limb response ⟶ *Focal brain damage, e.g.*
       (i.e. hemi/monoparesis)   *– tumour*
                                     – trauma
                                     – haematoma
                                     – encephalitis

[N.B. – *hepatic encephalopathy*
       – *hypoglycaemia*   } occasionally produce
       – *uraemia.*   asymmetrical responses]

Symmetrical limb responses
Reacting pupils   } ⟶ suggests a *metabolic encephalopathy*
Full eye movements   *or drug toxicity*
Subhyaloid/vitreous haemorrhage (on fundoscopy) ⟶ *Subarachnoid haemorrhage*

COMA AND IMPAIRED CONSCIOUS LEVEL

Investigations
The sequence of investigations depends on the clinical findings:

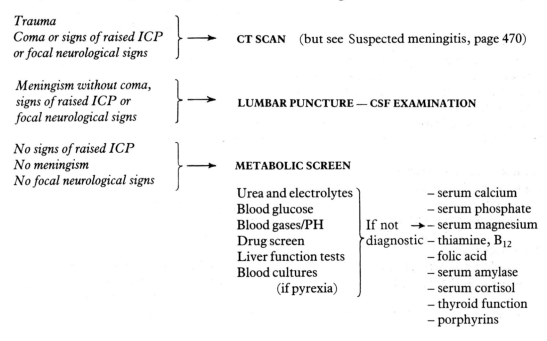

Trauma
Coma or signs of raised ICP ⟶ **CT SCAN** (but see Suspected meningitis, page 470)
or focal neurological signs

Meningism without coma,
signs of raised ICP or ⟶ **LUMBAR PUNCTURE — CSF EXAMINATION**
focal neurological signs

No signs of raised ICP
No meningism ⟶ **METABOLIC SCREEN**
No focal neurological signs

Urea and electrolytes — serum calcium
Blood glucose — serum phosphate
Blood gases/PH — serum magnesium
Drug screen   If not ⟶ — thiamine, B_{12}
Liver function tests   diagnostic — folic acid
Blood cultures — serum amylase
  (if pyrexia) — serum cortisol
— thyroid function
— porphyrins

In addition:
    SKULL X-RAY ——may reveal an unsuspected fracture, pineal shift, calcification or an osteolytic lesion.
    CHEST X-RAY ——may reveal a bronchial carcinoma.
    ELECTROENCEPHALOGRAPHY - may provide evidence of   – subclinical epilepsy
                                                    – herpes simplex encephalitis
                                                   – metabolic encephalopathy.

Prognosis
Although *conscious level examination* does not aid diagnosis, it plays an essential rôle in patient management and along with the *duration of coma, pupil response* and *eye movements* provides valuable prognostic information.

TRANSIENT LOSS OF CONSCIOUSNESS

Many conditions causing coma may also transiently affect a patient's conscious level. This results from:

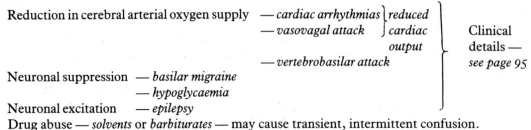

Reduction in cerebral arterial oxygen supply — *cardiac arrhythmias* ⎱ *reduced* ⎰ — *vasovagal attack* ⎰ *cardiac* ⎱ *output*
— *vertebrobasilar attack*

Clinical details — *see page 95*

Neuronal suppression — *basilar migraine*
— *hypoglycaemia*

Neuronal excitation — *epilepsy*

Drug abuse — *solvents* or *barbiturates* — may cause transient, intermittent confusion.

DIAGNOSTIC APPROACH

History

The patient's own description of the attack or that of an eyewitness may virtually establish the diagnosis. Prodromal features of pallor, nausea and sweating accompany *vasovagal attacks*. Clonic/tonic movements occur shortly after the onset of an *epileptic 'grand mal' attack* (but tonic movements can occur with a prolonged vasovagal attack or cardiac arrhythmia).

Palpitations, sweating, behavioural disturbances and seizures may precede loss of consciousness from *hypoglycaemia*. Vertigo and scintillating teichopsia often precede *basilar migraine*.

Electroencephalography (EEG) may reveal a focal disturbance – *epilepsy*.

Electrocardiography (ECG) may reveal a *cardiac arrythmia*.

Blood glucose may indicate *hypoglycaemia*.

If an eyewitness account and the above tests provide no evidence of the cause, proceed to:

1. **Telemetric EEG and ECG monitoring** over a 24-hour period.
2. **72-hour fast** – if symptoms appear, check **blood glucose** and **insulin** levels.

Often attacks of unconsciousness remain unexplained and possibly have a psychological or attention-seeking basis. The circumstances of the attack (e.g. during an argument), the non-stereotyped nature of the episode and the lack of personal trauma with repeated falls all suggest a 'functional' *non-organic* explanation.

CONFUSIONAL STATES AND DELIRIUM

Of all acute medical admissions, 5–10% present with a **confused verbal response,** i.e. disorientation in time and/or place. Most patients are easily distracted, have slowed thought processes and a limited concentration span. Some may lose interest in the examination to the point of drifting off to sleep.

Perceptual disorders (illusions and hallucinations) may accompany the confused state — **delirium.** This is often associated with withdrawal and lack of awareness or with restlessness and hyperactivity.

Primary neurological disorders contribute to only 10% of those patients presenting with an acute confusional state. In the elderly, postoperative disorientation is particularly common and multiple factors probably apply; in these patients the prognosis is good.

DIAGNOSTIC APPROACH

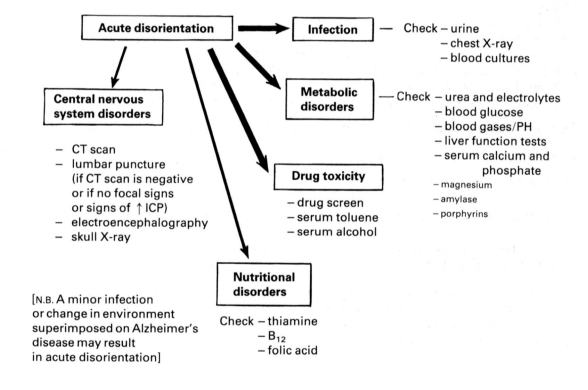

Acute disorientation → **Infection** — Check – urine
  – chest X-ray
  – blood cultures

Central nervous system disorders

– CT scan
– lumbar puncture
  (if CT scan is negative
  or if no focal signs
  or signs of ↑ICP)
– electroencephalography
– skull X-ray

Metabolic disorders — Check – urea and electrolytes
  – blood glucose
  – blood gases/PH
  – liver function tests
  – serum calcium and
    phosphate
  – magnesium
  – amylase
  – porphyrins

Drug toxicity

– drug screen
– serum toluene
– serum alcohol

Nutritional disorders

Check – thiamine
  – B_{12}
  – folic acid

[N.B. A minor infection or change in environment superimposed on Alzheimer's disease may result in acute disorientation]

87

EPILEPSY

Definitions

A seizure or epileptic attack is the consequence of a paroxysmal uncontrolled discharge of neurons within the central nervous system. The clinical manifestations range from a major motor convulsion to a brief period of lack of awareness.

The *prodrome* refers to mood or behavioural changes which may precede the attack by some hours.

The *aura* refers to the symptom immediately before loss of consciousness and will localise the attack to its point of origin within the nervous system.

The *ictus* refers to the attack or seizure itself.

The *postictal period* refers to the time immediately after the ictus during which the patient may be confused, disorientated and demonstrate automatic behaviour.

The stereotyped and uncontrollable nature of the attack is characteristic of epilepsy.

History

Epilepsy has been described since ancient times. The 19th century neurologist Hughlings-Jackson suggested 'a sudden excessive disorderly discharge of cerebral neurons' as the causation of the attack. Berger (1929) recorded the first electroencephalogram (EEG) and not long after, it was appreciated that certain seizures were characterised by particular EEG abnormalities.

Incidence and course

Epilepsy usually presents in childhood or adolescence but may occur for the first time at any age.

5% of the population suffer a single seizure at some time.

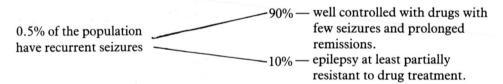

0.5% of the population have recurrent seizures

90% — well controlled with drugs with few seizures and prolonged remissions.

10% — epilepsy at least partially resistant to drug treatment.

6 years after diagnosis 40% of patients have had a substantial remission; after 20 years — 75%.

EPILEPSY IS A SYMPTOM OF NUMEROUS DISORDERS, BUT IN 50% OF SUFFERERS THE CAUSE REMAINS UNCLEAR DESPITE CAREFUL HISTORY TAKING, EXAMINATION AND INVESTIGATION.

EPILEPSY — CLASSIFICATION

The modern classification of the epilepsies is based upon the *nature* of the attack rather than the presence or absence of an underlying cause. The use of the electroencephalogram (EEG) has greatly increased our understanding of the source or 'point of origin' of any particular type of epileptic attack.

Attacks which begin **focally** from a single location within one hemisphere are thus distinguished from those of **generalised** nature which probably commence in deeper midline structures and project to both hemispheres simultaneously.

PARTIAL (focal, local) SEIZURES

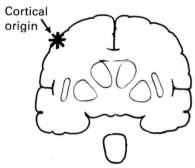

Cortical origin

Focal EEG abnormality

A. Simple partial seizures
— motor
— sensory

B. Complex partial seizures (when partial seizure is accompanied by any degree of impaired conscious level)

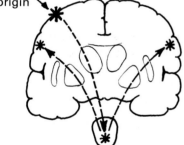

Cortical origin

C. Partial seizures evolving to tonic/clonic convulsion

Focal → generalised EEG abnormality

GENERALISED SEIZURES (convulsive or non-convulsive)

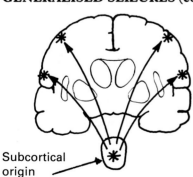

Subcortical origin

A. Absences
B. Myoclonic seizures
C. Clonic seizures
D. Tonic seizures
E. Tonic/clonic seizures
F. Atonic seizures

Generalised EEG abnormality

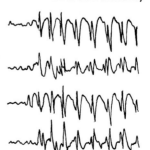

UNCLASSIFIED SEIZURES, e.g. infantile spasms

THE PARTIAL SEIZURES

SIMPLE MOTOR SEIZURES

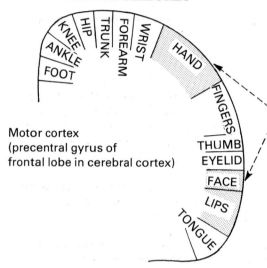

Motor cortex
(precentral gyrus of
frontal lobe in cerebral cortex)

These arise in the frontal motor cortex with movements occurring in contralateral face, trunk or limbs.

The **Jacksonian** motor seizure consists of a 'march' of involuntary movement from one muscle group to the next.

Movement is clonic (shaking) and usually begins in hand or face — these having the largest representative cortical area.

Motor seizures with the above 'march' are quite rare, usually they are less localised, involving many muscle groups simultaneously and are tonic (rigid) or clonic.

After a motor seizure the affected limb(s) may remain weak for some hours before return of function occurs — **Todd's paralysis.**

Adversive seizures

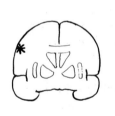

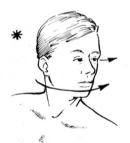

The patient is aware of movement of the head. Attacks often progress to loss of consciousness and tonic/clonic epilepsy.

The patient's eyes and head turn away from the site of the focal origin usually in the supplementary motor cortex of the frontal lobe with involvement of the frontal 'gaze centre'. Some doubt the localising value of such an attack.

SIMPLE SENSORY SEIZURES

These arise in the sensory cortex, the patient describing paraesthesia or tingling in an extremity or on the face sometimes associated with a sensation of distortion of body image. A 'march' similar to the Jacksonian motor seizure may occur. Motor symptoms occur concurrently — the limb appears weak without involuntary movement.

The representation of limbs, trunk, etc. in the post-Rolandic sensory cortex is similar to that of the motor cortex.

VISUAL, AUDITORY AND AUTONOMIC simple partial seizures occur, but are rare.

Motor and sensory seizures indicate structural brain disease, the focal onset localising the lesion. Full investigation is mandatory.

THE PARTIAL SEIZURES

COMPLEX PARTIAL SEIZURES

These attacks usually originate within the temporal lobe and are characterised by a complex aura (initial symptom) and some impairment of consciousness.

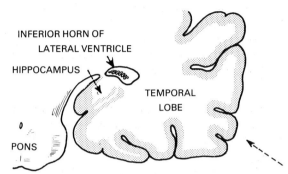

Complex partial seizures are generally synonymous with **psychomotor epilepsy** and **temporal epilepsy** (though motor, sensory and other partial seizures can be associated with impaired consciousness when propagated through the temporal lobe).

The seizure origin lies in the medial part of the temporal lobe, hippocampus or lateral surface of the lobe.

Coronal section through the pons showing medial aspect of the temporal lobe and hippocampus

The nature of the attack

The content of attacks may vary in an individual patient. Commonly encountered symptoms include:

Visceral disturbance: Gustatory (taste) and olfactory (smell) hallucinations, lip smacking, epigastric fullness, choking sensation, nausea, pallor, pupillary changes (dilatation), tachycardia.
Memory disturbance: Deja vu ('something has happened before'), jamais vu ('feeling of unfamiliarity'), depersonalisation, derealisation, flashbacks, formed visual or auditory hallucinations.
Motor disturbance: Fumbling movement, rubbing, chewing, semi-purposeful limb movements.
Affective disturbance: Displeasure, pleasure, depression, elation, fear.
A constellation of these symptoms associated with subtle clouding of consciousness characterises a complex partial seizure.

AUTOMATISM occurs during the state of clouding of consciousness either during or after the attack (postictal) and takes the form of involuntary, often complicated, motor activity. In ambulatory automatism, subjects may 'wander off'.

Confusion and headache after an attack are common. The whole episode may last for seconds but occasionally may be prolonged and a rapid succession or cluster of attacks may occur. Attacks show an increased incidence in adolescence and early adult life. A history of birth trauma or febrile convulsions in infancy may be obtained. Lesions in the hippocampus occur as a result of anoxia or from the convulsion itself and act as a source of further epilepsy. When surgery is carried out, hippocampal sclerosis is often found. Occasionally other pathologies are identified, such as hamartomas, vascular malformations and low-grade malignant astrocytomas.

PARTIAL SEIZURES EVOLVING TO TONIC/CLONIC CONVULSION

Seizure discharges have the capacity to spread from their point of origin and excite other structures. When spread occurs to the subcortical structures (thalamus and upper reticular formation) their excitation releases a discharge which spreads back to the whole cerebral cortex of both hemispheres, resulting in a tonic/clonic seizure. This chain of events is reflected in the electroencephalogram (EEG).

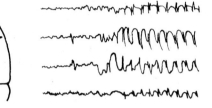

The symptoms (aura) before the tonic/clonic convulsion give a clue to the site of the initial discharge (simple partial or complex partial).

An eyewitness account is important as the aura may be forgotten by the patient because of retrograde amnesia. In some the aura are absent.

TONIC/CLONIC ATTACKS
Loss of consciousness; falls to the ground.

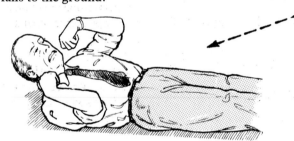

1. **Tonic phase (10 seconds)**
   Eyes open. Elbows flexed.
   Arms pronated. Legs extended.
   Teeth clenched. Pupils dilated.
   Breath held — cyanosis.
   Bowel/bladder control may be lost at the end of this phase.

2. **Clonic phase (1-2 minutes)**
   Tremor gives way to violent
        generalised shaking.
   Eyes roll backwards and forwards.
   Tongue may be bitten. Tachycardia develops.
   Breathing recommences at end of phase.

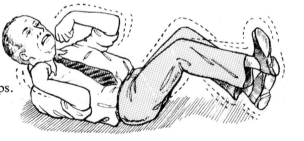

The patient then sleeps with stertorous respiration and cannot be roused. On regaining consciousness confusion and headache are present. He may feel exhausted for hours or even days afterwards. Muscles may ache as a result of violent movement and muscle damage occurs with elevation of the muscle enzyme creatinine phosphokinase (CPK). Trauma occurs frequently, either as a result of the fall, or as a result of the movements, e.g. posterior dislocation of the shoulder.

The differentiation of these attacks from hysteria will be discussed later.

GENERALISED SEIZURES

Generalised seizure attacks arise from subcortical structures and involve both hemispheres. Consciousness may be impaired and motor manifestations are bilateral.

ABSENCES (*Syn:* **Petit mal**)
Onset in childhood (between 4 and 12 years of age). Family history in 40% of patients.
The absence may occur many times a day with a duration of 5–15 seconds.
The patient stares vacantly, eyes may blink and myoclonic jerks occur.
Attacks may be induced by hyperventilation.
Frequent episodes lead to falling off in scholastic performance.
Attacks rarely present beyond adolescence.
In 30% of children, adolescence may bring tonic/clonic seizures (**Grand mal**).
Distinction of absences from complex partial seizures is easy; the latter are longer — 30 seconds or more — and followed by headache, lethargy, confusion and automatism.

The *ELECTROENCEPHALOGRAM (EEG)* is diagnostic.

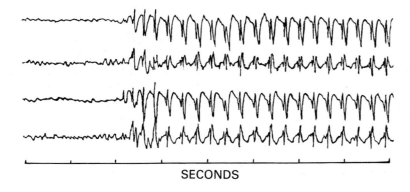

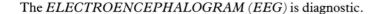
SECONDS

3 per second spike and wave activity occurs in all leads, persisting as long as the seizure. Hyperventilation evokes this appearance during recording. Similarly, photic stimulation — flashing a light in both eyes — may produce spike and wave discharge.

PETIT MAL STATUS
Long periods of clouding of consciousness with continuing 'spike and wave' activity on the EEG.

MYOCLONIC SEIZURES
Sudden, brief, generalised muscle contractions. They often occur in the morning and are occasionally associated with tonic/clonic seizures. Myoclonus also occurs in degenerative and metabolic disease (see page 186).

TONIC SEIZURES
Sudden sustained muscular contraction associated with immediate loss of consciousness.
Tonic episodes occur as frequently as tonic/clonic episodes in children and should alert the physician to a possible anoxic aetiology.
In adults, tonic attacks are rare.

GENERALISED SEIZURES

TONIC/CLONIC SEIZURES (*Syn:* **Grand mal**)
It is the absence of a focal onset which may distinguish this *primary* generalised seizure from that evolving from a partial seizure.

The *epileptic cry* must not be confused with an aura of focal onset. This results from tonic contraction of respiratory muscles with partial closure of vocal cords. The tonic phase is associated with rapid neuronal discharge. The clonic phase begins as neuronal discharge slows.

The *EEG* during an attack is, not surprisingly, marred by movement artefact. 10–14 Hz spike activity may be seen. When the seizure ends, the record may be 'silent' and then gradually pick up. Slow rhythm may persist for some hours — postictal changes.

The record between attacks may be normal or slow with occasional clinically silent bursts of seizure activity.

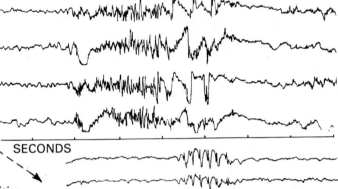

SECONDS

Again, hyperventilation or photic stimulation may bring out abnormalities.

SECONDS

ATONIC SEIZURES
These are characterised by a loss of muscle tone and a sudden fall. Consciousness may only be briefly lost. The EEG shows polyspike activity or low voltage fast activity.

UNCLASSIFIED SEIZURES

INFANTILE SPASMS

These occur in the first few months of life.

Repetitive shock-like flexion of neck and trunk with flexion of knees (Salaam attacks) characterise this disorder.
Infants will show a progressive mental deterioration unless attacks are controlled.
The EEG shows continuous irregular spike and wave activity called *hypsarrhythmia*. Steroids, if given early, may reduce the frequency and duration of infantile spasms. Two types of infantile spasm are recognised:

1. Of unknown etiology with normal development leading up to the onset.
2. With a definable cause — perinatal cerebral injury, congenital abnormality.

40% make a good recovery (attend normal school).

The **REFLEX EPILEPSIES** are a rare group of seizure disorders in which tonic/clonic or complex partial seizures are evoked by sensory stimuli. A primary generalised seizure induced by photic stimulation may be regarded as a reflex epilepsy, but the term is usually reserved for:

1. **Musicogenic epilepsy** in which certain musical themes or tones 'trigger' seizures.
2. **Reading epilepsy** in which reading a passage will evoke involuntary jaw movements followed by a seizure.
3. **Arithmetical epilepsy** in which performing calculations will 'trigger' seizures.

EPILEPSY – DIFFERENTIAL DIAGNOSIS

The diagnosis depends on the patient's and witnesses' account of the attacks.

Impairment of consciousness occurs in: **vasovagal syncope, cardiac arrhythmias, migraine** (basilar migraine), **hypoglycaemia, episodic confusion, narcolepsy.**

Hysterical and malingering **pseudoseizures** cause diagnostic difficulties especially when occurring in a patient who also has genuine epilepsy.

SYNCOPE (VASOVAGAL) ATTACKS

These attacks occur usually when the patient is standing and result from a global reduction of cerebral blood flow.

Prodromal pallor, nausea and sweating occur; if the patient sits down, the attack may pass off or proceed to a brief loss of consciousness.

Tonic and clonic movements may develop if impaired cerebral blood flow is prolonged ('anoxic' seizures).

Mechanism: Peripheral vasodilatation with drop in blood pressure followed by vagal overactivity with fall in heart rate.

Syncopal attacks occur in hot, crowded rooms (e.g. classroom) or in response to pain or emotional disturbance.

'Reflex' syncope from cardiac slowing may occur with carotid sinus compression. Similarly, cough syncope may result from vigorous coughing.

CARDIAC ARRHYTHMIAS

Seen in situations such as complete heart block (Adams–Stokes attacks).

Prolonged arrest of cardiac rate or critical reduction will progressively lead to loss of consciousness — tonic jerks — cyanosis/stertorous respiration — fixed pupils and extensor plantar responses.

On recovery of normal cardiac rhythm, the degree of persisting neurological damage depends upon the duration of the episode and the presence of pre-existing cerebrovascular disease. In suspected patients, electrocardiography is mandatory. Continuous (24 hours) ECG monitoring may be necessary.

MIGRAINE

The slow evolution of focal hemisensory or hemimotor symptoms in complicated migraine contrasts with the more rapid 'spread' of such manifestations in simple partial seizures.

HYPOGLYCAEMIA

Amongst other neuroglycopenic manifestations, seizures or intermittent behavioural disturbances may occur. A rapid fall of blood sugar is associated with symptoms of catecholamine release, e.g. palpitations, sweating, etc. In 'atypical' seizures such a metabolic cause should be excluded, preferably by blood sugar estimation when symptomatic.

EPISODIC CONFUSION

Intermittent confusional episodes in persons on drugs such as barbiturates or toxins such as solvent abuse.

PANIC ATTACKS

Hyperventilation can induce focal sensory symptoms.

NARCOLEPSY

Episodes of inappropriate sudden sleep may easily be confused with epilepsy (see page 103).

EPILEPSY – DIFFERENTIAL DIAGNOSIS

PSEUDOSEIZURES

A difficult distinction lies between genuine epilepsy and attention seeking, hysterical or malingering episodes in which violent shaking and feigned loss of consciousness occurs (pseudoseizures). Often known epileptics will also manifest such attacks.

The following aids distinction:

Pseudoseizures	Genuine seizures
Pupils remain unchanged	Pupils dilate
Blood pressure/heart rate do not alter	Blood pressure/heart rate increase
Plantar responses down going	Extensor plantar responses
May show facial cyanosis but not nail beds	Face and nail beds cyanosed

Biochemical tests

Po_2 and pH unaltered	Po_2 and pH lowered
Creatine phosphokinase normal	Creatine phosphokinase elevated
Serum prolactin levels normal	Marked elevation of serum prolactin

Electroencephalogram

Muscle artefact	Muscle artefact and seizure activity

Caution: The postictal confusional state may result in behaviour so bizarre that a pseudoseizure is wrongly suspected.

EPILEPSY – CAUSATION

Epilepsy is a symptom of disease rather than a disease itself. The investigation of epilepsy depends on knowledge of potential causes.

Partial seizures with or without **secondary generalisation.**

Newborn	Infancy	Childhood	Adolescence and adulthood
Hypocalcaemia	Febrile convulsions	Trauma	Trauma. Neoplasm. Withdrawal from drugs/alcohol. Arteriovenous malformation CNS infection.
Hypoglycaemia	Inborn errors of metabolism	Congenital defects	
Asphyxia	Congenital defects	Arteriovenous malformation	
Hyperbilirubinaemia	CNS infection	CNS infection	
Water intoxication			
Inborn errors of metabolism			
Trauma		**Late adult**	Trauma. Neoplasm. Drug/alcohol withdrawal. Vascular disease Degenerative disease CNS infection
Intracranial haemorrhage (Vit.K deficiency, thrombocytopenia, etc.)			

Once epilepsy has been 'triggered' by a specific cause at a given period it may persist throughout life, e.g. febrile convulsion in infancy or neonatal asphyxia may be the cause of complex partial seizures which reappear some years later.

Other general medical conditions may be associated with seizures, e.g. metabolic diseases, collagen vascular disorders.

EPILEPSY

Generalised epilepsies

There appears to be no clearly definable cause. Genetic factors play a role; concordance in monozygote twins is 75% for petit mal. An autosomal dominant gene would appear responsible for spike and wave abnormalities seen in the EEG's of parents and siblings of patients with generalised epilepsy. The defect is assumed to be metabolic though its nature is unknown.

EPILEPSY – INVESTIGATION

With an incidence of 0.5% of the population, selectivity in investigation is necessary. CT scanning could not realistically be carried out in all patients.

The concern of the clinician is that epilepsy may be symptomatic of a cerebral lesion. Investigations serve to define a cause and to aid diagnosis in difficult cases.

Routine Investigations

Haematology

Biochemistry (electrolytes, urea and calcium)

Skull X-ray

Chest X-ray

Electroencephalogram (EEG)

Computerised tomography (CT) scanning should be performed when seizures are:
– late in onset
– partial in type
– refractory in nature (to drug treatment)
– associated with abnormal clinical signs
or when epilepsy presents as status epilepticus

In doubtful cases the patient should not be labelled 'epileptic'.

Specialised neurophysiological investigations

Indicated if attacks of unconsciousness are frequent or persistent and the diagnosis remains unclear.

Sleep electroencephalography (EEG).

'Activated' EEG recording with procyclidine or insulin.

Telemetric EEG recording over 24–48 hours often combined with video recording of the patients (split screen display).

These investigations may reveal 'diagnostic' epileptic discharges.

Advanced investigations

These are reserved for cases of intractable epilepsy where surgery is considered.

Telemetric and foramen ovale EEG recording.

Specialised CT techniques, e.g. special temporal lobe slices.

Magnetic resonance imaging which will display low-grade gliomas and hamartomas often missed on CT scanning.

Positron emission tomography (PET) or single photon emission computed tomography (SPECT) which localise functional changes in cerebral blood flow and metabolism.

Long established investigations such as lumbar air encephalography (LAEG) and angiography are now rarely performed in the assessment of epilepsy.

EPILEPSY – TREATMENT

The majority of patients respond to drug therapy (anticonvulsants). In intractable cases surgery may be necessary.

Drug treatment should be simple, preferably using one anticonvulsant (monotherapy). Polytherapy is to be avoided especially as drug interactions occur between major anticonvulsants.

Treatment is aimed at rendering the patient 'fit free', though not always achieved. If the patient goes three years without an attack, withdrawal of therapy should be considered; an EEG should preferably be performed and should show no 'discharge'. Withdrawal should be carried out only if the patient is satisfied that a further fit would not ruin employment etc. (e.g. car driver). The risk of teratogenicity is well known (6%) especially with phenytoin, but withdrawing drug therapy in pregnancy is perhaps more risky to the fetus than continuation. All anticonvulsants probably have some risk of producing fetal abnormalities, though these are usually mild. Sodium valproate has been incriminated in neural tube defects — spina bifida.

A common problem in epilepsy clinics is non-compliance with drug therapy. The introduction of assay of blood anticonvulsant levels has led to:

1. Identification of non-compliers.
2. Tailoring of drug dose to patient's requirements.
3. The realisation of failure with therapeutic levels of one anticonvulsant and thus the logical change to another.

The commonest anticonvulsants in present clinical use are:

Carbamazepine	Sodium valproate	Clonazepam	Ethosuximide
Phenobarbitone	Primidone	Phenytoin	

Sodium valproate is the first-line drug in the treatment of the generalised epilepsies in adults. In childhood use ethosuximide.

Carbamazepine is the first-line drug in the treatment of partial seizures and partial seizures evolving to tonic/clonic seizures.

	Sodium valproate	Phenobarbitone	Phenytoin	Carbamazepine
Mode of action	Inhibitor of GABA transaminase and glutamate decarboxylase	Depressant effect on neuronal membranes	Membrane stabilizer. Prevents Na^+ influx	Related to tricyclic drugs. Action as phenytoin
Metabolised	Liver Protein bound. Short variable half-life	Liver or excreted in urine unchanged Long half-life (60 hours)	Liver Can saturate enzyme systems Long half-life	Liver. Enzyme inducer. Short half-life (10 hours).
Dose (ADULT)	2-3 × daily. 600 mg to 3 g total daily dose	Can be given as single dose, e.g. 90 mg at night	Can be given as single dose e.g. 150 – 400 mg at night	2-3 × daily. 600 mg to 1.2 g total daily dose
Side effects	Gastrointestinal upset Thrombocytopenia Drug-induced hepatitis Hair loss Tremor/chorea	Sedation.Depression Behavioural disturbance in children. Skin rashes Withdrawal seizures	Gum hypertrophy Acne.Coarsening of facial characteristics At toxic levels – nystagmus. – ataxia, diplopia – neuropathy	Gastrointestinal upset Ataxia Skin rash Agranulocytosis Antidiuretic effect

A large number of novel anticonvulsants are currently being evaluated — GABA agonists, Ca^+ channel blockers and glutamate antagonists.

EPILEPSY – SURGICAL TREATMENT

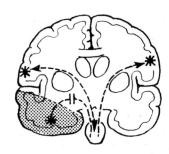

In some patients, despite adequate drug administration (checked by serum levels), recurrent seizures prevent a normal life style; of these a proportion may benefit from operation provided seizures arise from a single focus. Theoretically, removal of the focus abolishes the partial seizure and prevents progression to a generalised seizure.

Extensive EEG investigation, both before and often during operation, helps to localise the site of the primary focus.

CT or MRI scanning may reveal an underlying structural abnormality (e.g. tumour, AVM or hamartoma) increasing the likelihood of improvement after operative removal. The discovery of a structural abnormality may in itself indicate the need for operation. In many patients with a temporal focus, temporal lobectomy reveals scarring of the most medial aspect – 'medial temporal sclerosis'. It is not known whether this is the cause of the epilepsy or the result of anoxia during repeated attacks.

Operation is contraindicated in patients with severe mental retardation or with an underlying psychiatric problem.

Operative techniques

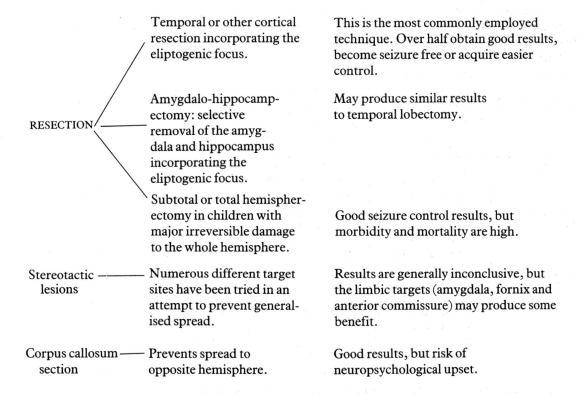

RESECTION	Temporal or other cortical resection incorporating the eliptogenic focus.	This is the most commonly employed technique. Over half obtain good results, become seizure free or acquire easier control.
	Amygdalo-hippocamp-ectomy: selective removal of the amygdala and hippocampus incorporating the eliptogenic focus.	May produce similar results to temporal lobectomy.
	Subtotal or total hemispher-ectomy in children with major irreversible damage to the whole hemisphere.	Good seizure control results, but morbidity and mortality are high.
Stereotactic lesions	Numerous different target sites have been tried in an attempt to prevent general-ised spread.	Results are generally inconclusive, but the limbic targets (amygdala, fornix and anterior commissure) may produce some benefit.
Corpus callosum section	Prevents spread to opposite hemisphere.	Good results, but risk of neuropsychological upset.

STATUS EPILEPTICUS

A succession of tonic/clonic convulsions, one after the other with a gap between each, is referred to as **serial epilepsy.**

When consciousness does not return between attacks the condition is then termed **status epilepticus.** This state may be life-threatening with the development of pyrexia, deepening coma and circulatory collapse.

Status epilepticus may occur with frontal lobe lesions, following head injury, on reducing drug therapy (especially phenobarbitone), with alcohol or other sedation withdrawal, drug intoxications (tricyclic antidepressants), infections, metabolic disturbances (hyponatraemia) or pregnancy.

TREATMENT

There is no completely satisfactory approach.
Death occurs in 5–10%.

NOTE: ALL DOSE REGIMES APPLY TO
ADULTS AND NOT TO CHILDREN

General

Establish an airway.

O_2 inhalation 10 litres/minute.

I.V. infusion: 500 ml 5% dextrose/0.9N saline.

Vital signs recorded regularly — especially temperature.

Prevent hyperthermia (sponging, etc.).

Specific

Diazepam 5 mg i.v. followed, after 2 minutes gap, by further 5 mg i.v.

Effective for 10–20 minutes then seizures may return.

Beware respiratory depression with repeated injections.

When the effect of bolus injection wears off, a continuous diazepam infusion can be used (50–100 mg of diazepam in 500 ml dextrose/saline).

If not controlled then proceed to longer acting drug.

Phenytoin does not depress respiration.

Loading dose: 15 mg/kg given slowly i.v. at rate of 50 mg/min in normal saline.

Monitor ECG and blood pressure — there is a risk of arrythmias and hypotension.

Contraindicated where known cardiac conduction defect or history of recent myocardial infarction.

Maintenance, 500 mg i.v. or orally, daily.

If condition persists 30 minutes after loading dose, phenobarbitone may be added, 200–300 mg i.v. given at rate of 50 mg/min.

Respiration should be monitored.

At this point seizures should be controlled.

120 mg phenobarbitone i.m. 4-hourly and 500 mg phenytoin i.v. daily should be given until oral therapy can be initiated.

Throughout treatment the patient should receive the previously established anticonvulsant treatment, especially when using drugs (e.g. diazepam) which have only a temporary effect.

STATUS EPILEPTICUS

Electrolytes as well as calcium and blood glucose should be checked initially and throughout. Blood gases should be estimated if clinically indicated.

Other drugs:
Chlormethiazole and paraldehyde may be used in resistant status. Thiopentone at non-anaesthetising dosage, i.e. 2 ml/min i.v. for 30–60 minutes or general anaesthesia with neuromuscular blockade is reserved for life-threatening refractory status.

Non-convulsive status (complex partial and petit mal) as well as simple partial status do not threaten life and respond well to i.v. diazepam or i.v. phenytoin.

Prognosis on withdrawal of drug treatment
Several factors increase the likelihood of relapse of epilepsy after drug withdrawal:
- epilepsy associated with known cerebral damage
- infantile onset.

Drug withdrawal should be performed slowly. Within 2 years of withdrawing treatment, 50% of persons will suffer a further attack.

Epilepsy and Pregnancy
The frequency of seizures may decrease in pregnancy. The patient may present with the first seizure during pregnancy (when investigation is limited) or during the puerperium. Tumours or arteriovenous malformations can enlarge in pregnancy and produce such seizures; however, these causes are rare and most attacks idiopathic. Cortical venous thrombosis and systemic lupus erythematosus should be considered as alternative explanations. Care must be taken when prescribing treatment in pregnancy (teratogenicity).

THE FEBRILE CONVULSION

Febrile convulsions occur in the immature brain as a response to high fever, probably as a result of water and electrolyte disturbance.

No particular infection can be incriminated.

Usually occurs between 6 months and 3 years of age.

Rare after 5 years of age.

Recurrent in 50% of patients.

Long-term follow up suggests a liability to develop seizures in later life (unassociated with fever) especially in males.

The duration of seizure, number of seizures and positive family history all increase risk.

Treatment is aimed at preventing a prolonged seizure by sponging the patient and using rectal diazepam.

The role of prophylaxis after one seizure is debatable.

DISORDERS OF SLEEP

PHYSIOLOGY

Sleep results from activity in certain sleep producing areas of the brain rather than from reduced sensory input to the cerebral cortex. Stimulation of these areas produces sleep; damage results in states of persistent wakefulness.

Pontine

reticular formation
raphe nuclei

Medullary

Two states of sleep are recognised:

1. **Rapid eye movement (REM) sleep**	2. **Non-rapid eye movement (non-REM) sleep**
Characterised by: Rapid conjugate eye movement	Absence of eye movement
Fluctuation of temperature, BP, heart rate and respiration	Stability of temperature, BP, heart rate and respiration
Muscle twitching	Absence of muscle twitching
Presence of dreams	Absence of dreams
Originates in: Pontine reticular formation	Midline pontine and medullary nuclei (raphe nuclei)
Mediated by: Noradrenaline	Serotonin

The **electroencephalogram** shows characteristic patterns which correspond to the type and depth of sleep.

REM sleep		a low voltage record with mixed frequencies, dominated by fast activity.
Non-REM sleep Drowsiness		a relatively low voltage record with slow rhythms, interrupted by alpha rhythm.
Intermediate		sharp waves evident in vertex leads (V waves).
Deep sleep		a high voltage record dominated by slow wave activity.

The sleep pattern

In adults non-REM and REM sleep alternate throughout the night.

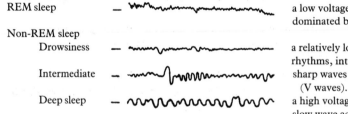

Non-REM   REM

60–90 min

Retiring   10–15 min

Rising

50%   REM   REM   20%

50%   Non-REM   Non-REM   80%

Neonates   Adults

The proportion of REM to non-REM varies with age. ———

In view of the important rôle of serotonin and noradrenaline in sleep, it is understandable that drugs may affect the duration and/or content of sleep.

DISORDERS OF SLEEP

NARCOLEPSY AND CATAPLEXY

Narcolepsy

An irresistible desire to sleep in inappropriate circumstances and places. Attacks occur suddenly and are of brief duration unless patient remains undisturbed.

Cataplexy

Sudden loss of postural tone. The patient crumples to the ground. Consciousness is preserved. Emotion – laughter or crying – can precipitate an attack.

The narcolepsy/cataplexy tetrad

Only 10% of patients manifest the complete tetrad

Sleep paralysis

On awakening, the patient is unable to move. This may last for 2–3 minutes.

Hypnagogic hallucinations

Vivid dreams or hallucinations occur as the patient falls asleep or occasionally when apparently awake.

Males are affected more than females.

Onset is in adolescence/early adult life. The disorder is life long, but becomes less troublesome with age. It may have a familial incidence, or may occur after head injury, with multiple sclerosis, or with hypothalamic tumours. The cause remains unknown, though the increased incidence of certain histocompatibility antigens (DR2) in sufferers does suggest an immunological basis.

Diagnosis

The diagnosis is dependent upon the clinical history. The electroencephalogram may help, showing a REM pattern with daytime sleep and at the onset of nocturnal sleep.

Treatment

Drugs which inhibit REM sleep may benefit:
- amphetamines and their derivatives, e.g. dexamphetamine sulphate, methylphenidate hydrochloride.
- other drugs are preferable but have a selective effect: clomipramine and mazindol for narcolepsy; fluvoxamine for cataplexy.

NIGHT TERRORS (pavor nocturnus)

These occur in children, shortly after falling asleep and during deep to intermediate non-REM sleep. The child awakes in a state of fright with a marked tachycardia, yet in the morning cannot recollect the attack. Such attacks are not associated with psychological disturbance, are self limiting and if necessary will respond to diazepam.

NIGHTMARES

These occur during REM sleep. Drug or alcohol withdrawal promotes REM sleep and is often associated with vivid dreams.

SOMNAMBULISM (sleep walking)

Sleep walking varies from just sitting up in bed to walking around the house with the eyes open, performing complex major tasks. Episodes occur during intermediate or deep non-REM sleep. In childhood, somnambulism is associated with night terrors and bed wetting, but not with psychological disturbance. In adults, there is an increased incidence of psychoneurosis.

103

DISORDERS OF SLEEP

SLEEP STARTS

On entering sleep, sudden jerks of the arms or legs commonly occur and are especially frequent when a conscious effort is made to remain awake, e.g. during a lecture. This is a physiological form of myoclonus.

HYPERSOMNIA

Lesions which affect the structures in the floor of the third ventricle may produce excessive sleepiness, e.g. tumours or encephalitis, and are often associated with diabetes insipidus.

Systemic disease such as myxoedema may result in hypersomnia, as may conditions which produce hypercapnia — chronic bronchitis, or primary muscle disease, e.g. dystrophia myotonica.

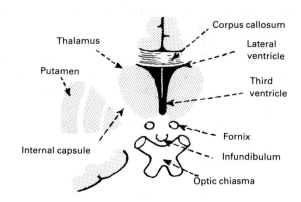

SLEEP APNOEA SYNDROMES

Respiratory rate fluctuates during REM sleep with occasional short episodes of apnoea. These are normal physiological events.

Sleep apnoea may also result from central reduction of respiratory drive or a mechanical obstruction of the airway.

Central causes:	Mechanical causes:
Brain stem medullary infarction or following cervical/foramen magnum surgery.	Obesity. Tonsillar enlargement. Myxoedema. Acromegaly.

When breathing ceases, the resultant hypercapnia and hypoxia eventually stimulate respiration.

Patients may present with daytime sleepiness, nocturnal insomnia and early morning headache. Snoring and restless movements are characteristic. In severe cases of sleep apnoea, hypertension may develop with right heart failure secondary to pulmonary arterial hypertension. Polycythaemia and left heart failure may ensue.

Treatment depends on aetiology. Mechanical airway obstruction should be relieved; drugs such as theophylline are occasionally helpful.

The *Pickwickian syndrome:* sleep apnoea associated with obesity, named after the Dickens' fat boy who repeatedly fell asleep.

HIGHER CORTICAL DYSFUNCTION

Specific parts of the cerebral hemispheres are responsible for a certain aspect of function. In normal circumstances these functions are integrated and the patient operates as a whole. Damage to part of the cortex will result in a characteristic disturbance of function. Interruption by disease of 'connections' between one part of the cortex and another will 'disconnect' function.

GENERAL ANATOMY

Brodmann, on the basis of histological differences, divided the cortex into 47 areas. Knowledge of these areas is not practical, though they are referred to often in some texts.

Six layers can be recognised in the cerebral cortex superficial to the junction with the underlying white matter.

The relative preponderance of each layer varies in different regions of the cortex and appears to be related to function.

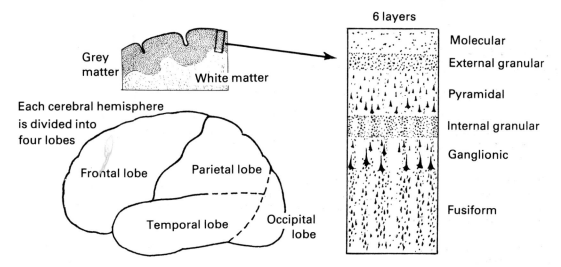

The frontal motor cortex, dominated by pyramidal rather than granular layers, is termed the AGRANULAR CORTEX.

The parietal sensory cortex, dominated by granular layers, is termed the GRANULAR CORTEX.

The largest cells of the agranular cortex are the giant cells of Betz. These give rise to some of the motor fibres of the corticospinal tract.

RIGHT AND LEFT HEMISPHERE FUNCTION

Unilateral brain damage reveals a difference in function between hemispheres. The left hemisphere is 'dominant' in right-handed people. In left-handed subjects the left hemisphere is dominant in the majority (up to 75%).

Hand preference may be hereditary, but in some cases disease of the left hemisphere in early life determines left-handedness.

HIGHER CORTICAL DYSFUNCTION

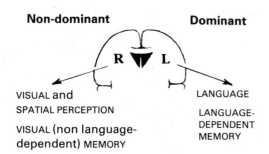

Non-dominant

Dominant

R L

VISUAL and SPATIAL PERCEPTION

VISUAL (non language-dependent) MEMORY

LANGUAGE

LANGUAGE-DEPENDENT MEMORY

Hemisphere dominance may be demonstrated by the injection of sodium amytal into the internal carotid artery. On the dominant side this will produce an arrest of speech for up to 30 seconds – the WADA TEST. Such a test may be important before temporal lobectomy for epilepsy when handedness/hemisphere dominance is in doubt.

FRONTAL LOBES

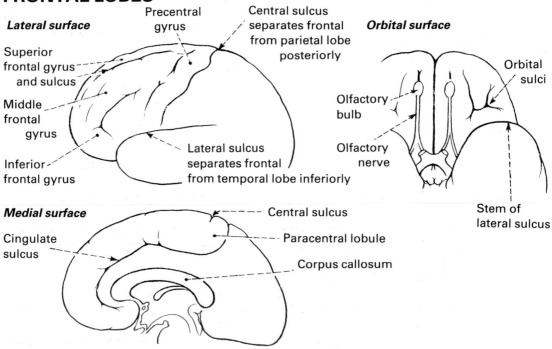

Lateral surface

Superior frontal gyrus and sulcus

Middle frontal gyrus

Inferior frontal gyrus

Precentral gyrus

Central sulcus separates frontal from parietal lobe posteriorly

Lateral sulcus separates frontal from temporal lobe inferiorly

Orbital surface

Olfactory bulb

Olfactory nerve

Orbital sulci

Stem of lateral sulcus

Medial surface

Cingulate sulcus

Central sulcus

Paracentral lobule

Corpus callosum

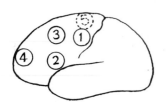

FRONTAL LOBE FUNCTION

1. Precentral gyrus — motor cortex contralateral movement — face, arm, leg, trunk.
2. Broca's area — dominant hemisphere — expressive centre for speech.
3. Supplementary motor area — contralateral head and eye turning.
4. Prefrontal areas — 'personality', initiative.
5. Paracentral lobule — cortical inhibition of bladder and bowel voiding.

FRONTAL LOBES

IMPAIRMENT OF FRONTAL LOBE FUNCTION

1. Precentral gyrus
Monoplegia or hemiplegia depending on extent of damage.

2. Broca's area (inferior part of dominant frontal lobe)
Results in Broca's dysphasia (see page 120)
(motor or expressive).

3. Supplementary motor area
Paralysis of head and eye movement to opposite side.
Head turns 'towards' diseased hemisphere
and eyes look in the same direction.

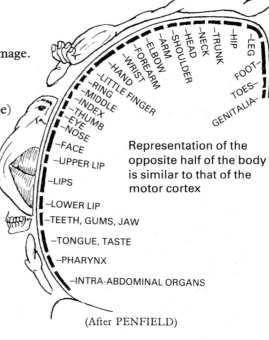

Representation of the opposite half of the body is similar to that of the motor cortex

(After PENFIELD)

4. Prefrontal areas (the vast part of the frontal lobes anterior to the motor cortex as well as undersurface — orbital — of frontal lobes)
Damage is often bilateral, e.g. infarction, following haemorrhage from anterior communicating artery aneurysm, neoplasm, trauma or anterior dementia, resulting in a change of personality with antisocial behaviour/loss of inhibitions.

Inappropriate jocularity (WITZELSUCHT).

The patient loses initiative and becomes disinterested and unconcerned.

An extreme of this state is AKINETIC MUTISM where, as a result of bilateral damage to the orbital surface of the frontal lobes, the patient appears awake and has normal ocular movement but does not speak, is incontinent and makes minimal motor response to painful stimulation. This state may also occur with hydrocephalus.

Pre-frontal lesions are also associated with:
      1. Primitive reflexes — grasp, pout, etc. (see page 123).
      2. Disturbance of gait — 'frontal ataxia'.
      3. Resistance to passive movements of the limbs — PARATONIA.

Unilateral lesions may show minor degrees of such change.

5. Paracentral lobule
Damage to the posterior part of the superior frontal gyrus results in incontinence of urine and faeces – 'loss of cortical inhibition'. This is particularly likely with ventricular dilatation and is an important symptom of normal pressure hydrocephalus.

107

PARIETAL LOBES

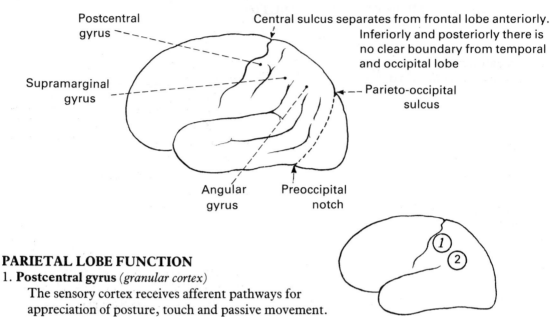

Postcentral gyrus

Central sulcus separates from frontal lobe anteriorly. Inferiorly and posteriorly there is no clear boundary from temporal and occipital lobe

Supramarginal gyrus

Parieto-occipital sulcus

Angular gyrus

Preoccipital notch

PARIETAL LOBE FUNCTION

1. **Postcentral gyrus** (*granular cortex*)
   The sensory cortex receives afferent pathways for appreciation of posture, touch and passive movement.
2. **Supramarginal and angular gyri** (*dominant hemisphere*) make up part of Wernicke's speech area.
   This is the receptive language area where auditory and visual aspects of comprehension are integrated.
3. The **non-dominant** parietal lobe is important in the concept of body image and the awareness of the external environment. The ability to construct shapes, etc. results from such visual/proprioceptive skills.
4. The **dominant** parietal lobe is implicated in the skills of handling numbers/calculation.
5. The **visual pathways** — the fibres of the optic radiation (lower visual field) — pass deep through the parietal lobe.

IMPAIRMENT OF PARIETAL LOBE FUNCTION

1. Disease of **either dominant or non-dominant** sensory cortex (postcentral gyrus) will result in contralateral disturbance of cortical sensation:
   Postural sensation disturbed.
   Sensation of passive movement disturbed.
   Accurate localisation of light touch may be disturbed.
   Discrimination between one and two points (normally 4 mm on finger tips) is lost.
   Appreciation of size, shape, texture and weight may be affected, with difficulty in distinguishing coins placed in hand, etc. (astereognosis).
   Perceptual rivalry (sensory inattention) is characteristic of parietal lobe disease. Presented with two stimuli, one applied to each side (e.g. light touch to the palm of the hand) simultaneously, the patient is only aware of that one contralateral to the normal parietal lobe. As the gap between application of stimuli is increased (approaching 2–4 seconds) the patient becomes aware of both.

2. **Supramarginal and angular gyri** — receptive dysphasia (see page 120).

PARIETAL LOBES

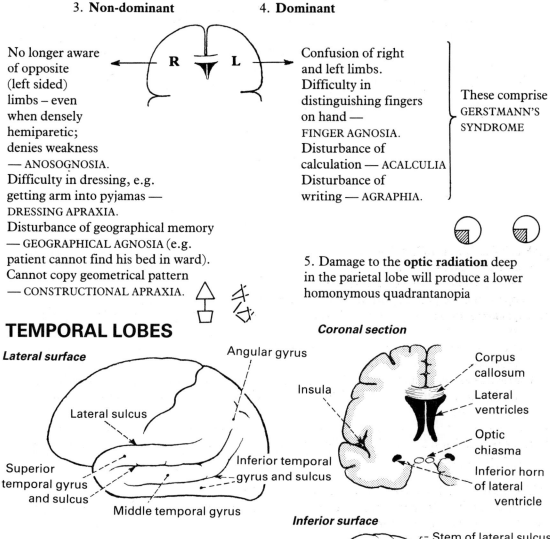

3. **Non-dominant**

No longer aware of opposite (left sided) limbs – even when densely hemiparetic; denies weakness — ANOSOGNOSIA.
Difficulty in dressing, e.g. getting arm into pyjamas — DRESSING APRAXIA.
Disturbance of geographical memory — GEOGRAPHICAL AGNOSIA (e.g. patient cannot find his bed in ward).
Cannot copy geometrical pattern — CONSTRUCTIONAL APRAXIA.

4. **Dominant**

Confusion of right and left limbs.
Difficulty in distinguishing fingers on hand — FINGER AGNOSIA.
Disturbance of calculation — ACALCULIA
Disturbance of writing — AGRAPHIA.

These comprise GERSTMANN'S SYNDROME

5. Damage to the **optic radiation** deep in the parietal lobe will produce a lower homonymous quadrantanopia

TEMPORAL LOBES

Lateral surface

Lateral sulcus

Angular gyrus

Superior temporal gyrus and sulcus

Inferior temporal gyrus and sulcus

Middle temporal gyrus

Coronal section

Insula

Corpus callosum

Lateral ventricles

Optic chiasma

Inferior horn of lateral ventricle

Inferior surface

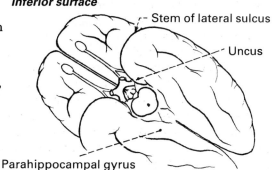

Stem of lateral sulcus

Uncus

Parahippocampal gyrus

Anteriorly, the temporal lobe is separated from the frontal lobe by the lateral sulcus. Posteriorly and superiorly, separation from occipital and parietal lobes is less clearly defined.

The lateral sulcus is deep and contains 'buried' temporal lobe. The buried island of cortex is referred to as the INSULA.

The temporal lobe also has a considerable inferior and medial surface in contact with the middle fossa.

109

TEMPORAL LOBES

TEMPORAL LOBE FUNCTION

1. The **auditory cortex** lies on the upper surface of the superior temporal gyrus, buried in the lateral sulcus (Heschl's gyrus).
   The **dominant** hemisphere is important in the hearing of language.
   The **non-dominant** hemisphere is important in the hearing of sounds, rhythm and music.
   Close to the auditory cortex labyrinthine function is represented.

2. The **middle and inferior temporal gyri** are concerned with learning and memory (see later).

3. The **limbic lobe:** the inferior and medial portions of the temporal lobe, including the hippocampus and parahippocampal gyrus.
   The sensation of olfaction is mediated through this structure as well as emotional/affective behaviour.
   Olfactory fibres terminate in the uncus.
   The limbic lobe or system also incorporates inferior frontal and medial parietal structures and will be discussed later.

4. The **visual pathways** pass deep in the temporal lobe around the posterior horn of the lateral ventricle.

IMPAIRMENT OF TEMPORAL LOBE FUNCTION

1. **Auditory cortex**
   Cortical deafness: Bilateral lesions are rare but may result in complete deafness of which the patient may be unaware.
   Lesions which involve surrounding association areas may result in difficulty in hearing spoken words (dominant) or difficulty in appreciating rhythm/music (non-dominant) — *AMUSIA*.
   Auditory hallucinations may occur in temporal lobe disease, e.g. complex partial seizures.

2. **Middle and inferior temporal gyri**
   Disturbance of memory/learning will be discussed later.
   Disordered memory may occur in complex partial seizures either after the event — postictal amnesia — or in the event – deja vu, jamais vu.

3. **Limbic lobe** damage may result in:
   Olfactory hallucination with complex partial seizures.
   Aggressive or antisocial behaviour.
   Inability to establish new memories (see later).

4. Damage to **optic radiation** will produce an upper homonymous quadrantanopia.

   Dominant hemisphere lesions are associated with Wernicke's dysphasia.

OCCIPITAL LOBE

The occipital lobe merges anteriorly with the parietal and temporal lobes.

On the medial surface the calcarine sulcus extends forwards and the parieto-occipital sulcus separates occipital and parietal lobes.

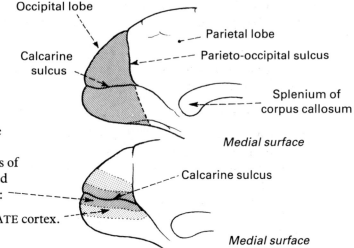

OCCIPITAL LOBE FUNCTION

The occipital lobe is concerned with the perception of vision (the visual cortex).

The visual cortex lies along the banks of the calcarine sulcus – this area is referred to as the STRIATE cortex:

above and below this lies the PARASTRIATE cortex.

The *striate* cortex is the primary visual cortex and when stimulated by visual input relays information to the *parastriate* — association visual cortex. This, in turn, connects with the parietal, temporal and frontal lobes both on the same side and on the opposite side (through the posterior part of the corpus callosum) so that the meaning of a visual image may be interpreted, remembered, etc.

The visual field is represented upon the cortex in a specific manner (page 136).

IMPAIRMENT OF OCCIPITAL LOBE FUNCTION

A cortical lesion will result in a homonymous hemianopia with or without involvement of the macula, depending on the posterior extent of the lesion.

When only the occipital pole is affected, a central hemianopic field defect involving the macula occurs with a normal peripheral field of vision.

Cortical blindness

Extensive bilateral cortical lesions of the striate cortex will result in cortical BLINDNESS. In this, the pupillary light reflex is normal despite the absence of conscious perception of the presence of illumination (light reflex fibres terminate in the midbrain).

Anton's syndrome

Involvement of both the striate and the parastriate cortices affects the interpretation of vision. The patient is unaware of his visual loss and denies its presence. This denial in the presence of obvious blindness characterises Anton's syndrome.

Cortical blindness occurs mainly in vascular disease (posterior cerebral artery), but also following hypoxia and hypertensive encephalopathy or after surviving tentorial herniation.

111

OCCIPITAL LOBE

Visual hallucinations are common in migraine when the occipital lobe is involved; also in epilepsy when the seizure source lies here.

Hallucinations of occipital origin are elementary — unformed — appearing as patterns (zig-zags, flashes) and fill the hemianopic field, whereas hallucinations of temporal lobe origin are formed, complex and fill the whole of the visual field.

Visual illusions also may occur as a consequence of occipital lobe disease. Objects appear smaller (MICROPSIA) or larger (MACROPSIA) than reality. Distortion of a shape may occur or disappearance of colour from vision.

These illusions are more common with non-dominant occipital lobe disease.

Prosopagnosia: the patient, though able to see a familiar face, e.g. a member of the family, cannot name it. This is usually associated with other disturbances of 'interpretation' and naming with intact vision such as colour agnosia (recognition of colours and matching of pairs of colours). Bilateral lesions at occipito-temporal junction are responsible.

HIGHER CORTICAL DYSFUNCTION THE DISCONNECTION SYNDROMES

Cortical function is described, on the previous pages, 'lobe by lobe'. These functions integrate by means of connections between hemispheres and lobes. Lesions of these connecting pathways disorganise normal function, resulting in recognisable syndromes — the disconnection syndromes. APRAXIA is a feature of some of these disorders. IDEOMOTOR APRAXIA — language in the form of a command cannot alone initiate and direct the performance of a learned motor task, e.g. "Shake your fist", "Wave good-bye with your hand" — though these tasks can be performed spontaneously. Apraxia is not associated with motor weakness or incoordination.

The connecting pathways may be divided into:

*Intra*hemispheric: lying in the subcortical white matter and linking parts of the same hemisphere.

*Inter*hemispheric: traversing the corpus callosum and linking related parts of the two hemispheres.

THE INTRAHEMISPHERIC DISCONNECTION SYNDROMES

1. Conduction Aphasia
Lesion of the arcuate fasciculus linking Wernicke's and Broca's speech areas.
Characterised by:
Fluent dysphasic speech. Good comprehension of written/spoken material. Poor repetition.

2. Pure word deafness
Lesion of the connection between the primary auditory cortex (Herschl's gyrus) and auditory association cortex.
Characterised by:
Impaired comprehension of spoken word. Self-initiated language is normal. The patient seems deaf, but audiometry is normal.

3. Buccal lingual and 'sympathetic' apraxia.
Involves the links between left and right association motor cortices in the subcortical region.
Characterised by:
Right brachiofacial weakness and apraxia of tongue, lip and left limb movements.

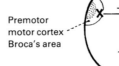

Premotor
motor cortex
Broca's area

THE INTERHEMISPHERIC DISCONNECTION SYNDROMES

1. Left side apraxia
Lesion of the anterior corpus callosum with interruption of the connections between the left and right association motor cortices.
Characterised by:
Apraxia of left sided limb movements.

2. Pure word blindness or alexia without agraphia
Lesion of the posterior corpus callosum and dominant occipital lobe with interruption of connections between the visual cortex and the angular gyrus/Wernicke's area.
Characterised by:
Inability to read, to name colours, to copy writing, but with normal spontaneous writing and the ability to identify colours.

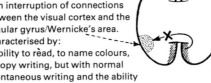

3. Agenesis of the corpus callosum

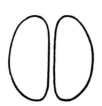

This is a developmental disorder with no connection between the two hemispheres.
Characterised by:
A failure to name an object presented visually or by touch to the non-dominant hemisphere. (The right and left visual fields cannot match presented objects.)

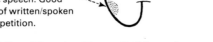

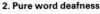

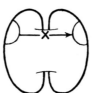

113

HIGHER CORTICAL DYSFUNCTION — MEMORY

Memory is the ability to retain and recall information and experiences.

It involves
- *Registration* – a confused patient cannot register new information.
- *Retention* – affected in disorders such as KORSAKOFF'S psychosis.
- *Recall* – rarely organically disordered.
- *Reproduction* – language dependent.

The limbic system contains structures important in memory.

The **hippocampus,** a deep structure in the temporal lobe, ridges the floor of the lateral ventricle. Fimbriae of the hippocampus connect this structure to the **fornix.**

There appears to be a loop from hippocampus→fornix→mamillary body→thalamus→cingulate gyrus →back to hippocampus.

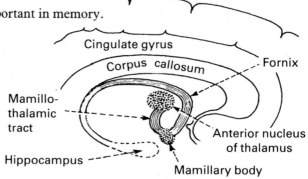

THE MEMORY PROCESS

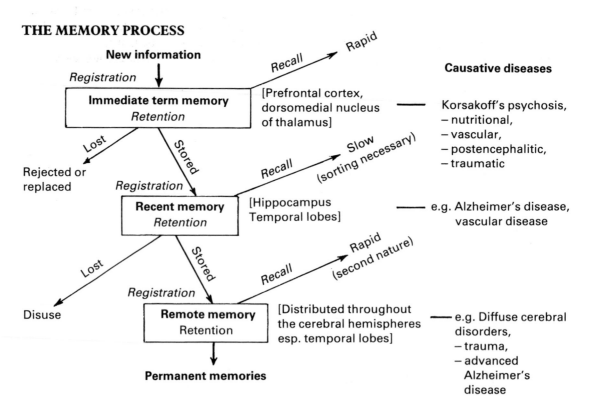

There is great individual variability between the extent of the lesion and the degree of memory disturbance.

HIGHER CORTICAL DYSFUNCTION — MEMORY

TESTS OF MEMORY (see Examination, page 8)

These aim to distinguish loss of immediate, recent or remote memory.

Disorders may be further classified into those which affect memories established before the injury or damage — RETROGRADE AMNESIA, and those established following the injury or damage — ANTEGRADE AMNESIA or POST-TRAUMATIC AMNESIA.

SPECIFIC DISORDERS OF MEMORY

Korsakoff's psychosis	*Lesion*	*Etiology*
An inability to acquire new memories, with some impairment of memory prior to onset of illness (retrograde amnesia).	Hippocampus and limbic structures, especially the dorsomedial nucleus of the thalamus.	Bilateral thalamic infarction. Herpes simplex encephalitis. Tuberculous meningitis. Vitamin B_1 deficiency. Third ventricular tumours.
Confabulation — a false description of present events and circumstances — is usually present		Dementias (posterior type) in which temporal lobes are involved early.

Transient global amnesia.

This is a condition of middle-late age in which total amnesia for recent events occurs with normal function during this period, i.e. the patient may go to work and behave normally or seem mildly disorientated. Recurrent attacks are uncommon. Episodes may last for some hours.

Pathogenesis is unknown, but presumed vascular (bilateral hippocampal) ischaemia seems probable. The condition appears benign.

DISORDERS OF SPEECH AND LANGUAGE

Introduction

Disturbed speech and language are important symptoms of neurological disease. The two are not synonymous. Language is a function of the dominant cerebral hemisphere and may be divided into (a) *emotional* — the instinctive expression of feelings representing the earliest forms of language acquired in infancy and (b) *symbolic or propositional* — conveying thoughts, opinions and concepts. This language is acquired over a 20-year period and is dependent upon culture, education and normal cerebral development.

An understanding of disorders of speech and language is essential, not just to the clinical diagnosis but also to improve communication between patient and doctor. All too often patients with language disorders are labelled 'confused' as a consequence of superficial evaluation.

DYSARTHRIA

Dysarthria is a *disturbance of articulation* in which the content of speech — language — is unaffected.

Mechanism of articulation

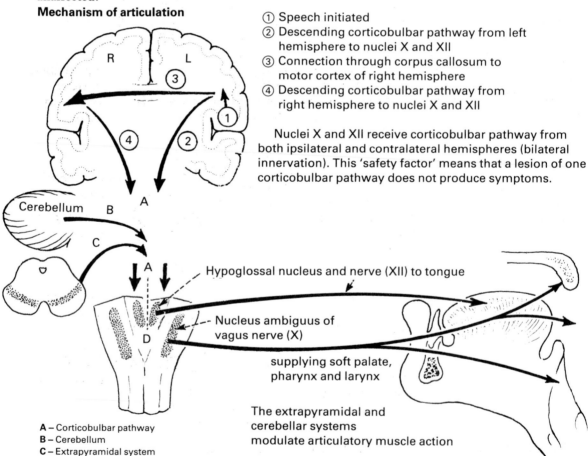

① Speech initiated
② Descending corticobulbar pathway from left hemisphere to nuclei X and XII
③ Connection through corpus callosum to motor cortex of right hemisphere
④ Descending corticobulbar pathway from right hemisphere to nuclei X and XII

Nuclei X and XII receive corticobulbar pathway from both ipsilateral and contralateral hemispheres (bilateral innervation). This 'safety factor' means that a lesion of one corticobulbar pathway does not produce symptoms.

Hypoglossal nucleus and nerve (XII) to tongue

Nucleus ambiguus of vagus nerve (X)

supplying soft palate, pharynx and larynx

The extrapyramidal and cerebellar systems modulate articulatory muscle action

A – Corticobulbar pathway
B – Cerebellum
C – Extrapyramidal system
D – Nuclei of lower motor neurons of X, XII cranial nerves

Muscles of expression, innervated by the facial nerve, play a role in articulation and weakness results in dysarthria.

DISORDERS OF SPEECH — DYSARTHRIA

DIAGNOSTIC APPROACH

Listen to spontaneous speech and ask the patient to read aloud. Observe:
lingual consonants –
'*ta ta ta*'
(made with the tongue),
labial consonants —
'*mm mm mm*'
(made with the lips),
guttural consonants —
'*ga ga ga*'
(laryngeal and pharyngeal/palatal).
Difficulty with articulation
= **DYSARTHRIA**

N.B. Beware misinterpretation, dialect or poorly fitting teeth.

Speech hoarse and strained; labial consonants especially affected.

Associated contralateral hemiparesis or dysphasia → SPASTIC DYSARTHRIA (Cortical origin)

Other signs of pseudobulbar palsy (impaired chewing, swallowing) → SPASTIC DYSARTHRIA (Corticobulbar origin)

Causative diseases
e.g. Middle cerebral artery occlusion.
Neoplasm.

e.g. Bilateral small vessel occlusion.
Motor neuron disease.

Speech slow and monotonous with abnormal separation of syllables —
'*scanning speech*'; at times may sound explosive —
Associated signs of cerebellar disease → ATAXIC DYSARTHRIA

(Lesion in cerebellar vermis and paravermis)

e.g. Multiple sclerosis, Hereditary ataxias.

Soft and monotonous with poor volume and little inflection —
Associated signs of extrapyramidal disease → HYPOKINETIC (slow) HYPERKINETIC (fast) DYSARTHRIA (Lesion of the extrapyramidal system)

e.g. Parkinson's disease.
Huntington's chorea.

Labial consonants first affected, later gutturals. *Nasal speech* and progression to total loss of articulation (*anarthria*).
Associated signs of l.m.n. weakness of X and XII → FLACCID DYSARTHRIA

(Involvement of X and XII nuclei or emergent nerves to muscles of articulation.)

e.g. Motor neuron disease.
Bulbar poliomyelitis.
Cranial polyneuritis.

Many diseases affect multiple sites and a 'mixed' dysarthria occurs.

For example, multiple sclerosis with corticobulbar and cerebellar involvement will result in a mixed spastic/ataxic dysarthria.

DISORDERS OF SPEECH — DYSPHONIA

Sound is produced by the passage of air over the vocal cords.

Respiratory disease or vocal cord paralysis results in a disturbance of this facility — **dysphonia.**
A complete inability to produce sound is referred to as **aphonia.**

DIAGNOSTIC APPROACH

If, despite attempts, there is deficient sound production then examine the vocal cords by *indirect laryngoscopy.*

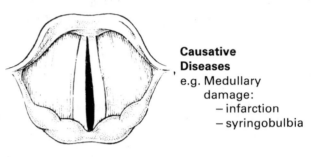

Causative Diseases
e.g. Medullary
    damage:
      – infarction
      – syringobulbia

Normal
abduction
of vocal cords –
'Ahh'

Mirror held
in posterior
pharynx

Paralysis of both vocal cords
Patient speaks in whispers
and inspiratory stridor is present.

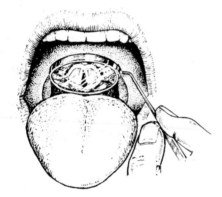

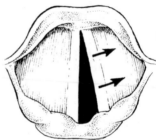

e.g. Recurrent laryngeal
    nerve palsy:
      – following thyroid
    surgery
      – bronchial neoplasm
      – aortic aneurysm

Spastic Dysphonia
Sounds as though speaking
while being strangled!
Similar to writer's cramp.
No known pathological cause

Paralysis of right vocal cord
which does not move with *'Ahh'*
while left abducts. When patient
says *'E'* normal cord will move
towards paralysed cord.
Voice is hoarse and nasal.

OTHER DISORDERS OF SPEECH

Mutism: An absence of any attempt at oral communication. It may be associated with bilateral frontal lobe or third ventricular pathology (see Akinetic mutism).

Echolalia: Constant repetition of words or sentences heard in severe dementing illness.

Palilalia: Repetition of last word or words of patient's speech. Heard in extrapyramidal disease.

Logorrhoea: Prolonged speech monologues; associated with Wernicke's dysphasia.

DISORDERS OF LANGUAGE – DYSPHASIA

Dysphasia is a loss of production or comprehension of spoken and/or written language.

Hand preference is associated with 'hemisphere dominance' for language. In right-handed people the left hemisphere is dominant; in left-handed people the left hemisphere is dominant in most, though 25% have a dominant right hemisphere.

The cortical centres for language reside in the dominant hemisphere.

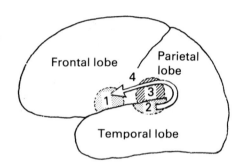

1 Broca's area
Executive or motor area for the production of language – lies in the inferior part of the frontal lobe on the lateral surface of the cerebral hemisphere abutting the mouth of the Sylvian fissure.

2 and 3 Receptive areas
Here the spoken word is understood and the appropriate reply or action initiated. These areas lie at the posterior end of the Sylvian fissure on the lateral surface of the hemisphere.

The temporal lobe receptive area (**2**) lies close to the auditory cortex of the transverse gyrus of the temporal lobe. The parietal lobe receptive area (**3**) lies within the angular gyrus.

Receptive and expressive areas must be linked in order to integrate function. The link is provided by (**4**), the **Arcuate fasciculus,** a fibre tract which runs forwards in the subcortical white matter.

Dysphasia may develop as a result of vascular, neoplastic, traumatic infective or degenerative disease of the cerebrum when language areas are involved.

119

DISORDERS OF LANGUAGE – DYSPHASIA

DIAGNOSTIC APPROACH

Listen to content and fluency of speech. Test comprehension, i.e. simple then complex commands

Non-fluent, hesitant speech; may be confined to a few repeated utterances or, in less severe cases, is of a 'telegraphic' nature with articles and conjunctions omitted.
Good comprehension.
Handwriting poor.
Look for coexisting right arm and face weakness.

→ BROCA'S DYSPHASIA
(Motor or expressive dysphasia)

Face Arm Trunk

Causative diseases

Vascular disease
Neoplasm
Trauma
Infective disease
Degenerative disease

Comprehension impaired.
Speech non-sensical but fluent.
  neologisms — non-existent words.
  paraphrasia — half right words.
Patient unaware of language problem.
Handwriting poor.

Differentiate from confused patient — construction of words and sentences is normal.

→ WERNICKE'S DYSPHASIA
(Sensory or receptive dysphasia)

Parietal
Temporal

Vascular disease
Neoplasm
Trauma
Infective disease
Degenerative disease

Non-fluent speech and impaired comprehension.
Often associated with hemiplegia/hemianaesthesia and visual field deficit.

→ GLOBAL DYSPHASIA
Damage involving a large area of the dominant hemisphere.

Vascular disease
Neoplasm
Trauma
Infective disease
Degenerative disease

Speech nonsensical but fluent (neologisms and paraphrasia) yet comprehension is normal.
Repetition is poor.

→ CONDUCTION DYSPHASIA

Vascular disease
Neoplasm
Trauma
Infective disease
Degenerative disease

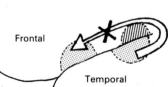

Frontal

Temporal

DEMENTIAS

Definition

Progressive deterioration of intellect, behaviour and personality as a consequence of diffuse disease of the cerebral hemispheres, maximally affecting the cerebral cortex and hippocampus.

Distinguish from *delirium* which is an acute disturbance of cerebral function with impaired conscious level, hallucinations and autonomic overactivity as a consequence of toxic, metabolic or infective conditions.

Dementia may occur at any age but is more common in the elderly, accounting for 40% of long-term psychiatric in-patients over the age of 65 years. A recent study shows an annual incidence rate of 187/100 000 persons. Dementia is a symptom of disease rather than a single disease entity. When occurring under the age of 65 years it is labelled 'presenile' dementia. This term is artificial and does not suggest a specific aetiology.

Clinical course:

The rate of progression depends upon the underlying cause.

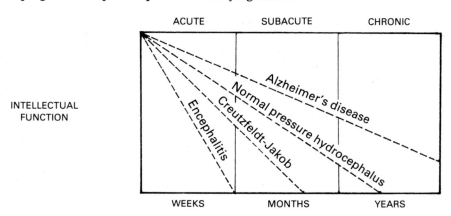

The duration of history helps establish the cause of dementia; Alzheimer's disease is slowly progressive over years, whereas encephalitis may be rapid over weeks. Dementia due to cerebrovascular disease appears to occur 'stroke by stroke'.

All dementias show a tendency to be accelerated by change of environment, intercurrent infection or surgical procedures.

Development of symptoms

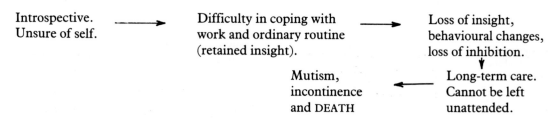

This initial phase of dementia may be inseparable from the *pseudodementia* of *depressive illness*.

121

DEMENTIAS — CLASSIFICATION

BASED ON CAUSE

Alzheimer's
Cerebrovascular
  Multi-infarct dementia
  Binswanger's disease
Neurodegenerative
  Pick's disease
  Huntington's chorea
  Parkinson's disease
Infectious
  Creutzfeld-Jakob disease
  HIV infection
  Viral encephalitis
  Progressive multifocal
    leucoencephalopathy
Normal pressure hydrocephalus

Nutritional
  Wernicke Korsakoff
    (thiamine deficiency)
  B_{12} deficiency
  Folate deficiency
Metabolic
  Hepatic disease
  Thyroid disease
  Parathyroid disease
  Cushing's syndrome
Chronic inflammatory
  Collagen vascular disease
   and vasculitis
  Multiple sclerosis
Trauma
  Head injury
  'Punch drunk' syndrome
Tumour
  e.g. Subfrontal meningioma

Alzheimer's disease accounts for 60% of all dementias; cerebrovascular disease 20%.

It is important to investigate all patients with dementia as many causes are treatable; in practice 10–15% can be reversed.

BASED ON SITE

Subdividing dementia depending upon the site of predominant clinical involvement is of questionable diagnostic value. However, many clinicians use this classification:

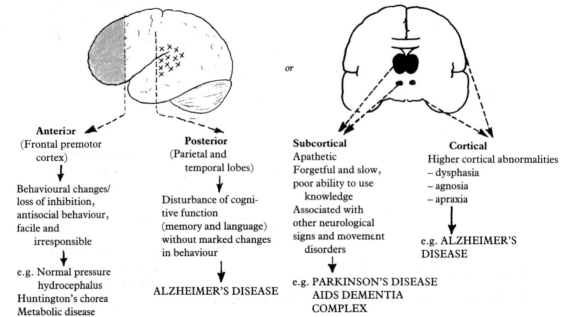

Anterior (Frontal premotor cortex) → Behavioural changes/loss of inhibition, antisocial behaviour, facile and irresponsible → e.g. Normal pressure hydrocephalus, Huntington's chorea, Metabolic disease

Posterior (Parietal and temporal lobes) → Disturbance of cognitive function (memory and language) without marked changes in behaviour → ALZHEIMER'S DISEASE

or

Subcortical Apathetic, Forgetful and slow, poor ability to use knowledge, Associated with other neurological signs and movement disorders → e.g. PARKINSON'S DISEASE, AIDS DEMENTIA COMPLEX

Cortical Higher cortical abnormalities – dysphasia – agnosia – apraxia → e.g. ALZHEIMER'S DISEASE

122

DEMENTIAS — HISTORY AND CLINICAL EXAMINATION

When obtaining a history from a demented person and relative establish:
- Rate of intellectual decline
- Impairment of social function
- General health and relevant disorders, e.g. stroke, head injury
- Nutrition status
- Drug history
- Family history of dementia.

Tests to assess intellectual function are designed to check:
- Memory
- Abstract thought
- Judgement
- Specific higher cortical functions

> A simple bedside battery of tests includes:
> - Age
> - Place of birth
> - Date of birth
> - School
> - Date
> - Time of day
> - Season of year
> - Prime Minister
> - Dates of World War II
> - Months backwards
> - Interpretation of proverbs
> - Following three stage commands
> - Read and obey instructions
> - Name objects
> - Copy design
> - Serial 7s
>
> In early dementia or pseudodementia a formal assessment from a clinical psychologist is advisable.

On neurological examination note:
- Focal signs
- Involuntary movements
- Pseudobulbar signs
- Primitive reflexes:

Pout reflex

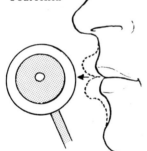

Tap lips with tendon hammer — a pout response is observed

Glabellar reflex

Patient cannot inhibit blinking in response to stimulation (tapping between the eyes)

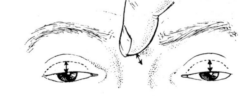

Grasp reflex

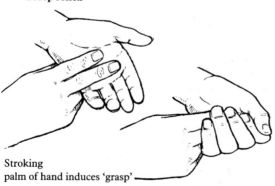

Stroking palm of hand induces 'grasp'

Palmomental reflex

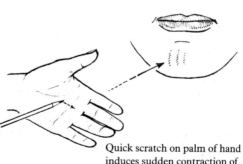

Quick scratch on palm of hand induces sudden contraction of mentalis muscle in face

Primitive reflexes are present in infancy and in aged people, as well as in dementia.

123

DEMENTIAS — SPECIFIC DISEASES

ALZHEIMER'S DISEASE
This is the commonest cause of dementia with an estimated half million sufferers in the UK. The disorder rarely occurs under the age of 45 years. The incidence increases with age. Familial cases are occasionally seen.

Pathology

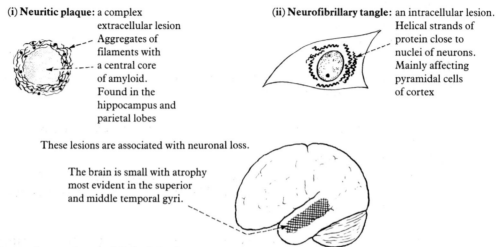

(i) Neuritic plaque: a complex extracellular lesion
Aggregates of filaments with a central core of amyloid. Found in the hippocampus and parietal lobes

(ii) Neurofibrillary tangle: an intracellular lesion. Helical strands of protein close to nuclei of neurons. Mainly affecting pyramidal cells of cortex

These lesions are associated with neuronal loss.

The brain is small with atrophy most evident in the superior and middle temporal gyri.

Diagnosis may be established during life by the early memory failure and slow progression and by excluding other causes.

CT scanning: aids diagnosis by excluding multiple infarction or a mass lesion.

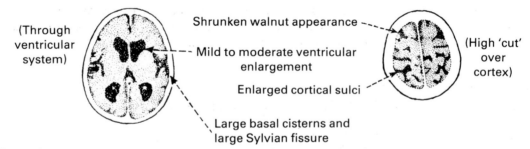

(Through ventricular system)

Shrunken walnut appearance

Mild to moderate ventricular enlargement

Enlarged cortical sulci

(High 'cut' over cortex)

Large basal cisterns and large Sylvian fissure

Causation
The cause of Alzheimer's disease is not known. An association with Down's syndrome suggests a disease locus on chromosome 21, and this has been confirmed in familial cases. Early research suggested selective lesions of neurotransmitter pathways occurred and a disorder of cholinergic innervation was postulated. It is now known that *many* neurotransmitter pathways are defective.

Treatment
No effective treatment exists. Transmitter augmentation therapy seems unlikely to be effective in view of the many neurotransmitters involved. A recent non-randomised study of the anticholinesterase THA claimed some limited success. Randomised trials are now in progress.

DEMENTIAS — SPECIFIC DISEASES

MULTI-INFARCT (arteriosclerotic dementia)
This is an overdiagnosed condition which accounts for less than 10% of cases of dementia.
Dementia occurs 'stroke by stroke', with progressive focal loss of function. Clinical features of
stroke profile — hypertension, diabetes, etc. — are present.
Diagnosis is obtained from the history and confirmed by CT scan.

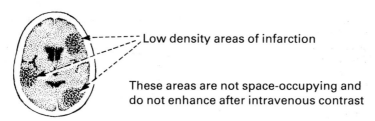

Low density areas of infarction

These areas are not space-occupying and
do not enhance after intravenous contrast

Treatment: Maintain adequate blood pressure control. Anti-platelet aggregants (aspirin).

AIDS DEMENTIA COMPLEX (see page 494)
Approximately two-thirds of persons with AIDS develop dementia, mostly due to AIDS
dementia complex. In some patients HIV is found in the CNS at postmortem. In others an immune
mechanism or an unidentified pathogen is blamed.
     Dementia is initially of a 'subcortical' type.
     CT shows atrophy; MRI shows increased T2 signal from white matter. Imaging excludes other
infections and neoplastic causes of intellectual decline.
     Treatment with Zidovudine (AZT) halts and partially reverses neuropsychological deficit.

METABOLIC DEMENTIA
General medical examination is important in suggesting underlying systemic disease. B_{12}
deficiency may produce dementia rather than subacute combined degeneration of the spinal cord.
     In alcoholics, consider not only Wernicke Korsakoff syndrome but also *chronic subdural
haematoma.*

NORMAL PRESSURE HYDROCEPHALUS
Normal pressure hydrocephalus (NPH) is the term applied to the triad of:

Dementia   occurring in conjunction with
Gait disturbance   *hydrocephalus* and *normal*
Urinary incontinence CSF pressure.

Two types occur:
     1. NPH with a *preceding cause* – subarachnoid haemorrhage
                              – meningitis
                              – trauma
                              – radiation-induced
(This must be distinguished from hydrocephalus with raised intracranial pressure associated
with these causes.)
     2. NPH with no known preceding cause – *idiopathic.*

DEMENTIAS — SPECIFIC DISEASES

NORMAL PRESSURE HYDROCEPHALUS (*contd*)

Aetiology is unclear. It is presumed that at some preceding period, impedence to normal CSF flow causes raised intraventricular pressure and ventricular dilatation. Compensatory mechanisms permit a reduction in CSF pressure yet the ventricular dilatation persists and causes symptoms:

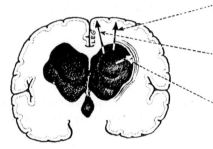

Pressure on frontal lobes ——————→ Dementia
(possibly related to decreased
cerebral blood flow).

Pressure on the cortical centre ——————→ Incontinence
for bladder and bowel control
in the paracentral lobe.

Pressure on the 'leg fibres' from ——————→ Gait disturbance
the cortex passing around the   and pyramidal
ventricle towards the internal capsule.   signs in the legs

Diagnosis is based on clinical picture plus CT scan evidence of ventricular enlargement.

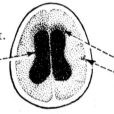

The lateral ventricles are often dilated more than the 3rd and 4th

Note the presence or absence of periventricular lucency (PVL) and width of cortical sulci

Normal pressure hydrocephalus must be differentiated from patients whose ventricular enlargement is merely the result of shrinkage of the surrounding brain, e.g. Alzheimer's disease. These patients do not respond to CSF shunting, whereas a proportion of patients with NPH (but not all) show a definitive improvement with shunting.

Investigations are designed to identify patients most likely to benefit from operation.

Numerous predictive tests have been assessed including:

ISOTOPE CISTERNOGRAPHY: a radioisotope injected into the cervical subarachnoid space does not pass over the hemispheres as expected but enters the ventricular system.

CSF INFUSION STUDIES: these note the intracranial pressure response to a volume of fluid infused into the ventricles or directly into the lumbar theca.

SULCAL WIDTH on CT scan: theoretically, the wider the sulci, the greater the atrophy, the poorer the response — but not consistent in practice.

The most reliable guides to response appear to be:
1. The presence of PERIVENTRICULAR LUCENCY on CT scan.
2. The presence of BETA WAVES for more than 5% of a 24-hour period of intraventricular pressure monitoring.

Beta waves

mmHg $\begin{matrix} 10 \\ 0 \end{matrix}$ ⌐⌐⌐ ～～～～～～～～ ⌐———⌐ 1 min

Operation: Ventriculo-peritoneal or ventriculo-atrial shunt (see page 362).

Results: The best response occurs in patients with a known preceding cause (e.g. subarachnoid haemorrhage), PVL on CT scan and beta waves on ICP monitoring.

DEMENTIAS — SPECIFIC DISEASES

TRAUMA

Reduction of intellectual function is common after severe head injury. Chronic subdural haematoma can also present as progressive demential, especially in the elderly.

Punch-drunk encephalopathy (dementia pugilistica) is the cumulative result of repeated cerebral trauma. It occurs in both amateur and professional boxers and is manifest by dysarthria, ataxia and extrapyramidal signs associated with 'subcortical' dementia. There is no treatment for this progressive syndrome.

TUMOUR presenting as dementia

Concern is always expressed at the possibility of dementia being due to intracranial tumour. This is rare, but may happen when tumours occur in certain sites.

Mental or behavioural changes occur in 50–70% of all brain tumours as distinct from dementia which is associated with **frontal lobe tumours** (and subfrontal tumours), **III ventricle tumours** and **corpus callosum tumours.**

Suspect in recent onset dementia with focal signs, e.g. subfrontal lesions may be associated with loss of smell (I cranial nerve involvement) and optic atrophy (II cranial nerve involvement).

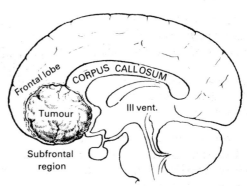

Other causes of dementia are considered in relevant sections.

DEMENTIA — DIAGNOSTIC APPROACH

It is neither practical nor essential to perform all the screening tests in every patient with dementia. The presenting features should guide investigations.

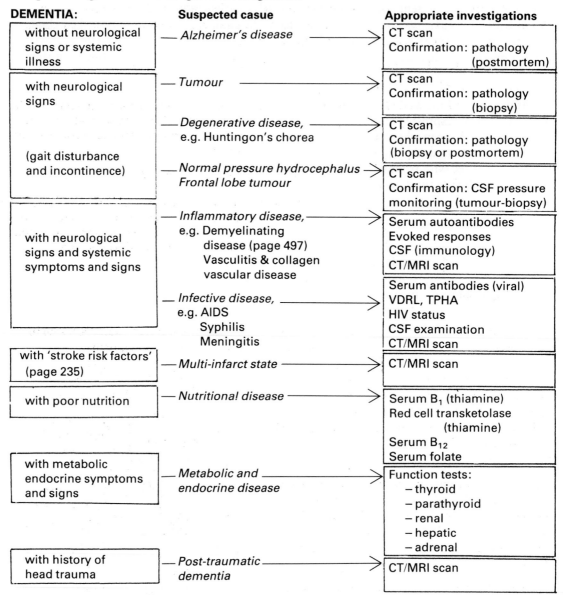

DEMENTIA:	Suspected casue	Appropriate investigations
without neurological signs or systemic illness	Alzheimer's disease	CT scan Confirmation: pathology (postmortem)
with neurological signs	Tumour	CT scan Confirmation: pathology (biopsy)
(gait disturbance and incontinence)	Degenerative disease, e.g. Huntingon's chorea	CT scan Confirmation: pathology (biopsy or postmortem)
	Normal pressure hydrocephalus Frontal lobe tumour	CT scan Confirmation: CSF pressure monitoring (tumour-biopsy)
with neurological signs and systemic symptoms and signs	Inflammatory disease, e.g. Demyelinating disease (page 497) Vasculitis & collagen vascular disease	Serum autoantibodies Evoked responses CSF (immunology) CT/MRI scan
	Infective disease, e.g. AIDS Syphilis Meningitis	Serum antibodies (viral) VDRL, TPHA HIV status CSF examination CT/MRI scan
with 'stroke risk factors' (page 235)	Multi-infarct state	CT/MRI scan
with poor nutrition	Nutritional disease	Serum B_1 (thiamine) Red cell transketolase (thiamine) Serum B_{12} Serum folate
with metabolic endocrine symptoms and signs	Metabolic and endocrine disease	Function tests: – thyroid – parathyroid – renal – hepatic – adrenal
with history of head trauma	Post-traumatic dementia	CT/MRI scan

Neuropsychometric testing is performed:
- to diagnose early dementia
- to separate true dementia from pseudodementia
- to monitor progress or trials of treatment.

When the reason for dementia is unclear, comprehensive investigation is essential to ensure that treatable nutritional, infective, metabolic and structural causes are not overlooked.

IMPAIRMENT OF VISION

ANATOMY AND PHYSIOLOGY

Anatomically the visual system is contained in the supratentorial compartment. It is composed of peripheral receptors in the retina, central pathways and cortical centres. The control of ocular movement and pupillary responses are closely integrated. The eye is the peripheral receptor organ concerned with the presentation of light stimuli to the retina.

The retina Three distinct layers of the retina are identified:

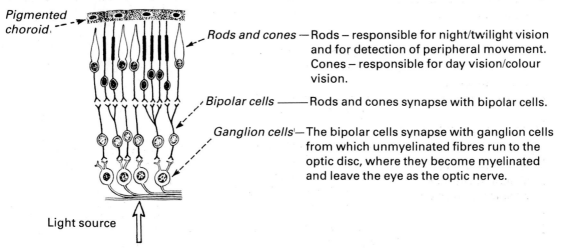

Pigmented choroid

Rods and cones — Rods – responsible for night/twilight vision and for detection of peripheral movement. Cones – responsible for day vision/colour vision.

Bipolar cells — Rods and cones synapse with bipolar cells.

Ganglion cells — The bipolar cells synapse with ganglion cells from which unmyelinated fibres run to the optic disc, where they become myelinated and leave the eye as the optic nerve.

Light source

The *macular region* of the retina is its most important area for visual acuity. Here, cones lie in the greatest concentration whereas rods are more numerous in the surrounding retina.

The optic nerve leaves the orbit through the *optic foramen* and passes posteriorly to unite with the opposite optic nerve at the *optic chiasma*. Here, partial decussation occurs (axons from ganglion cells on the nasal side of the retina cross over to the opposite side).

The *optic tract* consisting of ipsilateral temporal and contralateral nasal fibres passes to the *lateral geniculate body*. A few fibres leave the tract before the lateral geniculate body and pass to the *superior colliculus* (fibres concerned with pupillary light reflex).

Axons of cell bodies in the lateral geniculate body make up the *optic radiation*. This enters the hemisphere in the most posterior part of the internal capsule, courses deep in parietal and temporal lobes and terminates in the *calcarine cortex* of the occipital lobe.

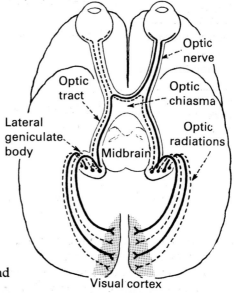

Optic nerve

Optic tract

Optic chiasma

Optic radiations

Lateral geniculate body

Midbrain

Visual cortex

IMPAIRMENT OF VISION

CLINICAL APPROACH AND DIFFERENTIAL DIAGNOSIS

Patients presenting with visual impairment require a systematic examination, not only of *vision*, but also of the *pupillary response, eye movements*, and, unless the cause clearly lies within the globe, a *full neurological examination.*

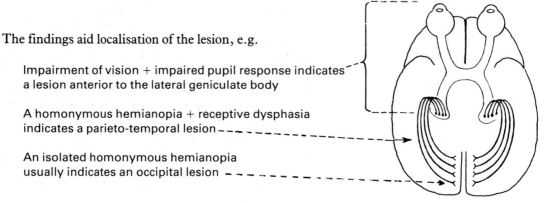

The findings aid localisation of the lesion, e.g.

Impairment of vision + impaired pupil response indicates a lesion anterior to the lateral geniculate body

A homonymous hemianopia + receptive dysphasia indicates a parieto-temporal lesion

An isolated homonymous hemianopia usually indicates an occipital lesion

Refractive errors are excluded by testing visual acuity through a pinhole or by correcting a lens deformity (page 9).

Four types of refractive error exist:

> **PRESBYOPIA** — failure of accommodation with age
> **HYPERMETROPIA** (long sightedness) — short eyeball
> **MYOPIA** (short sightedness) — long eyeball
> **ASTIGMATISM** — variation in corneal curvature

If this examination is normal, then the lesion lies in the retina, visual pathways or visual cortex.

Examine the globe and anterior chamber

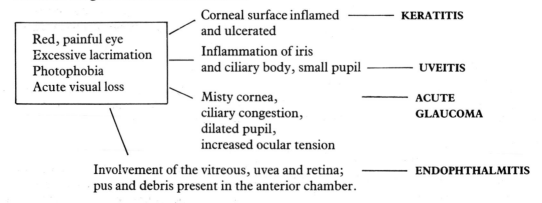

Red, painful eye
Excessive lacrimation
Photophobia
Acute visual loss

Corneal surface inflamed and ulcerated — **KERATITIS**

Inflammation of iris and ciliary body, small pupil — **UVEITIS**

Misty cornea, ciliary congestion, dilated pupil, increased ocular tension — **ACUTE GLAUCOMA**

Involvement of the vitreous, uvea and retina; pus and debris present in the anterior chamber. — **ENDOPHTHALMITIS**

Examine the lens with an ophthalmoscope

Opacification indicates CATARACT.

IMPAIRMENT OF VISION

CLINICAL APPROACH AND DIFFERENTIAL DIAGNOSIS *(contd)*

Examine the posterior segment of the eye with an ophthalmoscope.

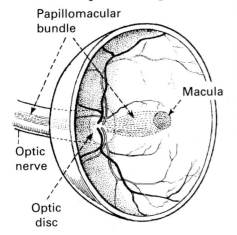

Papillomacular bundle

Macula

Optic nerve

Optic disc

Pupil dilatation may be required.

In the normal fundus, the *disc* is pale with a central cup and reddish-brown surrounding retina. Arteries and veins emerge from the optic disc. The *macula* is darker than the rest of the fundus and lies on the temporal side of the disc. One-third of all retinal fibres arise from the small macular region and pass to the optic nerve head (disc) as the *papillomacular bundle*. The macula is the region of sharpest vision (cone vision), whereas peripheral vision (rod vision) serves the purpose of perception of movement and directing central/macular vision. The optic nerve head contains no rods or cones and accounts for the physiological *blind spot* in normal vision. The macular fibres being so functionally active, are the most susceptible to damage and produce a specific defect in the visual field — a **scotoma**.

Retinal abnormality with acute impairment of vision

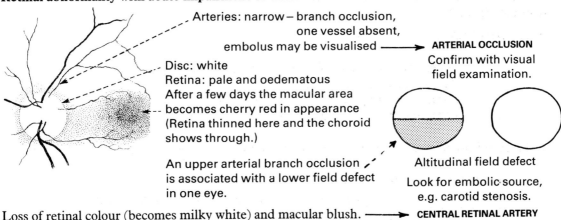

Arteries: narrow – branch occlusion, one vessel absent, embolus may be visualised ⟶ **ARTERIAL OCCLUSION**

Disc: white
Retina: pale and oedematous
After a few days the macular area becomes cherry red in appearance (Retina thinned here and the choroid shows through.)

An upper arterial branch occlusion is associated with a lower field defect in one eye.

Confirm with visual field examination.

Altitudinal field defect

Look for embolic source, e.g. carotid stenosis.

Loss of retinal colour (becomes milky white) and macular blush. ⟶ **CENTRAL RETINAL ARTERY** OCCLUSION

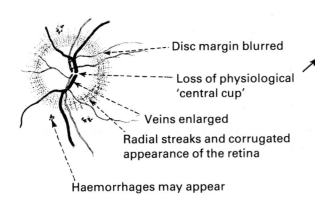

Disc margin blurred

Loss of physiological 'central cup'

Veins enlarged

Radial streaks and corrugated appearance of the retina

Haemorrhages may appear

Papillitis: *visual acuity severely affected* due to associated inflammation of the optic nerve (retrobulbar neuritis).

Papilloedema does not affect visual acuity (unless the macular area is affected by haemorrhage) although the blind spot is enlarged.

IMPAIRMENT OF VISION

CLINICAL APPROACH AND DIFFERENTIAL DIAGNOSIS *(contd)*

N.B. Distinguish:

HYPERMETROPIC patients who have a pale indistinct disc often difficult to differentiate from early papilloedema.

HYPERTENSIVE RETINOPATHY — superficial haemorrhages and 'cotton wool' exudates.

PSEUDOPAPILLOEDEMA — 'DRUSEN' — colloid bodies near the optic disc which raise the disc and blur the margin. This is a variant of normal.

Separation of the superficial retina from the pigment layer ⟶ **RETINAL DETACHMENT** (traumatic or spontaneous)

Retinal abnormalities with gradual impairment of vision

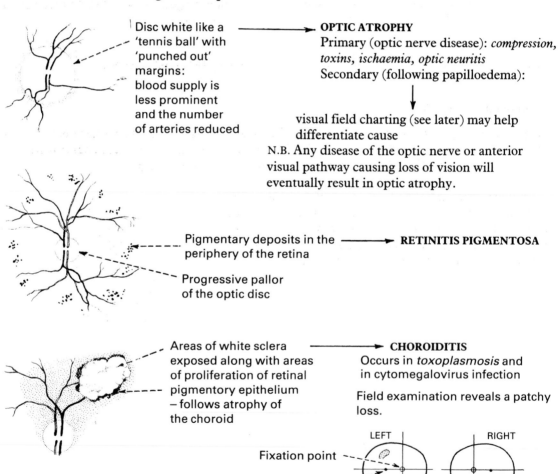

Disc white like a ⟶ **OPTIC ATROPHY**
'tennis ball' with
'punched out'
margins:
blood supply is
less prominent
and the number
of arteries reduced

Primary (optic nerve disease): *compression, toxins, ischaemia, optic neuritis*
Secondary (following papilloedema):

visual field charting (see later) may help differentiate cause

N.B. Any disease of the optic nerve or anterior visual pathway causing loss of vision will eventually result in optic atrophy.

Pigmentary deposits in the ⟶ **RETINITIS PIGMENTOSA**
periphery of the retina

Progressive pallor
of the optic disc

Areas of white sclera ⟶ **CHOROIDITIS**
exposed along with areas
of proliferation of retinal
pigmentory epithelium
– follows atrophy of
the choroid

Occurs in *toxoplasmosis* and in cytomegalovirus infection

Field examination reveals a patchy loss.

LEFT   RIGHT

Fixation point

Blind spot

IMPAIRMENT OF VISION

CLINICAL APPROACH AND DIFFERENTIAL DIAGNOSIS *(contd)*

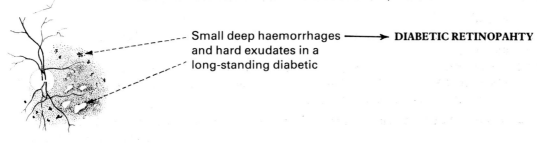

Small deep haemorrhages and hard exudates in a long-standing diabetic ⟶ **DIABETIC RETINOPAHTY**

Dark oval mass — possibly related to secondary retinal detachment — in middle aged patient ⟶ **MALIGNANT MELANOMA**

White mass behind the pupil — in infancy ⟶ **RETINOBLASTOMA**

Examine the visual fields

If ophthalmoscopic examination is normal, or if optic atrophy is evident, then visual field examination is essential. Visual confrontation is useful for detecting large defects, but smaller defects require visual field charting with a Goldmann perimeter (page 10).

In interpreting the physical findings of examination it is important to remember that the ocular system *reverses* the image. The nasal side of the fundus picks up the temporal image and vice versa. Damage, therefore, to the nasal side of the retina will produce a temporal visual field defect.

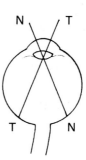

IMPAIRMENT OF VISION

CLINICAL APPROACH AND DIFFERENTIAL DIAGNOSIS *(contd)*

Central scotoma   Characteristic of most optic nerve lesions.

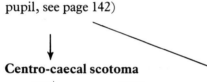

L   R

RETROBULBAR NEURITIS — associated papillitis may be evident on fundoscopy; may be first sign of *multiple sclerosis*.

OPTIC NERVE COMPRESSION

X-ray optic foramen ——— ***Orbital lesion*** (usually with
CT scan (orbital/intracranial)   – *tumour*   proptosis)
                                   – *granuloma*

Lesion within optic canal
– *tumour*, e.g. meningioma
– *granuloma*
– *hyperostosis*, e.g. Paget's disease, fibrous dysplasia

Intracranial lesions
– *tumour*, e.g. meningioma (chordoma, dermoid)
– *granuloma*, e.g. tuberculoma sarcoid (rare)
– *aneurysm*, e.g. anterior communicating, ophthalmic→angiography confirms

Pupil response may be impaired (Marcus-Gunn pupil, see page 142)

OPTIC NERVE GLIOMA   → CT scan → exploration
LEBER'S OPTIC ATROPHY — large bilateral scotoma

Centro-caecal scotoma

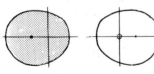

The scotoma extends to involve the blind spot. Characteristic of *toxic amblyopia* – alcohol, tobacco.

Arcuate scotoma

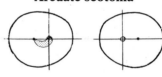

The scotoma extends from the blind spot following the course of nerve fibres.

Characteristic of *glaucoma;* seen also in small lesions close to the optic disc such as *choroiditis.*

Mononuclear blindness

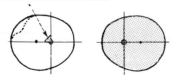

The end result of an inflammatory, vascular or compressive optic nerve lesion.

Direct pupillary response absent; consensual present.

Junctional scotoma

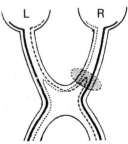

– indicates the presence of an *optic nerve lesion immediately anterior to the chiasma.*

Nasal fibres not only decussate in the chiasma, but also loop forward into the opposite optic nerve. This lesion emphasises the importance of examining the 'normal' eye in monocular impairment of vision.

IMPAIRMENT OF VISION

CLINICAL APPROACH AND DIFFERENTIAL DIAGNOSIS *(contd)*
Bitemporal hemianopia/quadrantanopia

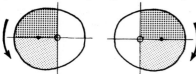
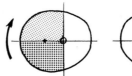
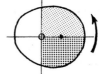

Involvement of the upper quadrants first indicates compression of the optic chiasma from below and suggests:
- **PITUITARY ADENOMA**
- **NASOPHARYNGEAL CARCINOMA**

Skull X-ray/CT scan

- **SPHENOID SINUS MUCOCELE**

Involvement of the lower quadrants first indicates compression of the optic chiasma from above and suggests:
- **CRANIOPHARYNGIOMA**
- **THIRD VENTRICULAR TUMOUR**

CT scan

The optic chiasma is closely associated with the pituitary fossa.

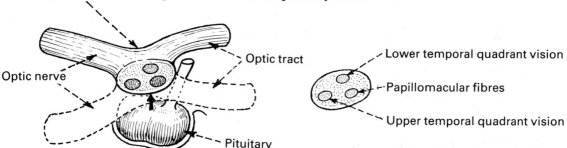

Optic tract

Optic nerve

Pituitary

Lower temporal quadrant vision

Papillomacular fibres

Upper temporal quadrant vision

Homonymous hemianopia

An incongruous homonymous hemianopia (i.e. one eye more affected that the other) suggests a compressive lesion of the **optic tract** near the chiasma.

- *vascular cause* (sudden onset)
- *tumour* (gradual onset)

CT scan

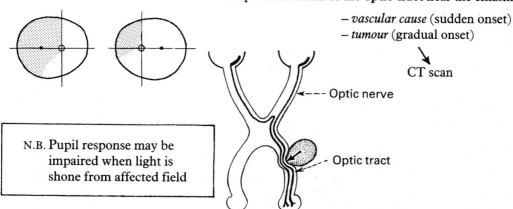

Optic nerve

Optic tract

N.B. Pupil response may be impaired when light is shone from affected field

The 'incongruous' defect occurs as a result of rotation of nasal and temporal fibres.

IMPAIRMENT OF VISION

CLINICAL APPROACH AND DIFFERENTIAL DIAGNOSIS (*contd*)
Congruous homonymous hemianopia (fields can be exactly superimposed)

Inferior quadrantanopia

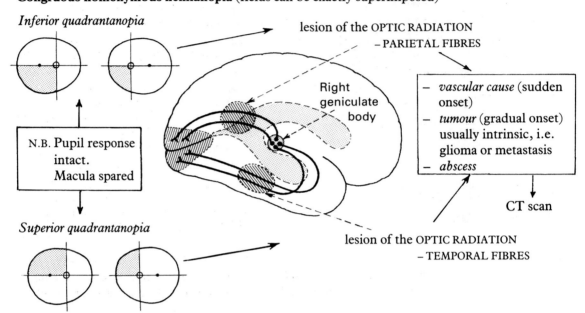

lesion of the OPTIC RADIATION
– PARIETAL FIBRES

Right geniculate body

- *vascular cause* (sudden onset)
- *tumour* (gradual onset) usually intrinsic, i.e. glioma or metastasis
- *abscess*

CT scan

N.B. Pupil response intact.
Macula spared

Superior quadrantanopia

lesion of the OPTIC RADIATION
– TEMPORAL FIBRES

At the temporo-parietal junction where fibres meet, lesions produce a complete 'homonymous hemianopia'.

Homonymous hemianopia with macular involvement

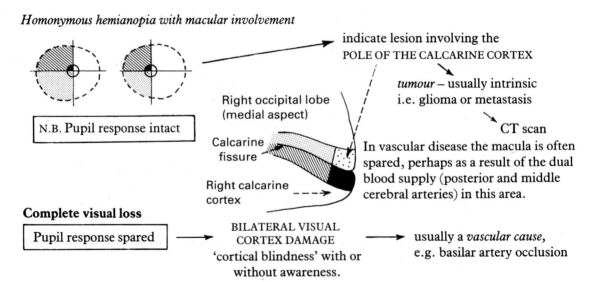

indicate lesion involving the
POLE OF THE CALCARINE CORTEX

tumour – usually intrinsic i.e. glioma or metastasis

CT scan

N.B. Pupil response intact

Right occipital lobe (medial aspect)

Calcarine fissure

Right calcarine cortex

In vascular disease the macula is often spared, perhaps as a result of the dual blood supply (posterior and middle cerebral arteries) in this area.

Complete visual loss

Pupil response spared → BILATERAL VISUAL CORTEX DAMAGE 'cortical blindness' with or without awareness. → usually a *vascular cause*, e.g. basilar artery occlusion

The interpretation of the visual image and its integration with other cortical functions is discussed under 'Higher cortical function'.

DISORDERS OF SMELL

OLFACTORY (I) cranial nerve conveys the sensation of smell.

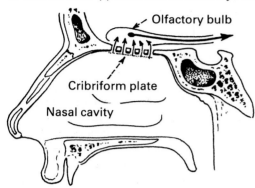

A number of fine nerves arising from receptor cells in the nasal mucosa pierce the *cribriform plate* of the ethmoid bone. These pass to the *olfactory bulb* where they synapse with neurons of the olfactory tract.

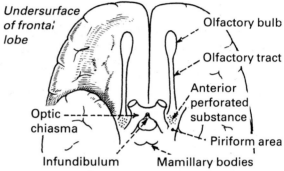

The neurons pass back in the olfactory tract to the *piriform area* of the temporal lobe and the *amygdaloid nucleus.*

Differential diagnosis

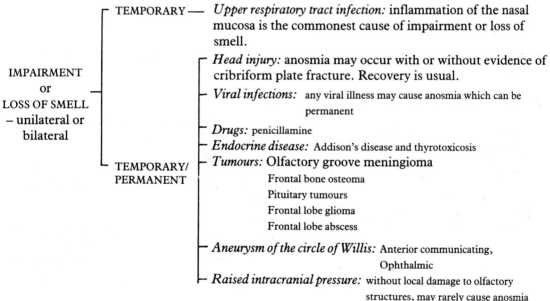

IMPAIRMENT
or
LOSS OF SMELL
– unilateral or
bilateral

TEMPORARY — *Upper respiratory tract infection:* inflammation of the nasal mucosa is the commonest cause of impairment or loss of smell.

TEMPORARY/
PERMANENT

Head injury: anosmia may occur with or without evidence of cribriform plate fracture. Recovery is usual.

Viral infections: any viral illness may cause anosmia which can be permanent

Drugs: penicillamine

Endocrine disease: Addison's disease and thyrotoxicosis

Tumours: Olfactory groove meningioma
Frontal bone osteoma
Pituitary tumours
Frontal lobe glioma
Frontal lobe abscess

Aneurysm of the circle of Willis: Anterior communicating, Ophthalmic

Raised intracranial pressure: without local damage to olfactory structures, may rarely cause anosmia

OLFACTORY
HALLUCINATIONS — Complex partial seizures — *Temporal lobe disease* (hippocampus pirifirm area)

PUPILLARY DISORDERS

ANATOMY/PHYSIOLOGY

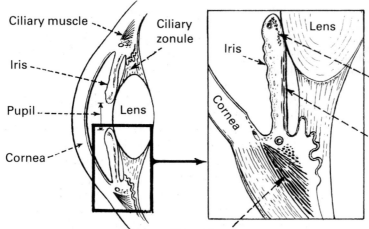

The iris controls the size of the pupil. It contains two groups of smooth muscle fibre:

1. *Sphincter pupillae;* a circular constrictor, innervated by the *parasympathetic* nervous system.
2. *Dilator pupillae;* a radial dilator, innervated by the *sympathetic* nervous system.

The ciliary muscle, innervated by the parasympathetic, controls the degree of convexity of the lens through the ciliary zonule.

Pathway of pupillary constriction and the light reflex (parasympathetic)

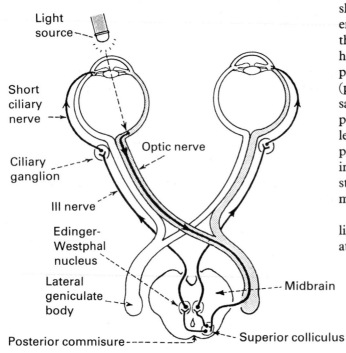

A stimulus, such as a bright light shone in the left eye, will send an afferent impulse along the **optic nerve** to the midbrain (superior colliculus); here a second order fibre passes to the *Edinger Westphal nucleus* (part of the III nerve nucleus) on the same and opposite side (through the posterior commissure). Efferent fibres leave in the **oculomotor nerve,** pass to the ciliary ganglion and thence, in the short ciliary nerve, to the constrictor fibres of the sphincter pupillae muscle.

If all pathways are intact, shining a light in one eye will constrict *both pupils* at an equal rate and to a similar degree.

PUPILLARY DISORDERS

Pathway of pupillary dilatation (sympathetic)

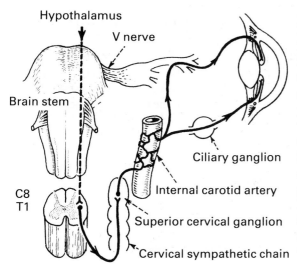

Sympathetic fibres descend from the hypothalamus through the lateral aspect of the brain stem into the spinal cord. The pupillary fibres pass out in the anterior roots of C8 and T1, enter the sympathetic chain and, in the superior cervical ganglion, give rise to postganglionic fibres which ascend on the wall of the internal carotid artery to enter the cranium. The fibres eventually leave the intracranial portion of the internal carotid artery and pass directly through the ciliary ganglion to the iris or join the cranial nerves III, IV, V and VI, running to the eye and iris. Sudomotor fibres (concerned with sweating) run up the external carotid artery to the dermis of the face.

Interruption of sympathetic supply affects:
1. Pupillary dilatation
2. Levator palpebrae muscle (30% supplied by sympathetic)
3. Vasoconstrictor fibres to orbit, eyelid and face.

Mechanism of accommodation

When gaze is focused on a near object the medial rectus muscles contract, producing convergence, the ciliary muscles contract enabling the lens to produce a more convex shape and the pupil constricts (accommodation for near vision).

The pathway is poorly understood but must involve the visual cortex, Edinger-Westphal nuclei and both medial rectus components of the III nerve nucleus in the midbrain.

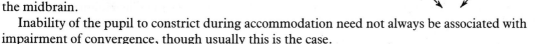

Inability of the pupil to constrict during accommodation need not always be associated with impairment of convergence, though usually this is the case.

PUPILLARY DISORDERS

PUPIL DILATATION – CAUSES
III nerve lesion

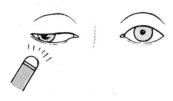

Examination of the light reflex (page 11) distinguishes lesions of the optic (II) and oculomotor (III) nerves.

Failure of the pupil to constrict when light is shone into either the affected or the contralateral eye indicates a III nerve lesion.

Look for — **ptosis** — 70% of levator palpebrae muscle is supplied by the oculomotor nerve

        — **impaired eye movements.**

Causes of a III nerve lesion are described on page 149.

In comatose patients, pupil dilatation and failure to react to light is the simplest way of detecting a III nerve lesion; after head injury or in patients with raised intracranial pressure this is an important sign of transtentorial herniation.

The tonic pupil — Adie's pupil

This is a benign condition usually affecting young women. Onset is usually acute and unilateral in 80%.

The pupil dilates and the patient complains of mistiness in the affected eye.

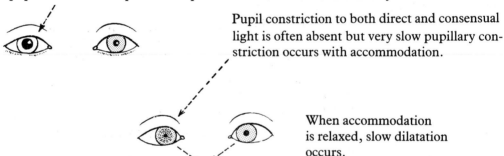

Pupil constriction to both direct and consensual light is often absent but very slow pupillary constriction occurs with accommodation.

When accommodation is relaxed, slow dilatation occurs.

Occasionally the pupil appears completely unreactive to both light and accommodation. When the pupil is associated with reduced or absent limb reflexes this is termed the **Holmes-Adie** syndrome.

Diagnosis: confirmed by pupillary response to pilocarpine (0.1% or 0.05%)—the tonic pupil will constrict (denervation hypersensitivity); the normal eye is not affected.

The cause is unknown; the lesion probably lies in the midbrain or ciliary ganglion.

Drugs

Mydriatic drops
Amphetamine } overdose produces large unreactive pupils.

N.B. Pupils are often large in childhood and may fluctuate in size in response to fatigue and excitement.

PUPILLARY DISORDERS

PUPIL CONSTRICTION – CAUSES *(contd)*
Horner's syndrome

Lesion

MYOSIS: the affected pupil is smaller than the opposite pupil. It does not dilate when the eye is shaded.

PTOSIS: the affected eyelid droops and may be slightly raised voluntarily. Ptosis is less marked than with a III nerve palsy.

DISTURBANCE OF SWEATING: depends on the site of the lesion. Absence of sweating occurs when the lesion is proximal to fibre separation along the internal and external carotid arteries.

Horner's syndrome may result from sympathetic damage at the following sites:

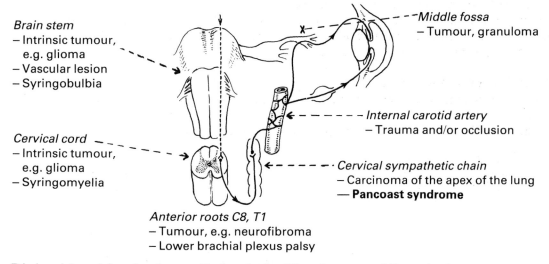

Brain stem
– Intrinsic tumour,
   e.g. glioma
– Vascular lesion
– Syringobulbia

Middle fossa
– Tumour, granuloma

Internal carotid artery
– Trauma and/or occlusion

Cervical cord
– Intrinsic tumour,
   e.g. glioma
– Syringomyelia

Cervical sympathetic chain
– Carcinoma of the apex of the lung
— **Pancoast syndrome**

Anterior roots C8, T1
– Tumour, e.g. neurofibroma
– Lower brachial plexus palsy

Distinguish peripheral and central lesions by instilling drugs, e.g. 1% cocaine in eyes.

Preganglionic lesions	**Postganglionic lesion**
Right sided Horner's	Right sided Horner's

Cocaine acts at the adrenergic nerve endings and, by preventing adrenaline uptake, causes pupil dilatation when the lesion is preganglionic.

When the lesion is postganglionic, cocaine has little effect because there are no nerve endings on which the drug may act.

Investigative approach: depends on associated signs. Chest X-ray is mandatory.

PUPILLARY DISORDERS

PUPIL CONSTRICTION – CAUSES *(contd)*

The Argyll-Robertson pupil

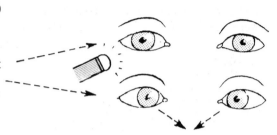

A *small pupil, irregular* in shape, which does not react to light but does react to accommodation.

It responds inadequately to pupillary dilator drugs.

Argyll-Robertson pupils are usually synonymous with *syphilitic infection*, but they may also result from *any midbrain lesion — neoplastic, vascular, inflammatory or demyelinative.*

The Argyll-Robertson pupil has also been described in *diabetes* and in *alcoholic neuropathy* as well as following infectious mononucleosis. The lesion could lie in the midbrain, involving fibres passing to the Edinger-Westphal nucleus, in the posterior commissure or, alternatively, in the ciliary ganglion. A central lesion seems most likely.

Investigative approach: – look for associated signs of neurosyphilis
– blood serology — VDRL, TPHA.

Drugs: *Opiate* overdosage produces small unreactive pupils.

N.B. In the elderly the pupils become small.

OTHER PUPILLARY DISORDERS

Failure of accommodation and convergence

Impaired accommodation and convergence are of limited diagnostic value since other clinical features are usually more prominent.

Causes: – extrapyramidal disease, e.g. Parkinson's
– tumours of the pineal region.

The Marcus Gunn pupil (pupillary escape)

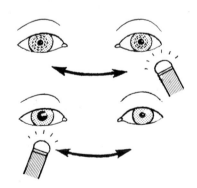

Illumination of one eye normally produces pupillary constriction with a degree of waxing and waning (hippus).

When afferent transmission in the optic nerve is impaired, this 'escape' becomes more evident.

If the light source is 'swung' from eye to eye, dwelling 4 seconds on each, the affected pupil may eventually, paradoxically, dilate — a 'Marcus Gunn' pupil.

The swinging light test is a sensitive test of optic nerve damage.

DIPLOPIA — IMPAIRED OCULAR MOVEMENT

Diplopia or double vision results from impaired ocular movement.

RELATED ANATOMY AND PHYSIOLOGY

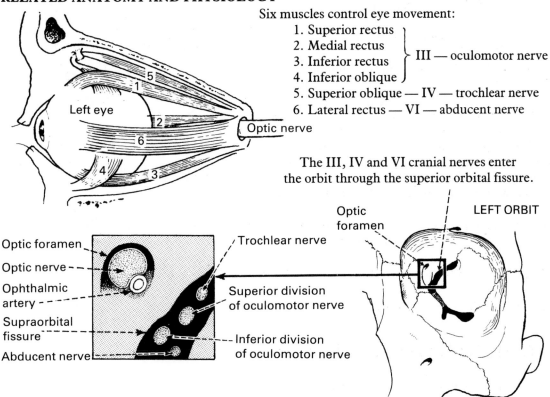

Six muscles control eye movement:

1. Superior rectus
2. Medial rectus
3. Inferior rectus
4. Inferior oblique
  } III — oculomotor nerve
5. Superior oblique — IV — trochlear nerve
6. Lateral rectus — VI — abducent nerve

The III, IV and VI cranial nerves enter the orbit through the superior orbital fissure.

LEFT ORBIT

Optic foramen

Optic foramen
Optic nerve
Ophthalmic artery
Supraorbital fissure
Abducent nerve

Trochlear nerve
Superior division of oculomotor nerve
Inferior division of oculomotor nerve

The line of action of individual ocular muscles

Eye movements result from a continuous interplay of all the ocular muscles, but each muscle has a direction of maximal efficiency. The oblique muscles move the eye up and down when it is turned in. The superior and inferior recti move the eye up and down when it is turned out.

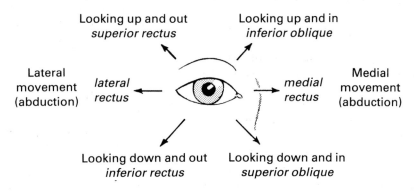

Looking up and out
superior rectus

Looking up and in
inferior oblique

Lateral movement (abduction)
lateral rectus

Medial movement (abduction)
medial rectus

Looking down and out
inferior rectus

Looking down and in
superior oblique

Eye movements are examined in the six different directions of gaze representing individual muscle action.

143

DIPLOPIA — IMPAIRED OCULAR MOVEMENT

The line of action of individual ocular muscles (contd)

As a result of the angle of insertion into the globe, the inferior and superior recti and the oblique muscles also have a rotatory or torsion effect.

When the eye is turned out, the oblique muscles rotate the globe; when turned in, the inferior or superior recti rotate the globe.

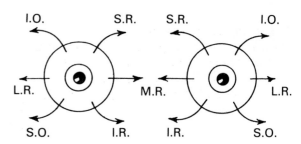

OCULOMOTOR (III) nerve

The oculomotor nucleus lies in the *ventral periaqueductal grey matter* at the level of the *superior colliculus*. Nerve fibres pass through the *red nucleus* and *substantia nigra* and emerge medial to the *cerebral peduncle*.

The nucleus has a complex structure:

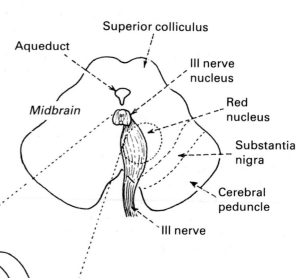

Perlia's nuclei (parasympathetic) concerned with convergence and accommodation.
Edinger – Westphal nuclei (pupil constriction)
 Medial rectus and inferior oblique
 Inferior rectus
 Superior rectus
Caudal nucleus of Perlia (levator of eyelid)

The nucleus is a paired structure which lies close to the midline, the portion representing the medial rectus abutting its neighbour. It has a complex structure:

DIPLOPIA — IMPAIRED OCULAR MOVEMENT

III nerve *(contd)*

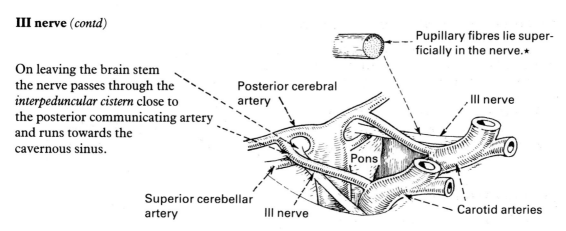

Pupillary fibres lie superficially in the nerve.★

On leaving the brain stem
the nerve passes through the
interpeduncular cistern close to
the posterior communicating artery
and runs towards the
cavernous sinus.

Posterior cerebral
artery

III nerve

Pons

Superior cerebellar
artery

III nerve

Carotid arteries

★This in part explains early pupillary involvement with III nerve compression and pupillary sparing with nerve infarction in hypertension and diabetes.

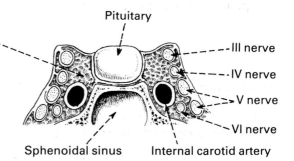

The nerve runs within the lateral wall of the
cavernous sinus

and then finally through the *superior
orbital fissure* into the *orbit*.
Here it divides into:
1. Superior branch to the levator of the
eyelid and the superior rectus.
2. Inferior branch to the inferior oblique,
medial and inferior recti.

Pituitary

III nerve

IV nerve

V nerve

VI nerve

Sphenoidal sinus

Internal carotid artery

TROCHLEAR (IV) nerve

This nerve supplies the *superior oblique muscle* of the eye.
The nucleus lies in the midbrain at the level of the
inferior colliculus, near the ventral *periaqueductal
grey matter.* The nerve passes laterally and dorsally
around the central grey matter and decussates
in the dorsal aspect of the brain stem in close
proximity to the *anterior medullary velum* of
the cerebellum.

Emerging from the brain stem the nerve
passes laterally around the *cerebral
peduncle* and pierces the dura to lie in
the lateral wall of the *cavernous sinus.*
Finally, it passes through the *superior
orbital fissure* into the orbit.

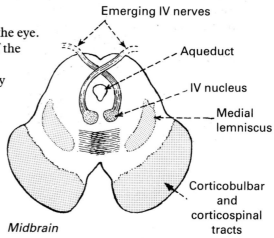

Emerging IV nerves

Aqueduct

IV nucleus

Medial
lemniscus

Corticobulbar
and
corticospinal
tracts

Midbrain

145

DIPLOPIA — IMPAIRED OCULAR MOVEMENT

ABDUCENS (VI) nerve

This nerve supplies the *lateral rectus muscle* of the eye.

The nucleus lies in the floor of the IV ventricle within the lower portion of the *pons*. The axons pass ventrally through the pons without decussating.

Note the close association of the VI and VII nuclei.

Emerging from the brain stem the nerve runs up anterior to the pons for approximately 15 mm before piercing the dura overlying the *basilar portion* of the *occipital bone*.

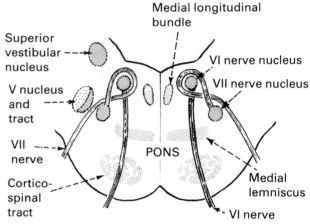

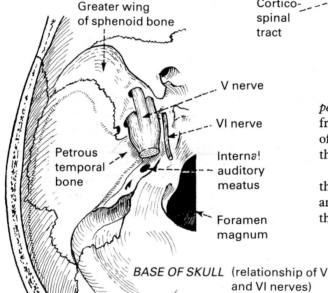

BASE OF SKULL (relationship of V and VI nerves)

Under the dura the nerve runs up the *petrous portion* of the *temporal bone* and from its apex passes on to the lateral wall of the *cavernous sinus* and finally through the *superior orbital fissure*.

Note the long intracranial course and the proximity of the VI to the V cranial and greater superficial petrosal nerves at the apex of the petrous temporal bone.

DIPLOPIA

When the eyes fix on an image, impairment of movement of one eye results in projection of the image upon the macular area in the normal eye and to one side of the macula in the paretic eye; two images of the single object are thus perceived.

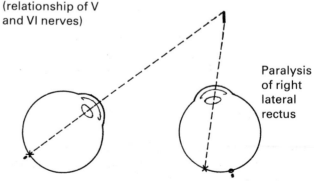

The image seen by the paretic eye is the *false image;* that seen by the normal eye is the *true image*. The false image is always *outermost;* this may lie in the vertical or the horizontal plane.

146

DIPLOPIA — IMPAIRED OCULAR MOVEMENT

CLINICAL ASSESSMENT

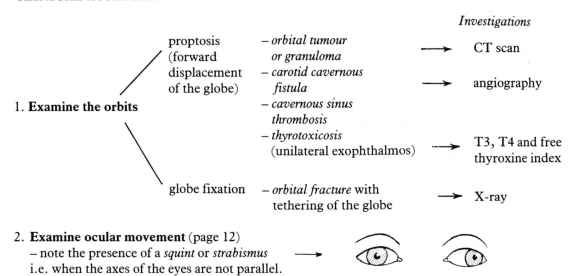

Investigations

1. Examine the orbits

proptosis (forward displacement of the globe)

– *orbital tumour or granuloma* ⟶ CT scan

– *carotid cavernous fistula* ⟶ angiography

– *cavernous sinus thrombosis*

– *thyrotoxicosis* (unilateral exophthalmos) ⟶ T3, T4 and free thyroxine index

globe fixation

– *orbital fracture* with tethering of the globe ⟶ X-ray

2. Examine ocular movement (page 12)
 – note the presence of a *squint* or *strabismus* ⟶
 i.e. when the axes of the eyes are not parallel.

Differentiate

Concomitant squint — an ocular disorder. The eyes adopt an abnormal position in relation to each other and the deviation is constant in all directions of gaze. Such squints are usually 'convergent' and develop in the first few years of life before binocular vision is established. Suppression of vision from one eye (*amblyopia ex anopsia*) results in *absence of diplopia*. Occasionally patients subconsciously alternate vision from one eye to the other, retaining equal visual function in both – *strabismus alternans*. Correction of an underlying hypermetropia with convex lenses may offset the tendency for the eyes to converge.

Paralytic squint:
 – Affected eye shows limited movement.
 – Angle of eye deviation and diplopia greatest when looking in the direction controlled by the weak muscle.
 – Diplopia is always present.
 – The patient may assume a head tilt posture to minimise the diplopia. Paralytic squint results from disturbance of function of nerves or muscles.

III NERVE LESION

In the primary position, the affected eye deviates laterally (due to unopposed action of the lateral rectus) and **ptosis** and **pupil dilatation** are evident.

(Ptosis may be complete, unlike the partial ptosis of a Horner's syndrome which disappears on looking up.)

DIPLOPIA — IMPAIRED OCULAR MOVEMENT

IV NERVE LESION

The eyes appear conjugate in the primary position.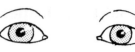

Testing eye movements reveals defective depression of the adducted eye.

Symptomatically the patient complains of double vision when looking downwards, e.g. when descending stairs or reading, and the head may tilt to the opposite side to minimise the diplopia.

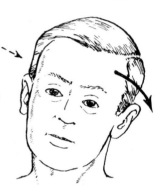

A IV nerve palsy is difficult to detect when associated with a III nerve palsy. If inward rotation (intorsion) is absent on looking downwards when the eye is abducted, then a IV nerve palsy coexists with the III nerve palsy.

VI NERVE LESION

The eyes appear conjugate in the primary position.

On looking to the paralysed side (right) there is failure of abduction of the affected eye.

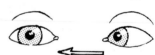

Diplopia is horizontal (true and fake image side by side) and is present only when looking to the paralysed side and is maximal at the extreme of binocular lateral vision.

NOTE: In partial oculomotor palsies, the patient may be aware of diplopia, although eye movements appear normal. When this occurs:
- check diplopia is 'true' by noting its disappearance on covering one eye.
- determine the direction of maximal image displacement and the eye responsible for the outermost image (see page 13).

This information is sufficient to differentiate a III, IV and VI nerve lesion.

OCULAR MUSCLES

If the limitation of eye movement is not restricted to one muscle, or group of muscles with a common innervation, and affects both eyes, look for:
- involvement of extraocular muscles (levator palpebrae superioris, orbicularis oculi)
- signs of fatigue on repeated testing

myasthenia gravis
ocular myopathy

DIPLOPIA — IMPAIRED OCULAR MOVEMENT

CAUSES OF III NERVE LESION

Midbrain

When BILATERAL → oculomotor nucleus

When III nerve lesion is associated with

    TREMOR → red nucleus

    or

    CONTRALATERAL HEMIPARESIS → cerebral peduncles
(WEBER'S SYNDROME)

Infarction, demyelination, intrinsic tumour, e.g. glioma, basilar aneurysm compression

Orbital fissure/orbit

Look for PROPTOSIS and associated involvement of the IV, VI and FIRST DIVISION of the V NERVES
– *Orbital tumour, granuloma,*
– *Periosteitis*

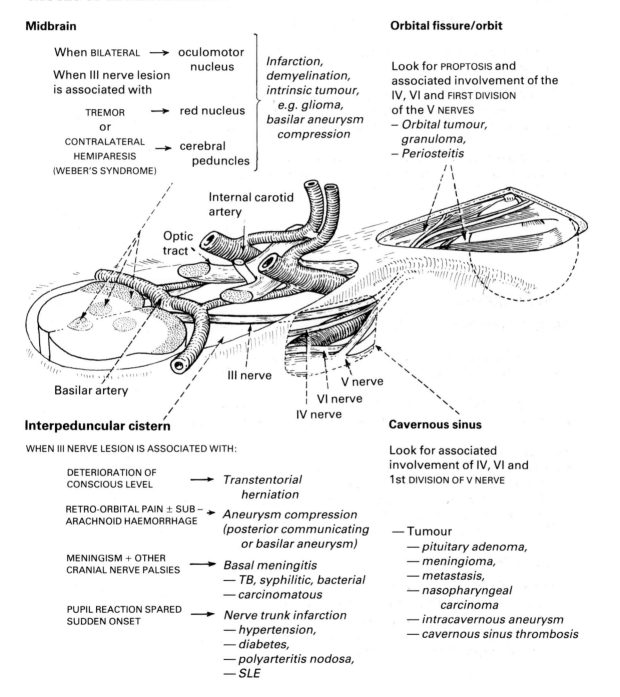

Internal carotid artery

Optic tract

Basilar artery

III nerve

V nerve

VI nerve

IV nerve

Interpeduncular cistern

WHEN III NERVE LESION IS ASSOCIATED WITH:

DETERIORATION OF CONSCIOUS LEVEL → *Transtentorial herniation*

RETRO-ORBITAL PAIN ± SUB–ARACHNOID HAEMORRHAGE → *Aneurysm compression (posterior communicating or basilar aneurysm)*

MENINGISM + OTHER CRANIAL NERVE PALSIES → *Basal meningitis*
— TB, syphilitic, bacterial
— carcinomatous

PUPIL REACTION SPARED SUDDEN ONSET → *Nerve trunk infarction*
— hypertension,
— diabetes,
— polyarteritis nodosa,
— SLE

Cavernous sinus

Look for associated involvement of IV, VI and 1st DIVISION OF V NERVE

— Tumour
    — *pituitary adenoma,*
    — *meningioma,*
    — *metastasis,*
    — *nasopharyngeal carcinoma*
    — *intracavernous aneurysm*
    — *cavernous sinus thrombosis*

DIPLOPIA — IMPAIRED OCULAR MOVEMENT

CAUSES OF IV NERVE LESION

Midbrain

When IV nerve lesion is associated with:

CONTRALATERAL HEMIPARESIS, CONTRALATERAL HEMISENSORY LOSS } intrinsic midbrain lesion } *infarction, demyelination, intrinsic tumour, e.g. glioma*

Orbital fissure orbit Cavernous sinus } *Causes as for III nerve lesion*

Proximity to anterior medullary velum and superior vermis } *cerebellar tumour, e.g. medulloblastoma*

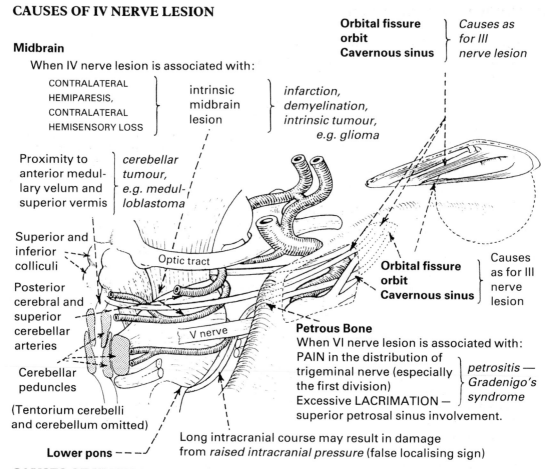

Superior and inferior colliculi

Optic tract

Posterior cerebral and superior cerebellar arteries

V nerve

Cerebellar peduncles

(Tentorium cerebelli and cerebellum omitted)

Lower pons ‒ ‒ ‒

Orbital fissure orbit Cavernous sinus } Causes as for III nerve lesion

Petrous Bone
When VI nerve lesion is associated with:
PAIN in the distribution of trigeminal nerve (especially the first division) } *petrositis — Gradenigo's syndrome*
Excessive LACRIMATION — superior petrosal sinus involvement.

Long intracranial course may result in damage from *raised intracranial pressure* (false localising sign)

CAUSES OF VI NERVE LESION

When VI nerve lesion is associated with:

CONTRALATERAL HEMIPARESIS, CONTRALATERAL HEMISENSORY LOSS, LOWER MOTOR NEURON VII LESION } nuclear or intramedullary lesion } *infarction, demyelination, intrinsic tumour, e.g. glioma*

NOTE: Infective or carcinomatous meningitis and nerve trunk infarction may also involve the IV and VI nerves, although less often than the III nerve.

Investigative approach

Impaired ocular movement from III, IV or VI nerve lesions requires full investigation with *straight X-rays, conventional or dynamic CT scan* and, where appropriate, *CSF cytology.* Unexplained III nerve lesions require *angiography;* only in elderly hypertensive or diabetic patients with pupillary sparing may angiography be omitted.

When myopathy or myasthenia gravis is suspected then appropriate investigations — receptor antibodies, EMG studies and occasionally muscle biopsy — may be necessary.

DISORDERS OF GAZE

ANATOMY AND PHYSIOLOGY

Two cortical centres of ocular control are recognised:
1. Middle gyrus of frontal lobe (frontal eye field).
2. Occipital cortex.

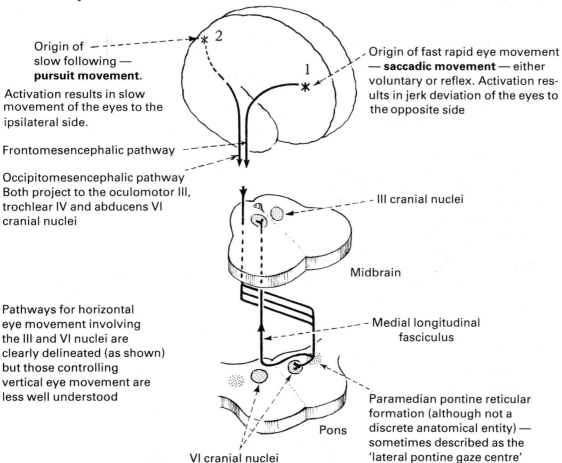

Origin of slow following — **pursuit movement.**
Activation results in slow movement of the eyes to the ipsilateral side.

Origin of fast rapid eye movement — **saccadic movement** — either voluntary or reflex. Activation results in jerk deviation of the eyes to the opposite side

Frontomesencephalic pathway

Occipitomesencephalic pathway
Both project to the oculomotor III, trochlear IV and abducens VI cranial nuclei

III cranial nuclei

Midbrain

Pathways for horizontal eye movement involving the III and VI nuclei are clearly delineated (as shown) but those controlling vertical eye movement are less well understood

Medial longitudinal fasciculus

Paramedian pontine reticular formation (although not a discrete anatomical entity) — sometimes described as the 'lateral pontine gaze centre'

Pons

VI cranial nuclei

Note that the cortical descending pathways from one side activate the ipsilateral III nucleus and the contralateral VI nucleus thus swinging the direction of gaze to the opposite side.

It is important to distinguish between **saccadic** and **pursuit** movement. When following an object a slow pursuit movement maintains the image on the macular area of the retina. To fixate on a new object, rapid saccadic movement aligns the new target on the macular area. When locked in to the new target, pursuit movement maintains fixation.

Eye movement occurs voluntarily in a conjugate (parallel) manner in any direction. Eye movements also occur reflexly to labyrinthine stimulation.

DISORDERS OF GAZE

Gaze disorders usually follow vascular episodes (infarct or haemorrhage) but may also occur in traumatic, inflammatory or neoplastic disease.

CONJUGATE DEVIATION OF THE EYES
Occurring during a seizure

Eyes deviate towards the affected limbs in a jerking fashion.

 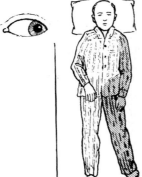

Indicates an epileptic focus in the frontal lobe contralateral to the direction of eye deviation. →

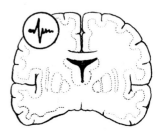

Accompanying a hemiparesis

Tonic deviation of the eyes *away* from the hemiparetic limb.

  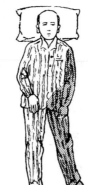

Indicates a lesion in the frontal lobe *ipsilateral* to the direction of eye deviation. →

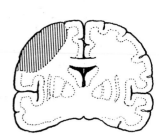

Tonic deviation of the eyes *towards* the hemiparetic limb.

  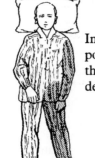

Indicates a lesion in the pons *contralateral* to the direction of eye deviation. →

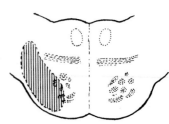

DISORDERS OF GAZE

PARINAUD'S SYNDROME

A syndrome characterised by impaired ocular motility and pupillary responses.

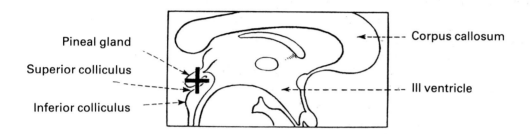

The lesion affects the midbrain tectum (✚)
>   — Upward gaze and convergence are lost
>   — The pupils may dilate and the response to light and accommodation is impaired.

Causes:

> Third ventricular tumours.
> Pineal region tumours.
> Hydrocephalus.
> Wernicke's encephalopathy.
> Encephalitis.

INTERNUCLEAR OPHTHALMOPLEGIA (ataxic nystagmus)

This disorder, due to damage to the medial longitudinal bundle, is dealt with on page 182. It is an *internuclear* disorder of eye movement.

OCULAR APRAXIA
Bilateral prefrontal motor cortex damage will produce this unusual finding in which the patient does not move the eyes voluntarily to command, yet has a full range of random eye movement.

FACIAL PAIN AND SENSORY LOSS

The fifth cranial nerve subserves facial sensation and innervates the muscles of mastication.

Anatomy

The anatomical arrangement of the trigeminal central connections are complex.

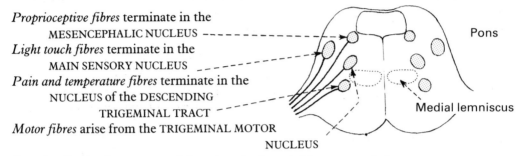

Proprioceptive fibres terminate in the
    MESENCEPHALIC NUCLEUS
Light touch fibres terminate in the
    MAIN SENSORY NUCLEUS
Pain and temperature fibres terminate in the
    NUCLEUS of the DESCENDING
        TRIGEMINAL TRACT
Motor fibres arise from the TRIGEMINAL MOTOR
           NUCLEUS

Pons

Medial lemniscus

Longitudinal arrangement of the trigeminal nuclei (sensory paths)

The separate location of the main sensory nucleus and nucleus of the descending trigeminal tract account for **dissociated sensory loss,** i.e. a low pontine or medullary lesion will result in loss of pain and temperature sensation with pre-servation of light touch.

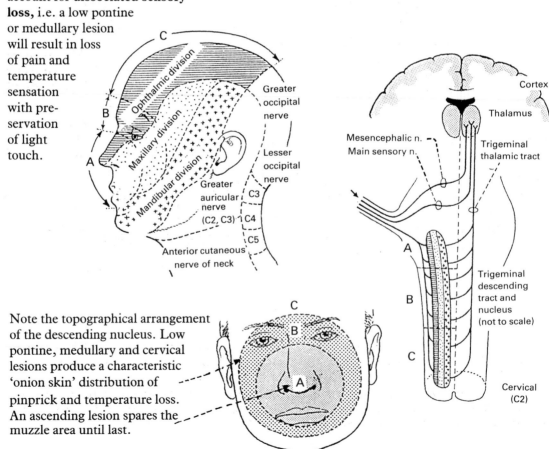

Note the topographical arrangement of the descending nucleus. Low pontine, medullary and cervical lesions produce a characteristic 'onion skin' distribution of pinprick and temperature loss. An ascending lesion spares the muzzle area until last.

FACIAL PAIN AND SENSORY LOSS

The peripheral course of the V nerve

The nerve roots emerge from the lateral aspect of the brain stem at the midpontine level and run to the Gasserian ganglion. This contains the bipolar sensory nuclei and lies on the apex of the petrous bone in the middle fossa. It gives off the three divisions of the trigeminal nerve. Each division exits through its own foramen and supplies a specific area of the face.

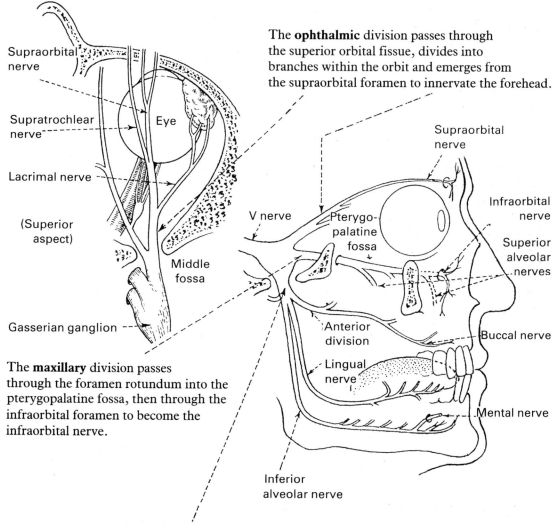

The **ophthalmic** division passes through the superior orbital fissue, divides into branches within the orbit and emerges from the supraorbital foramen to innervate the forehead.

The **maxillary** division passes through the foramen rotundum into the pterygopalatine fossa, then through the infraorbital foramen to become the infraorbital nerve.

The **mandibular** division exits from the foramen ovale. The anterior trunk incorporates the motor division of the V nerve, innervating the muscles of mastication — masseter, pterygoids and temporalis — as well as innervating the cheek and gums (buccal nerve).

The lingual branch of the posterior trunk innervates the anterior two-thirds of the tongue (and is joined by the chordi tympani from the facial nerve carrying salivary secretomotor fibres and taste from the anterior two-thirds of the tongue).

FACIAL PAIN AND SENSORY LOSS

EXAMINATION OF FACIAL SENSATION
This should include examination of the *corneal reflex* and *masticatory muscle function* (page 14).

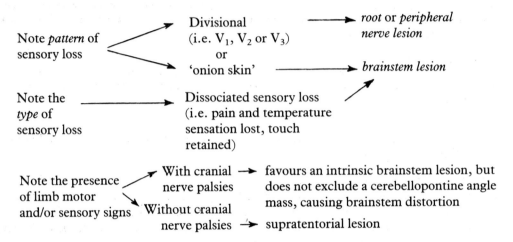

Note *pattern* of sensory loss

→ Divisional (i.e. V_1, V_2 or V_3) → root or *peripheral nerve lesion*

or

→ 'onion skin' → *brainstem lesion*

Note the *type* of sensory loss → Dissociated sensory loss (i.e. pain and temperature sensation lost, touch retained)

Note the presence of limb motor and/or sensory signs

→ With cranial nerve palsies → favours an intrinsic brainstem lesion, but does not exclude a cerebellopontine angle mass, causing brainstem distortion

→ Without cranial nerve palsies → supratentorial lesion

CAUSES OF V NERVE LESIONS

Pons
When associated with other cranial nerve lesions and long tract signs:
— *vascular*
— *neoplastic*
— *demyelination*
— *syringobulbia* (especially dissociated sensory loss)

(Tentorium cerebelli omitted)

Orbital fissure
Orbit
Cavernous sinus

First division of V nerve ± III, IV and VI nerve palsies } (*see III nerve lesions, page 149*).

Petrous apex
associated VI nerve palsy
— *petrositis (Gradenigo's syndrome)*

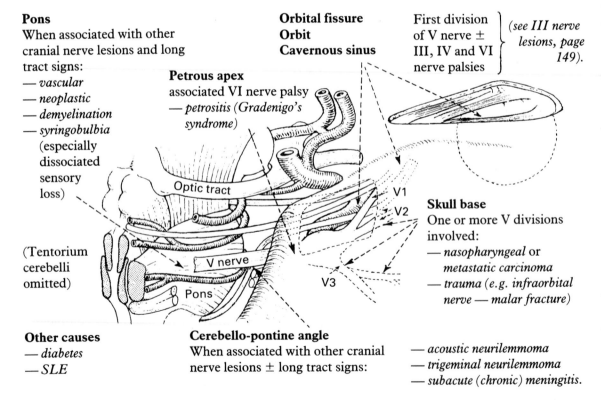

Optic tract

V nerve

Pons

V1
V2
V3

Skull base
One or more V divisions involved:
— *nasopharyngeal* or *metastatic carcinoma*
— *trauma (e.g. infraorbital nerve — malar fracture)*

Other causes
— *diabetes*
— *SLE*

Cerebello-pontine angle
When associated with other cranial nerve lesions ± long tract signs:

— *acoustic neurilemmoma*
— *trigeminal neurilemmoma*
— *subacute (chronic) meningitis.*

FACIAL PAIN AND SENSORY LOSS

Herpes zoster infection
Herpes zoster may affect the Gasserian ganglion, causing inflammation and nerve cell necrosis. Herpetic skin eruptions result and cover either the whole trigeminal area or one individual division — usually the ophthalmic division. Rarely trigeminal motor paralysis occurs. 'Scarring' in the ganglion after recovery probably explains postherpetic neuralgia.
Management: Acyclovir prevents dissemination in immunocompromised patients. Local application of idoxuridine accelerates healing and reduces pain.

Trigeminal neuropathy:
This painful condition causes a progressive sensory loss in one or more trigeminal divisions with trophic ulceration of the nasal ala. Such sensory disturbance may occur in systemic lupus erythematosus but usually the cause is unexplained. The condition runs a slow protracted course.

Gradenigo's syndrome:
Infection involving the inferior petrosal sinus (usually extending from the middle ear) may produce V and VI nerve damage causing diplopia, facial pain and sensory loss.

NEUROPATHIC KERATITIS
Corneal anaesthesia from a central or peripheral V nerve lesion may lead to a neuropathic keratitis. The corneal surface becomes hazy, ulcerated and infected and blindness may follow.

Patients with absent corneal sensation should wear a protective shield, attached to the side of spectacles, when out of doors.

FACIAL PAIN — DIAGNOSTIC APPROACH

Pain in the face may result from many different disorders and often presents as a diagnostic problem to the neurologist or neurosurgeon.

Consider:

1. Site of pain

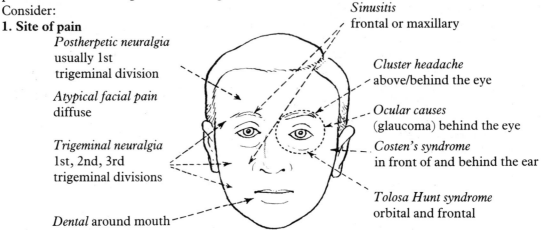

Postherpetic neuralgia
usually 1st
trigeminal division

Atypical facial pain
diffuse

Trigeminal neuralgia
1st, 2nd, 3rd
trigeminal divisions

Dental around mouth

Sinusitis
frontal or maxillary

Cluster headache
above/behind the eye

Ocular causes
(glaucoma) behind the eye

Costen's syndrome
in front of and behind the ear

Tolosa Hunt syndrome
orbital and frontal

2. Quality of pain

Trigeminal neuralgia	— sharp, stabbing, shooting, paroxysmal
Atypical facial pain	— dull, persisting
Postherpetic neuralgia	— dull, burning, persisting, occasional paroxysm
Dental	— dull
Sinusitis	— sharp, boring, worse in the morning
Ocular	— dull, throbbing
Costen's syndrome	— severe aching, aggravated by chewing
Cluster headache	— sharp, intermittent

3. Associated symptoms/signs

Trigeminal neuralgia	— often no neurological deficit, but occasional blunting of pinprick over involved region
Atypical facial pain	— accompanying features of depressive illness
Postherpetic neuralgia	— evidence of scarring associated with sensory loss
Dental	— swelling of lips/face
Sinusitis	— puffy appearance around eyes, tenderness to percussion over involved sinus
Ocular	— glaucoma: associated visual symptoms — blurring/haloes/loss
Costen's syndrome	— tenderness over temporomandibular joints
Cluster headache	— associated lacrimation/rhinorrhoea

Attention to site, quality and associated symptoms and signs should result in the diagnosis.

FACIAL PAIN — TRIGEMINAL NEURALGIA

TRIGEMINAL NEURALGIA (tic douloureux)

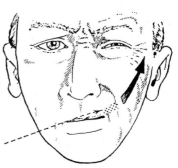

Trigeminal neuralgia is characterised by paroxysmal attacks of severe, short, sharp, stabbing pain affecting one or more divisions of the trigeminal nerve. The pain involves the second or third divisions more often than the first; it rarely occurs bilaterally, and never simultaneously on each side. Paroxysmal attacks last for several days or weeks; they are often superimposed on a more constant ache. When the attacks settle, the patient may remain pain free for many months.

Chewing, speaking, washing the face, tooth-brushing, cold winds, or touching a specific 'trigger spot', e.g. upper lip or gum, may all precipitate an attack of pain.

Trigeminal neuralgia more commonly affects females and patients over 50 years of age.

Aetiology
In many patients the cause remains unexplained, as do the long periods of remission. Trigeminal pain may be symptomatic of disorders which affect the nerve root or its entry zone.

Root or root entry zone compression — *tumours* of the cerebellopontine angle lying against the V nerve roots, e.g. meningioma, epidermoid cyst, frequently present with trigeminal pain.
— *arterial vessels* often abut and sometimes clearly indent the trigeminal nerve roots.

Demyelination — a lesion in the pons should be considered in a 'young' person with trigeminal neuralgia. Trigger spots are rare. Remission occurs infrequently and the response to drug treatment is poor.

Management
Drug therapy
CARBAMAZEPINE proves effective in most patients (and helps confirm the diagnosis). Provided toxicity does not become troublesome, i.e. drowsiness, ataxia, the dosage is increased until pain relief occurs (600–1600 mg/day). When remission occurs, drug treatment can be discontinued.

If pain control is limited, other drugs — CLONAZEPAM, PHENYTOIN — may benefit.

Persistence of pain on full drug dosage or an intolerance of the drugs, indicates the need for more radical measures.

FACIAL PAIN — TRIGEMINAL NEURALGIA

MANAGEMENT (*contd*)
Operative therapy

Peripheral nerve techniques:
Nerve block with alcohol or phenol
provides temporary relief (up to two years).
Avulsion of the supra- or infraorbital
nerves gives more prolonged
pain relief.

**Trigeminal ganglion/
root injection:**
Alcohol or phenol injection
into the trigeminal ganglion
effectively produces pain relief,
but area control is limited
and the risk of corneal anaesthesia, ulceration and scarring
is high.
Glycerol injection into Meckel's
cave usually produces good pain
relief with minimal sensory
damage.

Trigeminal root section:
Through either a subtemporal (extra- or intradural) or posterior fossa approach, the appropriate trigeminal root is identified and
divided.

Microvascular decompression:
Exploration of the cerebellopontine
angle reveals blood vessels in contact with the trigeminal nerve root or
root entry zone in the majority of patients.
Separation of these structures and insertion
of a non absorbable sponge produces pain
relief in most patients, without the
associated problems of nerve destruction.

Radiofrequency thermocoagulation:
The site of facial 'tingling' produced by electrical stimulation of a needle inserted into the trigeminal ganglion,
accurately identifies the location of the needle tip. When
the site of tingling corresponds to the trigger spot or site of
pain origin, radiofrequency thermocoagulation under general anaesthetic, produces a permanent lesion — usually
resulting in analgesia of the appropriate area with retention
of light touch.

Results and complications

Pain relief — accurate comparison of the wide variety of techniques used for trigeminal
neuralgia is difficult; all but peripheral nerve avulsion appear to produce similar results.
Approximately 80–85% of patients remain pain free for a 5-year period. Results of peripheral nerve
avulsion are less satisfactory with pain recurring in 50% within 2 years.

Dysaesthesia/Anaesthesia dolorosa — this troublesome sensory disturbance follows any
destructive technique to nerve or root in 5–30% of patients. Microvascular decompression avoids
this problem and as yet the incidence appears very low with glycerol injection.

Corneal anaesthesia — this occurs most frequently following phenol or alcohol injection into the
trigeminal ganglion, but is also a problem when root section or thermocoagulation involves the first
division.

Mortality — microvascular decompression and open root section carry a low mortality rate (1–
3%), but this must not be ignored when comparing results with safer methods.

Treatment selection: This largely depends on the surgeon's personal preference and experience.

V_1 *pain* — microvascular decompression or perhaps glycerol injection provides minimal risk of
sensory loss and corneal ulceration.

V_2 *and* V_3 *pain* — in addition to the above, thermocoagulation provides good results.

Frail and elderly patients tolerate glycerol injection and thermocoagulation more easily than
other procedures.

160

FACIAL PAIN — OTHER CAUSES

Temporomandibular joint dysfunction (Costen's syndrome)

Aching pain occurring around the ear, aggravated by chewing; due to malalignment of one temporomandibular joint as a consequence of dental loss with altered 'bite' or involvement of the joint in rheumatoid arthritis.
This condition requires dental treatment with realignment.

Raeder's syndrome (the paratrigeminal syndrome)

Pain and sensory loss in 1st and 2nd trigeminal divisions, maximal around the eye and associated with a sympathetic paresis (ptosis and small pupil). Sweating in the lower face is preserved. Associated with lesions of the middle fossa, e.g. nasopharyngeal carcinoma, granulomas.

Tolosa Hunt syndrome

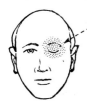

Intermittent attacks of severe orbital pain with the development of ocular palsies and loss of 1st division trigeminal sensation.
Caused by granulomas (or osteitis) involving the superior orbital fissure or cavernous sinus.

Atypical facial pain

The patient, often a young or middle-aged woman, experiences a dull, persistent pain, spreading diffusely over one or both sides of the face. These symptoms often result from an underlying depression and may respond well to antidepressant therapy.

Herpes zoster

Frequently affects the trigeminal territory, especially the ophthalmic division producing a painful 'herpetic rash' and often involving the cornea. The acute symptoms may resolve but lead to a chronic postherpetic neuralgia which slowly improves. Surgical procedures such as trigeminal root section do not help. The incidence of postherpetic neuralgia is not influenced by treatment with antiviral agents (acyclovir) in the acute phase.

'Cluster' headaches — see page 68.

FACIAL WEAKNESS

Related anatomy

The facial (VII) nerve contains mainly motor fibres supplying the muscles of facial expression, but also visceral efferent (parasympathetic) and visceral afferent (taste) fibres.

The motor nucleus lies in the lower pons medial to the descending nucleus and tract of the Vth cranial nerve. Axons from the motor nucleus wind around the nucleus of the VIth cranial nerve. The facial nerve and its visceral root *(nervus intermedius)* exit from the lateral aspect of the brain stem and cross the cerebellopontine angle immediately adjacent to the VIII cranial nerve. They enter the internal auditory meatus and, passing through the facial canal of the temporal bone, lie in close proximity to the inner ear and tympanic membrane. The facial nerve gives off several branches before exiting from the skull through the stylomastoid foramen.

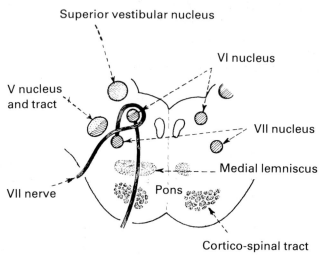

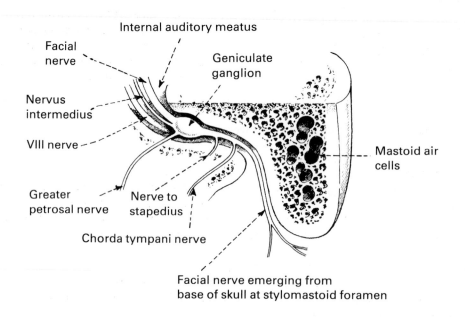

FACIAL WEAKNESS

Visceral efferent and visceral afferent fibres arise and terminate in the superior salivary nucleus and nucleus/tractus solitarius respectively.

They run together as nervus intermedius and accompany the facial nerve to the internal auditory meatus. The parasympathetic fibres (visceral efferent) pass in the greater petrosal nerve to the sphenopalatine ganglion and thence to the lacrimal gland to produce tears.

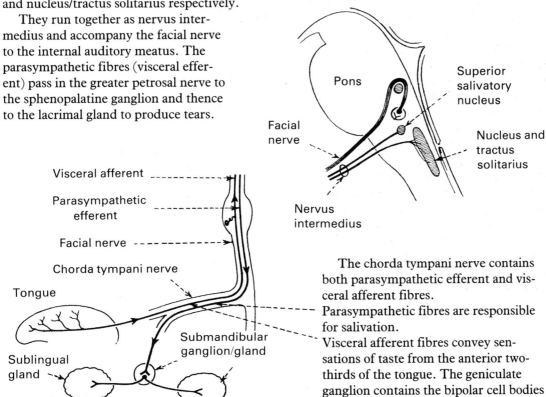

The chorda tympani nerve contains both parasympathetic efferent and visceral afferent fibres.
Parasympathetic fibres are responsible for salivation.
Visceral afferent fibres convey sensations of taste from the anterior two-thirds of the tongue. The geniculate ganglion contains the bipolar cell bodies of these afferent fibres.

Supranuclear control of facial muscles
The muscles in the lower face are controlled by the contralateral hemisphere, whereas those in the upper face receive control from both hemispheres (bilateral representation). Hence a lower motor neuron lesion paralyses all facial muscles on that side, but an upper motor neuron (supranuclear) lesion paralyses only the muscles in the lower half of the face on the opposite side.

Clinical examination of the facial nerve (see page 15)
In addition to examining for facial weakness and taste impairment, also note whether the patient comments on reduced lacrimation or salivation on one side, or hyperacusis (exaggeration of sounds due to loss of the stapedius reflex).

FACIAL WEAKNESS

LESION, LOCALISATION AND CAUSE
Note the *distribution:*

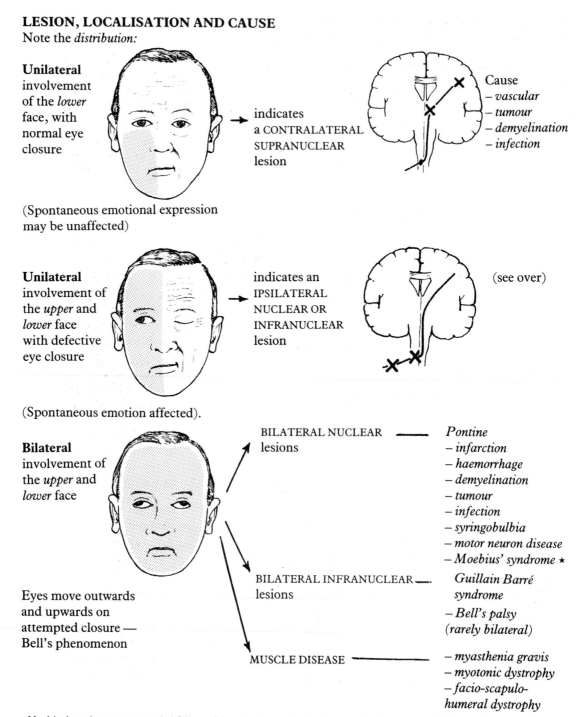

Unilateral involvement of the *lower* face, with normal eye closure

indicates a CONTRALATERAL SUPRANUCLEAR lesion

Cause
– *vascular*
– *tumour*
– *demyelination*
– *infection*

(Spontaneous emotional expression may be unaffected)

Unilateral involvement of the *upper* and *lower* face with defective eye closure

indicates an IPSILATERAL NUCLEAR OR INFRANUCLEAR lesion

(see over)

(Spontaneous emotion affected).

Bilateral involvement of the *upper* and *lower* face

BILATERAL NUCLEAR lesions

Pontine
– *infarction*
– *haemorrhage*
– *demyelination*
– *tumour*
– *infection*
– *syringobulbia*
– *motor neuron disease*
– *Moebius' syndrome* ★

BILATERAL INFRANUCLEAR lesions

Guillain Barré syndrome

– *Bell's palsy (rarely bilateral)*

Eyes move outwards and upwards on attempted closure — Bell's phenomenon

MUSCLE DISEASE

– *myasthenia gravis*
– *myotonic dystrophy*
– *facio-scapulo-humeral dystrophy*

★Moebius' syndrome: a congenital failure of the development of the facial and abducens nuclei (bilateral).

164

FACIAL WEAKNESS

NUCLEAR / INFRANUCLEAR LESIONS
The following features (if present) help in lesion location:

– VI nerve palsy ⟶ **Pons**
– contralateral   – *vascular*
   limb weakness   – *demyelination*
                  – *tumour*
                  – *encephalitis*
                  – *syringobulbia*
                  – *motor neuron*
                     disease

– V, VIII, (IX, X, XI) ⟶ **Cerebellopontine**
   nerve palsies   **angle or internal**
– loss of taste, salivation,   **auditory meatus**
   and lacrimation   – *acoustic tumours*
– hyperacusis   – *meningioma*
                        – *epidermoid*
                        – *glomus jugulare*
                           tumour

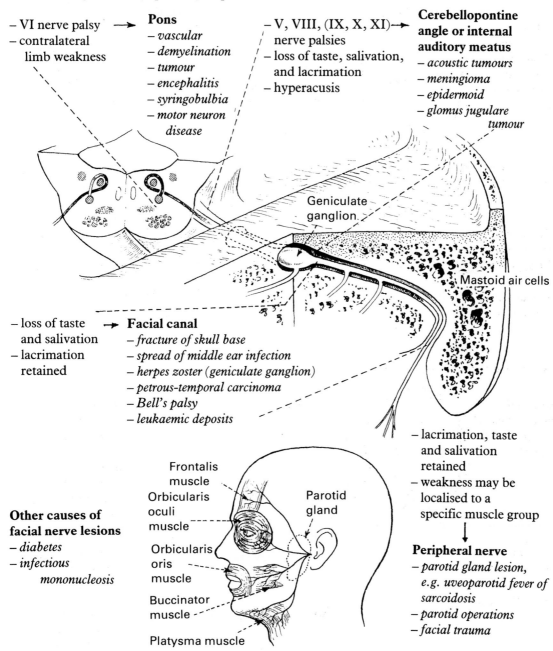

Geniculate ganglion

Mastoid air cells

– loss of taste ⟶ **Facial canal**
   and salivation   – *fracture of skull base*
– lacrimation   – *spread of middle ear infection*
   retained   – *herpes zoster (geniculate ganglion)*
                     – *petrous-temporal carcinoma*
                     – *Bell's palsy*
                     – *leukaemic deposits*

– lacrimation, taste
   and salivation
   retained
– weakness may be
   localised to a
   specific muscle group
              ↓

Frontalis muscle

Orbicularis oculi muscle

Parotid gland

Orbicularis oris muscle

Buccinator muscle

Platysma muscle

Other causes of facial nerve lesions
– *diabetes*
– *infectious mononucleosis*

Peripheral nerve
– *parotid gland lesion,*
   e.g. uveoparotid fever of
   sarcoidosis
– *parotid operations*
– *facial trauma*

BELL'S PALSY

Bell's palsy is an acute paralysis of the face related to 'inflammation' and swelling of the facial nerve within the facial canal or at the stylomastoid foramen. It is usually unilateral, rarely bilateral, and may occur repetitively. In some, a family history of the condition is evident.

Aetiology

Uncertain, but may be associated with viral infections, e.g. herpes simplex; epidemics of Bell's palsy occur sporadically.

Symptoms

Pain of variable intensity behind an ear precedes weakness, which develops over a 48-hour period.

Impairment of taste, hyperacusis and salivation depend on the extent of inflammation and will be lost in more severe cases. Lacrimation is seldom affected.

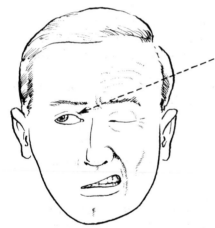

On attempting to close the eyes and show the teeth, the one eye does not close and the eyeball rotates upwards and outwards — Bell's phenomenon (normal eyeball movement on eye closure).

Treatment

During the acute stage protect the exposed eye during sleep.

Prednisolone given in high dosage in the acute stage (40–60 mg per day for 5 days) may reduce inflammation, but there is no conclusive evidence of benefit.

Prognosis

Most patients (80%) recover in 4–8 weeks without treatment. In the remainder, residual facial asymmetry may require corrective surgery. Incomplete paralysis indicates a good prognosis. In patients with complete paralysis, electrical absence of denervation on electromyography is an optimistic sign.

Occasionally aberrant reinnervation occurs — movement of the angle of the mouth on closing the eyes or lacrimation when facial muscles contract (crocodile tears).

OTHER FACIAL NERVE DISORDERS

RAMSAY HUNT SYNDROME

Herpes zoster infection of the geniculate (facial) ganglion causes sudden severe facial weakness with a typical zoster vesicular eruption within the external auditory meatus. Pain is a major feature and may precede the facial weakness, and serosanguinous fluid may discharge from the ear.

Deafness may result from VIII involvement. Occasionally, other cranial nerves from V–XII are also affected.

Treatment

Antiviral agents (acyclovir) may help.

HEMIFACIAL SPASM

This condition is characterised by unilateral clonic spasms beginning in the orbicularis oculi and spreading to involve other facial muscles.

Onset usually occurs in middle to old age and women are preferentially affected.

The aetiology remains unknown but 'irritation' from an adjacent blood vessel (or from a tumour) may cause demyelination and 'short-circuiting' within the nerve. Occasionally hemifacial spasm follows a Bell's palsy.

The clinician must distinguish hemifacial spasm from milder habit spasms or tics which tend to be familial, and also from 'focal' seizures selectively affecting the face.

Progression may eventually result in facial paralysis.

Investigations

A CT scan of the posterior fossa excludes the presence of a cerebellar pontine angle lesion.

Treatment

Drugs — Anxiolytics and carbamazepine may produce some benefit but are of no lasting value. When spasm is confined to orbicularis oculi, local infiltration with botulinum toxin is helpful.

Surgery — Posterior fossa exploration and microvascular decompression i.e. dissecting blood vessels off the facial nerve roots and root entry zone, gives excellent results (cure rate 80%), but carries the risk of producing deafness and rarely brainstem damage. Alternative, less successful treatments include phenol injection or partial section of the facial nerve; these methods inevitably cause some facial weakness.

TONIC FACIAL SPASM

Less common than hemifacial spasm. Occurs with cerebellar pontine angle lesions. It produces tonic elevation of the corner of the mouth with narrowing of the eye. The diagnosis is confirmed by CT scanning and treatment is surgical.

FACIAL MYOKYMIA

A rare condition seen most often in multiple sclerosis. Flickering of facial muscles results from spontaneous discharge in the facial motor nucleus. Other brainstem signs are present. The facial movements respond to carbamazepine.

167

DEAFNESS, TINNITUS AND VERTIGO

Deafness, tinnitus and vertigo result from disorders affecting the auditory and vestibular apparatus or their central connections transmitted through the VIII cranial nerve.

MECHANISMS OF AUDITORY AND VESTIBULAR FUNCTION

Auditory function: the cochlea converts sound waves into action potentials in cochlear neurons. Sound waves are transmitted by the tympanic membrane and the ossicles to the oval window, setting up waves in the perilymph of the cochlea. The action of the waves on the spiral organ (of Corti) generates action potentials in the cochlear division of the VIII cranial nerve.

Vestibular function: the vestibular system responds to rotational and linear acceleration (including gravity) and along with a visual and proprioceptive input maintains equilibrium and body orientation in space. Inertia of the endolymph within the semicircular canals during rotational acceleration displaces the cupola, activates the hair cells and transmits action potentials to the vestibular division of the VIII cranial nerve. Linear acceleration results in displacement of the otoliths within the utricle or saccule. This distorts the hair cells and increases or decreases the frequency of action potentials in the vestibular division of the VIII cranial nerve.

CENTRAL CONNECTIONS

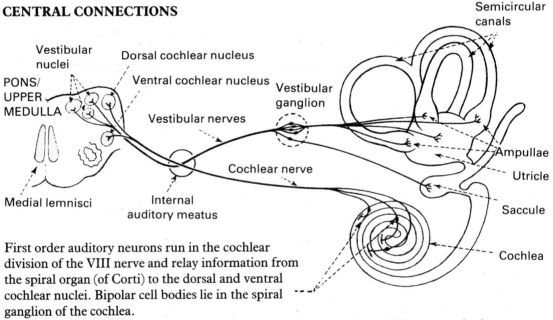

First order auditory neurons run in the cochlear division of the VIII nerve and relay information from the spiral organ (of Corti) to the dorsal and ventral cochlear nuclei. Bipolar cell bodies lie in the spiral ganglion of the cochlea.

First order vestibular neurons lie in the vestibular division of the VIII nerve and relay information from the utricle, saccule and semicircular canals to the vestibular nuclei (superior, inferior, medial and lateral). Bipolar cell bodies lie in the vestibular ganglion.

The cochlear (acoustic) and vestibular divisions travel together through the petrous bone to the internal auditory meatus where they emerge to pass through the subarachnoid space in the cerebellopontine angle, each entering the brain stem separately at the pontomedullary junction.

DEAFNESS, TINNITUS AND VERTIGO

CENTRAL CONNECTIONS (*contd*)

Auditory: From the cochlear nucleus, second order neurons either pass upwards in the lateral lemniscus to the ipsilateral inferior colliculus or decussate in the trapezoid body and pass up in the lateral lemniscus to the contralateral inferior colliculus.

Third order neurons from the inferior colliculus on each side run to the medial geniculate body on both sides.

Fourth order neurons pass through the internal capsule and auditory radiation to the auditory cortex.

The bilateral nature of the connections ensures that a unilateral central lesion will not result in lateralised hearing loss.

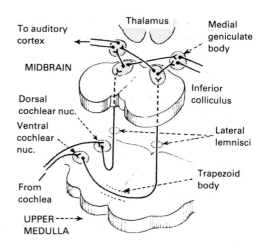

Vestibular:

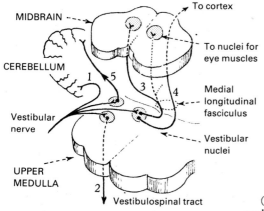

1. Directly to cerebellum.
2. Second order neurons arise in the vestibular nucleus and descend in the ipsilateral vestibulospinal tract.
3. Second order neurons project to the oculomotor nuclei (III, IV, VI) through the medial longitudinal fasciculus.
4. Second order neurons project to the cortex (temporal lobe). The pathway is unclear.
5. Second order neurons project to the cerebellum.

(There is a bilateral feedback loop to the vestibular nuclei from the cerebellum through the fastigial nucleus.)

DEAFNESS: Two types of hearing loss are recognised:

1. *Conductive deafness:* failure of sound conduction to the cochlea.

2. *Sensorineural deafness:* failure of action potential production or transmission due to disease of the cochlea, cochlear nerve or cochlear central connections.

Further subdivision into cochlear and retrocochlear deafness helps establish the causative lesion.

TINNITUS: a sensation of noise of ringing, buzzing, hissing or singing quality.

Tinnitus may be (i) continuous or intermittent, (ii) unilateral or bilateral, (iii) high or low pitch.

As a rule, when hearing loss is accompanied by tinnitus, conductive deafness is associated with low pitch tinnitus — sensorineural deafness is associated with high pitch tinnitus, except Meniere's disease where tinnitus is low pitch.

VERTIGO: an illusion of rotatory movement due to disturbed orientation of the body in space. The sufferer may sense that the environment is moving. Vertigo may result from disease of the labyrinth, vestibular nerve or their central connections.

DEAFNESS, TINNITUS AND VERTIGO

Clinical examination

Examination of the external auditory meatus, tympanic membrane and eye movements (for nystagmus) and Weber's and Rinne's tests (page 16) provide valuable information, but more detailed neuro-otological tests (pages 60, 61) are usually required to determine the exact nature of the auditory or vestibular dysfunction and to locate the lesion site. The results of these tests may indicate the need for further investigation (e.g. CT scan).

Causes of deafness

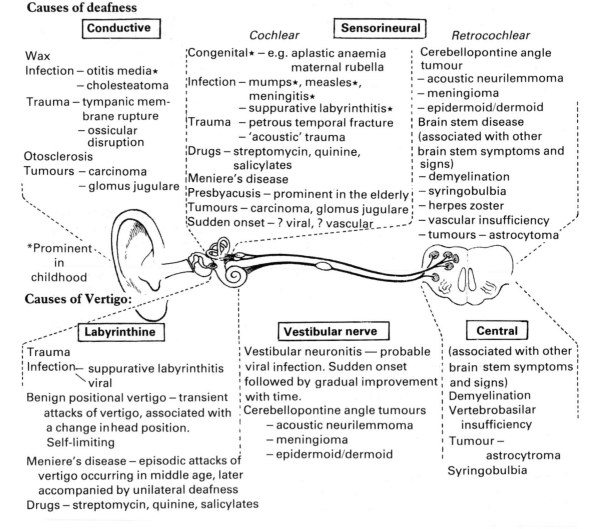

Conductive

Wax
Infection – otitis media*
    – cholesteatoma
Trauma – tympanic mem-
    brane rupture
    – ossicular
    disruption
Otosclerosis
Tumours – carcinoma
    – glomus jugulare

Cochlear

Sensorineural

Congenital* – e.g. aplastic anaemia
    maternal rubella
Infection – mumps*, measles*,
    meningitis*
    – suppurative labyrinthitis*
Trauma – petrous temporal fracture
    – 'acoustic' trauma
Drugs – streptomycin, quinine,
    salicylates
Meniere's disease
Presbyacusis – prominent in the elderly
Tumours – carcinoma, glomus jugulare
Sudden onset – ? viral, ? vascular

Retrocochlear

Cerebellopontine angle
tumour
– acoustic neurilemmoma
– meningioma
– epidermoid/dermoid
Brain stem disease
(associated with other
brain stem symptoms and
signs)
– demyelination
– syringobulbia
– herpes zoster
– vascular insufficiency
– tumours – astrocytoma

*Prominent
in
childhood

Causes of Vertigo:

Labyrinthine

Trauma
Infection – suppurative labyrinthitis
    viral
Benign positional vertigo – transient
    attacks of vertigo, associated with
    a change in head position.
    Self-limiting
Meniere's disease – episodic attacks of
    vertigo occurring in middle age, later
    accompanied by unilateral deafness
Drugs – streptomycin, quinine, salicylates

Vestibular nerve

Vestibular neuronitis — probable
viral infection. Sudden onset
followed by gradual improvement
with time.
Cerebellopontine angle tumours
    – acoustic neurilemmoma
    – meningioma
    – epidermoid/dermoid

Central

(associated with other
brain stem symptoms
and signs)
Demyelination
Vertebrobasilar
    insufficiency
Tumour –
    astrocytroma
Syringobulbia

Causes of tinnitus

Any lesion causing deafness may also cause tinnitus. Occasionally patients perceive a vibratory noise inside the head, transmitted from an arteriovenous malformation or carotid stenosis.

In addition, patients with non-specific disease, e.g. anaemia, fever, hypertension, occasionally complain of tinnitus.

DISORDERS OF THE LOWER CRANIAL NERVES

NINTH (GLOSSOPHARYNGEAL) CRANIAL NERVE

This is a mixed nerve with motor, sensory and parasympathetic functions.

1. Motor fibres to stylopharyngeus muscle arise in the nucleus ambiguus.

2. Preganglionic parasympathetic fibres arise in the inferior salivatory nucleus and pass to the otic ganglion. From there postganglionic fibres innervate the parotid gland.

3. General somatic sensory fibres innervate the area of skin behind the ear, pass to the superior ganglion and end in the nucleus and tract of the trigeminal nerve.

4. Sensory fibres innervate the posterior part of the tongue (taste), pharynx, eustachian tube and carotid body/sinus and terminate centrally in the nucleus solitarius. The cell bodies lie in the inferior ganglion.

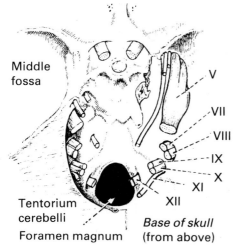

The IX nerve emerges as 5 or 6 rootlets from the medulla, dorsal to the olivary nucleus and passes with the vagus and accessory nerves through the jugular foramen in the neck.

Within the neck the nerve lies in close proximity to the internal carotid artery and internal jugular vein.

The superior and inferior ganglia lie in the jugular foramen, the otic ganglion in the neck below the foramen ovale.

Clinical examination (see page 17)

Disorders of the glossopharyngeal nerve

Glossopharyngeal palsy from either medullary or nerve root lesions does not occur in isolation. When associated with X and XI cranial nerve lesions, this constitutes the *jugular foramen syndrome.* Lesions producing this syndrome are listed on page 175.

GLOSSOPHARYNGEAL NEURALGIA

Short, sharp, lancinating attacks of pain, identical to trigeminal neuralgia in nature but affecting the posterior part of the pharynx or tonsillar area. The pain often radiates towards the ear and is triggered by swallowing. Reflex bradycardia and syncope can occur. As with trigeminal neuralgia, carbamazepine often provides effective relief — if not, section of the glossopharyngeal nerve in the tonsillar fossa or intracranial section of the IX nerve roots give good results.

DISORDERS OF THE LOWER CRANIAL NERVES

TENTH (VAGUS) CRANIAL NERVE
This is a mixed nerve with motor, sensory and parasympathetic functions.

The central connections are complex though similar to those of the glossopharyngeal nerve.

1. Motor fibres supplying the pharynx, soft palate and larynx arise in the nucleus ambiguus.

2. Preganglionic parasympathetic fibres arise in the dorsal motor nucleus. Postganglionic fibres supply the thoracic and abdominal viscera.

3. Afferent fibres from the pharynx, larynx and external auditory meatus have cell bodies in the jugular ganglion and end in the nucleus and tract of the trigeminal nerve.

4. Afferent fibres from abdominal and thoracic viscera have cell bodies in the nodose ganglion and end in the nucleus solitarius. Taste perception in the pharynx ends similarly.

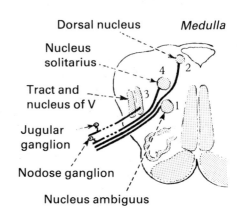

The nerve emerges from the brain stem as a series of converging rootlets. It exits from the cranial cavity by the jugular foramen where both ganglia lie.

Extracranial branches:

Motor and sensory supply to the pharynx

Superior laryngeal branch to the laryngeal muscles

Recurrent laryngeal branch

Supply to thoracic and abdominal viscera

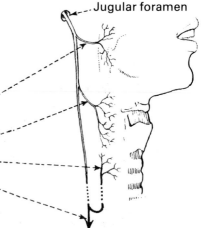

Disorders of the vagus nerve cause:
Palatal weakness
Unilateral — minimal symptoms.
Bilateral — nasal regurgitation of fluid, nasal quality of speech.
Pharyngeal weakness
Pharyngeal muscles are represented by the middle part of the nucleus ambiguus.
Unilateral — pharyngeal wall droops on the affected side.
Bilateral — marked dysphagia.
Laryngeal weakness
Motor fibres arise in the lowest part of the nucleus ambiguus.
Fibres to *tensors of the vocal cords* pass in *superior laryngeal nerves*.
Fibres to *adductors and abductors of the vocal cords* are supplied by the *recurrent laryngeal nerves*.

DISORDERS OF THE LOWER CRANIAL NERVES

Clinical examination (see page 17)

Direct examination of the vocal cords helps identification of the lesion site.

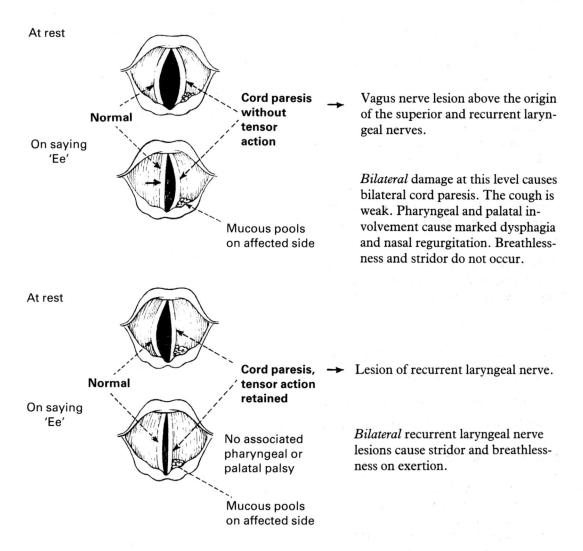

At rest

Normal

On saying 'Ee'

Cord paresis without tensor action → Vagus nerve lesion above the origin of the superior and recurrent laryngeal nerves.

Mucous pools on affected side

Bilateral damage at this level causes bilateral cord paresis. The cough is weak. Pharyngeal and palatal involvement cause marked dysphagia and nasal regurgitation. Breathlessness and stridor do not occur.

At rest

Normal

On saying 'Ee'

Cord paresis, tensor action retained → Lesion of recurrent laryngeal nerve.

No associated pharyngeal or palatal palsy

Mucous pools on affected side

Bilateral recurrent laryngeal nerve lesions cause stridor and breathlessness on exertion.

173

DISORDERS OF THE LOWER CRANIAL NERVES

ELEVENTH (ACCESSORY) CRANIAL NERVE
This is a purely motor nerve supplying the sternomastoid and trapezius muscles.

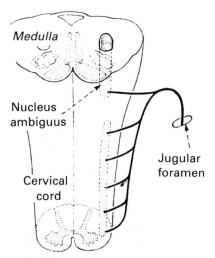

The cranial portion of the accessory nerve arises from the lowest part of the nucleus ambiguus in the medulla.

The spinal part arises in the ventral grey matter of the upper five cervical segments, ascends alongside the spinal cord and passes through the foramen magnum. After joining with the cranial portion it exits as the accessory nerve through the jugular foramen.

The *supranuclear connections* act on the ipsilateral sternomastoid (turning the head to the contralateral side) and on the contralateral trapezius. This results in:
– head turning away from the relevant hemisphere during a seizure
– head turning towards the relevant hemisphere with cerebral infarction.

Clinical examination (see page 18)

TWELFTH (HYPOGLOSSAL) CRANIAL NERVE
This is a purely motor nerve which supplies the intrinsic muscles of the tongue.

The nucleus lies in the floor of the IV ventricle and fibres pass ventrally to leave the brain stem lateral to the pyramidal tract.

Since each nucleus is bilaterally innervated, a unilateral supranuclear lesion will not produce signs or symptoms. A bilateral supranuclear lesion results in a thin pointed (spastic) tongue which cannot be protruded.

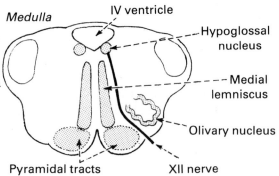

A lesion of the hypoglossal nerve results in atrophy and deviation of the tongue to the weak side (see page 18).

CAUSES OF LOWER CRANIAL NERVE LESIONS

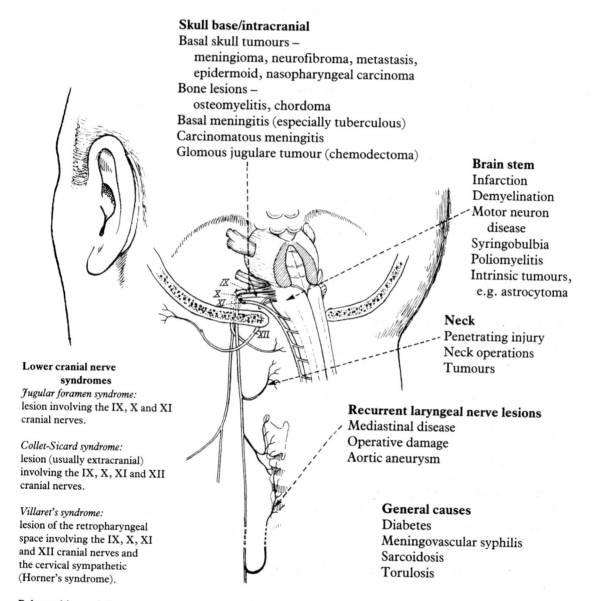

Skull base/intracranial
Basal skull tumours –
    meningioma, neurofibroma, metastasis,
    epidermoid, nasopharyngeal carcinoma
Bone lesions –
    osteomyelitis, chordoma
Basal meningitis (especially tuberculous)
Carcinomatous meningitis
Glomous jugulare tumour (chemodectoma)

Brain stem
Infarction
Demyelination
Motor neuron
    disease
Syringobulbia
Poliomyelitis
Intrinsic tumours,
    e.g. astrocytoma

Neck
Penetrating injury
Neck operations
Tumours

**Lower cranial nerve
    syndromes**
Jugular foramen syndrome:
lesion involving the IX, X and XI
cranial nerves.

Collet–Sicard syndrome:
lesion (usually extracranial)
involving the IX, X, XI and XII
cranial nerves.

Villaret's syndrome:
lesion of the retropharyngeal
space involving the IX, X, XI
and XII cranial nerves and
the cervical sympathetic
(Horner's syndrome).

Recurrent laryngeal nerve lesions
Mediastinal disease
Operative damage
Aortic aneurysm

General causes
Diabetes
Meningovascular syphilis
Sarcoidosis
Torulosis

Polyneuritis cranialis
Multiple cranial nerve palsies of unknown aetiology which spontaneously remit. The diagnosis is dependent upon exclusion
of other possible causes. Occasionally it occurs in association with postinfectious polyneuropathy.

CEREBELLAR DYSFUNCTION

Anatomy

The cerebellum lies in the posterior fossa, posterior to the brain stem, separated from the cerebrum above by the tentorium cerebelli.

The cerebellum consists of two laterally placed hemispheres and the midline structure — the vermis.

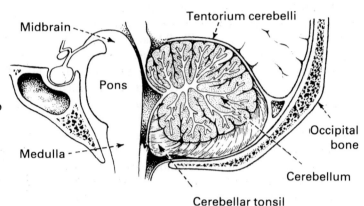

Three major phylogenetic subdivisions of the cerebellum are recognised, but are of little clinical value.

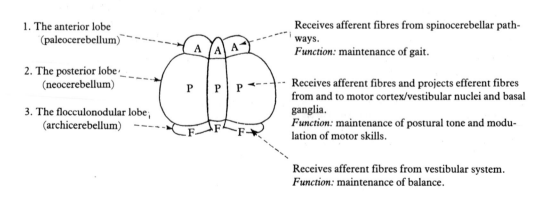

1. The anterior lobe (paleocerebellum) — Receives afferent fibres from spinocerebellar pathways.
Function: maintenance of gait.

2. The posterior lobe (neocerebellum) — Receives afferent fibres and projects efferent fibres from and to motor cortex/vestibular nuclei and basal ganglia.
Function: maintenance of postural tone and modulation of motor skills.

3. The flocculonodular lobe (archicerebellum) — Receives afferent fibres from vestibular system.
Function: maintenance of balance.

CEREBELLAR DYSFUNCTION

The cerebellar cortex is made up of three cell layers. The middle or Purkinje layer contains Purkinje cells. These are the only neurons capable of transmitting efferent impulses. Deep within the cerebellar hemispheres in the roof of the 4th ventricle, lie four paired nuclei separated by white matter from the cortex.

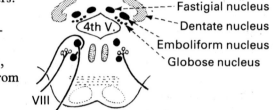

The efferent system

The Purkinje cells give rise to all efferent axons. These pass either to the deep nuclei of the cerebellum and thence to the brain stem, or to the vestibular nuclei of the brain stem. From there fibres relay back to the cerebral cortex and thalamus, or project into the spinal cord, influencing motor control.

The afferent system

Connections between the vestibular system and the cerebellum are described on page 169.

The spinocerebellar pathways form a major afferent input. These transmit 'subconscious' proprioception from muscles, joints and skin — especially of the lower limbs.

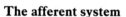

THE DORSAL SPINOCEREBELLAR TRACT   THE VENTRAL SPINOCEREBELLAR TRACT

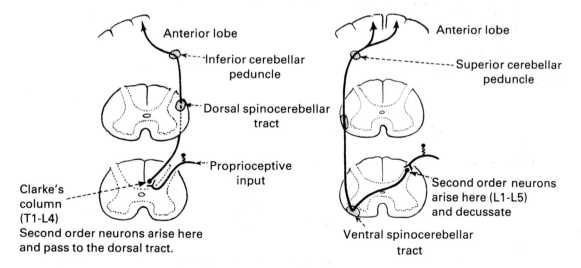

The cerebellar peduncles: Three peduncles connect the cerebellum to the brain stem:
  Superior peduncle — afferent and efferent fibres.
  Middle peduncle — afferent fibres only.
  Inferior peduncle — afferent and efferent fibres.

177

SYMPTOMS AND SIGNS OF CEREBELLAR DYSFUNCTION

The close relationship of structures within the posterior fossa makes the identification of exclusively cerebellar symptoms and signs difficult. Disease of the brain stem and its connections may produce identical results.

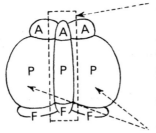

Damage to midline structures
— vermis (and flocculonodular lobe)
Results in: disturbance of equilibrium with unsteadiness on standing, walking and even sitting (truncal ataxia). The patient's gait is broad based and reeling. Eye closure does not affect balance (see Romberg's test). Tests of vestibular function, e.g. calorics, may be impaired.

Damage to hemisphere structures
— always produces signs *ipsilateral to the side of the lesion.*

Results in: a loss of the normal capacity to modulate fine voluntary movements. Errors or inaccuracies cannot be corrected. The patient complains of impaired limb co-ordination and certain signs are recognised:

Ataxia of extremities with unsteadiness of gait towards the side of the lesion.
Dysmetria: a breakdown of movement with the patient 'overshooting' the target when performing a specific motor task, e.g. finger-to-nose test.
Dysdiadochokinesia: a failure to perform a rapid alternating movement.
Intention tremor: a tremor which increases as the limb approaches its target.

Rebound phenomenon: the outstretched arm swings excessively when displaced.

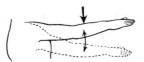

'Pendular' reflexes: the leg swings backwards and forwards when the knee jerk is elicited.

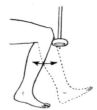

Eye movements
Nystagmus results from disease affecting cerebellar connections to the vestibular nuclei.
In unilateral disease, amplitude and rate increase when looking towards the diseased side.
Other ocular signs may occur, e.g. ocular dysmetria — an 'overshoot' when the eyes voluntarily fixate.

SYMPTOMS AND SIGNS OF CEREBELLAR DYSFUNCTION

Disturbance of speech
Scanning dysarthria may occur with speech occasionally delivered with sudden unexpected force —
explosive speech. Whether dysarthria results from hemisphere or midline vermis disease remains
debatable.
   Dysarthria, like nystagmus, is an inconsistent finding in cerebellar disease.

Titubation
Titubation is a rhythmic 'nodding' tremor of the head from side to side or to and fro, usually
associated with distal limb tremor. It appears to be of little localising value.

Head tilt
Abnormal head tilt suggests a lesion of the anterior vermis. Note that a IV (trochlear) cranial nerve
palsy and tonsillar herniation also produce this abnormal posture.

Involuntary movements
Myoclonic jerks and choreiform involuntary movements occur with extensive cerebellar disease
involving the deep nuclei.

ASSOCIATED NON-CEREBELLAR SIGNS AND SYMPTOMS: These arise from:
   – obstructive hydrocephalus
   –cranial nerve involvement
   – brain stem involvement.
(Extensor spasms from brain stem damage may be wrongly described as 'cerebellar fits'.)

CLASSIFICATION OF CEREBELLAR DYSFUNCTION

The following disorders are dealt with in their specific sections.

Developmental
   – agenesis
   – Dandy-Walker malformation
   – Arnold-Chiari malformations
   – Von Hippel Lindau disease.
Demyelinative
   – multiple sclerosis.
Degenerative
   – ataxia telangiectasia
   – Friedreich's ataxia, etc.
Neoplastic
   – astrocytoma, medulloblastoma,
      haemangioblastoma, metastasis
   – non-metastatic cerebellar degeneration.

Infectious
   – abscess formation
   – acute cerebellitis
   – acute disseminated encephalomyelitis
   – Guillain Barré variant.
Metabolic
   – myxoedema
   – non-metastatic manifestation of malignancy
   – alcohol (vitamin B_1 deficiency)
   – inborn disorders of metabolism.
Vascular
   – cerebellar haemorrhage
   – cerebellar infarction.
Drugs/toxins
   – alcohol
   – phenytoin.

179

NYSTAGMUS

Nystagmus is defined as an involuntary 'to and fro' movement of the eyes in a horizontal, vertical, rotatory or mixed direction. The presence and characteristics of such movements help localise to the site of neurological disease.

Nystagmus may be *pendular* — equal velocity and amplitude in all directions,
or *jerk* — with a fast phase (specifying the direction) and a slow phase.

The normal maintenance of ocular posture and alignment of the eyes with the environment depends upon:

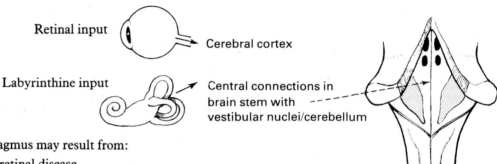

Retinal input — Cerebral cortex

Labyrinthine input — Central connections in brain stem with vestibular nuclei/cerebellum

Nystagmus may result from:
- retinal disease
- labyrinthine disease, or
- disorders affecting the cerebellum or a substantial portion of the brain stem.

Examination for nystagmus
'Nystagmoid' movements of the eyes are present in many people at extremes of gaze.
Nystagmus present with the eyes deviated less than 30° from the midline is abnormal.

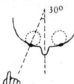

When nystagmus is present only with the eyes deviated to one side — *1st degree nystagmus*.
With eyes deviated to one side and in the midline position also — *2nd degree nystagmus*.
When present in all directions of gaze — *3rd degree nystagmus*.
If nystagmus is detected, note the type (jerk or pendular), direction (of fast phase) and degree.

Nystagmus suppressed by visual fixation may appear in darkness, but this requires specialised techniques (electronystagmography — see page 62) to demonstrate.

RETINAL OR OCULAR nystagmus
Physiological: following moving objects beyond the limits of gaze — opticokinetic nystagmus.
Pathological: occurs when vision is defective. Fixation is impaired and the eyes vainly search.

Nystagmus is:
Rapid
Pendular (lacks slow and fast phase)
Increased when looking to sides
Persistent throughout lifetime

Occurs in *congenital cataract, congenital macular defect, albinism.*

NYSTAGMUS

VESTIBULAR nystagmus

Nystagmus arises from:
- natural stimulation of the vestibular apparatus — rotational or linear acceleration.
- artificially removing or increasing the stimulus from one labyrinth (e.g. caloric testing).
- damage to vestibular apparatus or the vestibular nerve.

Creates an imbalance between each side resulting in a slow drift of the eyes towards the damaged side (or side with the reduction in stimulus) followed by a fast compensatory movement to the opposite side.

Physiological

(i) Rotational acceleration produces nystagmus in the plane of rotation.

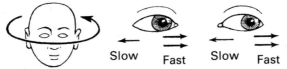

Slow   Fast   Slow   Fast

Slow phase in a direction tending to maintain the visual image.
Fast phase in the opposite direction.

(ii) Caloric testing sets up convection currents in the lateral semicircular canal producing a horizontal nystagmus (see page 62).

Pathological

Damage to labyrinth or vestibular nerve.

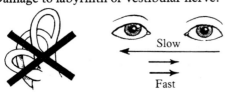

Slow

Fast

Slow phase to side of lesion.
Quick or fast phase to normal side.
Rotatory component often present.
Turning eyes away from the side of the lesion increases amplitude but does not change direction of nystagmus.
In severe cases, the nystagmus is 3rd degree and gradually settles to 1st degree with recovery.
Enhanced by loss of ocular fixation.
Vertigo accompanies nystagmus.

Often associated with tinnitus and hearing loss. Vertigo and nystagmus settle simultaneously.

Occurs in acute labyrinthine disease — *Ménière's disease, vestibular neuronitis, vascular disease.*

POSITIONAL nystagmus: this may occur in labyrinthine disease in association with vertigo when the patient assumes a certain posture.

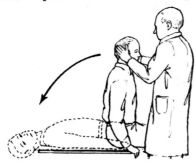

To elicit, suddenly reposition the patient:

After a delay of several seconds, nystagmus develops often with a rotatory component. With repeated testing, the nystagmus fatigues.

181

NYSTAGMUS

CENTRAL NERVOUS SYSTEM nystagmus

Central nystagmus arises from damage to the central vestibular connections in the vestibular nuclei and brain stem. The nystagmus may be horizontal, vertical, rotatory or dissociated (present in one eye only).

> The direction (fast phase) is determined by direction of gaze (multidirectional).
> Vertigo is seldom present.
> Signs of other nuclear or tract involvement in brain stem should be evident.

Central nystagmus occurs in *vascular disease, demyelination, neoplasms, nutritional disease (Wernicke's encephalopathy), alcohol intoxication and drug toxicity, e.g. phenytoin.*

Posterior fossa lesions may produce *positional nystagmus.* This may be distinguished from labyrinthine disease by:

> Absence of delay before onset, lack of fatiguing with repetitive testing, and a tendency to occur with any rather than one specific head movement.

Although nystagmus often occurs in cerebellar disease, the rôle of the cerebellum in its production remains unclear. *The fast phase tends to occur to the side of the cerebellar damage (i.e. the opposite of labyrinthine disease).*

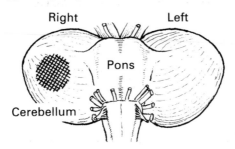

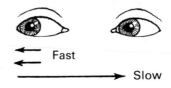

Rebound nystagmus occurs where the eyes 'overshoot' on return to the midline.

INTERNUCLEAR OPHTHALMOPLEGIA (Ataxic nystagmus)

The median longitudinal fasciculus links, among other structures, the innervation of the lateral rectus with the contralateral medial rectus muscle in order to coordinate horizontal gaze. A lesion of this fasciculus will cause *dissociate nystagmus.*

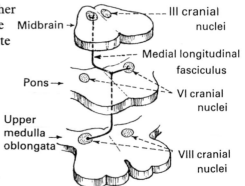

direction of gaze to R   *direction of gaze to L*

Nystagmus in abducting eye   No adduction   *then*   No adduction   Nystagmus in abducting eye

Eyes no longer move as one and nystagmus is present in one eye but not the other.

NYSTAGMUS

In unilateral medial longitudinal fasciculus lesions the eye fails to adduct towards the affected side.

N.B. Internuclear ophthalmoplegia differs from a bilateral III nerve or nuclear lesion in that the pupil is not affected and when testing eye movements individually, some adduction occurs.

OTHER VARIETIES OF CENTRAL NERVOUS SYSTEM NYSTAGMUS

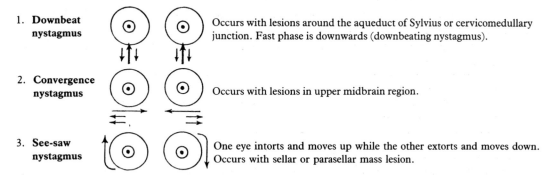

1. **Downbeat nystagmus**

Occurs with lesions around the aqueduct of Sylvius or cervicomedullary junction. Fast phase is downwards (downbeating nystagmus).

2. **Convergence nystagmus**

Occurs with lesions in upper midbrain region.

3. **See-saw nystagmus**

One eye intorts and moves up while the other extorts and moves down. Occurs with sellar or parasellar mass lesion.

A group of confusing terms are used to describe abnormal, involuntary eye movements seen in cerebellar/brain stem disease:

Ocular bobbing — fast drift downwards, slow drift upwards; seen with large pontine lesions. (Horizontal eye movements are absent.)

Opsoclonus — rapid conjugate jerks of eyes; made worse by movement. The movements are random.

Oscillopsia is a term used to describe the patient's awareness of jumping of the environment as a consequence of rapid jerking eye movements.

CONGENITAL nystagmus

This is a mixed pendular/jerk nystagmus present from birth. A family history may be present. Recognition is important to obviate unnecessary investigations.

TREMOR

Tremor is commonly encountered in clinical practice. Diagnosis depends on examination of the character of the tremor as well as the presence of other specific features.

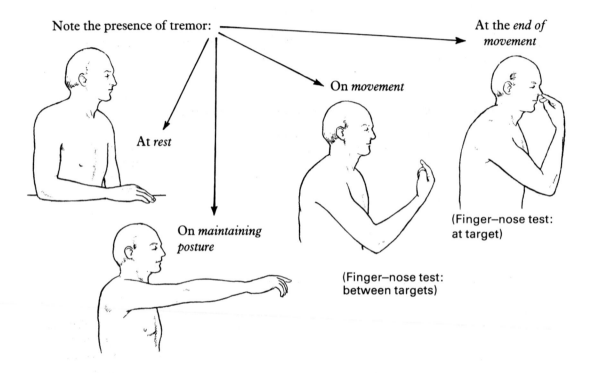

Note the presence of tremor:

At the *end of movement*

On *movement*

At *rest*

On *maintaining posture*

(Finger–nose test: at target)

(Finger–nose test: between targets)

Observe:
- the *rate* (slow, <5 per second), (rapid, >5 per second).
- the *amplitude* (fine or coarse).
- the *distribution:* face, head, trunk; limbs — distal, proximal.

All tremors disappear during sleep.

Physiological tremor is evident on maintaining a fixed posture, fast in rate, fine in character, distal in distribution and non-disabling.

Pathological tremor occurs at rest or with movement, slow in rate, coarse in character, proximal or distal and often asymmetrical in distribution. This tremor is socially and physically disabling.

TREMOR

CHARACTERISTICS OF PATHOLOGICAL TREMOR
Tremor at rest

'Pill-rolling' tremor, decreasing
with movement.
Rate: 3–7 per second.
Amplitude: coarse.
Distribution: distal limbs.

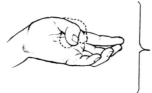

PARKINSONIAN TREMOR

Tremor on maintaining posture and throughout range of movement

Tremor absent at rest, when the limb is relaxed, but
present on maintaining a fixed posture and during
movement.
Rate: 10–14 per second.

POSTURAL TREMOR
Probably an exaggeration of
physiological tremor.

Seen in: – *thyrotoxicosis,*
           – *liver disease,*
           – *drug* and *alcohol withdrawal.*

A specific type of postural tremor occurs with a slower rate.

Occurs with:

Rate: 8 per second.
Slow insidious onset.
Distribution:
  Upper limbs involved, lower limbs rarely.
  Titubation (tremor of the head on the trunk) present.
  May involve the jaw, lips and tongue.

FAMILIAL TREMOR — often Mendelian
                    dominant.
ESSENTIAL TREMOR — no family
                    history.
SENILE TREMOR —   develops
                    in old age.

   The tremor may progress until handwriting becomes impossible and feeding difficult. Alcohol
may temporarily abort the tremor; beta blockers may produce an improvement.

Tremor during and maximal at the end of movement

Tremor absent at rest; present during movement and
maximal on approaching target, e.g. finger–nose test.
Rate: 4–6 per second.
Amplitude: coarse.
Distribution: Proximal and distal.
              Titubation may occur.

CEREBELLAR TREMOR
('intention tremor')

Extremely severe tremor — sufficient to interrupt
movement and throw patient off balance.

→

MIDBRAIN TREMOR
due to disease involving the
cerebellar/red nucleus connections,
e.g. *multiple sclerosis.*

185

MYOCLONUS

Myoclonus is a shock-like contraction of muscles which occurs irregularly and asymmetrically. Such jerks occur repetitively in the same muscle groups and range from a flicker in a single muscle to contraction in a group of muscles sufficient to displace the affected limb.

Pathophysiology

The precise nature of myoclonus remains unclear. Several forms exist, some clearly related to epilepsy; others may be associated with damage to inhibitory mechanisms in the brainstem reticular formation. Myoclonus may result from pathological changes affecting a variety of different sites including the motor cortex, cerebellum and spinal cord.

Clinical features

Myoclonic movements when repetitive vary in frequency between 5–60/minute. The muscles of the face, oral cavity and limbs are preferentially affected. The movements disappear during sleep and may be accentuated or precipitated by visual, auditory or tactile stimulation. Repetitive stimulation may result in a crescendo of myoclonus which resembles a seizure.

Causes

Myoclonus occurs in many rare disorders of the nervous system. Three groups of disorder are recognised:

Progressive myoclonus

Familial disorders:
 – Lafora body disease
 – Tay Sach's disease
 – Gaucher's disease
 – Ramsay Hunt syndrome
 – Benign polymyoclonus
Degenerative disease:
 – Subacute sclerosing panencephalitis
 – Alzheimer's disease
 – Creutzfeldt-Jakob disease

Epilepic disorders in which myoclonus occurs

Hypsarrhythmia
Generalised seizures:
 – associated with petit mal
 – during prodrome of grand mal
 – photosensitive myoclonus
Lennox Gastaut syndrome
(atypical petit mal, drop attacks
and mental retardation)

Metabolic disease associated with transient myoclonus

 — Hyponatraemia
 — Hypocalcaemia
 — Renal, hypoxic, hepatic encephalopathy

Palatal myoclonus — an unusual myoclonic disorder with rapid regular movements of the soft palate and occasionally of the pharyngeal and facial musculature. Palatal movements occur at a rate of 120–140/minute. This disorder is associated with degenerative changes in the olivary and dentate nuclei.

Treatment
Benzodiazepine drugs such as clonazepam may suppress myoclonic movements.

DISORDERS OF STANCE AND GAIT

The normal gait is characterised by an erect posture, moderately sized steps and the medial malleoli of the tibia 'tracing' a straight line.

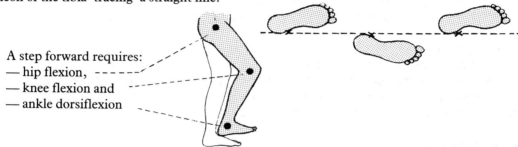

A step forward requires:
— hip flexion,
— knee flexion and
— ankle dorsiflexion

Co-ordination ensures fluidity of movement.

Antigravity reflexes maintain the erect posture. They depend upon spinal cord and brain stem connections to produce extension.

ASSESSMENT OF STANCE AND GAIT

In a patient complaining of disturbance of walking, careful assessment indicates the likely site of the causative lesion.

Watch the patient:
— walking
— performing *tandem gait* — heel to toe walking,
— standing with heels together with (a) eyes open, (b) eyes closed — this (Romberg's test) distinguishes cerebellar from sensory ataxia.

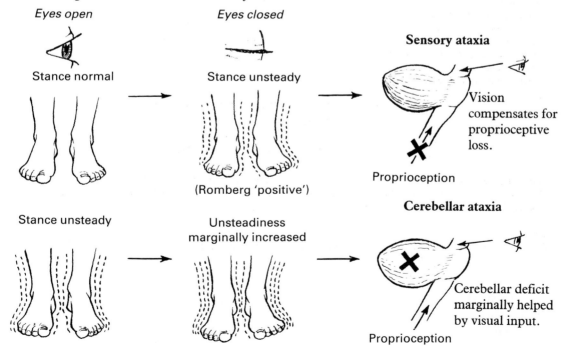

Eyes open | Eyes closed | **Sensory ataxia**

Stance normal | Stance unsteady | Vision compensates for proprioceptive loss.

(Romberg 'positive') | Proprioception

Stance unsteady | Unsteadiness marginally increased | **Cerebellar ataxia**

Cerebellar deficit marginally helped by visual input.

Proprioception

SPECIFIC DISORDERS OF STANCE AND GAIT

ATAXIC GAIT

1. Cerebellar The feet are separated widely when
standing or walking.
Steps are jerky and unsure, varying in size.
The trunk sways forwards.
In mild cases: Tandem gait (heel-toe walking)
is impaired; the patient falling to one or both sides.

2. Sensory

Disturbed conscious or unconscious proprioception due to interruption of afferents in peripheral nerves or spinal cord (posterior columns, spinocerebellar tracts).

The gait appears normal when the eyes are open although the feet usually 'stamp' on the ground. Examination reveals a positive Romberg's test and impaired joint position sensation.

HEMIPLEGIC GAIT

The leg is extended and the toes forced downwards.
When walking, abduction and circumduction at the hip
prevent the toes from catching on the gound.

In paraplegia, strong adduction at the hips can produce a
scissor-like posture of the lower limbs.
In mild weakness, the gait may appear normal, but excessive wear
occurs at the outer front aspect of the patient's shoe sole.

Hemiplegic gait

PARKINSONIAN (festinating) GAIT

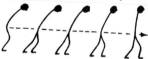

The patient adopts a flexed, stooping posture. To initiate walking, he leans forwards and then hurries (festinates) to 'catch up' on himself. The steps are short and shuffling.

STEPPAGE GAIT

Lower motor neuron weakness of pretibial and
peroneal muscles produces
this gait disorder. The patient
lifts the affected leg high
so that the toes clear the ground.

When bilateral, it resembles
a high-stepping horse.

MYOPATHIC (waddling) GAIT

Characteristic of muscle disease. Trunk and pelvic muscle weakness result in a sway-back, pot-bellied appearance with difficulty in pelvic 'fixation' when walking.

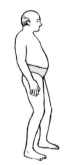

FRONTAL LOBE GAIT

Disturbance of connections between frontal cortex, basal ganglia and cerebellum produces this characteristic disturbance. The gait is wide based (feet wide apart). Initiation is difficult, the feet often seem 'stuck' to the floor. There is a tendency to fall backwards. Power and sensation are normal.

HYSTERICAL GAIT

Characterised by its bizarre nature.

Numerous variations are seen. The hallmark is inconsistency supported by the lack of
neurological signs. Close observation is essential.

LIMB WEAKNESS

Limb weakness results from damage to the **motor system** at any level from the motor cortex to muscle.

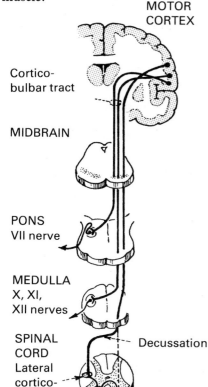

MOTOR CORTEX

Cortico-bulbar tract

MIDBRAIN

PONS
VII nerve

MEDULLA
X, XI,
XII nerves

SPINAL CORD
Lateral cortico-spinal tract

Decussation

The anterior cortico-spinal tract carries only 20% of the descending fibres and decussates at segmental level.

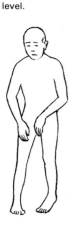

UPPER MOTOR NEURON WEAKNESS

MUSCLE TONE
Hypertonicity develops after a period (a few days or weeks) of 'neural shock'. Passive movements produce a 'clasp knife' quality, i.e. sudden 'give' towards the end of movement.
Clonus — present.

MUSCLE FASCICULATION
Absent.

MUSCLE WASTING
Absent — but, in the long term, disuse atrophy results.

REFLEXES
— **Tendon** — exaggerated.
— **Superficial** — depressed or absent (abdominal, cremasteric).
— **Plantar response** — extensor.

DISTRIBUTION
In general, whole limb or limbs are involved, e.g. monoplegia, hemiplegia, paraplegia.

Weakness shows a PREDILECTION for certain muscle groups in a PYRAMIDAL DISTRIBUTION, i.e.

upper limbs — extensor weakness > flexor weakness

lower limbs — flexor weakness > extensor weakness

This results in the *'spastic' posture* with the arm and the wrist flexed and the leg extended. In upper motor neuron lesions, SKILLED movements, e.g. fastening buttons, are always more affected than unskilled movements.

N.B. *Dual innervation* from each hemisphere results in sparing of the upper face, muscles of mastication, the palate and tongue with a unilateral upper motor neuron lesion.

189

LIMB WEAKNESS

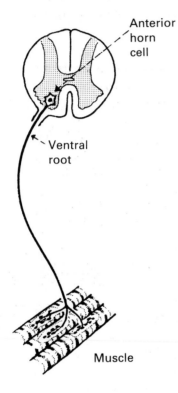

Anterior horn cell

Ventral root

Muscle

LOWER MOTOR NEURON WEAKNESS

MUSCLE TONE
Hypotonicity with diminished resistance to passive stretch.
Clonus — absent.

MUSCLE FASCICULATION
Present — irregular, non-rhythmical contractions of groups of motor units. More prevalent in anterior horn cell disease than in nerve root damage.

MUSCLE WASTING
Wasting becomes evident in the paretic muscle within 2–3 weeks of the onset.

REFLEXES
— **Tendon** — depressed or absent.
— **Superficial** — unaffected (abdominal, cremasteric).
— **Plantar response** — flexor.

DISTRIBUTION
Either — muscle groups involved in distribution of a spinal segment/root, plexus or peripheral nerve,
    or — generalised limb involvement affecting proximal or distal muscles or following a specific distribution, e.g. facioscapulohumeral dystrophy.

LIMB WEAKNESS

LESION LOCALISATION

The foregoing clinical features readily distinguish weakness of an upper motor neuron, lower motor neuron or mixed pattern. Combining these findings with other neurological signs enables localisation of the lesion site.

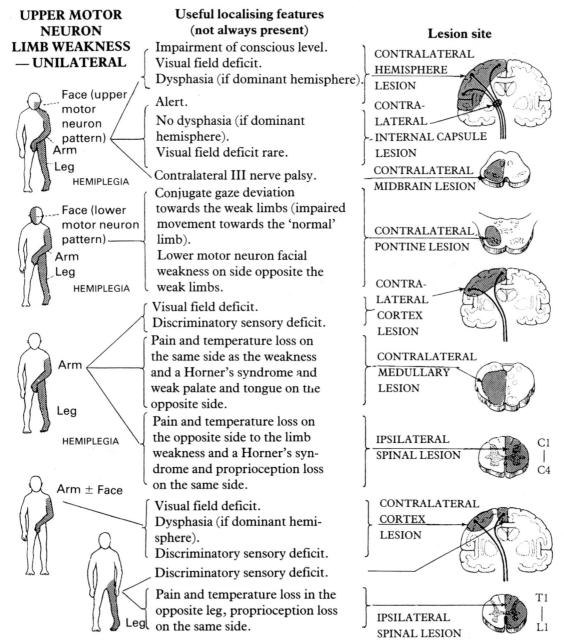

UPPER MOTOR NEURON LIMB WEAKNESS — UNILATERAL

Useful localising features (not always present)

Lesion site

Face (upper motor neuron pattern)
Arm
Leg
HEMIPLEGIA

Impairment of conscious level.
Visual field deficit.
Dysphasia (if dominant hemisphere).

CONTRALATERAL HEMISPHERE LESION

Alert.
No dysphasia (if dominant hemisphere).
Visual field deficit rare.

CONTRA-LATERAL INTERNAL CAPSULE LESION

Contralateral III nerve palsy.

CONTRALATERAL MIDBRAIN LESION

Face (lower motor neuron pattern)
Arm
Leg
HEMIPLEGIA

Conjugate gaze deviation towards the weak limbs (impaired movement towards the 'normal' limb).
Lower motor neuron facial weakness on side opposite the weak limbs.

CONTRALATERAL PONTINE LESION

Arm
Leg
HEMIPLEGIA

Visual field deficit.
Discriminatory sensory deficit.

CONTRA-LATERAL CORTEX LESION

Pain and temperature loss on the same side as the weakness and a Horner's syndrome and weak palate and tongue on the opposite side.

CONTRALATERAL MEDULLARY LESION

Pain and temperature loss on the opposite side to the limb weakness and a Horner's syndrome and proprioception loss on the same side.

IPSILATERAL SPINAL LESION
C1 — C4

Arm ± Face

Visual field deficit.
Dysphasia (if dominant hemisphere).
Discriminatory sensory deficit.

CONTRALATERAL CORTEX LESION

Leg

Discriminatory sensory deficit.

Pain and temperature loss in the opposite leg, proprioception loss on the same side.

IPSILATERAL SPINAL LESION
T1 — L1

MONOPLEGIA

LIMB WEAKNESS

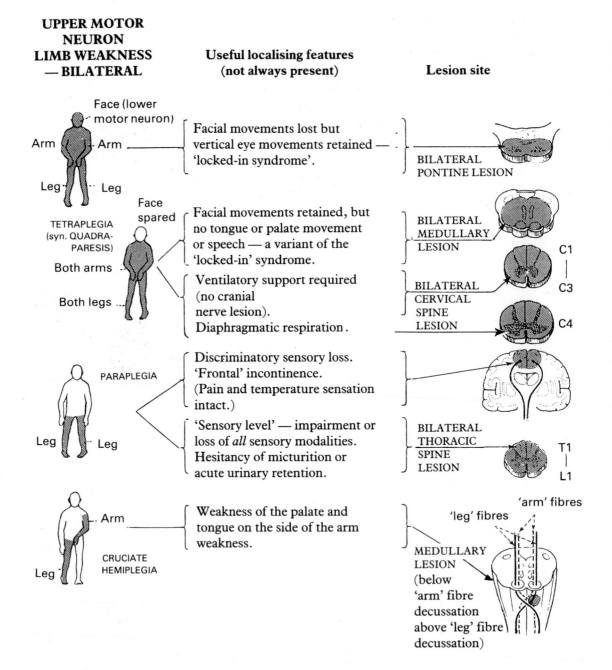

UPPER MOTOR NEURON LIMB WEAKNESS — BILATERAL

Useful localising features (not always present)

Lesion site

Face (lower motor neuron)

Arm — Arm

Leg — Leg

TETRAPLEGIA (syn. QUADRA-PARESIS)

Face spared

Both arms

Both legs

Facial movements lost but vertical eye movements retained — 'locked-in syndrome'.

BILATERAL PONTINE LESION

Facial movements retained, but no tongue or palate movement or speech — a variant of the 'locked-in' syndrome.

BILATERAL MEDULLARY LESION

Ventilatory support required (no cranial nerve lesion). Diaphragmatic respiration.

BILATERAL CERVICAL SPINE LESION

C1 — C3

C4

PARAPLEGIA

Leg — Leg

Discriminatory sensory loss. 'Frontal' incontinence. (Pain and temperature sensation intact.)

'Sensory level' — impairment or loss of *all* sensory modalities. Hesitancy of micturition or acute urinary retention.

BILATERAL THORACIC SPINE LESION

T1 — L1

CRUCIATE HEMIPLEGIA

Arm

Leg

Weakness of the palate and tongue on the side of the arm weakness.

'arm' fibres

'leg' fibres

MEDULLARY LESION (below 'arm' fibre decussation above 'leg' fibre decussation)

LIMB WEAKNESS

MIXED UPPER AND LOWER MOTOR NEURON WEAKNESS — UNILATERAL OR BILATERAL

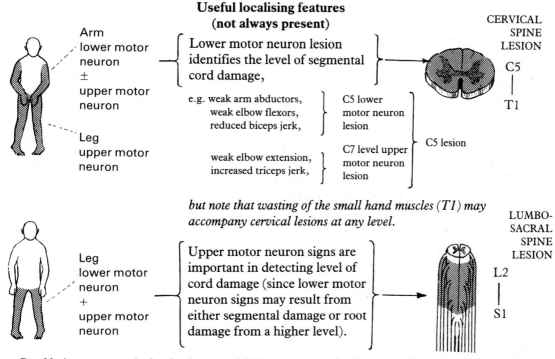

Arm
lower motor
neuron
±
upper motor
neuron

Leg
upper motor
neuron

Useful localising features (not always present)

Lower motor neuron lesion identifies the level of segmental cord damage,

e.g. weak arm abductors, weak elbow flexors, reduced biceps jerk, } C5 lower motor neuron lesion

weak elbow extension, increased triceps jerk, } C7 level upper motor neuron lesion

} C5 lesion

CERVICAL SPINE LESION

C5
|
T1

but note that wasting of the small hand muscles (T1) may accompany cervical lesions at any level.

Leg
lower motor
neuron
+
upper motor
neuron

Upper motor neuron signs are important in detecting level of cord damage (since lower motor neuron signs may result from either segmental damage or root damage from a higher level).

LUMBO-SACRAL SPINE LESION

L2
|
S1

N.B. *Dual lesions, e.g. cervical + lumbar spondylosis may cause mixed (umn and lmn) signs in both arm and leg.*

LOWER MOTOR NEURON LIMB WEAKNESS — UNILATERAL OR BILATERAL

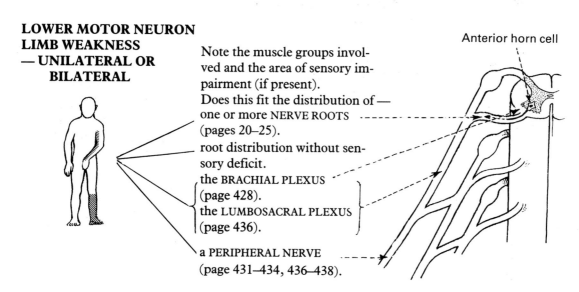

Note the muscle groups involved and the area of sensory impairment (if present).
Does this fit the distribution of —
one or more NERVE ROOTS (pages 20–25).
root distribution without sensory deficit.
the BRACHIAL PLEXUS (page 428).
the LUMBOSACRAL PLEXUS (page 436).
a PERIPHERAL NERVE (page 431–434, 436–438).

Anterior horn cell

LIMB WEAKNESS

**LOWER MOTOR NEURON
LIMB WEAKNESS
— BILATERAL** (*contd*)

Note the muscle groups
involved and area of sensory impairment
(as above).

DISTAL muscle groups involved ———————— POLYNEURO-
PATHY

reflexes absent
or diminished

PROXIMAL muscle groups involved

reflexes
present

MYOPATHY

SPECIFIC muscle groups involved. — FACIOSCAPULOHUMERAL
DYSTROPHY

NEUROMUSCULAR
JUNCTION

**LIMB WEAKNESS
— VARIABLE INTENSITY**

Fatigue with repetitive effort

HYSTERIA

LESION SITE	DIFFERENTIAL DIAGNOSIS	PRELIMINARY INVESTIGATIONS
Cerebral hemispheres, midbrain, pons, medulla	*Vascular* *Tumour* *Infection*	CT scan
Spinal cord	*Demyelination* *Demyelination*	Visual evoked potentials CSF oligoclonal bands MRI scan
	Spondylosis/disc disease *Tumour* *Infection* *Vascular*	Straight X-ray Myelography MRI scan
Anterior horn cell (± spinal cord)	*Motor neuron disease* (*progressive muscular atrophy*)	Electromyography (EMG)
Nerve roots	*Spondylosis/disc disease* *Tumour*	Myelography
Plexus/peripheral nerves	*Peripheral neuropathy* *Trauma* *Tumour infiltration*	EMG Nerve conduction studies
Neuromuscular junction	*Myasthenia gravis* *Myasthenic syndrome*	EMG, Tensilon test
Muscle	*Myopathy* *Dystrophy*	EMG, Muscle biopsy

SENSORY IMPAIRMENT

ANATOMY AND PHYSIOLOGY

The sensory system relays information from both the external and the internal environment.

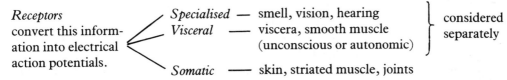

Receptors convert this information into electrical
action potentials.

Specialised — smell, vision, hearing
Visceral ——— viscera, smooth muscle
         (unconscious or autonomic)
} considered
separately

Somatic ——— skin, striated muscle, joints

Cutaneous receptors are of several types and, while overlap does occur, each has some specific
purpose.

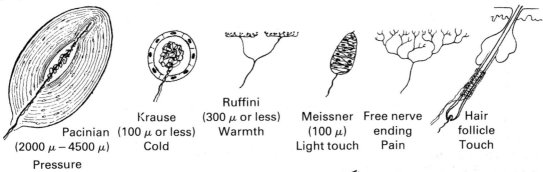

Pacinian
(2000 μ – 4500 μ)
Pressure

Krause
(100 μ or less)
Cold

Ruffini
(300 μ or less)
Warmth

Meissner
(100 μ)
Light touch

Free nerve
ending
Pain

Hair
follicle
Touch

Muscle and tendon receptors
These receptors along with
those of pressure and touch
provide information on body
and limb position — proprioception.

Muscle spindle

Golgi
tendon organ

Repetitive stimulation of most receptors results in a reduction in the action potential frequency —
ADAPTATION.

CENTRAL CONNECTIONS

Sensory neurons (bipolar cells) relay information to the
spinal cord via the dorsal root to the dorsal root entry zone.
The anatomical and physical characteristics of the neurons
vary depending on the information they carry,
as do the central pathways:

Cell bodies
lie in the
dorsal root
ganglia

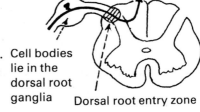

Dorsal root entry zone

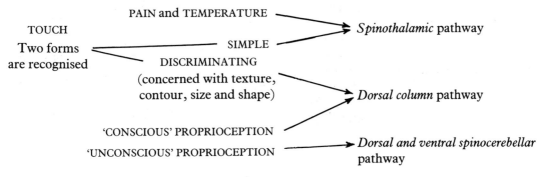

PAIN and TEMPERATURE ———————→ *Spinothalamic* pathway

TOUCH
Two forms
are recognised

SIMPLE ———→

DISCRIMINATING
(concerned with texture,
contour, size and shape) ————→ *Dorsal column* pathway

'CONSCIOUS' PROPRIOCEPTION ————→

'UNCONSCIOUS' PROPRIOCEPTION ————→ *Dorsal and ventral spinocerebellar*
pathway

195

SENSORY IMPAIRMENT

SPINOTHALAMIC PATHWAY

1. Fibres enter the root entry zone and pass up or down for several segments in *Lissauer's* tract before terminating in the dorsal aspect of the dorsal horn.
2. *Second order neurons* synapse locally and cross the midline and run up the *spinothalamic* tract and *lateral lemniscus* to terminate in the posterolateral nucleus of the *thalamus*. Throughout its course, the fibres lie in a *somatotopic arrangement* with sacral fibres outermost. In the brain stem the lateral lemniscus gives off collateral branches to the *reticular formation,* which projects widely to the cerebral cortex and limbic system and is joined by fibres from the contralateral nucleus and tract of the trigeminal nerve.
3. From the thalamus, *third order neurons* project to the *parietal cortex*.

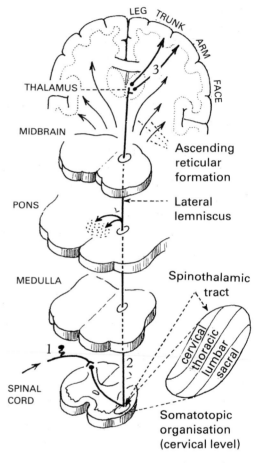

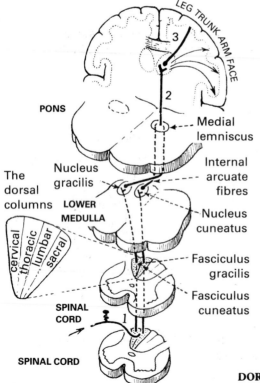

DORSAL COLUMN PATHWAY

1. Fibres enter in the root entry zone and run up-wards in the *dorsal columns* to the *lower medulla* where they terminate in the *nucleus gracilis* and *nucleus cuneatus*.
2. *Second order neurons* decussate as the *internal arcuate fibres* and pass upwards in the *medial lemniscus*. Maintaining a *somatotopic arrangement*, they terminate in the ventral posterolateral thalamus.
3. *Third order neurons* arise in the thalamus and project to the *parietal cortex*.

DORSAL AND VENTRAL SPINOCEREBELLAR PATHWAYS:
see Cerebellar dysfunction, page 177.

SENSORY IMPAIRMENT

EXAMINATION OF THE SENSORY SYSTEM: see page 21

CLINICAL FEATURES

Sensory disturbance may result in:

NEGATIVE symptoms: 'a loss of feeling'
'a deadness'.

POSITIVE symptoms: 'a pins and needles sensation'
'a burning feeling'.

Lesions of the PERIPHERAL NERVES or NERVE ROOTS may produce 'negative' or 'positive' symptoms.

SPINOTHALAMIC TRACT lesions —
seldom produce pain but usually a *lack of awareness of pain and temperature.*
This may result in:
— trophic changes: cold
blue extremities
hair loss
brittle nails
— painless burns
— joint deformation (Charcot's joints).

DORSAL COLUMN lesions —
produce a *discriminatory type of sensory loss.*
— impaired two point discrimination
— astereognosis (failure to discriminate objects held in the hand).
— sensory ataxia (disturbed proprioception).

Lesions of the PARIETAL CORTEX also produce a *discriminatory type of sensory loss.* Minor lesions produce *sensory inattention* (perceptual rivalry) — with bilateral simultaneous limb stimulation, the stimulus is only perceived on the unaffected side.

LESION LOCALISATION

The pattern of the sensory deficit aids lesion localisation.

Sensory deficit	Useful localising features (if present)	Lesion site

HEMISENSORY LOSS

'Discriminatory' sensory deficit.
Sensory inattention (perceptual rivalry)
Only minimal pain and temperature loss

LESION OF CONTRALATERAL PARIETAL CORTEX

or selective deficit in face, arm, trunk or leg.

SELECTIVE CORTICAL LESION

Loss of all sensory modalities including pain and temperature in the face, arm, trunk and leg.

CONTRALATERAL THALAMIC LESION

SENSORY IMPAIRMENT

LESION LOCALISATION *(contd)*

Sensory deficit	Useful localising features (if present)	Lesion site

FACIAL SENSORY LOSS   HEMISENSORY LOSS

Loss of all modalities in the limbs (depending on the extent of the lesion).
Loss of pain and temperature on the opposite side of the face with or without 'muzzle' area sparing and a lateral gaze palsy towards that side.

CONTRALATERAL PONTINE LESION

(Ipsilateral to the facial sensory loss)

As above — but lateral gaze normal.
Weakness of palate and tongue on side opposite to the limb sensory deficit.

CONTRALATERAL MEDULLARY LESION

CONTRALATERAL SPINOTHALAMIC TRACT LESION

Loss of pain, temperature and light touch below a specific dermatome level (may spare sacral sensation).

(Partial spinothalamic tract lesion)

Loss of all modalities at one or several dermatome levels.

Loss of pain and temperature below a specific dermatome level.

Loss of proprioception and 'discriminatory' touch up to similar level and limb weakness.

BROWN-SEQUARD SYNDROME

(Partial cord lesion)

Bilateral loss of all modalities.
Bilateral leg weakness.

COMPLETE CORD LESION

'SUSPENDED' SENSORY LOSS

Bilateral loss of pain and temperature.
Preservation of proprioception and 'discriminatory' sensation.

CENTRAL CORD LESION

SENSORY IMPAIRMENT

LESION LOCALISATION (contd)

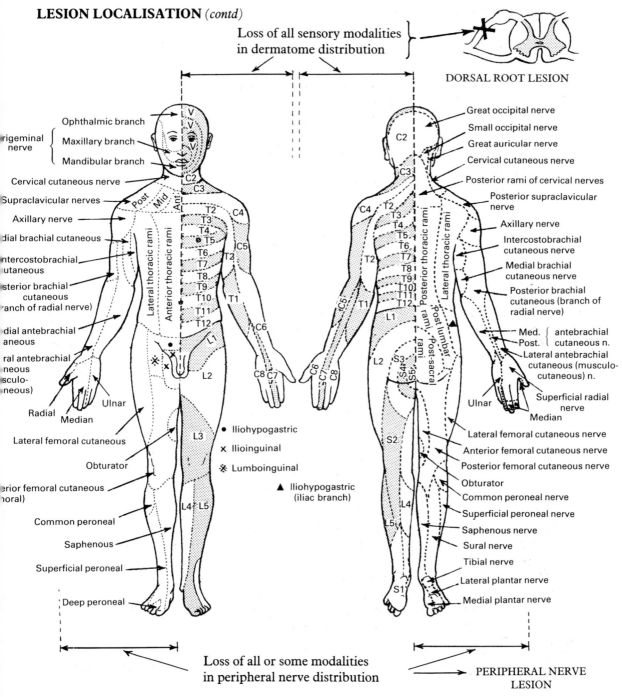

Loss of all sensory modalities in dermatome distribution

DORSAL ROOT LESION

Loss of all or some modalities in peripheral nerve distribution

PERIPHERAL NERVE LESION

DIFFERENTIAL DIAGNOSIS — as for limb weakness — page 194.

PAIN

Peripheral receptors of pain — free nerve endings lying in skin or other organs — are the distal axons of sensory neurons. Such unmyelinated or only thinly myelinated axons are of small diameter. The termination and central connections of these axons are described on page 196.

The type of stimulus required to activate free endings varies, e.g. in muscle — ischaemia, in abdominal viscera — distension.

Certain substances — bradykinins, prostaglandins, histamine — may stimulate free nerve endings.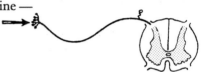

These substances are released in damaged tissue.

CONTROL OF SENSORY (PAIN) INPUT

The Gate control theory

A relay system in the posterior horn of the spinal cord modifies pain input. This involves interneuronal connections within the substantia gelatinosa (a layer of the posterior horn which extends throughout the whole length of the spinal cord on each side).

An afferent impulse arriving at the posterior horn in *thick myelinated fibres* has an inhibitory effect in the region of the substantia gelatinosa.

An afferent impulse arriving in *thin myelinated or unmyelinated fibres* (i.e. transmitting pain) has an excitatory effect in the region of the substantia gelatinosa.

The overall interaction of these inhibitory or excitatory effects determines the activity of second order neurons of the spinothalamic pathway.

A reduction in activity of large sensory fibres 'opens' the gate. Stimulation of large sensory fibres theoretically 'closes' the gate.

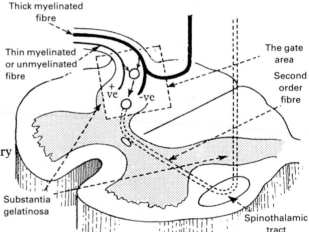

Cross section of the spinal cord: the gate area connections

In addition to these segmental influences, higher centres also control the gate region and form part of a feed-back loop.

Pain perception

The awareness of pain is brought about by projection from the thalamus to cerebral cortex. Personality, mood and neuroticism all influence the intensity of pain perception. Diffuse projections through Lissauer's tract and the reticular core of the spinal cord white matter to the reticular formation and limbic system probably contribute to the unpleasant, emotionally disturbing aspects of pain.

PAIN

NEUROTRANSMITTER SUBSTANCES

Evidence based on both human and animal studies has shown that an endogenous system, lying within the central nervous system can induce a degree of analgesia. Electrical stimulation of certain sites, such as the periaqueductal grey matter, can inhibit pain perception.

Receptor sites for endogenous opiates have been found in the posterior horns and thalamus as well as at several other sites. The endogenous substances which bind to these sites are called *encephalins* or *endorphins*.

Substance P, a polypeptide, found predominantly around free nerve ending receptors and in the spinal cord posterior horns, is the likely primary transmitter of pain.

DRUG TREATMENT

Sites of potential drug action:

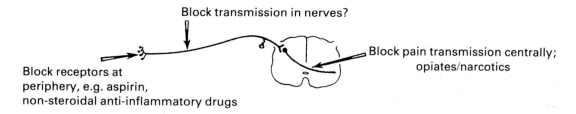

Block transmission in nerves?

Block receptors at periphery, e.g. aspirin, non-steroidal anti-inflammatory drugs

Block pain transmission centrally; opiates/narcotics

Drug selection in pain treatment depends on the severity, cause and the expected duration of the pain, i.e. *acute* pain — less than 2 weeks duration, e.g. postoperative,
post-traumatic,
renal colic.

chronic pain — *benign* origin, e.g. postherpetic neuralgia
phantom limb pain
chronic back pain.

— *malignant* origin.

1. In acute pain drug therapy ranges from *mild analgesics* — aspirin, paracetamol — to *narcotic agents* — morphine, heroin. *Tranquillisers* may also help.

2. In chronic pain of benign origin, narcotics and sedatives must be avoided. In these patients, depression usually plays a rôle and the clinician must not underestimate the value of *antidepressants.*
Anticonvulsants — carbamazepine appears to benefit many patients, although its mode of action in pain relief remains unknown.

3. In chronic pain from terminal malignancy, patients often require *strong narcotics* — morphine, heroin. Frequent administration of small doses provides the greatest effect.

PAIN — TREATMENT

CENTRAL TECHNIQUES

STEREOTACTIC THALAMOTOMY: The spinoreticular system appears largely responsible for the unpleasant aspects of pain sensation. Stereotactic obliteration of the spinoreticular relay nuclei in the thalamus (page 369) may help patients with intractable pain from malignancy involving the head, neck or brachial plexus, sites where other methods of pain control are limited.

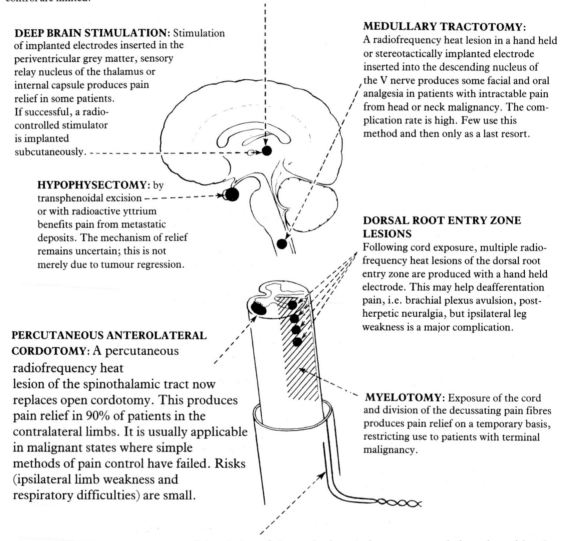

DEEP BRAIN STIMULATION: Stimulation of implanted electrodes inserted in the periventricular grey matter, sensory relay nucleus of the thalamus or internal capsule produces pain relief in some patients. If successful, a radio-controlled stimulator is implanted subcutaneously. - - - - - - - -

HYPOPHYSECTOMY: by transphenoidal excision - - - - - - - or with radioactive yttrium benefits pain from metastatic deposits. The mechanism of relief remains uncertain; this is not merely due to tumour regression.

MEDULLARY TRACTOTOMY: A radiofrequency heat lesion in a hand held or stereotactically implanted electrode inserted into the descending nucleus of the V nerve produces some facial and oral analgesia in patients with intractable pain from head or neck malignancy. The complication rate is high. Few use this method and then only as a last resort.

DORSAL ROOT ENTRY ZONE LESIONS
Following cord exposure, multiple radio-frequency heat lesions of the dorsal root entry zone are produced with a hand held electrode. This may help deafferentation pain, i.e. brachial plexus avulsion, post-herpetic neuralgia, but ipsilateral leg weakness is a major complication.

PERCUTANEOUS ANTEROLATERAL CORDOTOMY: A percutaneous radiofrequency heat lesion of the spinothalamic tract now replaces open cordotomy. This produces pain relief in 90% of patients in the contralateral limbs. It is usually applicable in malignant states where simple methods of pain control have failed. Risks (ipsilateral limb weakness and respiratory difficulties) are small.

MYELOTOMY: Exposure of the cord and division of the decussating pain fibres produces pain relief on a temporary basis, restricting use to patients with terminal malignancy.

DORSAL COLUMN STIMULATION: Stimulation of electrodes inserted percutaneously into the epidural space may benefit patients with chronic pain, unresponsive to non-invasive techniques. A trial with exteriorised electrodes permits evaluation, prior to implanting a radiocontrolled stimulator.

PAIN — TREATMENT

PERIPHERAL TECHNIQUES

NERVE BLOCKS: Injections of agents into peripheral nerves or roots abolishes pain in the appropriate dermatome; motor and sympathetic function are also lost. Local anaesthetics produce a temporary effect; neurolytic agents, e.g. phenol, alcohol, give permanent results.

– *Intraspinal* phenol or hypertonic saline for chronic pain usually used in patients with terminal malignancy.

– *Epidural* local anaesthetic produces temporary analgesia. Narcotic infusion appears useful for controlling postoperative pain and intractable pain in patients with terminal malignancy.

– *Sympathetic Ganglion or Trunk*
 — anaesthetics or neurolytic
 agent often helps causalgic pain
 (see page 204).

– *Paravertebral or Peripheral Nerve*
 — local anaesthetics may benefit temporary pain states, e.g. fractured rib, but neurolytic agents often cause a painful neuritis.

DORSAL RHIZOTOMY:
Division of the dorsal roots via a laminectomy has a high failure rate and provides only short lasting benefit. Now seldom performed.

ACUPUNCTURE:

Insertion and rotation of needles in specific cutaneous points appears to produce slight analgesia in acute pain. Long-term results in chronic pain are disappointing. Although endorphin release occurs, the rôle of the placebo effect remains unclear.

DENERVATION OF THE FACET JOINTS:
A percutaneous radiofrequency heat lesion applied to the posterior ramus of the spinal nerves exiting from the intervertebral foramen, denervates the facet joints. A preliminary test injection of local anaesthetic serves as a useful diagnostic procedure.

 This technique relieves facet joint pains in the majority of patients, but as the nerve regenerates, pain returns unless preventative measures are adopted.

TRANSCUTANEOUS ELECTRICAL NERVE STIMULATION (TENS):
Prolonged electrical stimulation over the affected site often alleviates pain of peripheral origin. This technique acts either by stimulating large diameter fibres, thus closing the 'gate' at the dorsal root entry zone or via higher centres.

PAIN SYNDROMES

Pain is not primarily a pathological phenomenon, but serves a protective function. Conditions with loss of pain perception exemplify this, resulting in frequent injuries, burns and subsequent mutilations, e.g. syringomyelia, hereditary sensory neuropathy, congenital insensitivity to pain.

Pathological conditions do, however, cause pain — as a symptom of cancer, injury or other disease.

The following conditions produce characteristic pain syndromes.

CAUSALGIA

Causalgia is an incomplete peripheral nerve injury producing intense, continuous, burning pain. Touching the limb aggravates the pain, and the patient resents any interference or attempt at limb mobilisation. The skin becomes red, warm and swollen.

Theoretical mechanism

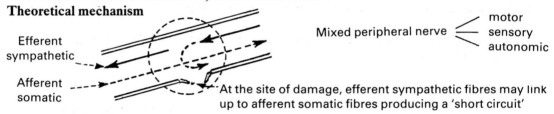

Causalgia only occurs with damage to peripheral nerves containing a large number of sympathetic fibres and responds in part to sympathetic blockade (pharmacological or surgical).

POSTHERPETIC NEURALGIA

Following activation of a latent infection with varicella zoster virus lying dormant in the dorsal root or gasserian ganglion, the patient develops a burning, constant pain with severe, sharp paroxysmal twinges over the area supplied by the affected sensory neurons. Touch exacerbates the pain. Thick myelinated fibres are preferentially damaged, possibly opening the 'gate'.

Treatment of postherpetic neuralgia is particularly difficult. Carbamazepine and/or antidepressants may help. Ethylchloride spray over the affected area provides temporary relief and percutaneous cordotomy benefits some patients. Dorsal root entry zone lesions in this condition await evaluation.

THALAMIC PAIN

Thalamic stimulation may produce or abolish pain depending upon the electrode site. A vascular accident which involves the inhibitory portion of the thalamus may result in pain — the thalamic syndrome.

Clinical features: Hemianaesthesia at onset precedes the development of pain contralateral to the lesion. The pain is burning and diffuse, and exacerbated by the touch of clothing.

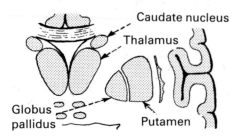

Treatment: Drug treatment gives poor results. A stereotactic procedure although increasing the sensory deficit may help.

Paradoxically the thalamic syndrome may occur following a thalamic stereotactic procedure for movement disorders.

PAIN SYNDROMES

PHANTOM LIMB PAIN

Following amputation of a limb, 10% of patients develop pain with a continuous persistent burning quality, caused by neuroma formation in the stump. The patient 'feels' the pain arising from some point on the missing limb (the pain input projects through pathways which retain the topographical image of the absent limb).

Treatment: as for postherpetic neuralgia — no specific treatment.

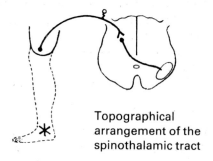

Topographical arrangement of the spinothalamic tract

VISCERAL AND REFERRED PAIN

Deep visceral pain is dull and boring; it is the consequence of distension or traction on free nerve endings.

Referred pain of a dull quality relates to a specific area of the body surface — often hypersensitive to touch.

The basis of referred pain

The visceral afferents converge upon the same cells in the posterior horns as the somatic efferents. The patient 'projects' pain from the viscera to the area supplied by corresponding somatic afferent fibres.

A knowledge of the source of referred pain is important in diagnosis and treatment.

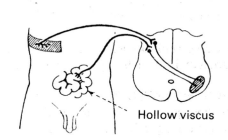

Hollow viscus

SITES OF REFERRED PAIN FROM SPECIFIC ORGANS

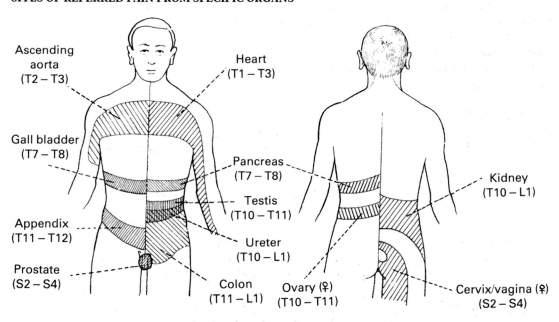

Ascending aorta (T2 – T3)

Heart (T1 – T3)

Gall bladder (T7 – T8)

Pancreas (T7 – T8)

Kidney (T10 – L1)

Appendix (T11 – T12)

Testis (T10 – T11)

Prostate (S2 – S4)

Ureter (T10 – L1)

Colon (T11 – L1)

Ovary (♀) (T10 – T11)

Cervix/vagina (♀) (S2 – S4)

205

LIMB PAIN

Pain may arise from any anatomical structure within the limb. Each produces characteristic features:

BONE – diffuse, aching pain
± palpable mass.

JOINTS – pain localised to affected joint.
– tenderness on palpation.
– movements restricted and painful.
– wasting of surrounding muscles may follow.

MUSCLES – pain localised to specific muscle
± wasting and weakness
± palpable mass.

TENDONS – pain localised to swollen, tender tendon sheath.

BLOOD VESSELS – pain brought on by exertion (claudication), relieved by rest.
– pain at rest in pale, pulseless limb (occlusion).
– pain associated with paraesthesia and digital pallor (Raynaud's).

NERVE ROOT – pain increased by coughing or by movement
± associated neurological deficit

PLEXUS OR PERIPHERAL NERVE — burning pain
± sweating, cyanosis and oedema of extremity,
± associated neurological deficit.

CAUSES OF UPPER LIMB PAIN

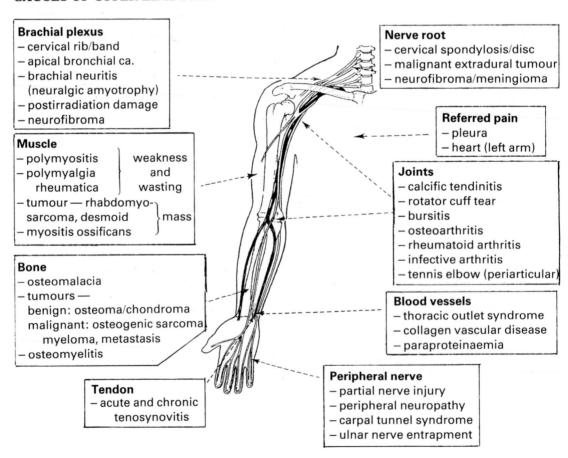

Brachial plexus
– cervical rib/band
– apical bronchial ca.
– brachial neuritis
 (neuralgic amyotrophy)
– postirradiation damage
– neurofibroma

Muscle
– polymyositis
– polymyalgia
 rheumatica   } weakness and wasting
– tumour — rhabdomyo-
 sarcoma, desmoid   } mass
– myositis ossificans

Bone
– osteomalacia
– tumours —
 benign: osteoma/chondroma
 malignant: osteogenic sarcoma,
  myeloma, metastasis
– osteomyelitis

Tendon
– acute and chronic
 tenosynovitis

Nerve root
– cervical spondylosis/disc
– malignant extradural tumour
– neurofibroma/meningioma

Referred pain
– pleura
– heart (left arm)

Joints
– calcific tendinitis
– rotator cuff tear
– bursitis
– osteoarthritis
– rheumatoid arthritis
– infective arthritis
– tennis elbow (periarticular)

Blood vessels
– thoracic outlet syndrome
– collagen vascular disease
– paraproteinaemia

Peripheral nerve
– partial nerve injury
– peripheral neuropathy
– carpal tunnel syndrome
– ulnar nerve entrapment

LIMB PAIN

CAUSES OF LOWER LIMB PAIN

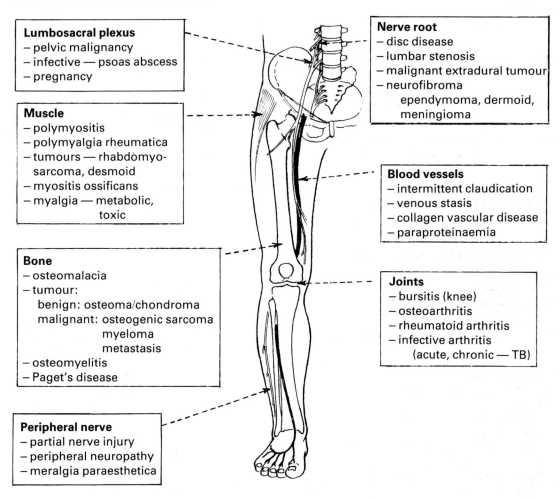

Lumbosacral plexus
– pelvic malignancy
– infective — psoas abscess
– pregnancy

Muscle
– polymyositis
– polymyalgia rheumatica
– tumours — rhabdòmyo-
   sarcoma, desmoid
– myositis ossificans
– myalgia — metabolic,
      toxic

Bone
– osteomalacia
– tumour:
   benign: osteoma/chondroma
   malignant: osteogenic sarcoma
            myeloma
            metastasis
– osteomyelitis
– Paget's disease

Peripheral nerve
– partial nerve injury
– peripheral neuropathy
– meralgia paraesthetica

Nerve root
– disc disease
– lumbar stenosis
– malignant extradural tumour
– neurofibroma
      ependymoma, dermoid,
      meningioma

Blood vessels
– intermittent claudication
– venous stasis
– collagen vascular disease
– paraproteinaemia

Joints
– bursitis (knee)
– osteoarthritis
– rheumatoid arthritis
– infective arthritis
      (acute, chronic — TB)

Meralgia paraesthetica: burning, tingling pain over the outer aspect of the thigh, increased when standing or by walking, due to a localised neuritis of the lateral cutaneous nerve of the thigh. A patch of sensory impairment may be evident over the outer aspect of the thigh.

Ekbom's syndrome: (syn. restless legs syndrome): intolerable tingling, burning sensation or pain in both legs, occurring only when sitting or lying down and relieved by walking; no associated neurological abnormality.

Investigation of limb pain depends on the suspected cause and may include straight X-rays, myelography, nerve conduction studies and EMG.

MUSCLE PAIN

The basis of muscle pain is usually ischaemia. Reduction of blood flow results in the accumulation of prostaglandins, histamine, serotonin and other substances which, along with a fall in pH, probably stimulate free nerve ending receptors. Swelling of muscle fibres will similarly evoke pain.

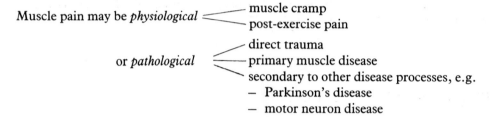

Muscle pain may be *physiological*
— muscle cramp
— post-exercise pain

or *pathological*
— direct trauma
— primary muscle disease
— secondary to other disease processes, e.g.
   — Parkinson's disease
   — motor neuron disease

DISORDERS OF MUSCLE RESULTING IN PAIN
Pain occurs in conditions in which muscle fibres are actively damaged, or blood supply and metabolism are significantly impaired.

Inflammatory myopathies: (see page 454)

Polymyalgia rheumatica
Proximal severe shoulder girdle pain occurring in elderly people, often associated with giant cell arteritis. The ESR is elevated but EMG and muscle enzyme estimations are normal. Muscle biopsy shows loss of type II muscle fibres. Non-steroidal anti-inflammatory drugs (NSAID) are effective. Where gaint cell arteritis co-exists, steroids produce a dramatic response.

BENIGN MYALGIC ENCEPHALOMYELITIS (ME) this puzzling disorder, often occurring in epidemics, is characterised by exercise-induced muscle pain.

DRUG INDUCED
Drugs — opiates, antimitotics (vincristine), cimetidine and clofibrate may cause severe pain and muscle tenderness, with elevated muscle enzymes and breakdown products (myoglobin) in the urine from extensive muscle necrosis. Recovery is usually complete. Alcohol abuse (binge drinking) can produce a similar picture.

IDIOPATHIC PAROXYSMAL MYOGLOBINURIA
Intermittent episodes of muscle cell damage with myoglobin in the urine, occurring spontaneously or precipitated by exercise. Drugs and alcohol should be excluded. Recovery between attacks is complete.

MALIGNANT HYPERPYREXIA
Characterised by a sudden rise in body temperature while undergoing a general anaesthetic, usually with halothane. Cardiac failure may result in death. In survivors, muscle pain due to extensive necrosis with myoglobinuria follows. Certain hereditary myopathic disorders, e.g. myotonic dystrophy, central core disease, show a tendency to develop this severe problem.

DISORDERS OF MUSCLE METABOLISM
The enzyme deficiency disorders (page 459) are characterised by the development of muscle pain following moderate exertion and relieved by rest.

MUSCLE PAIN

METABOLIC BONE DISEASE
Osteomalacia (common in immigrants with dietary vit. D deficiency) causes muscle weakness, diffuse muscle pain and a waddling gait. Muscle wasting is absent and EMG and muscle enzymes are normal.

Muscle biopsy shows the same fibre type loss as seen in polymyalgia rheumatica.

Confirmation of diagnosis requires serum vit.D estimation. Osteomalacia secondary to renal disease, malabsorption syndrome, hyperparathyroidism and chronic anticonvulsant medication may produce a similar picture.

DIAGNOSTIC APPROACH TO MUSCLE PAIN

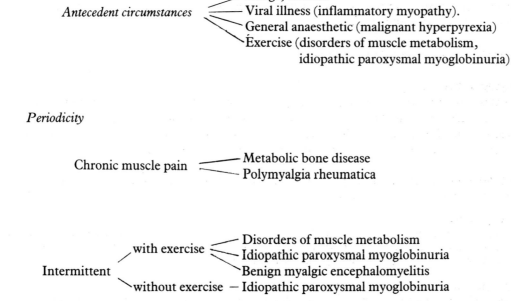

Antecedent circumstances
- Drugs, alcohol
- Viral illness (inflammatory myopathy).
- General anaesthetic (malignant hyperpyrexia)
- Exercise (disorders of muscle metabolism, idiopathic paroxysmal myoglobinuria)

Periodicity

Chronic muscle pain
- Metabolic bone disease
- Polymyalgia rheumatica

Intermittent
- with exercise
  - Disorders of muscle metabolism
  - Idiopathic paroxysmal myoglobinuria
  - Benign myalgic encephalomyelitis
- without exercise — Idiopathic paroxysmal myoglobinuria

A large number of patients referred with muscle pain remain undiagnosed even after extensive investigation.

BRAIN DEATH

The advent of improved intensive care facilities and more aggressive resuscitation techniques has led to an increase in numbers of patients with irreversible brain damage in which tissue oxygenation is maintained by a persistent heart beat and artificial ventilation.

In recent years, a government working party has published guidelines for the diagnosis of brain death which, when fulfilled, indicate that recovery is impossible. In these patients, organs may be removed for transplantation before discontinuing ventilation.

The tests are designed to detect failure of *brain stem* function, but certain *preconditions* must first be met.

Preconditions

Depressant drugs must not contribute towards the patient's clinical state — if in doubt allow an adequate time interval to elapse to eliminate any possible persistent effect.

Hypothermia must not be a primary cause — ensure that temperature is not less than 35 °C.

Severe *metabolic* or *endocrine* disturbance must be excluded as a possible cause of the patient's condition.

The patient must be on a ventilator as a result of inadequate spontaneous respiration or respiratory arrest — if a neuromuscular blocking drug has been used, exclude a prolonged effect by observing a muscle twitch on nerve stimulation, e.g. electrical stimulation of the median nerve should cause a thumb twitch.

The cause of the patient's condition must be established and this must be compatible with irreversible brain damage, e.g. severe head injury, spontaneous intracerebral haematoma. *If in doubt, delay brain death testing.*

BRAIN DEATH TESTS

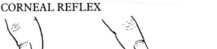

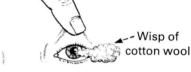

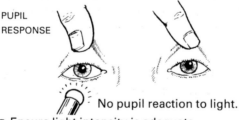

PUPIL RESPONSE

CORNEAL REFLEX

- - Wisp of cotton wool

No pupil reaction to light.

N.B. Ensure light intensity is adequate.

No orbicularis oculi contraction in response to corneal stimulation.

VESTIBULO-OCULAR REFLEX

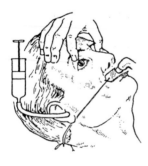

No eye movements occur when 50 ml of iced water are slowly injected into the external meatus. (Ensure that the external meatus is not occluded with wax or blood.) In coma with preserved brain stem function, the eyes tonically deviate towards the tested ear after a delay of 20 seconds.

Maximal response is obtained with the head raised 30° from the horizontal.

GAG REFLEX

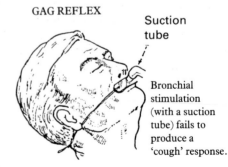

Suction tube

Bronchial stimulation (with a suction tube) fails to produce a 'cough' response.

BRAIN DEATH

MOTOR RESPONSE

No motor response in the face or in the muscles supplied by cranial nerves in response to a painful stimulus, e.g. supraorbital pain.

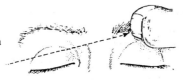

N.B. Limb responses are of no value in testing brain stem integrity. Movements can occur in response to limb or trunk stimulation (especially in the legs), tendon reflexes may persist in a patient with brain stem death but intact cord function. Conversely, limb movements and reflexes may be absent in a patient with an intact brain stem and spinal cord damage.

RESPIRATORY MOVEMENTS

No respiratory movements are observed when the patient is disconnected from the ventilator. During this test, anoxia is prevented by passing 6 litres O_2 per minute down the endotracheal tube. This should maintain adequate PO_2 levels for up to 10 minutes.

N.B. Ensure that apnoea is not a result of a low PCO_2. This should be greater than 6.65 kPa (50 mmHg).

Clinician's status

Recommendations state that these tests should be carried out by two doctors, both with expertise in the field; one of consultant status, the other of consultant or senior registrar status. The doctors may carry out the tests individually or together.

Test repetition and timing

The test should be repeated but the interval should be left to the discretion of the clinician. The initial test may be performed within a few hours of the causal event, but in most instances is delayed for 12–24 hours, or longer if there is any doubt about the preconditions.

Timing of death

Certification of death occurs when brain death is established, i.e. at the time of the second test. Old concepts of death occurring at the time the heart ceases to beat are no longer applicable.

Supplementary investigations

Electroencephalography (EEG) is of no value in diagnosing brain death. Some patients with the potential to recover show a 'flat' trace whereas, in others with irreversible brain stem damage, electrical activity can occasionally be recorded from the scalp electrodes.

Similarly, angiography or cerebral blood flow measurement are of no additional value to the clinical tests described above, provided the preconditions are fulfilled.

In some countries these tests are used as 'legal' rather than clinical criteria of brain death.

LOCALISED NEUROLOGICAL DISEASE AND ITS MANAGEMENT
A. INTRACRANIAL

HEAD INJURY

INTRODUCTION
Many patients attend accident and emergency departments with head injury. Approximately 300 per 100 000 of the population per year require hospital admission; of these 9 per 100 000 die, i.e. 5000 patients per year in Britain. Some of these deaths are inevitable, some are potentially preventable.

The principal causes of head injury include road traffic accidents, falls, assaults, injuries occurring at work, in the home and during sports. The relative frequency of each cause varies between different age groups and from place to place throughout the country.

Head injuries from road traffic accidents are most common in young males; alcohol is frequently involved. Road traffic accidents, although only constituting about 25% of all patients with head injury, are the cause of more serious injuries. This cause contributes to 60% of the deaths from head injury; of these, half die before reaching hospital.

In the UK many measures have been introduced to reduce the incidence, such as seat belt and crash helmet legislation. Once a head injury has occurred, nothing can alter the impact damage. The aim of head injury management is to minimise damage arising from secondary complications.

PATHOLOGY
Brain damage occurs both at impact and as a result of the development of secondary complications.

IMPACT DAMAGE is of two types, which may coexist:
1. Cortical contusions and lacerations
These may occur under or opposite (contre-coup) the site of impact, but most commonly involve the frontal and temporal lobes. Contusions are usually multiple and may occur bilaterally. Multiple contusions do not in themselves contribute to depression of conscious level, but this may arise when bleeding into the contusions produces a space-occupying haematoma.

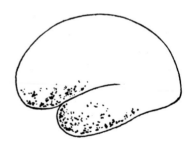

2. Diffuse white matter lesions
This type of brain damage occurs as a result of mechanical shearing following deceleration, causing disruption and tearing of axons. Depending on the severity of injury it may cause immediate mild to severe depression of conscious level and even death.

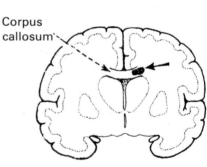

Corpus callosum

Superior cerebellar peduncle

Pons

The *macrosopic* appearance may appear entirely normal but in some patients pathological sections reveal small intracerebral haematomas, particularly in the corpus callosum or in the superior cerebellar peduncle.

HEAD INJURY

Diffuse white matter lesions *(contd)*
Microscopic evidence of neuronal damage depends on the duration of survival and on the severity of the injury. After a few days, retraction balls and microglial clusters are seen in the white matter.

 Retraction balls reflect axonal damage. Note only axons in one plane are involved, indicating the direction of the 'shear'

Microglial clusters (hyper-trophied microglia) are found diffusely throughout the white matter

If the patient survives 5 weeks or more after injury then appropriate staining demonstrates Wallerian degeneration of the long tracts and white matter of the cerebral hemispheres. Even a minor injury causing a transient loss of consciousness produces some neuronal damage. Since neuronal regeneration cannot occur, the effects of repeated minor injury are cumulative.

SECONDARY BRAIN DAMAGE may occur at any time after the initial impact. Impact damage is unavoidable, but secondary brain damage caused by haematoma, brain swelling, brain shift, ischaemia and infection may be preventable and this must be the aim of head injury management.

1. Intracranial haematoma
Intracranial bleeding may occur either outside (extradural) or within the dura (intradural).

Intradural lesions usually consist of a mixture of both subdural and intracerebral haematomas although pure subdurals occur in a proportion. Brain damage is caused directly or indirectly as a result of tentorial or tonsillar herniation.

Incidence of haematoma:
Extradural — 16%
Intradural:
pure subdural — 22%
intracerebral
±subdural — 54%
Extra- + Intradural— 8%

Extradural
A skull fracture tearing the middle meningeal vessels bleeds into the extradural space. This usually occurs in the temporal or temporoparietal region.

Occasionally extradural haematomas are caused by a ruptured sagittal or transverse sinus.

Dura

Intracerebral ± subdural (burst lobe)
Contusions in the frontal and temporal lobes often lead to bleeding into the brain substance, usually associated with an overlying subdural haematoma.

'Burst lobe' is a term some-times used to describe the ap-pearance of intracerebral haematoma mixed with necrotic brain tissue, ruptur-ing out into the subdural space.

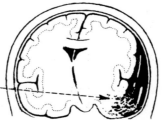

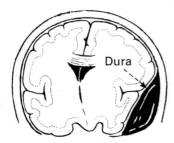

Dura

Subdural
In some patients impact may rupture bridging veins from the cortical surface to the venous sinuses producing a pure subdural haematoma with no evidence of under-lying cortical contusion or laceration.

HEAD INJURY

SECONDARY BRAIN DAMAGE (*contd*)

2. Cerebral swelling
This may occur with or without intracranial haematoma.
It results from either vascular engorgement or an increase in
extra- or intracellular fluid, the exact causative mechanisms
in different injuries remaining unknown.

3. Tentorial/tonsillar herniation (syn. 'cone')
It is unlikely the high intracranial pressure
alone directly damages neuronal tissue, but brain
damage occurs as a result of tonsillar or tentorial
herniation (see page 77). A progressive increase
in intracranial pressure due to a supratentorial
haematoma initially produces midline shift.
Herniation of the medial temporal lobe through
the tentorial hiatus follows (*lateral tentorial
herniation*), causing midbrain compression and
damage. Uncontrolled lateral tentorial herniation
or diffuse bilateral hemispheric swelling will result
in *central tentorial herniation*. Herniation of the
cerebellar tonsils through the foramen magnum
(*tonsillar herniation*) and consequent lower brainstem compression may follow central tentorial
herniation or may result from the infrequently
occurring traumatic posterior fossa haematoma.

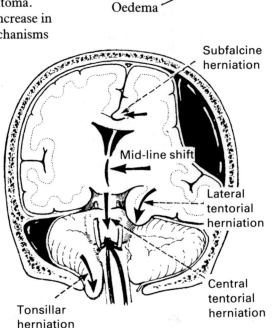

4. Cerebral ischaemia
Cerebral ischaemia commonly occurs after severe head
injury and is caused by either hypoxia or impaired cerebral
perfusion. In the normal subject, a fall in blood pressure
does not produce a drop in cerebral perfusion since 'autoregulation' results in cerebral vasodilatation. After head
injury, however, autoregulation is often defective and
hypotension may have more drastic effects.

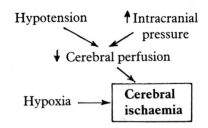

5. Infection

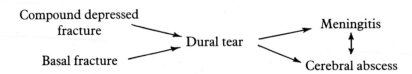

The presence of a dural tear provides a potential route for infection. This seldom occurs within 48
hours of injury and may develop after several months or years.

HEAD INJURY — CLINICAL ASSESSMENT

MULTIPLE INJURY — PRIORITIES OF ASSESSMENT

Patients admitted in coma with multiple injuries require urgent care and the clinician must be aware of the priorities of assessment and management.

Airway

Check for obstruction and use oropharyn-geal airway or endotracheal tube.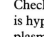

Breathing

Administer oxygen and check respiratory movements are adequate; if not, ventilate.

Chest/abdominal injury

Examine chest for possible flail segment or haemo/pneumothorax. Examine abdomen for possible bleeding; if in doubt, use peritoneal lavage. (X-ray chest and abdomen).

Circulation

Check pulse and blood pressure. If patient is hypotensive, replace blood loss with plasma substitute followed by whole blood when available.

Head/spinal injury

Assess conscious level and focal signs. Consider possibility of spinal injury. (X-ray skull and spine, CT scan).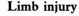

Limb injury

Examine limbs for lacerations and fractures. (X-ray.)

When intracranial haematoma is suspected, a CT scan is essential, especially before clinical signs are masked by a general anaesthetic required for the management of limb or abdominal injuries. However, if difficulty occurs in maintaining blood pressure, then urgent laparotomy or thoracotomy would take precedence over further investigation of a possible intracranial haematoma.

HEAD INJURY — ASSESSMENT

Some patients may describe the events leading to and following head injury, but often the doctor depends on descriptions from witnesses.

Points to determine:

Period of loss of consciousness: Relates to severity of diffuse brain damage and may range from a few seconds to several weeks.

Period of post-traumatic amnesia: This is the period of permanent amnesia occurring after head injury. It also reflects the severity of damage and in severe injuries may last several weeks. (Period of retrograde amnesia, i.e. amnesia for events before the injury is of less value since it bears no relation to the severity of injury and may improve with time).

Cause and circumstances of the injury: The patient may collapse, or crash his vehicle as a result of some preceding intracranial event, e.g. subarachnoid haemorrhage or epileptic seizure. The more 'violent' the injury, the greater the risk of associated extracranial injuries.

Presence of headache and vomiting: These are common symptoms after head injury. If they persist, the possibility of intracranial haemorrhage must be considered.

HEAD INJURY — CLINICAL ASSESSMENT

EXAMINATION

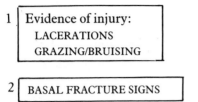

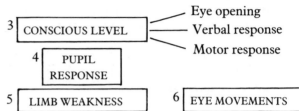

1 | Evidence of injury:
LACERATIONS
GRAZING/BRUISING

3 | CONSCIOUS LEVEL ——— Eye opening
— Verbal response
— Motor response

4 | PUPIL RESPONSE

2 | BASAL FRACTURE SIGNS

5 | LIMB WEAKNESS

6 | EYE MOVEMENTS

1. Lacerations and bruising

The presence of these features confirms the occurrence of a head injury, but traumatic intracranial haematoma can occur in patients with no external evidence of injury.

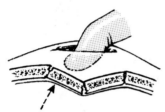

Always explore deep lacerations with a gloved finger for evidence of a *depressed fracture*.

Beware of falling into the trap of diagnosing a depressed fracture when only scalp haematoma is present.

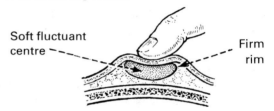

Soft fluctuant centre ---

Firm rim

Consider the possibility of a hyperextension injury to the cervical spine if frontal laceration or bruising is present.

2. Basal skull fracture

Clinical features indicate the presence of a basal skull fracture which may not be evident on routine skull X-ray or even on specific views of the skull base. If present, a potential route of infection exists with the concomitant risk of meningitis.

ANTERIOR FOSSA FRACTURE

CSF rhinorrhoea

Bilateral periorbital haematoma

Subconjunctival haemorrhage

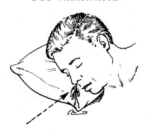

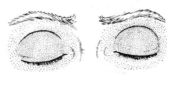

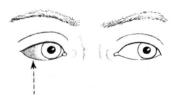

If the nasal discharge contains glucose, then the fluid is CSF rather than mucin.

Bruising limited to the orbital margins indicates blood tracking from behind.

Bruising under conjunctiva extending to posterior limits of the sclera indicates blood tracking from orbital cavity.

HEAD INJURY — CLINICAL ASSESSMENT

Basal skull fracture *(contd)*

PETROUS FRACTURE

Bleeding from the external auditory meatus or CSF otorrhoea:

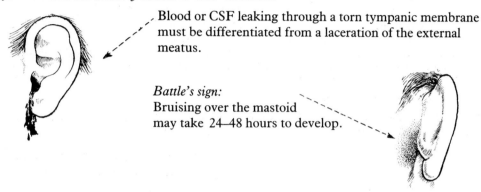

Blood or CSF leaking through a torn tympanic membrane must be differentiated from a laceration of the external meatus.

Battle's sign:
Bruising over the mastoid
may take 24–48 hours to develop.

Patients with signs of basal fracture require prophylactic antibiotic treatment for at least seven days or if a CSF leak is present for seven days after this has stopped (see page 225).

3. Conscious level

Assess patient's conscious level in terms of *eye opening, verbal* and *motor response* on admission (see page 5) and record at regular intervals thereafter. An observation chart incorporating these features is essential and clearly shows the trend in the patient's condition. Deterioration in conscious level indicates the need for immediate investigation and action where appropriate.

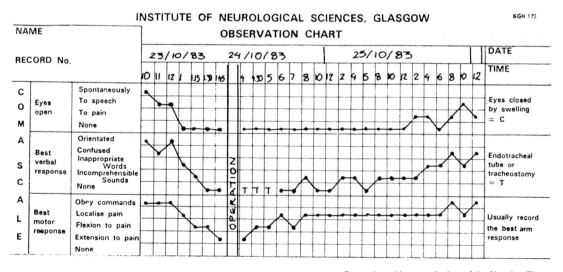

INSTITUTE OF NEUROLOGICAL SCIENCES, GLASGOW

OBSERVATION CHART

SGH 172

HEAD INJURY — CLINICAL ASSESSMENT

4. Pupil response

The light reflex (page 138) tests optic (II) and oculomotor (III) nerve function. Although II nerve dysfunction after head injury is important to record and may result in permanent visual impairment, it is the III nerve function which is the most useful indicator of an expanding intracranial lesion. Herniation of the medial temporal lobe through the tentorial hiatus directly damages the III nerve resulting in pupil dilatation with impaired or absent reaction to light. The *pupil dilates on the side of the expanding lesion* and is an important localising sign. With a further increase in intracranial pressure, bilateral III nerve palsies may occur.

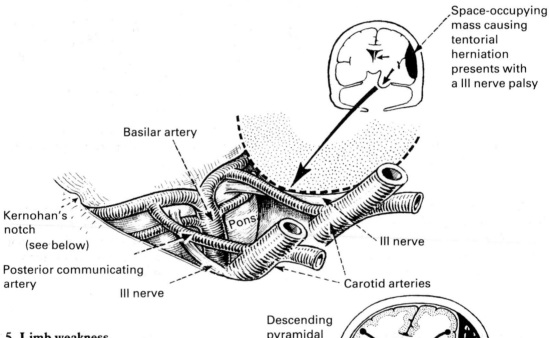

Space-occupying mass causing tentorial herniation presents with a III nerve palsy

Basilar artery

Kernohan's notch (see below)

Pons

III nerve

Posterior communicating artery

III nerve

Carotid arteries

5. Limb weakness

Determine limb weakness by comparing the response in each limb to painful stimuli (page 30). Hemiparesis or hemiplegia usually occurs in the limbs contralateral to the side of the lesion but may also occur in the ipsilateral limbs. This is due to indentation of the contralateral cerebral peduncle by the edge of the tentorium cerebelli (Kernohan's notch). Limb deficits are therefore of limited value in localising the site of the lesion.

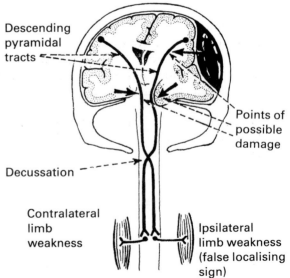

Descending pyramidal tracts

Points of possible damage

Decussation

Contralateral limb weakness

Ipsilateral limb weakness (false localising sign)

HEAD INJURY — CLINICAL ASSESSMENT

6. Eye movements

The presence or absence of abnormal eye movements is of limited value in immediate management, but provides a useful prognostic guide.

Eye movements may occur spontaneously, or can be elicited reflexly (page 30) by head rotation (oculocephalic reflex) or by caloric stimulation (oculovestibular reflex).

SPONTANEOUS
OCULOCEPHALIC
(Doll's eye)
REFLEX
OCULOVESTIBULAR REFLEX

Fast
corrective
phase (often absent in the
comatose patient)

Iced water

Abnormal eye movements may result from: brainstem dysfunction, damage to the nerves supplying the extraocular muscles or damage to the vestibular apparatus. Absent eye movements relate to low levels of responsiveness and indicate a gloomy prognosis.

Vital signs

At the beginning of the century, the eminent neurosurgeon Harvey Cushing noted that a rise in intracranical pressure led to a rise in blood pressure and a fall in pulse rate and produced abnormal respiratory patterns. In the past, much emphasis has been placed on close observation of these vital signs in patients with head injury. These changes, however, may not occur and when present are usually preceded by deterioration in conscious level. This last observation is therefore more relevant.

Cranial nerve lesions

Basal skull fracture or extracranial injury can result in damage to the cranial nerves. Evidence of this damage must be recorded but, with the exception of a III nerve lesion, does not usually help immediate management. Full cranial nerve examination is difficult in the comatose patient and this can await patient co-operation.

Clinical assessment cannot reliably distinguish the type or even the site of intracranial haematoma, but is invaluable in indicating the need for further investigation and in providing a baseline against which any change can be compared.

HEAD INJURY — INVESTIGATIVE APPROACH

IN THE ACCIDENT AND EMERGENCY DEPARTMENT

X-ray the skull if:
(plus cervical spine, chest, abdomen, pelvis and limbs if required)

– conscious level is impaired at the time of examination or if the patient has lost consciousness at any time since the injury
– neurological symptoms or signs are present
– CSF leak from the nose (rhinorrhoea) or ear (otorrhoea)
– penetrating injury is suspect
– significant scalp bruising or swelling
– patient assessment is difficult (e.g. alcohol intoxication).

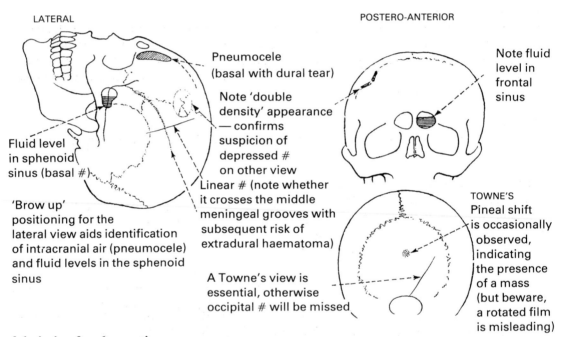

LATERAL

Pneumocele
(basal with dural tear)

Note 'double density' appearance
— confirms suspicion of depressed # on other view

Fluid level in sphenoid sinus (basal #)

Linear # (note whether it crosses the middle meningeal grooves with subsequent risk of extradural haematoma)

'Brow up' positioning for the lateral view aids identification of intracranial air (pneumocele) and fluid levels in the sphenoid sinus

A Towne's view is essential, otherwise occipital # will be missed

POSTERO-ANTERIOR

Note fluid level in frontal sinus

TOWNE'S
Pineal shift is occasionally observed, indicating the presence of a mass (but beware, a rotated film is misleading)

Admission for observation

Patients at risk of developing secondary complications (e.g. intracranial haematoma) require admission, i.e. patients with:
– a depressed conscious level (including confusion)
– focal neurological signs
– a skull fracture (base or vault)
– transitory loss of consciousness or post-traumatic amnesia if unsupervised at home.

IF IN DOUBT, ADMIT.

Risk of intracranial haematoma (requiring removal) in adult attending A & E departments after head injury.		
No skull #	— orientated	1 in 6000
No skull #	— not orientated	1 in 120
Skull #	— orientated	1 in 32
Skull #	— not orientated	1 in 4

Adapted with permission Mendelow et al 1983 ii: 1173–1176 British Medical Journal

HEAD INJURY — INVESTIGATIVE APPROACH

Neurosurgical referral/CT scan

IMMEDIATE
- Skull # with – confusion, or neurological symptoms or signs or epilepsy.
- Coma (with or without skull #), i.e. not obeying commands, no eye opening, no speech
- Deterioration in level of consciousness (e.g. confused verbal response ⟶ no verbal response).

DELAYED
- Persistent confusion or focal signs of > 8 hours duration.
- Compound depressed skull # (refer within 12 hours)
- Persistent CSF leak of > 7 days duration.

Transfer to the neurosurgical unit

Prior to the transfer, ensure that resuscitation is complete, and that more immediate problems have been dealt with (see page 217). Insert an oropharyngeal airway or intubate if necessary. Ventilate if the blood gases are inadequate ($P_{O_2} < 60$ mmHg or $P_{CO_2} > 45$ mmHg). If the patient's conscious level is deteriorating, an intravenous bolus infusion of 100 ml of 20% mannitol should 'buy time' by temporarily reducing the intracranial pressure.

CT scan in head injury

Scans must extend from the posterior fossa to the vertex, otherwise haematomas in these sites will be missed.

EXTRADURAL haematoma
—area of increased density, convex inwards. - - - - - - - - - -
Spread limited by dural adhesion to skull

- - - - - Midline shift with compression of ipsilateral ventricle

The contralateral ventricle often dilates due to obstruction at the foramen of Munro

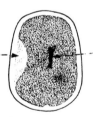

SUBDURAL haematoma — area of increased density spreading around surface of cerebral hemisphere. Subdural haematomas become isodense with brain 10–20 days following injury and hypodense thereafter.

'Burst' temporal lobe

'Burst' frontal lobe

INTRACEREBRAL haematoma —
'BURST LOBE' (± subdural haematoma)
— appears as an irregular area of increased density (blood clot) surrounded by area of low density (oedematous brain).

- - - - - overlying subdural haematoma

HEAD INJURY — INVESTIGATIVE APPROACH

CT scan in head injury (*contd*)
Whether a haematoma is present or not, look at the *basal cisterns.*

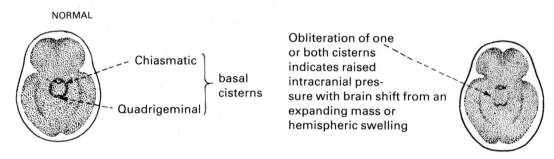

With *diffuse shearing injuries,* small haematomas may be seen on CT scan scattered throughout the white matter, particularly in the corpus callosum or in the superior cerebellar peduncle.

If *hydrocephalus* is present on the upper scan cuts, look carefully for a haematoma (extradural, subdural or intracerebral) in the posterior fossa, compressing and obstructing the 4th ventricle.

In the absence of CT scanning, ANGIOGRAPHY shows displacement of vessels and gives a useful guide to the haematoma site. Failing this, bilateral burr holes are placed in frontal, temporal and parietal sites; even in experienced hands, however, this exploratory approach will miss 30% of intracranial haematomas.

Further investigation may be required to exclude other coincidental or contributory causes of the head injury, e.g. drugs, alcohol, postictal state, encephalitis (Cause of coma, see page 82).

HEAD INJURY — MANAGEMENT

Management aims at preventing the development of secondary brain damage from intracranial haematoma, ischaemia, raised intracranial pressure with tentorial or tonsillar herniation and infection.
— Ensure the *airway is patent* and that *blood oxygenation is adequate. Intubation* is advisable in patients 'flexing to pain' or worse. *Artificial ventilation* may be required if respiratory movements are depressed or lung function is impaired, e.g. 'flail' segment, aspiration pneumonia, pulmonary contusion or fat emboli. Hypoxia can cause direct cerebral damage, but in addition causes vasodilatation resulting in an increase in cerebral blood volume with subsequent rise in ICP.
— A *space-occupying haematoma requires urgent evacuation* (see over). If the patient's conscious level is deteriorating, give an initial or repeat i.v. bolus of mannitol (100 ml of 20%).
— Scalp *lacerations* require cleaning, inspection to exclude an underlying depressed fracture and suturing.
— *Correct hypovolaemia* following blood loss — but avoid fluid overload as this may aggravate cerebral oedema. In adults, 2 litres/day of fluid is sufficient. Commence nasogastric fluids or oral fluids when feasible.

HEAD INJURY — MANAGEMENT

– Administer *prophylactic antibiotics* (e.g. penicillin and sulphadimidine) if clinical findings suggest a basal fracture. If a CSF leak persists for more than 7 days, operation is required. N.B. Although most clinicians still use antibiotics in patients with basal skull fracture, their value remains controversial as some believe they merely encourage growth of resistant organisms.
– *Anticonvulsants* (e.g. phenytoin) must be given intravenously if seizures occur; further seizures and in particular status epilepticus significantly increase the risk of cerebral anoxia.
– Consider *treatment of raised ICP*, when cerebral swelling occurs in the absence of a haematoma or in the postoperative period following removal of a haematoma (see below). *Brain protective agents*, e.g. Nimodipine, await evaluation. [*Steroids:* it is now well established that steroids, even in megadosage, are of no benefit in the management of the head-injured patient.]

INTRACRANIAL HAEMATOMA

Most intracranial haematomas require urgent evacuation — evident from the patient's clinical state combined with the CT scan appearance of a space-occupying mass.

Extradural haematoma

Using the CT scan the position of the extradural haematoma is accurately delineated and a 'horse shoe' craniotomy flap is turned over this area, allowing complete evacuation of the haematoma. For low temporal extradural haematomas, a 'question mark' flap may be more suitable. If patient deterioration is rapid, a burr hole and craniectomy positioned centrally over the haematoma may provide temporary relief, but this seldom provides adequate decompression.

Scalp flap

Bone flap overlying extradural haematoma

Subdural/intracerebral haematoma ('burst lobe')

Subdural and intracerebral haematomas usually arise from lacerations on the under-surface of the frontal and/or temporal lobes. Again the CT scan is useful in demonstrating the exact site. A 'question mark' flap permits good access to both frontal and temporal 'burst' lobes. The subdural collection is evacuated and any underlying intracerebral haematoma is removed along with necrotic brain.

N.B. Burr holes are insufficient to evacuate an acute subdural haematoma or to deal with any underlying cortical damage.

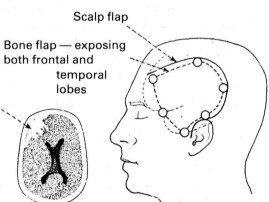

Scalp flap

Bone flap — exposing both frontal and temporal lobes

HEAD INJURY — MANAGEMENT

INTRACRANIAL HAEMATOMA (*contd*)

Conservative management of traumatic intracranial haematomas

Not all patients with traumatic intracranial haematomas deteriorate. In some, the haematomas are small and clearly do not require evacuation. In others, however, the decision to operate or not proves difficult, e.g. the CT scan may reveal a moderate-sized haematoma with minimal or no mass effect in a conscious but confused patient.

If conservative management is adopted, careful observation in a neurosurgical unit is essential. Any deterioration indicates the need for operation. In this group of patients, intracranial pressure monitoring may serve as a useful guide. An intracranial pressure of 30 mmHg or more suggests that haematoma evacuation is required as the likelihood of subsequent deterioration with continued conservative management would be high.

DIFFUSE BRAIN DAMAGE/NEGATIVE CT SCAN

A proportion of patients have no intracranial haematoma on CT scan or have only a small haematoma causing no mass effect.

In these patients, coma or impairment of conscious level may be due to:

– *diffuse shearing injury* — suspect if no improvement in conscious level since the impact.

– *cerebral ischaemic damage*
– *cerebral swelling*
– *fat emboli*
– *meningitis*

suspect if deterioration is delayed — a patient who talks after impact does not have a significant shearing injury.

Several of these factors may coexist and may also contribute to brain damage in patients with intracranial haematoma.

The management principles outlined above apply; in particular it is essential to ensure that respiratory function is adequate.

Fat emboli usually occur one or two days after injury and may be related to fracture manipulation; deterioration of respiratory function usually accompanies cerebral damage and most patients require ventilation.

Meningitis may occur several days after injury in the presence of basal fractures, but this is rare when prophylactic antibiotics are given.

Cerebral swelling may occur at any time after injury and cause a rise in intracranial pressure.

HEAD INJURY — MANAGEMENT

TREATMENT OF RAISED INTRACRANIAL PRESSURE (ICP)

Treatment of raised intracranial pressure (*in the absence of any identifiable cause, e.g. haematoma or* ↑ P_{CO_2}) is a controversial topic in head injury management. Some believe that active reduction of an elevated ICP significantly reduces management mortality and morbidity. Others feel that if brain damage is severe enough to cause a rise in ICP, then artificially reducing the ICP to normal levels does not alter the extent of the damage, or improve outcome. In adults, there is as yet no conclusive evidence that active ICP reduction improves mortality or morbidity. In children, however, the pathogenesis of raised ICP may differ; some studies suggest that cerebral vasodilatation with a subsequent increase in cerebral blood volume is a major factor, rather than an increase in brain water content (cerebral oedema). If so, treatment of raised ICP may well benefit.

PATIENT SELECTION: Consider patients with a 'flexion' motor response or worse (a response of 'localising' to pain signifies a milder degree of injury and spontaneous recovery is likely). Insert a ventricular catheter and monitor ICP. If ICP is high (e.g. > 30 mm Hg) this may be reduced by:

– *hyperventilation*, reducing the P_{CO_2} to 3.5 kPa ⎫
– *repeated mannitol infusion* ⎬ see page 80.
– *CSF drainage* ⎭

These artificial methods of ICP reduction are maintained until the level falls spontaneously to within normal limits. In many patients, this treatment fails to produce a sustained effect and the ICP returns to previous levels or continues to rise unabated until death ensues.

Some clinicians use barbiturate therapy when the ICP fails to respond to other measures, but its value remains unproven.

Repeat CT scanning
Indications:
Delayed deterioration in clinical state ⎫
          or ⎬ in patients with diffuse injury or following evacuation of an intracranial haematoma
Failure to improve after 48 hours ⎭

Occasionally, small areas of 'insignificant' contusion on an initial CT scan may develop into a space-occupying haematoma requiring evacuation. Following haematoma evacuation, recollection may occur in 5–10% of cases.

227

DEPRESSED SKULL FRACTURE

This injury is caused by a blow from a sharp object. Since diffuse 'deceleration' damage is minimal, patients seldom lose consciousness.

SIMPLE DEPRESSED FRACTURE (closed injury)
There is no overlying laceration and no risk of infection. Operation is not required except for cosmetic reasons. Removal of any bone spicules imbedded in brain tissue does not reverse neuronal damage.

COMPOUND DEPRESSED FRACTURE (open injury)
A scalp laceration is related to (but does not necessarily overlie) the depressed bone segments. Failure to detect a compound depressed fracture with an associated dural tear is likely to result in meningitis or cerebral abscess.

Investigation
Double density appearance on *skull X-ray* suggests depression but tangential views may be required to establish the diagnosis. Impairment of conscious level or the presence of focal signs indicate the need for a *CT scan* to exclude underlying extradural haematoma or severe cortical contusion.

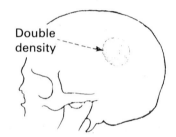

Double density

Tangential view

Management

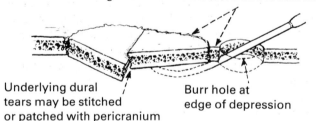

Bone edges nibbled away until fragments can be elevated and removed.

Underlying dural tears may be stitched or patched with pericranium

Burr hole at edge of depression

The aim of treatment is prevention of infection. The wound is debrided and the fragments elevated within 24 hours from injury. Bone fragments are either removed or replaced after washing with antiseptic. Antibiotics are not essential unless the wound is excessively dirty.

If the venous sinuses are involved in the depressed fracture, then operative risks from excessive bleeding may outweigh the risk of infection and antibiotic treatment alone is given.

Complications
Most patients make a rapid and full recovery, but a few develop complications:
Infection occurs when treatment is delayed, or debridement inadequate, and may lead to meningitis or abscess formation.
Epilepsy: Early epilepsy (in the first week) occurs in 10% of patients with depressed fracture. Late epilepsy develops in 15% overall, but is especially common when the dura is torn, when focal signs are present, when post-traumatic amnesia exceeds 24 hours or when early epilepsy has occurred (the risk ranges from 3 – 70%, depending on the number of the above factors involved). Elevation of the bone fragments does not alter the incidence of epilepsy.

DELAYED EFFECTS OF HEAD INJURY

EPILEPSY
Post-traumatic epilepsy
Post-traumatic epilepsy may be categorised into two types:
early — occurring in the first week from injury, *late* — occurring after the first week from injury.

Early epilepsy
Early epilepsy occurs in 5% of patients admitted to hospital with non-missile (i.e. deceleration) injuries. It is particularly frequent in the first 24 hours after injury. Focal seizures are as common as generalised seizures. Status epilepticus occurs in 10%.

    The risk of early epilepsy is high in – children
                       – patients with prolonged post-traumatic amnesia
                       – patients with an intracranial haematoma
                       – patients with a compound depressed fracture .

Late epilepsy
Late epilepsy also occurs in about 5% of all patients admitted to hospital after head injury. It usually presents in the first year, but in some the first attack occurs as long as 10 years from the injury. Usually seizures are generalised, but temporal lobe epilepsy (complex partial seizures) occurs in 20%. Late epilepsy is prevalent in patients with – early epilepsy
                                        – intracranial haematoma
                                      – compound depressed fracture.

    Prophylactic anticonvulsants appear to be of little benefit in preventing the development of an epileptogenic focus. Management is discussed on page 98.

CEREBROSPINAL FLUID (CSF) LEAK
After head injury a basal fracture may cause a fistulous communication between the CSF space and the paranasal sinuses or the middle ear. Profuse CSF leaks (rhinorrhoea or otorrhoea) are readily detectable, but brain may partially plug the defect and the leak may be minimal or absent. Failure to protect these patients with antibiotics may result in meningitis. When this is associated with anterior fossa fractures, it is usually pneumococcal; when associated with fractures through the petrous bone, a variety of organisms may be involved.
Clinical signs of a basal fracture have previously been described (page 218). The patient may comment on a 'salty taste' in his mouth. Anosmia suggests avulsion of the olfactory bulb from the cribriform plate.

Management

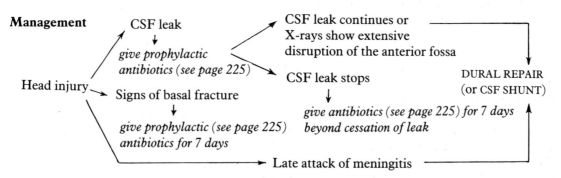

DELAYED EFFECTS OF HEAD INJURY

CSF LEAK (*contd*)
Preoperative investigations

X-ray or tomography of the anterior fossa or petrous bone may help identify the fracture site.

CT cisternography — CT scanning after running contrast injected into the lumbar theca, up to the basal cisterns may identify the exact site of the leak.

CSF isotope infusion studies combined with pledget insertion into the nasal recesses may also be of value, but results can be misleading.

Operation

As fractures of the anterior fossa often extend across the midline, a bifrontal exploration is required. The dural tear is repaired with fascia lata or lyophilised dural substitute. A CSF leak through the middle ear requires a subtemporal approach.

Failure to repair a CSF fistula may result from impaired CSF absorption with an intermittent or persistent elevation of ICP. In these patients a CSF shunt may be of benefit.

POSTCONCUSSIONAL SYMPTOMS

Even after relatively minor head injury, patients may have persistent symptoms of:

- headache, dizziness and increased irritability
- difficulty in concentration and in coping with work
- fatigue and depression.

This condition was once thought to have a purely psychological basis, but it is now recognised that in an injury of sufficient severity to cause loss of consciousness, or a period of post-traumatic amnesia, some neuronal damage occurs; studies show a distinct delay in information processing in these patients, requiring several weeks to resolve. Vestibular 'concussion' (end-organ damage) may contribute to the symptomatology ('dizziness' and vertigo).

CUMULATIVE BRAIN DAMAGE

The effects of repeated neuronal damage are cumulative; when this exceeds the capacity for compensation, permanent evidence of brain damage ensues. The 'punch-drunk' state is well recognised in boxers, but recent reports suggest that dementia may also occur from repeated head injury in jockeys.

DELAYED EFFECTS OF HEAD INJURY

CRANIAL NERVE DAMAGE

Cranial nerve damage occurs in about one-third of patients with severe head injury, but treatment is seldom of benefit. These lesions may contribute towards the patient's residual disability.

Nerve	Cause of damage	Clinical problem	Management	Prognosis
I	Usually associated with anterior fossa fracture and CSF rhinorrhoea	Anosmia	Nil	Recovery often occurs in a few months
II	Optic nerve usually damaged in the optic foramen. Chiasmal damage occasionally occurs. [N.B. Visual loss may also occur from damage to the globe, occipital cortex or optic radiations]	Visual loss or field defect in one eye Bitemporal hemianopia.	Nil. Local eye/orbital damage may need treatment	Recovery seldom occurs
III IV VI	IÍI nerve damage usually results from tentorial herniation but can also occur in fractures involving the superior orbital fissure or cavernous sinus. IV nerve damage is uncommon. VI nerve damage is usually associated with fractures of the petrous or sphenoid bones	Pupil inequality, ptosis and disturbance of ocular movements	Nil [other than removing cause of tentorial herniation]	Recovery usually occurs
V	Occasionally follows petrous or sphenoid fractures	Facial analgesia / anaesthesia	Nil	Usually permanent
VII	Associated with petrous fracture	Immediate or delayed facial palsy	Otologists occasionally recommend decompression. Early steroid therapy may benefit	Immediate lesions have a poor prognosis; delayed lesions usually recover
VIII	Petrous fracture may damage: – nerve – cochlea – ossicles Haemotympanum may result	Vertigo, 'dizziness', hearing loss, tinnitus	Ossicular damage may benefit from operation	Vestibular symptoms usually improve after several weeks. Nerve deafness is usually permanent. Conductive deafness from haemotympanum should gradually improve
IX, X XI, XII	Associated with very severe basal fractures or extracranial injury	Patient seldom survives primary damage		

231

DELAYED EFFECTS OF HEAD INJURY

OUTCOME AFTER SEVERE HEAD INJURY

Head injury remains a major cause of death, especially in the young. Of those patients who survive the initial impact and remain in coma for at least 6 hours, approximately 40% die within 6 months. The extent of recovery in the remainder depends on the severity of injury. Residual disabilities include both mental (impaired intellect, memory and behavioural problems) and physical defects (hemiparesis and dysphasia). Most recovery occurs within the first 6 months after injury, but improvement may continue for years. *Physiotherapy* and *occupational therapy* play an important role not only in minimising contractures and improving limb power and function but also in stimulating patient motivation.

Outcome is best assessed in terms of *dependence*. Even after severe injury most survivors regain an independent existence and may return to their premorbid social and occupational activities. Inevitably some remain severely disabled requiring long-term care, but fortunately few are left in a persistent vegetative state with no awareness or ability to communicate with their environment.

Prognostic features
The duration of coma relates closely to the severity of injury and to the final outcome, but in the early stages after injury the clinician must rely on other features — age, eye opening, verbal and motor responses, pupil response and eye movements.

CHRONIC SUBDURAL HAEMATOMA

Subdivision of subdural haematomas into acute and subacute forms serves no practical purpose. Chronic subdural haematoma however is best considered as a separate entity, differing both in presentation and management.

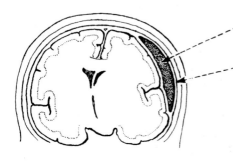

Chronic subdural haematoma — fluid may range from a faint yellow to a dark brown colour

A membrane grows out from the dura to envelop the haematoma

Chronic subdural haematomas occur predominantly in *infancy* and in the *elderly*. Trauma is the likely cause, although a history of this is not always obtained.

Predisposing factors

- Cerebral atrophy
- Low CSF pressure
  (after a shunt or fistula)   cause stretching of
                                    bridging veins
- Alcoholism
- Coagulation disorder

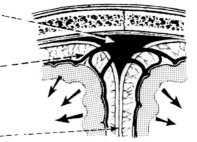

Sagittal sinus

Falx

Breakdown of protein within the haematoma and a subsequent rise in osmotic pressure was originally believed to account for the gradual enlargement of the untreated subdural haematoma. Recent studies showing equality of osmotic pressures in blood and haematoma fluid cast doubt on this theory and recurrent bleeding into the cavity is now known to play an important role.

Clinical features tend to be non-specific.

- Dementia.
- Deterioration in conscious level, occasionally with fluctuating course.
- Symptoms and signs of raised ICP.
- Focal signs occasionally occur, especially limb weakness. This may be ipsilateral to the side of the lesion, i.e. a false localising sign (see page 220).

CHRONIC SUBDURAL HAEMATOMA

Diagnosis

An *isotope brain scan* reliably detects chronic subdural haematomas, showing an area of increased uptake over the cortical surface.

Most patients with suspected chronic subdural haematoma are referred for a *CT scan*. Appearances depend on the time between injury and scan.

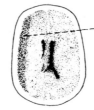

Injury > 3 weeks old: low density seen over hemisphere convexity

With injuries 1–3 weeks old, the subdural haematoma may be isodense with brain tissue.

If CT scan shows midline shift without any obvious extra- or intracerebral lesion, look at the shape of the ventricles.

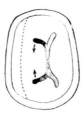

Extracerebral collection, i.e. chronic subdural haematoma, causes approximation of frontal and occipital horns

Separation of the frontal and occipital horns suggests an intrinsic lesion, e.g. encephalitis rather than a surface collection

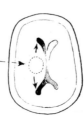

Management

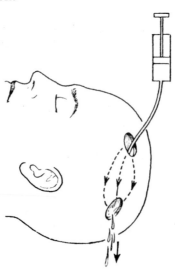

Adult

The haematoma is evacuated through two or three burr holes and the cavity is irrigated with saline. Drains may be left in the subdural space and nursing in the head-down position may help prevent recollection.

Craniotomy with excision of the membrane is seldom required.

In patients who have no depressed conscious level, conservative treatment with steroids over several weeks may result in resolution.

Infants

The haematoma is evacuated by repeated needle aspiration through the anterior fontanelle. Persistent subdural collections require a subdural peritoneal shunt. As in adults, craniotomy is seldom necessary.

CEREBROVASCULAR DISEASES

Vascular diseases of the nervous system are amongst the most frequent causes of admission to hospital. The annual rate of stroke in the UK varies regionally between 150–200/100 000.

Better control of hypertension, reduced incidence of heart disease and a greater awareness of all risk factors have combined to reduce the frequency of 'stroke'. Despite this, stroke still ranks third behind heart disease and cancer as a cause of death in affluent societies.

RISK FACTORS

Prevention of cerebrovascular disease is more likely to reduce death and disability than any medical or surgical advance in management. Prevention depends upon the identification of risk factors and their correction.

Hypertension

Hypertension is a major factor in the development of thrombotic cerebral infarction and intracranial haemorrhage.

There is no critical blood pressure level; the risk is related to the height of blood pressure and increases throughout the whole range from normal to hypertensive.

Systolic hypertension (frequent in the elderly) is also a significant factor and not as harmless as previously thought.

Cardiac disease

Cardiac enlargement, failure and arrhythmias, as well as rheumatic heart disease, mitral valve prolapse and, rarely, cardiac myxoma are all associated with an increased risk of stroke.

Diabetes

The risk of cerebral infarction is increased twofold in diabetes. More effective treatment of diabetes has not reduced the frequency of atherosclerotic sequelae.

Heredity

Close relatives are at only slightly greater risk than non-genetically related family members of a stroke patient. Diabetes and hypertension show familial propensity thus clouding the significance of pure hereditary factors.

Blood lipids, smoking, diet/obesity, soft water

These factors are much less significant than in the genesis of coronary artery disease.

Race

Alterations in life style, diet and environment probably explain the geographical variations more than racial tendencies.

Haematocrit

A high blood haemoglobin concentration (or haematocrit level) is associated with an increased incidence of cerebral infarction. Other haematological factors, such as decreased fibrinolysis, are important also.

Oral contraceptives

The evidence of pill-related stroke is inconclusive. A recent prospective study has suggested an increased risk of subarachnoid haemorrhage rather than thromboembolic stroke.

235

CEREBROVASCULAR DISEASE — MECHANISMS

'Stroke' is a generic term, lacking pathological meaning. Cerebrovascular diseases can be defined as those in which brain disease occurs secondary to a pathological disorder of blood vessels (usually arteries) or blood supply.

1. Occlusion by thrombus or embolus.

Whatever the mechanism, the resultant effect on the brain is either:
    ischaemia/infarction, or
    haemorrhagic disruption.

2. Rupture of vessel wall.

3. Disease of vessel wall.

4. Disturbance of normal properties of blood.

Of all strokes: — 85% are due to INFARCTION
               — 15% are due to HAEMORRHAGE.

CEREBROVASCULAR DISEASE – NATURAL HISTORY

Approximately one-third of all 'strokes' are fatal. The age of the patient, the anatomical size of the lesion, the degree of deficit and the underlying cause all influence the outcome.

Immediate outcome
In cerebral haemorrhage, mortality approaches 70%.
    Cerebral infarction fares better, with an immediate mortality of less than 25%, fatal lesions being large with associated oedema and brain shift.
    Embolic infarction carries a better outcome than thrombotic infarction.
    Fatal cases of infarction die either at onset or else, more commonly, after the first week from cardiovascular or respiratory complications.
    The level of consciousness on admission to hospital gives a good indication to immediate outcome. The deeper the conscious level the graver the prognosis.

Long-term outcome
The prognosis following infarction due to thrombosis or embolisation from diseased neck vessels or heart is dependent on the progression of the underlying atherosclerotic disease. Recurrent cerebral infarction, symptoms of coronary artery disease and/or peripheral vascular disease may ensue.
    The long-term prognosis following survival from haemorrhage depends upon the cause and the treatment.
    Recent studies report a cumulative reinfarction rate of 40% after 5 years for men and 20% for women.

CEREBROVASCULAR DISEASE — PATHOPHYSIOLOGY

Standard techniques of cerebral blood flow (CBF) measurement provide information on both global and regional flow in patients with cerebral ischaemia or infarction. Recent availability of positron emission tomography (PET), recording oxygen and glucose metabolism, as well as blood flow and blood volume, gives a more detailed and accurate understanding of pathophysiological changes after stroke.

Changes in cerebral infarction

ISCHAEMIC HEMISPHERE

NON-ISCHAEMIC HEMISPHERE

Reduction in global CBF

Mild reduction in global CBF — perhaps due to transneuronal depression of metabolism in the unaffected hemisphere — diaschisis.

In the infarcted area and its surroundings, more subtle changes of regional cerebral blood flow (rCBF) are detected.

In the normal brain, cerebral blood flow to a particular part varies depending on the metabolic requirements, i.e. the supply of O_2 and glucose is 'coupled' to the tissue needs. After infarction, between areas of reduced flow and areas of luxury perfusion, lie areas of *relative luxury perfusion* where reduced flow exceeds the tissue requirements, i.e. 'uncoupling' of flow and metabolism has occurred.

Areas of *reduced flow* are bordered by areas of increased flow — *luxury perfusion* — due to vasodilatation of arteriolar bed in response to lactic acidosis.

These changes in rCBF are transient and revert to normal within days of the onset. The degree of disturbance of rCBF correlates with outcome. Flow of < 28 ml/min/100g results in the development of the morphological changes of infarction.

Pathophysiology of ischaemia

Progression from *reversible ischaemia* to infarction depends upon the *degree* and *duration* of the reduced blood flow.

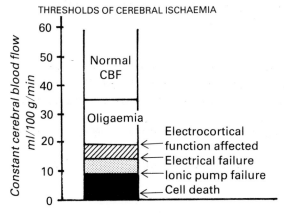

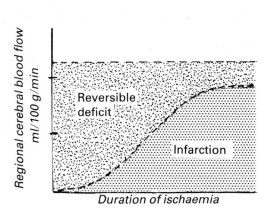

CEREBROVASCULAR DISEASE — PATHOPHYSIOLOGY

Ischaemic cascade
A significant fall in cerebral blood flow produces a cascade of events which, if unchecked, lead to the production and accumulation of toxic compounds and cell death.

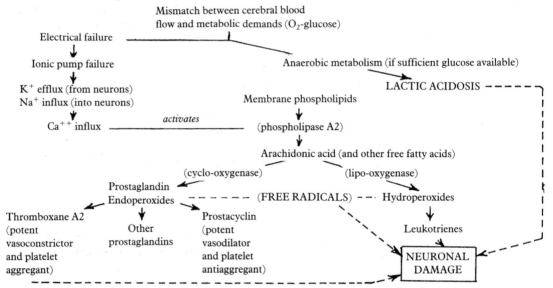

Role of neurotransmitters
Recent research has shown that one of the amino acid excitatory neurotransmitters, Glutamate, in *excess* is a powerful Neurotoxin, playing an important role in ischaemic brain damage.

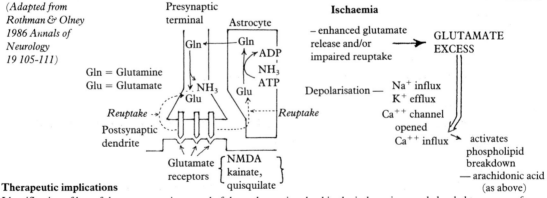

Therapeutic implications
Identification of harmful neurotransmitters and of the pathways involved in the ischaemic cascade has led to a surge of interest in *brain protective agents* —

Ca^{++} *antagonists:* unsuccessful in preventing 'vasospasm', recent studies of Nimodipine in patients with SAH have shown a significant reduction in ischaemic complications. This drug acts by opening up the collateral circulation and by blocking Ca^{++} influx.

Glutamine antagonists (e.g. NMDA antagonist — 'MK801'): significantly reduces ischaemia in animal studies. Toxicity has as yet prevented clinical trials.

Barbiturates: these reduce cerebral metabolism, thereby reducing neuronal requirements. They also block free radical production. The dosage required to lower metabolism produces significant hypotension and benefits remain unproven.

Thromboxane A2 inhibitors
Prostacyclin   } Early studies suggest that these agents may produce
Free radical scavengers } some benefit in reducing ischaemia.

CEREBROVASCULAR DISEASE — CAUSES

OCCLUSION (Atheromatous/thrombotic)

1. Large vessel occlusion or stenosis.

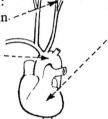

2. Branch vessel occlusion or stenosis.

3. Perforating vessel occlusion (lacunar infarction)

EMBOLISATION from:

1. Atheromatous plaque in the extracranial arteries or from the aortic arch.

2. The heart:
   – rheumatic heart disease
   – ischaemic heart disease
   – bacterial endocarditis
   – atrial myxoma
   – prosthetic valves
   – prolapsing mitral valve.

3. Miscellaneous:
   – fat emboli
   – air emboli
   – tumour emboli.

DISEASES OF THE VESSEL WALL

Arteritis
{
rheumatoid vasculitis
systemic lupus erythematosus (SLE)
polyarteritis nodosa
giant cell arteritis — temporal arteritis
Takayashu's arteritis

granulomatous vasculitis
}

Miscellaneous
{
syphilitic vasculitis
fibromuscular hyperplasia
sarcoidosis
}

{
Wegener's granulomatosis
granulomatous angiitis of the nervous system
}

DISEASES OF BLOOD

Coagulopathies
Haemoglobinopathies
Idiopathic and thrombotic thrombocytopenic purpura
Hyperviscosity syndromes, e.g. polycythaemia, thrombocythaemia

VENOUS THROMBOSIS

Venous thrombosis may occur with infection and dehydration or in association with arterial occlusion when related to oestrogen excess.

HAEMORRHAGE

1. Intracerebral haemorrhage (or intra-parenchymal haemorrhage) due to:
   Hypertension. Aneurysm. Neoplasm. Trauma
   Anticoagulant therapy Septicaemia
   Anticoagulant therapy. Septicaemia
   Disseminated intravascular coagulopathy
   Thrombotic thrombocytopaenic purpura
   Coagulation disorders, e.g. haemophilia

2. Subarachnoid haemorrhage due to:
   Aneurysm
   Arteriovenous malformation
   Trauma
   Tumour
   Anticoagulant therapy
   Coagulation disorders, e.g. haemophilia

239

OCCLUSIVE AND STENOTIC CEREBROVASCULAR DISEASE

PATHOLOGY
The normal vessel wall comprises:

Intima: a single endothelial cell lining.

Media: fibroblasts and smooth muscle with collagen support and elastic tissue.

Adventitia: mainly composed of thick collagen fibres.

Within brain and spinal cord tissue the adventitia is usually very thin and the elastic lamina between media and adventitia less apparent.

The intima is an important barrier to leakage of blood and constituents into the vessel wall. In the development of the atherosclerotic plaque, damage to the endothelium of the intima is the primary event.

The atherosclerotic plaque
Following intimal damage:

Intimal cells
Smooth muscle cells laden with
 cholesterol, lipids, phospholipids
Collagen and elastic fibres
} build up subintimally.

Haemorrhage may occur within the plaque or the plaque may ulcerate into the lumen of the vessel forming an intraluminal mural thrombus. Either way, the lumen of the involved vessel is narrowed (stenosed) or blocked (occluded).

The plaque itself may give rise to emboli. Cholesterol is present partly in crystal form and fragments following plaque rupture may be sufficiently large to occlude the lumen of distal vessels. The cholesterol esters, lipids and phospholipids each play a role in the aggregation of such emboli.

The carotid bifurcation in the neck is a frequent site at which the atheromatous plaque causes stenosis or occlusion.

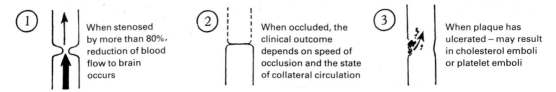

(1) When stenosed by more than 80%, reduction of blood flow to brain occurs

(2) When occluded, the clinical outcome depends on speed of occlusion and the state of collateral circulation

(3) When plaque has ulcerated – may result in cholesterol emboli or platelet emboli

Platelet emboli arise from thrombus developed over the damaged endothelium. This thrombus is produced partly by platelets coming into contact with exposed collagen fibres. Endothelial cells synthesise PROSTACYCLIN which is a potent vasodilator and inhibitor of platelet aggregation. THROMBOXANE A2, synthesised by platelets, has opposite effects. In thrombus formation these two PROSTAGLANDINS actively compete with each other.

CLINICAL SYNDROMES — LARGE VESSEL OCCLUSION

OCCLUSION OF THE INTERNAL CAROTID ARTERY — may present in a 'stuttering' manner due to progressive narrowing of the lumen or recurrent emboli.

The degree of deficit varies — occlusion may be asymptomatic and identified only at autopsy, or a catastrophic infarction may result.

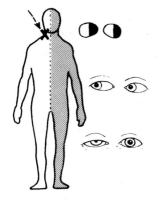

In the most extreme cases there may be:

    Slow mentation → deterioration of conscious level

    Homonymous hemianopia of the contralateral side

    Contralateral hemiplegia

    Contralateral hemisensory disturbance

    Gaze palsy to the opposite side — eyes deviated to the side of the lesion

A partial Horner's syndrome may develop on the side of the occlusion (involvement of sympathetic fibres on the internal carotid wall).

Occlusion of the dominant hemisphere side will result in a global aphasia.

Examination of the neck will reveal:

    Absent carotid pulsation at the angle of the jaw with poorly conducted heart sounds along the internal carotid artery.

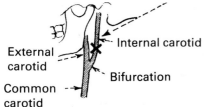

Prodromal symptoms prior to occlusion may take the form of monocular blindness — AMAUROSIS FUGAX and transient hemisensory or hemimotor disturbance

(see page 253).

The origins of the vessels from the aortic arch are such that an *innominate artery occlusion* will result not only in the clinical picture of carotid occlusion but will produce diminished blood flow and hence blood pressure in the right arm.

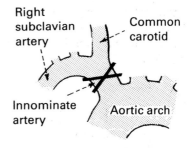

The outcome of carotid occlusion depends on the collateral blood supply primarily from the circle of Willis, but, in addition, the external carotid may provide flow to the *anterior and middle cerebral arteries* through meningeal branches and retrogradely through the ophthalmic artery to the *internal carotid artery*.

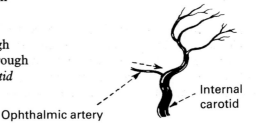

241

CLINICAL SYNDROMES — LARGE VESSEL OCCLUSION

ANTERIOR CEREBRAL ARTERY

Anatomy

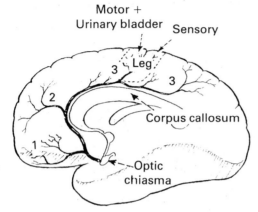

Medial surface of right cerebral hemisphere

The anterior cerebral artery is a branch of the internal carotid and runs above the optic nerve to follow the curve of the corpus callosum. Soon after its origin the vessel is joined by the anterior communicating artery. Deep branches pass to the anterior part of the internal capsule and basal nuclei.

Cortical branches supply the medial surface of the hemisphere:
1. Orbital
2. Frontal
3. Parietal.

Clinical features

The anterior cerebral artery may be occluded by embolus or thrombus. The clinical picture depends on the site of occlusion (especially in relation to the anterior communicating artery) and anatomical variation, e.g. both anterior cerebral arteries may arise from one side by enlargement of the anterior communicating artery.

Occlusion proximal to the anterior communicating artery is normally well tolerated because of the cross flow.

Distal occlusion results in weakness and cortical sensory loss in the contralateral lower limb with associated incontinence. Occasionally a contralateral grasp reflex is present.

Proximal occlusion when both anterior cerebral vessels arise from the same side results in 'cerebral' paraplegia with lower limb weakness, sensory loss, incontinence and presence of grasp, snout and palmomental reflexes.

Bilateral frontal lobe infarction may result in *akinetic mutism* (page 107) or deterioration in conscious level.

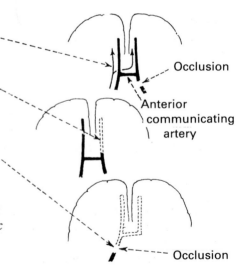

CLINICAL SYNDROMES — LARGE VESSEL OCCLUSION

MIDDLE CEREBRAL ARTERY

Anatomy

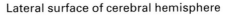

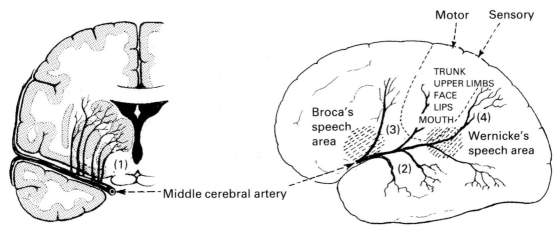

The middle cerebral artery is the largest branch of the internal carotid artery. It gives off (1) deep branches (perforating vessels — lenticulostriate) which supply the anterior limb of the internal capsule and part of the basal nuclei. It then passes out to the lateral surface of the cerebral hemisphere at the insula of the lateral sulcus. Here it gives off cortical branches (2) temporal, (3) frontal, (4) parietal.

Clinical features
The middle cerebral artery may be occluded by embolus or thrombus. The clinical picture depends upon the site of occlusion and whether dominant or non-dominant hemisphere is affected.

Occlusion at the insula

All cortical branches are involved —
Contralateral hemiplegia (leg relatively spared)
Contralateral hemianaesthesia and hemianopia
Aphasia (dominant)
Neglect of contralateral limbs and
Dressing difficulty (non-dominant).

When cortical branches are affected individually, the clinical picture is less severe, e.g. involvement of parietal branches alone may produce Wernicke's dysphasia with no limb weakness or sensory loss.

The deep branches (perforating vessels) of the middle cerebral artery may be a source of haemorrhage or small infarcts (lacunes — see later).

243

CLINICAL SYNDROMES — LARGE VESSEL OCCLUSION

VERTEBRAL ARTERY OCCLUSION

Anatomy

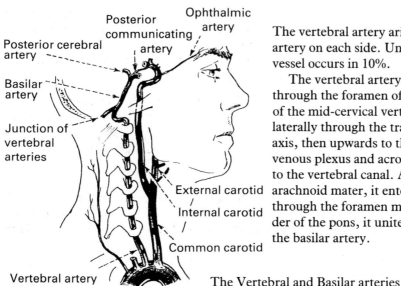

The Vertebral and Basilar arteries

The vertebral artery arises from the subclavian artery on each side. Underdevelopment of one vessel occurs in 10%.

The vertebral artery runs from its origin through the foramen of the transverse processes of the mid-cervical vertebrae. It then passes laterally through the transverse process of the axis, then upwards to the atlas accompanied by a venous plexus and across the suboccipital triangle to the vertebral canal. After piercing the dura and arachnoid mater, it enters the cranial cavity through the foramen magnum. At the lower border of the pons, it unites with its fellow to form the basilar artery.

The vertebral artery and its branches supply the medulla and the inferior surface of the cerebellum before forming the basilar artery.

Clinical features

Occlusion of the vertebral artery, when low in the neck, is compensated by anastomotic channels.

When one vertebral artery is hypoplastic, occlusion of the other is equivalent to basilar artery occlusion.

Only the posterior inferior cerebellar artery (PICA) depends solely on flow through the vertebral artery. Vertebral artery occlusion may therefore present as a PICA syndrome (page 248).

The close relationship of the vertebral artery to the cervical spine is important. Rarely, damage at intervertebral foramina or the atlanto-axial joints following subluxation may result in intimal damage, thrombus formation and embolisation.

Vertebral artery compression during neck extension may cause symptoms of intermittent vertebrobasilar insufficiency.

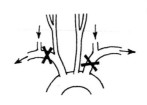

✗ Stenosis of the proximal left or right subclavian artery may result in retrograde flow down the vertebral artery on exercising the arm. This is commonly asymptomatic and demonstrated incidentally by Doppler techniques or angiography. Occasionally symptoms of vertebrobasilar insufficiency arise — *subclavian 'steal' syndrome*. Surgical reconstruction or bypass of the subclavian artery may be indicated.

CLINICAL SYNDROMES — LARGE VESSEL OCCLUSION

BASILAR ARTERY OCCLUSION

Anatomy

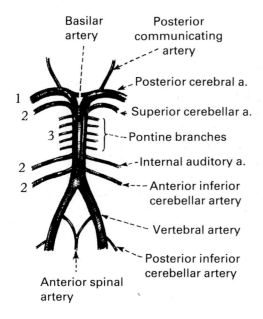

Basilar artery
Posterior communicating artery
Posterior cerebral a.
Superior cerebellar a.
Pontine branches
Internal auditory a.
Anterior inferior cerebellar artery
Vertebral artery
Posterior inferior cerebellar artery
Anterior spinal artery

The basilar artery supplies the brain stem from medulla upwards and divides eventually into posterior cerebral arteries as well as posterior communicating arteries which run forward to join the anterior circulation (circle of Willis).

Branches can be classified into:
1. Posterior cerebral arteries
2. Long circumflex branches
3. Paramedian branches.

Clinical features
Prodromal symptoms are common and may take the form of diplopia, visual field loss, intermittent memory disturbance and a whole constellation of other brain stem symptoms:
- vertigo
- ataxia
- paresis
- paraesthesia

The *complete basilar syndrome* following occlusion consists of:
- impairment of consciousness → coma
- bilateral motor and sensory dysfunction
- cerebellar signs
- cranial nerve signs indicative of the level of occlusion.

The clinical picture is variable. Occasionally basilar thrombosis is an incidental finding at autopsy.

'Top of basilar' occlusion: This results in lateral midbrain, thalamic, occipital and medial temporal lobe infarction. Abnormal movements (hemiballismus) are associated with visual loss, pupillary abnormalities, gaze palsies, impaired conscious level and disturbances of behaviour.

Paramedian perforating vessel occlusion gives rise to the 'LOCKED-IN' SYNDROME (page 249) and LACUNAR infarction (page 250).

CLINICAL SYNDROMES — LARGE VESSEL OCCLUSION

POSTERIOR CEREBRAL ARTERY

Anatomy

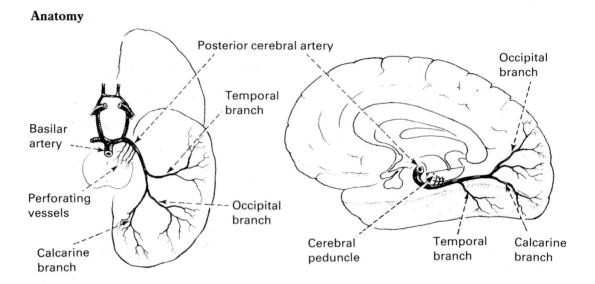

Undersurface of left cerebral hemisphere   Medial surface of right hemisphere

The posterior cerebral arteries are the terminal branches of the basilar artery. Small perforating branches supply midbrain structures, choroid plexus and posterior thalamus. Cortical branches supply the undersurface of the temporal lobe — temporal branch; and occipital and visual cortex — occipital and calcarine branches.

Clinical features

Proximal occlusion by thrombus or embolism will involve perforating branches and structures supplied:

> *Midbrain syndrome* — III nerve palsy with contralateral
> > hemiplegia — WEBER'S SYNDROME.
>
> *Thalamic syndromes* — chorea or hemiballismus with hemisensory disturbance.

Occlusion of cortical vessels will produce a different picture with visual field loss (homonymous hemianopia) and sparing of macular vision (the posterior tip of the occipital lobe, i.e. the macular area, is also supplied by the middle cerebral artery).

Posterior cortical infarction in the dominant hemisphere may produce problems in naming colours and objects.

CLINICAL SYNDROMES — BRANCH OCCLUSION

BASILAR ARTERY – LONG CIRCUMFLEX BRANCH OCCLUSION
Anatomy

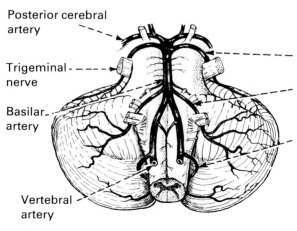

Posterior cerebral artery

Trigeminal nerve

Basilar artery

Vertebral artery

The cerebellum is supplied by three paired blood vessels:

1. Superior cerebellar artery ⎫
2. Anterior inferior cerebellar artery ⎬ arise from basilar artery
⎭

3. Posterior inferior cerebellar artery (PICA) which arises from the vertebral artery.

It can be seen that a vascular lesion in the territory of these vessels will produce, not only cerebellar, but also brain stem symptoms and signs localising to:

      (a) superior pontine,
      (b) inferior pontine and
      (c) medullary levels.

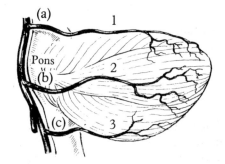

(a)
Pons
(b)
(c)
1
2
3

Clinical features

Superior cerebellar artery syndrome results in:

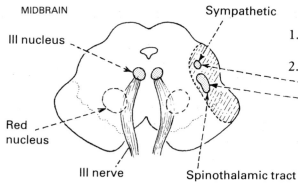

MIDBRAIN

Sympathetic

III nucleus

Red nucleus

III nerve

Spinothalamic tract

1. *Cerebellum* —
   disturbed gait, limb ataxia.
2. *Brain stem* —
   ipsilateral Horner's syndrome,
   contralateral sensory loss —
   pain/temperature (including face).

CLINICAL SYNDROMES — BRANCH OCCLUSION

Clinical features (*contd*)

Anterior inferior cerebellar artery syndrome results in:

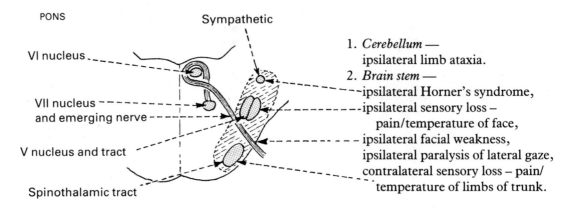

1. *Cerebellum* —
   ipsilateral limb ataxia.
2. *Brain stem* —
   ipsilateral Horner's syndrome,
   ipsilateral sensory loss –
   pain/temperature of face,
   ipsilateral facial weakness,
   ipsilateral paralysis of lateral gaze,
   contralateral sensory loss – pain/
   temperature of limbs of trunk.

Posterior inferior cerebellar artery syndrome (lateral medullary syndrome) results in:

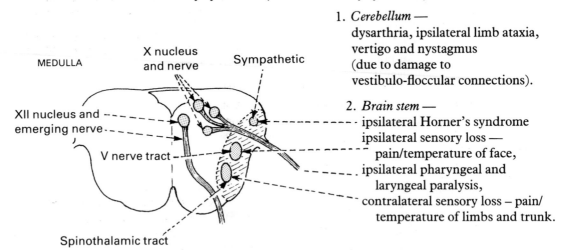

1. *Cerebellum* —
   dysarthria, ipsilateral limb ataxia,
   vertigo and nystagmus
   (due to damage to
   vestibulo-floccular connections).

2. *Brain stem* —
   ipsilateral Horner's syndrome
   ipsilateral sensory loss —
   pain/temperature of face,
   ipsilateral pharyngeal and
   laryngeal paralysis,
   contralateral sensory loss – pain/
   temperature of limbs and trunk.

CLINICAL SYNDROMES — BRANCH OCCLUSION

BASILAR ARTERY – PARAMEDIAN BRANCH OCCLUSION

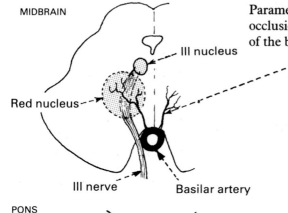

Paramedian branch occlusion is produced by occlusion of the penetrating midline branches of the basilar artery.

At the midbrain level damage to the nucleus or the fasciculus of the oculomotor nerve (III) will result in a complete or partial III nerve palsy; damage to the red nucleus (outflow from opposite cerebellar hemisphere) will also produce contralateral tremor — referred to as BENEDIKT'S SYNDROME.

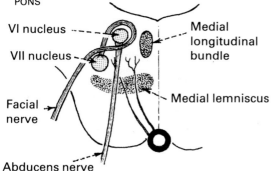

At the pontine level an abducens nerve (VI) palsy will occur with ipsilateral facial (VII) weakness and contralateral sensory loss — light touch, proprioception (medial lemniscus damage) when the lesion is more basal.

Abducens and facial palsy may be accompanied by contralateral hemiplegia — MILLARD-GUBLER SYNDROME.

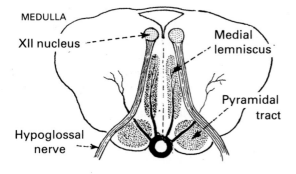

At the medullary level, bilateral damage usually occurs and results in the 'LOCKED-IN' SYNDROME. The patient is paralysed and unable to talk, although some facial and eye movements are preserved. Spinothalamic sensation is retained, but involvement of the medial lemniscus produces loss of 'discriminatory' sensation in the limbs. The syndrome usually follows basilar artery occlusion and carries a grave prognosis.

CLINICAL SYNDROMES — PERFORATING VESSEL OCCLUSION

LACUNAR INFARCTION

Lacunes are small fluid filled cavities 0.5–1.5 cm in diameter. They are found in basal ganglia, internal capsule and pons and are believed to represent small infarctions produced by occlusion of the small penetrating branches of the major intracranial arteries.

Lacunes are usually found in poorly controlled hypersensitive patients. Perforating vessels may occlude due to fibrin deposition, lipohyalinosis, microatheroma or embolism.

Lacunar infarction accounts for 10% of all strokes. Lacunes are frequently multiple and often found incidentally on high definition imaging.

Several distinct lacunar syndromes are recognised:

1. Pure motor hemiplegia
(60%)

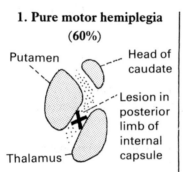

2. Pure sensory stroke
(10%)

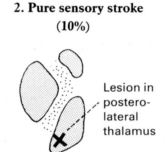

3. Dysarthria, clumsy hand
(20%)

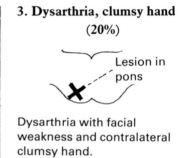

Dysarthria with facial weakness and contralateral clumsy hand.

4. Ipsilateral ataxia (arm/leg)
with leg weakness (rare)

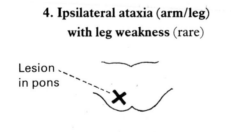

5. Severe dysarthria with
facial weakness (rare)

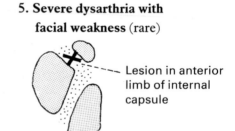

6. Multiple lacunar infarction 'etat lacunaire'

The patient acquires a shuffling gait — 'marche à petits pas' — with features of pseudobulbar palsy and dementia.

The control of hypertension following initial lacunar infarction is essential to reduce the likelihood of further episodes.

Aspirin and other antiplatelet drugs do not have a protective effect against recurrence.

EMBOLISATION

Unlike thrombotic infarction, embolic infarction is very sudden in onset. The clinical picture depends upon the vessel involved. Anterior, middle or posterior cerebral artery branch occlusion is often presumed embolic in origin as thrombotic occlusion beyond the first main intracranial branches is unusual.

The diagnosis of embolic infarction depends upon:

1. The identification of an embolic source, e.g. cardiac disease, carotid disease.
2. The clinical picture of sudden onset, with depression of consciousness if major vessel occlusion occurs.

Focal seizures are frequent at the onset and may persist for some time after the acute ischaemic episode.

EMBOLI ORIGINATING FROM THE INTERNAL CAROTID ARTERY AND AORTA

Emboli from these sites are the commonest of non-cardiac origin. The majority of all cerebral emboli arise from ulcerative plaques in the carotid arteries (see page 240). Emboli commonly produce *transient ischaemic attacks (TIA)* as well as *infarction*.

Symptoms are referrable to the eye (retinal artery) and to the anterior and middle cerebral arteries, and take the form of:

Visual loss — permanent or transient, i.e. *amaurosis fugax*.
Hemisensory and hemimotor disturbance.
Disturbance of higher function, e.g. dysphasia.
Focal or generalised seizures.

Emboli arising from the aorta (atheromatous plaque or aortic aneurysm) may involve both hemispheres and manifestations of limb and systemic embolisation may become apparent.

EMBOLISATION

EMBOLI OF CARDIAC ORIGIN

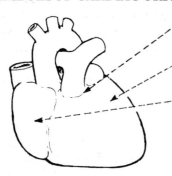

The heart represents a major source of cerebral emboli.

Valvular heart disease: rheumatic heart disease with mitral stenosis and atrial fibrillation.

Ischaemic heart disease: myocardial infarction with mural thrombus formation.

Arrhythmias: especially when of sinoatrial origin.

Bacterial endocarditis may give rise to septic cerebral embolisation with ischaemia → infection → abscess formation. Neurological signs will occur in 30% of all cases of bacterial endocarditis, *S. aureus* and *streptococci* being the offending organisms in the majority.

Non-bacterial endocarditis (marantic endocarditis): associated with malignant disease due to fibrin and platelet deposition on heart valves.

Atrial myxoma is a rare cause of recurrent cerebral embolisation. Bihemisphere episodes with a persistently elevated ESR should arouse suspicion which may be confirmed by cardiac ultrasound.

Mitral valve prolapse is a cause of embolisation, again confirmed by cardiac ultrasound.

Patent foramen ovale may result in paradoxical embolisation; suspect in patient with deep venous thrombosis who develops cerebral infarction.

EMBOLI FROM OTHER SOURCES

Fat emboli: following fracture, especially of long bones and pelvis, fat appears in the bloodstream and may pass into the cerebral circulation, usually 3–6 days after trauma. Emboli are usually multiple and signs are diffuse.

Air emboli follow injury to neck/chest, or follow surgery. Rarely, air emboli complicate therapeutic abortion. Again the picture is diffuse neurologically. Onset is acute; if the patient survives the first 30 minutes, prognosis is excellent.

Nitrogen embolisation or decompression sickness (the 'bends') produces a similar picture. If the patient survives, neurological disability may be profound.

Tumour emboli result in metastatic lesions; the onset is usually slow and progressive. Acute stroke-like presentation may occur, followed weeks or months later by the mass effects.

Lung
Melanoma
Testicular tumours
Lymphoblastic leukaemia   } commonly metastasise to brain.
Prostate
Breast
Renal

The clinical features of embolic vascular occlusion have already been discussed under Clinical syndromes.

TRANSIENT ISCHAEMIC ATTACKS (TIA's)

Transient ischaemic attacks are episodes of focal neurological symptoms due to inadequate blood supply to the brain. Attacks are sudden in onset, resolve within 24 hours or less and leave no residual deficit. Episodes which last longer than 24 hours but settle within 1 week are called *reversible ischaemic neurological deficits* (RINDs). These disorders are important as warning episodes or precursors of cerebral infarction.

Before diagnosing TIA's, consider other causes of transient neurological dysfunction — migraine, partial seizures, hypoglycaemia.

The pathogenesis of transient ischaemic attacks

A reduction of cerebral blood flow below 20–30 ml 100 g/min produces neurological symptoms. The development of infarction is a consequence of the *degree* of reduced flow and the *duration* of such a reduction. If flow is restored to an area of brain within the critical period, ischaemic symptoms will reverse themselves. TIAs may be due to:

1. Reduced flow through a vessel:

a fall in perfusion pressure, e.g. cardiac dysrhythmia associated with localised stenotic cerebrovascular disease

– the *haemodynamic* explanation.

2. Blockage of the passage of flow by embolism:

arising from plaques in aortic arch/extracranial vessels or from the heart

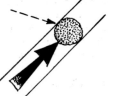

– the *embolic* explanation.

Both mechanisms occur. Emboli are accepted as the cause of the majority of TIAs.

The symptomatology of TIAs

Anterior (90%)
Carotid territory
  hemiparesis,
  hemisensory disturbance,
  dysphasia,
  monocular blindness
    (amaurosis fugax)

Posterior (7%)
Vertebrobasilar territory
  loss of consciousness
  bilateral limb motor/sensory
         dysfunction
  binocular blindness
  vertigo, tinnitus,   } not singly, but in
  diplopia, dysarthria } combination
             with each other

In 3%, transient ischaemic attacks are difficult to fit convincingly into either anterior or posterior circulation, e.g. dysarthria with hemiparesis.

The natural history of TIAS

Following a TIA, between 5–10% of patients will develop infarction in each year of follow-up, irrespective of the territory involved. The risk of infarction is probably at its greatest in the first 3–6 months after the initial TIA. Not all patients who develop cerebral infarction have had a warning TIA.

STENOTIC/OCCLUSIVE CEREBROVASCULAR DISEASE — INVESTIGATIONS

1. CONFIRM THE DIAGNOSIS
Computerised tomography (CT scan)
Ideally, all patients should have a CT scan, but this is rarely possible in view of the frequency of stroke.

In practice, a CT scan is performed if:
 – there is doubt about the diagnosis
 – symptoms progress
 – conscious level is depressed   ?haemorrhage or tumour
 – neck stiffness is present   ?cerebral haemorrhage (see page 258)
or prior to any invasive investigation.

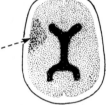

Infarction is evident as a low-density lesion which conforms to a vascular territory, i.e. usually wedge shaped. It is not immediately visible on CT but in most patients becomes apparent in 4–7 days.

CT scan also identifies:
 — the site and size of the infarct, providing a prognostic guide
 — the presence of haemorrhagic infarction where bleeding occurs into the infarcted area
 — intracerebral haemorrhage or tumour.

Magnetic resonance imaging (MRI)
T1 prolongation (i.e. hypointensity in relation to white and grey matter) occurs within a few hours of onset of ischaemic symptoms. Intracranial vessel occlusions show an absence of a 'signal void'. Posterior circulation strokes (lacunes) are more readily identified than with CT.

2. DEMONSTRATE THE SITE OF PRIMARY LESION
(a) Non-invasive investigation
Ultrasound — B-mode and doppler: assesses extra- and intracranial vessels (page 42). A normal study precludes the need for angiography.

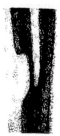

Internal carotid stenosis

Cardiac ultrasound: this often reveals a cardiac embolic source in young people with stroke, e.g. prolapsed mitral valve, patent foramen ovale.

(b) Invasive investigation
Often *cerebral angiography* is required as the definitive investigation, when the patient management is likely to be influenced by the result. There is no place for angiography in recent completed stroke due to either thrombosis or infarction until at least 1–2 weeks have elapsed. In the elderly or poor-risk patient, investigations to demonstrate the site of the primary lesion may be inappropriate.

STENOTIC/OCCLUSIVE DISEASE — INVESTIGATIONS

Indication for angiography

1. With suspected *extracranial* vascular disease
   - a recovered stroke patient at further risk
   - following TIAs/RINDs
   } if ultrasound positive.

2. With suspected *intracranial* vascular disease.

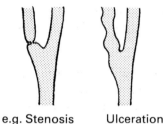

Angiography identifies the site and nature of the disease in intra- and extracranial vessels, and indicates the degree of collateral circulation.

e.g. Stenosis   Ulceration

Suspected carotid disease: demonstrate both carotids, intracranial vessels, the aortic arch and origins of the vertebrals. Approximately two-thirds of patients with carotid territory attacks will have angiographic abnormality.

Suspected vertebrobasilar disease: note the intracranial vessels and the course of the vertebral artery through the cervical foramina where osteophytic encroachment may occur. Note that proximal subclavian occlusion may result in retrograde flow down the vertebral arteries into the subclavian arteries, and cause TIAs aggravated by arm exercise — *subclavian steal* (page 244).

3. IDENTIFY FACTORS WHICH MAY INFLUENCE TREATMENT AND OUTCOME

General investigations identify conditions which may predispose towards premature cerebrovascular disease. These are essential in all patients.

Chest X-ray — cardiac enlargement — hypertension/valvular heart disease

ECG –   — ventricular enlargement and/or arrhythmias — hypertension/embolic disease
              recent myocardial infarct — embolic disease
              sinoatrial conduction defect — embolic disease/output failure

Blood glucose — diabetes mellitus

Serum lipids and cholesterol — hyperlipidaemia

ESR —
Auto-antibodies — } vasculitis/collagen vascular disease

Urine analysis — polyarteritis, thrombocytopenia

Full blood count — polycythaemia, thrombocytopenia

} See inflammatory vasculitis and blood diseases (pages 260, 263).

VDRL-TPHA — neurosyphilis

Note drug history — oral contraceptives, amphetamines, opiates

Cervical spine X-ray — atlanto-axial subluxation

Following the interpretation of these preliminary investigations, more detailed studies may be required, e.g.

- echo cardiography
- cardiac catheterisation } cardiac embolic source
- blood cultures ———— subacute bacterial endocarditis
- sickle cell screen
- plasma electrophoresis } haematological disorder
- viscosity studies

CEREBRAL INFARCTION — MANAGEMENT

THE ACUTE STROKE

Clinical history, examination and investigation will separate infarction and haemorrhage. Once the nature of the 'stroke' has been confidently defined, treatment should be instigated.

Treatment aims

- Prevent progression of present event
- Prevent immediate complication
- Prevent the development of subsequent events
- To rehabilitate the patient.

General measures

Infarction

Around the edge of an infarct, ischaemic tissue is at risk, but is potentially recoverable. This compromised but viable tissue must be protected by ensuring a good supply of glucose and oxygen. Factors which might adversely affect this must be maintained — hydration, oxygenation, blood pressure. To this end, treat chest infections and cardiac failure/dysrhythmias.

Specific measures

The following are generally ineffective, or are as yet inadequately evaluated.

Treatment of oedema

The degree of concomitant oedema relates to the magnitude of infarction. Oedema develops early and may cause ventricular displacement and transtentorial herniation with secondary brain stem damage. Controversy exists as to whether oedema is vasogenic or cytotoxic (as associated with metabolic encephalopathies), or a mixture of the two. Its effective treatment should lower morbidity and mortality but steroids and hyperosmolar agents (e.g. mannitol) have been used with little effect on outcome. The poor response probably reflects the 'mixed' nature of the oedema.

Anticoagulant therapy

The use of anticoagulants to minimise the extent or reduce the risk of further infarction should in most cases be discouraged. Bleeding can occur into an infarct (haemorrhagic infarction) and anticoagulants may precipitate this. There are, however, exceptions to this rule:

In patients with a known cardiac source of emboli, the risk of recurrent embolic infarction is high and anticoagulant therapy should be commenced once CT scan and lumbar puncture have ruled out haemorrhagic infarction. In chronic valvular disease, treatment is long term; following myocardial infarction (with mural thrombus), 6 months. With mitral valve prolapse, antiplatelet drugs will suffice. In atrial fibrillation unassociated with valvular heart disease, the place of anticoagulants is uncertain.

Anticoagulants are also often used in the management of 'stroke in evolution'. The neurological deficit fluctuates but gradually worsens over some hours. The gradual progression is considered due to increasing thrombus formation with progressive 'silting' of collateral vessels. Studies of anticoagulant therapy produce conflicting results probably because of other potential mechanisms, e.g. collateral perfusion failure.

CEREBRAL INFARCTION — MANAGEMENT

Specific measures *(contd)*

Fibrinolytic agents
Studies of streptokinase or urokinase have proved disappointing with an increased risk of
conversion to haemorrhagic infarction.

Decreasing blood viscosity
Improving hydration and venesection lower the haematocrit and reduce blood viscosity, thereby
increasing cerebral blood flow (to a greater extent than the oxygen carrying capacity is reduced).
Preliminary studies of venesection have produced encouraging results. Plasma expanders, low
molecular weight dextran and drugs that effect red blood cell deformity (pentoxifylline) lower
blood viscosity but seem of less value.

Drugs to increase the microcirculation
These treatments aim to improve blood flow in the small precapillaries and arterioles (150–200
micron range) and maintain viability of ischaemic tissue, but vasodilator agents, vasopressor
therapy and drugs such as aminophylline and naloxone have proved disappointing. Clinical trials
are currently assessing therapies which may influence the *ischaemic process*, e.g. *calcium antagonists*
(e.g. nimodipine and isradipine), *prostacyclin* (PGA2) and *selective glutamate antagonists* (MK 801).

Prevention of further stroke
The recognition of risk factors and their correction to minimise the risk of further events forms a
necessary and important step in long-term treatment.
- Control hypertension
- Emphasise the need to stop cigarette smoking
- Correct lipid abnormality
- Give platelet antiaggregation drugs (aspirin)
      to reduce the rate of reinfarction
- Remove or treat embolic source
- Treat inflammatory or vascular inflammatory diseases
- Stop thrombogenic drugs, e.g. oral contraceptives.

TRANSIENT ISCHAEMIC ATTACKS — MANAGEMENT

The aim of treatment is to prevent subsequent cerebral infarction.
Establish diagnosis and exclude other pathologies causing transient neurological symptoms, e.g. migraine.
Establish which vessel is involved ⟨ carotid territory
vertebrobasilar artery.

Correct predisposing condition.
Examine patient for evidence of extracranial vascular disease:

    Palpate carotids, upper limb pulses. Auscultate the neck for bruits.
    Check blood pressure in both arms. Examine heart.

The role of the various available treatments still remains unclear.

Medical treatment

General   Reduce risk factors as described (page 235).

Specific   *Antiplatelet agents:* several studies indicate that aspirin is a useful prophylactic in patients with TIAs. The recent UK TIA aspirin trial compared placebo with aspirin 1200 mg and aspirin 300 mg per day. Results showed no difference between the high and low dose, but both treatment groups showed an 18% reduction in end points (vascular and non-vascular events and mortality). Examination of individual end points — disabling stroke and vascular deaths, showed no significant benefit. Despite the possibility that aspirin might predispose to haemorrhagic stroke, the authors recommend that a patient requiring prophylaxis for cerebrovascular or cardiovascular disease should receive aspirin (300 mg per day), provided no contraindications exist (e.g. peptic ulcer).*
Anticoagulation: There is no evidence that anticoagulated TIA patients do more favourably than control groups, though studies are small and not all double blind; their role therefore remains unproven.

Surgical treatment

The purpose of investigation is to define a surgically amenable lesion. However, the role of surgery is unclear. Generally, stenotic lesions are treated by *carotid endarterectomy* to restore normal perfusion pressure and remove the embolic source. The advantage of operative removal of an ulcerative lesion compared to antiplatelet drugs to minimise the risk of emboli has yet to be determined. The decision to operate may be influenced by the experience of the operator, the general condition of the patient and the quality of anaesthetic and postoperative care. A European multicentre randomised trial of endarterectomy compared with the best medical treatment (aspirin) is currently in progress. Most surgery is confined to the carotid territory, though osteophytic vertebral artery compression, subclavian steal syndrome and vertebral artery origin stenosis are all amenable to surgery.

Superficial temporal to middle cerebral artery anastomosis (anterior circulation)
Extracranial-intracranial (EC-IC) bypass aims at enhancing the collateral circulation in patients with carotid or middle cerebral artery occlusion to lessen the likelihood of further ipsilateral infarction. A recent randomised multicentre international study, however, demonstrated that 'bypass was not superior to conservative treatment'. Despite many criticisms of the trial, this procedure has generally been abandoned. With the development of noninvasive techniques for assessing the intracranial collateral circulation, it is still possible that, with improved patient selection, this operation could gain favour in the future.

*1988 British Medical Journal 296: 307–308.

HYPERTENSION AND CEREBROVASCULAR DISEASE

Next to age, the most important factor predisposing to cerebral infarction or haemorrhage is hypertension. The risk is equal in males and females and is proportional to the height of blood pressure (diastolic and systolic).

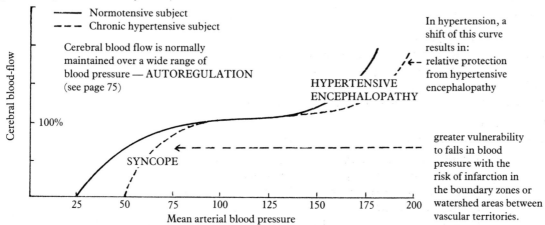

— Normotensive subject
- - - Chronic hypertensive subject

Cerebral blood flow is normally maintained over a wide range of blood pressure — AUTOREGULATION (see page 75)

HYPERTENSIVE ENCEPHALOPATHY

In hypertension, a shift of this curve results in:
← relative protection from hypertensive encephalopathy

100%

SYNCOPE

greater vulnerability to falls in blood pressure with the risk of infarction in the boundary zones or watershed areas between vascular territories.

Cerebral blood-flow

25   50   75   100   125   150   175   200

Mean arterial blood pressure

The pathological effects of sustained hypertension are:
– Charcot Bouchard microaneurysms → INTRACEREBRAL HAEMORRHAGE (from perforating vessels)
– Accelerated atheroma and thrombus formation → INFARCTION (large vessels)
– Hyalinosis and fibrin deposition → INFARCTION (lacunes — small vessels)

HYPERTENSIVE ENCEPHALOPATHY

An acute, usually transient, cerebral syndrome precipitated by sudden severe hypertension. The excessive blood pressure may be due to *malignant hypertension* from any cause, or uncontrolled hypertension in *glomerulonephritis, pregnancy* (eclampsia) or *phaeochromocytoma*.

The mechanism is complex:

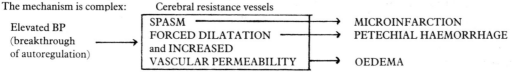

Cerebral resistance vessels

Elevated BP (breakthrough of autoregulation) →

SPASM → MICROINFARCTION
FORCED DILATATION → PETECHIAL HAEMORRHAGE
and INCREASED
VASCULAR PERMEABILITY → OEDEMA

Clinical features: Headache and confusion precede convulsions and coma. Papilloedema with haemorrhages and exudates are invariably found. Proteinuria and signs of renal and cardiac failure are common.
Diagnosis: CT scanning shows widespread white matter low attenuation and excludes other pathology.
Treatment: a precipitous fall in blood pressure can result in retinal damage and watershed infarction. Gradually reduce blood pressure with i.v. nitroprusside or hydralazine. Reserve peritoneal dialysis for resistant cases.
N.B. *With treatment full recovery is usual. Without treatment death occurs.*

BINSWANGER'S ENCEPHALOPATHY (Subcortical arteriosclerotic encephalopathy — SAE)

A *rare* disorder in which progressive dementia and pseudobulbar palsy are associated with diffuse hemisphere demyelination. The CT scan shows areas of periventricular low attenuation, often also involving the external capsule. The pathological changes were previously attributed to chronic diffuse oedema, but the recent finding of a high plasma viscosity in these patients suggests that this, in conjunction with hypertensive small vessel disease, could produce chronic ischaemic change in central white matter.

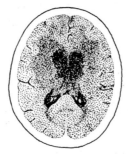

Subclinical forms of this disease may exist as this CT scan appearance is occasionally found in asymptomatic patients.

DISEASES OF THE VESSEL WALL

VASCULITIC AND COLLAGEN VASCULAR DISEASES
These disorders have systemic as well as neurological features. Occasionally only the nervous system is diseased.

Collagen vascular diseases:
> – Systemic lupus erythematosus
> – Rheumatoid arthritis
> – Other connective tissue disorders.

Vasculitis
> – Systemic necrotising vasculitis
>>   – polyarteritis nodosa
>>   – allergic angiitis
> – Granulomatous vasculitis
>>   – Wegener's granulomatosis
> – Giant cell arteritis
>>   – polymyalgia rheumatica
>>   – Takayasu's arteritis
>>   – granulomatous angiitis of nervous system
>>   – temporal arteritis (giant cell arteritis).

All the above conditions can result in 'stroke' (infarction or haemorrhage).

Mechanism
An immune basis for these disorders is likely.

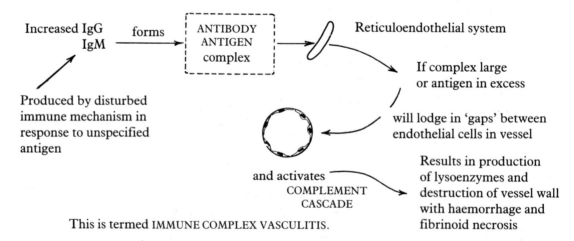

This is termed IMMUNE COMPLEX VASCULITIS.

Indirect immunofluorescent microscopy on biopsy material will demonstrate the presence of immune complexes.

In giant cell arteritis and granulomatous vasculitis, cellular immune mechanisms are probably to blame and vessels are directly attacked. A reaction of antigen with sensitised lymphocytes results in lymphokine release — attracted mononuclear cells release lysosomal enzymes with resultant granuloma formation.

DISEASES OF THE VESSEL WALL

VASCULITIS AND COLLAGEN VASCULAR DISEASES *(contd)*

CLINICAL PRESENTATIONS, DIAGNOSIS, MANAGEMENT

Systemic lupus erythematosus: in 75% of patients nervous system involvement occurs and may predate systemic manifestation.

– Psychiatric change
– Dementia
– Seizures
– HEMIPLEGIA
– Cranial or peripheral nerve involvement
– SPINAL stroke
– Involuntary movements.

INVESTIGATIONS

Blood

Elevated ESR
Circulating antibodies to nucleoproteins
 e.g. anti-DNA (ANA)
Elevated immunoglobulins
Depressed serum complement levels.

Other

EEG – diffuse disturbance
CT scan – multiple small intraparenchymal
 haemorrhages or infarcts
CSF – protein elevated (Ig), mononuclear
 cells, ANA, depressed complement
 levels
Angiography – vessels have beaded appearance
Skin/lymph node or renal biopsy.

PATHOLOGY

The predominant CNS finding is microvascular injury with hyalinisation, perivascular lymphocytosis, endothelial proliferation and thrombosis. Active vasculitis is rare.

TREATMENT

Corticosteroids in moderate dosage. In patients with severe or fulminant disease, immunosuppressants and plasma exchange may help.

Polyarteritis nodosa

Neurological involvement is common (80%):

– HEMIPLEGIA — microinfarction
– INTRACRANIAL HAEMORRHAGE — aneurysm formation
– SPINAL INFARCTION or HAEMORRHAGE
– Peripheral nerve involvement
– 'Cogan's' syndrome

{ interstitial keratitis
deafness
vertigo }

progressing to
→ seizures/stroke/coma

INVESTIGATIONS

Blood

Elevated ESR
Anaemia
Leukopenia
Eosinophilia
Positive RA latex test.

Other

Biopsy — Skin/renal/sural nerve
Microscopy — necrotic vessel,
 — lumen diminished,
 — leucocytes and eosinophils in
 necrotic media and adventitia
Positive indirect immunofluorescent microscopy.

TREATMENT

Steroids and immunosuppressant therapy have dramatically improved outcome (83% 5-year survival).

DISEASES OF THE VESSEL WALL

VASCULITIS AND COLLAGEN VASCULAR DISEASES *(contd)*

Allergic angiitis

Caused by immune complex deposition in vascular basement membrane. Neurological involvement in 30% of cases.

Systemic symptoms: fever   Followed by system involvement, e.g.
         rash ⟶   cardiopulmonary
         arthralgia   gastrointestinal
                     nervous system — neuropathy, STROKE-LIKE SYNDROME.

Causation: *Investigation:*

                               Other

Bacterial or viral   *Blood*   Biopsy — skin
   infection   ⟶ Elevated ESR   ⟶ Small arteries/veins affected
Underlying neoplasia   Anaemia   with marked inflammatory cell
                    Leukopenia   infiltration

Treatment: Remove or treat cause, and early high-dose steroids → rapid improvement.

Granulomatous vasculitis/Wegener's granulomatosis

Twice as common in males aged 20–50 years.   may invade from paranasal sinuses
A granuloma in upper or lower   into base of skull — chiasmal com-
respiratory tract with   pression, cranial nerve palsies,
associated glomerulonephritis   diabetes insipidus
                                STROKE-LIKE SYNDROME – brain granuloma
                                or vasculitis

Diagnosis: *Treatment:*
    Clinically   Cyclophosphamide produces
    Elevated ESR   remission, but 5-year
    Radiological findings (chest and sinuses)   survival is poor.
    Elevated immunoglobulins
    Impaired renal function.

Takayasu's disease

Aortic arch syndrome. Uncommon outside Asia. Presents in young adults or children. It is an arteritis affecting major branches — lymphocyte infiltration. When healing takes place, fibrosis narrows the vessels further.
    Systemic symptoms, fever, malaise and arthralgia are common.
    Transient ischaemia.
    Strokes.
    Coronary artery involvement; cardiac symptoms.
Diagnosis: suspected by absence of pulses in limbs and neck. Confirmed by angiography. Steroids are useful in the initial stages. There are no guidelines for surgical intervention.

Granulomatous angiitis of the nervous system

A rare vasculitis of unknown aetiology. Only the central nervous system is involved. Fever/headache/STROKE-LIKE SYNDROME/progressive encephalopathy.

Diagnosis: *Treatment:*
    Difficult   Prognosis is dismal, though
    Laboratory findings helpful   steroids and immunosuppressants
    — EEG and CT scan — non-specific   may produce brief remission
    — CSF lymphocytosis
    Meningeal biopsy diagnostic

Giant cell arteritis (syn: temporal arteritis) (see page 69)

DISEASE OF THE BLOOD

Disorders of the blood may manifest themselves as 'stroke-like' syndromes. Examination of the peripheral blood film is an important investigation in cerebrovascular disease. Where indicated, more extensive haematological investigation is necessary.

Disseminated intravascular coagulation (DIC)

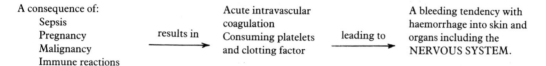

A consequence of:
  Sepsis
  Pregnancy   *results in* ⟶
  Malignancy
  Immune reactions

Acute intravascular coagulation
Consuming platelets   *leading to* ⟶
and clotting factor

A bleeding tendency with haemorrhage into skin and organs including the NERVOUS SYSTEM.

Neurological involvement — a diffuse fluctuating encephalopathy, subarachnoid or subdural haemorrhage.

Diagnosis confirmed by — low platelet count — prolonged prothrombin time and reduced fibrinogen levels.

Treatment
Heparin. Fresh frozen plasma/vitamin K. Treatment of underlying cause.

HAEMOGLOBINOPATHIES
These are genetically determined disorders in which abnormal haemoglobin is present in red blood cells.

Sickle cell disease
This disorder is common in Negro populations and also occurs sporadically throughout the Mediterranean and Middle East region.
    The patient is of small stature, usually with chronic leg ulcers, cardiomegaly and hepatosplenomegaly. When arterial oxygen saturation is reduced, 'sickling' will occur, manifested clinically by abdominal pain/bone pain.

Neurological involvement — hemiparesis, optic atrophy, subarachnoid haemorrhage.

Diagnosis is confirmed in vitro by the 'sickling' of cells when O_2 tension is reduced and by haemoglobin electrophoresis.

Treatment
Analgesics for pain
O_2 therapy, or hyperbaric O_2.

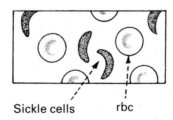

Sickle cells   rbc

263

DISEASES OF THE BLOOD

Polycythaemia

Both polycythaemia rubra vera (primary) and secondary polycythaemia may result in *neurological* involvement — increased viscosity results in reduced cerebral blood flow and an increased tendency towards thrombosis.

Headaches, visual blurring and vertigo are common neurological symptoms.

Transient ischaemic attacks and thrombotic cerebral infarction occur.

Diagnosis

Hb and PCV are elevated.

Primary polycythaemia is confirmed by increased red cell count, white blood count and platelets.

Secondary polycythaemia — respiratory, renal or congenital heart disease are causal.

Treatment

Venesection with replacement of volume with low molecular weight dextran.

Antimitotic drugs may also be used.

Hypergammaglobulinaemia

An increase in serum gamma globulin may arise as a primary event or secondary to leukaemia, myeloma, amyloid.

Neurological involvement develops in 20% of cases — due to increased viscosity.

Clinical features are similar to those of polycythaemia — peripheral nervous system involvement may also occur.

Diagnosis is confirmed by protein electrophoresis.

Treatment — underlying cause — plasmapheresis.

Thrombotic thrombocytopenic purpura (syn: Moschkowitz's syndrome)

This is a fibrinoid degeneration of the subintimal structures of small blood vessels. Lesions occur in all organs including the brain.

Clinical features — fever with purpura and multiorgan involvement and neurological features of diffuse encephalopathy or massive intracranial haemorrhage.

Haemolytic anaemia, haematuria and thrombocytopenia are the main laboratory features.

Treatment

Heparin, steroids and platelet inhibitors may be of value.

Thrombocytopenia

Whether idiopathic, drug-induced or due to myeloproliferative disorders, this condition may be associated with intracranial haemorrhage.

Thrombocytosis

This is an elevation in platelet count above 800 000 per mm^3. It may be part of a myeloproliferative disorder, or 'reactive' to chronic infection. Patients present with recurrent thrombotic episodes.

Treatment

Plasmapheresis and antimitotic drugs may be necessary.

Hyperfibrinogenaemia

Serum fibrinogen is occasionally elevated in people with cerebrovascular disease. This enhances coagulation and raises blood viscosity. Infection, pregnancy, malignancy and smoking all raise fibrinogen and may explain the increased risk of cerebral infarction. Arvin (Malayan viper venom) acutely lowers serum levels.

CEREBROVASCULAR DISEASE — VENOUS THROMBOSIS

The venous sinuses play an important role in CSF absorption with arachnoid villi penetrating in particular the sagittal sinus.

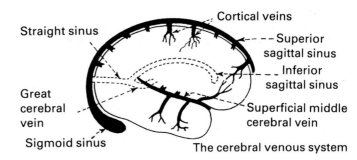

The cerebral venous system

Cerebral venous thrombosis is associated with several disorders:
- Head trauma
- Infection (middle ear and paranasal sinuses)
- Dehydration
- Pregnancy and puerperium
- Oral contraception
- Haematological disease, e.g. polycythaemia
- Malignant meningitis
- Miscellaneous disorders, e.g. polyarteritis nodosa.

Two anatomical types of venous thrombosis occur, though overlap is usual:

1. CORTICAL THROMBOPHLEBITIS

Cortical venous occlusion causes underlying infarction and haemorrhage and may produce subarachnoid blood.

Clinical features: Focal neurological signs with or without partial or generalised seizures. When infection is present symptoms and signs of sinusitis or otitis media coexist.

Treatment: Antibiotics to eradicate infection. Anticonvulsants.

2. DURAL SINUS OCCLUSION

(a) Cavernous sinus thrombosis

This commonly results from infection on the face spreading through the angular vein into the cavernous sinus.

Sphenoid, frontal and ethmoid sinuses may also act as infective sources.

Clinical features: The clinical picture is characteristic with fevers, rigors, headache and involvement of III, IV, VI cranial nerves as well as the ophthalmic division of V. Blockage of venous drainage results in oedema of the periorbital structures and forehead.

Treatment: Adequate and appropriate antibiotics, with surgical drainage of sinuses if this is the source of infection.

(b) Superior sagittal sinus thrombosis

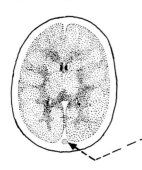

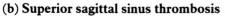

Usually results from extension of cortical thrombophlebitis. Anterior occlusion may be asymptomatic.
Posterior occlusion results in paralysis, seizures, visual disturbance and disordered CSF absorption with raised intracranial pressure and papilloedema.

CT scan shows the characteristic delta sign — a filling defect within the sinus after contrast administration.

Treatment: Antibiotics if infection. Anticonvulsants. CSF pressure monitoring and drainage.

265

CEREBROVASCULAR DISEASE — UNUSUAL FORMS

ABNORMALITIES OF EXTRACRANIAL VESSELS

Fibromuscular dysplasia

This disease involves intracranial as well as extracranial vessels which appear like a 'string of beads'. The patient presents with infarction as a result of thrombotic occlusion or haemorrhage from an associated saccular aneurysm, of which there is an increased risk.

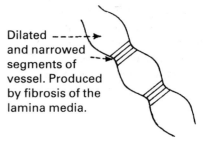

Dilated and narrowed segments of vessel. Produced by fibrosis of the lamina media.

Spontaneous arterial dissection

Extracranial and intracranial dissections are an underdiagnosed cause of stroke in young persons. Spontaneous dissections occur in Marfan's syndrome, fibromuscular dysplasia, migraine and hypertension. Pathological examination often reveals cystic degeneration or necrosis of the media.

Trauma to carotid and vertebral vessels

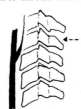

A direct blow to the neck, a sustained tight grip around the neck or a hyperextension injury may produce an intimal tear of the extracranial vessels. This may lead to dissection and occlusion.

The vertebral arteries are particularly susceptible to trauma in view of their close relationship to the cervical spine at intervertebral foramina, the atlanto-axial joint and the occipito-atlantal joint.

Angiography will confirm, and exploration and/or anticoagulant therapy may halt thrombus formation.

Cervical rib

Pressure from a cervical rib can result in aneurysmal formation in the subclavian artery with endothelial damage, thrombus formation and embolisation down the arm or retrograde thrombus spread and embolisation to the vertebral and common carotid arteries.

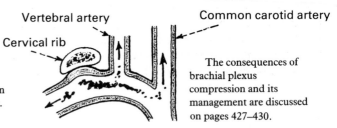

Vertebral artery

Common carotid artery

Cervical rib

Subclavian artery

The consequences of brachial plexus compression and its management are discussed on pages 427–430.

Inflammatory vessel occlusion

Infection in structures close to the carotid artery can result in inflammatory change in the vessel wall and secondary thrombosis. In children, infection in the retropharyngeal fossa (tonsillar infection) may cause cerebral infarction. Meningitis (especially pneumococcal) may result in secondary arteritis and occlusion of intracerebral vessels as they cross the subarachnoid space.

Moyamoya disease

Bilateral occlusion of the carotid artery at the siphon is followed by the development of a fine network of collateral arteries and arterioles at the base of the brain. This may be a congenital or acquired disorder. Children present with alternating hemiplegia, adults with subarachnoid haemorrhage. There is no specific treatment though some use surgical revascularisation procedures.

266

CEREBROVASCULAR DISEASE — INTRACEREBRAL HAEMORRHAGE

By definition, 'intracerebral haemorrhage' occurs within the brain substance, but rupture through to the cortical surface may produce associated 'subarachnoid' bleeding. When the haemorrhage occurs deep in the hemisphere, rupture into the ventricular system is common.

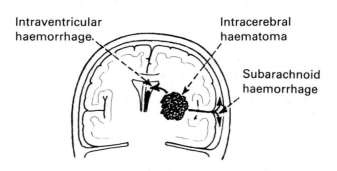

Intraventricular haemorrhage.

Intracerebral haematoma

Subarachnoid haemorrhage

CAUSES

Aneurysm
Arteriovenous malformation
Trauma
Hypertension

Blood dyscrasias
Vasculitis
Anticoagulant therapy
Drug abuse, e.g. cocaine
Idiopathic

In autopsy series, hypertension accounts for 40–50% of patients dying from non-traumatic haematomas. Aneurysms and arteriovenous malformations make up about 30%. In hypertensive patients, hyalinisation within the walls of small cerebral vessels results in the formation of *'microaneurysms'*. These are small outpouchings or local ectatic dilatations less than 1 mm in size, as initially described by Charcot and Bouchard. They tend to arise on intraparenchymal perforating vessels; rupture therefore occurs within the brain substance. In normotensive patients without any evident underlying pathology the cause remains unknown, but *cryptic arteriovenous malformations* are suspect especially in younger patients (i.e. less than 40 years) and when the haematoma is 'lobar' (i.e. frontal, temporal, parieto-occipital). In these patients, the haematoma may temporarily or permanently obliterate the lesion. Reinvestigation following haematoma resolution occasionally reveals previously undetected malformations.

PATHOLOGICAL EFFECTS

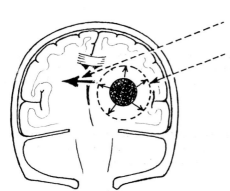

Space-occupying effect — brain shift.

48 hours after the bleed, the haematoma directly affects the adjacent brain substance producing a layer of necrosis surrounded by perivascular bleeding.

Oedema is seldom a prominent feature.

Haematoma resolution occurs in 4–8 weeks, leaving a cystic cavity.

267

INTRACEREBRAL HAEMORRHAGE

SITES
In hypertensive patients, up to 70% occur in the basal ganglia/thalamic region.

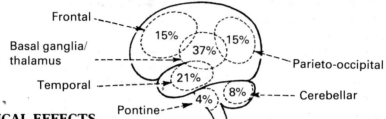

CLINICAL EFFECTS

SUPRATENTORIAL HAEMATOMA

Mass effect: Sudden onset of headache followed by either a rapid loss of consciousness or a gradual deterioration in conscious level over 24–48 hours.

Focal signs: Hemiparesis, hemisensory loss and homonymous hemianopia are common. The patient may be aware of limb weakness developing prior to losing consciousness.
A III nerve palsy indicates transtentorial herniation.

CEREBELLAR HAEMATOMA

— Sudden onset of headache with subsequent effects developing either acutely or subacutely —
Cerebellar and brainstem symptoms and signs, e.g. severe ataxia, dysarthria, nystagmus, vertigo and vomiting
CSF obstruction → hydrocephalus with symptoms and signs of ↑ ICP.

PONTINE HAEMATOMA

— Sudden loss of consciousness
Quadraplegia
Respiratory irregularities → slowed respiration
Pinpoint pupils, pyrexia
Skewed/dysconjugate eye movements
Death often follows.

INVESTIGATIONS
A CT scan determines the exact site and size of the haematoma and excludes other pathologies.

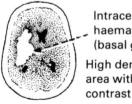

Intracerebral haematoma (basal ganglia)

High density area without contrast enhancement

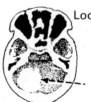

Look for hydrocephalus on higher cuts

Cerebellar haematoma

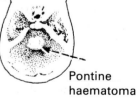

Pontine haematoma

Angiography
Indications:
– when the CT scan suggests a possible arteriovenous malformation (AVM) or aneurysm
– the 'young' patient, e.g. 40 years.
– prior to any operative intervention.

In patients with 'negative' angiography, managed conservatively, a late CT scan with contrast (double dose) following haematoma reabsorption may demonstrate a small enhancing AVM.

INTRACEREBRAL HAEMORRHAGE

MANAGEMENT

Supratentorial haematoma

In 1961 a controlled study of conservative versus operative evacuation of intercerebral haematomas (through a craniotomy flap) showed no difference in outcome (McKissock et al) and as a result many surgeons adopted a conservative approach.

More recent studies suggest that in selected patients, operative decompression is worthwhile. In general, haematoma evacuation is indicated in patients who deteriorate or fail to improve as a result of the 'mass' effect, especially when the lesion lies superficially; operation will not benefit moribund patients, i.e. patients extending to painful stimuli with no pupil reaction.

PROGNOSIS

Poor prognostic features

– Large, deep lesions (basal ganglia/thalamic)
– Depth of conscious level (flexion or extension to painful stimuli).

Good prognostic factors

– small superficial lesions (i.e. frontal, temporal or parieto-occipital)
– conscious patients or patients localising to painful stimuli.

The overall mortality ranges from 50–65% (90% if the patient is in coma).

Cerebellar haematoma:

Small haematomas causing minimal effects may be managed conservatively. Otherwise, urgent evacuation through a suboccipital craniectomy is required. Relief of brain stem compression may be life saving and operative morbidity is low.

The overall mortality is approximately 30%.

Pontine haemorrhage

The mortality from pontine haemorrhage is high. A conservative approach is usually adopted although some advocate operative exploration.

INTRAVENTRICULAR HAEMORRHAGE

Haemorrhage into the ventricles causes a sudden loss of consciousness. With a large bleed, death may follow from the pressure transmission from within the ventricular system. Blood in the ventricles does not in itself cause damage and, following clot resolution, complete recovery may occur.

No treatment is required; attempts at flushing out the ventricles usually fail. If the blood 'cast' causes obstructive hydrocephalus, then ventricular drainage (although hampered by the presence of blood) is indicated.

SUBARACHNOID HAEMORRHAGE (SAH)

Intracranial vessels lie in the *subarachnoid* space and give off small perforating branches to the brain tissue. Bleeding from these vessels or from an associated aneurysm occurs primarily into this space. Some intracranial aneurysms are imbedded within the brain tissue and their rupture causes intracerebral bleeding with or without subarachnoid haemorrhage.

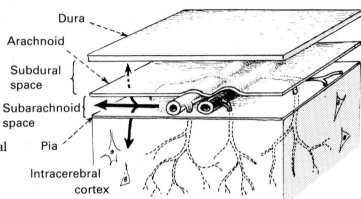

Occasionally the arachnoid layer gives way and a subdural haematoma results.

INCIDENCE

Subarachnoid haemorrhage occurs in approximately 10–15 per 100 000 per year.

CAUSE

Cerebral aneurysms are the most frequent cause of subarachnoid haemorrhage, with arteriovenous malformations accounting for 6%.

In many patients detailed investigation fails to reveal a source of the haemorrhage. Hypertension may account for some. Cryptic arteriovenous malformations or small thrombosed aneurysms may contribute to the remainder.

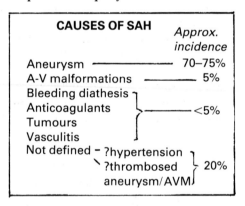

SYMPTOMS AND SIGNS

The severity of the symptoms is related to the severity of the bleed.

Severe *headache* of instantaneous onset (often described as a 'blow to the head') may drop the patient to his knees. A transient or prolonged *loss of consciousness* or *epileptic seizure* may immediately follow. Nausea and *vomiting* commonly occur. Symptoms continue for many days.

Occasionally, the headache is mild and may represent a 'warning leak' of blood before a major bleed.

SUBARACHNOID HAEMORRHAGE

SYMPTOMS AND SIGNS *(contd)*

Signs of meningism develop after 3 – 12 hours

Neck stiffness is present on passive neck flexion.

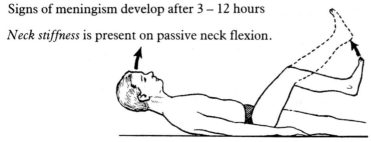

Kernig's sign: stretching nerve roots by extending the knee causes pain.

Coma or *depression of conscious level* may result from the direct effect of the subarachnoid haemorrhage or from the mass effect of an associated intracerebral haematoma.

Focal damage from a haematoma will produce *focal signs*, e.g. limb weakness, dysphasia. The presence of a III nerve palsy indicates either transtentorial herniation or direct nerve damage from a posterior communicating artery or basilar artery aneurysm.

Epilepsy frequently occurs and may mask other features.

Fundus examination may reveal *papilloedema* or a *subhyaloid or vitreous haemorrhage* caused by the sudden rise in intracranial pressure.

A *'reactive hypertension'* commonly develops, i.e. a rise in BP in patients with no evidence of pre-existing hypertension, and takes several days to return to normal levels.

Pyrexia is also a common finding; if severe and fluctuating, it may reflect ischaemic hypothalamic damage.

INVESTIGATIVE APPROACH

Lumbar puncture establishes the diagnosis of subarachnoid haemorrhage, but in patients with a mass lesion, lumbar puncture could precipitate transtentorial herniation.

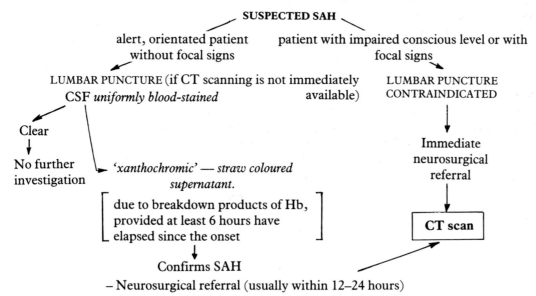

SUBARACHNOID HAEMORRHAGE

INVESTIGATIVE APPROACH (*contd*)

Age limit for neurosurgical referral: Since mortality and morbidity increase with age, the traditional limit for aneurysm surgery is 65 years. With modern anaesthetic and operative techniques, however, this no longer applies. Some surgeons consider patients over the age of 70 for further investigation with a view to direct or indirect operation (see below), provided their clinical state is satisfactory.

CT scan

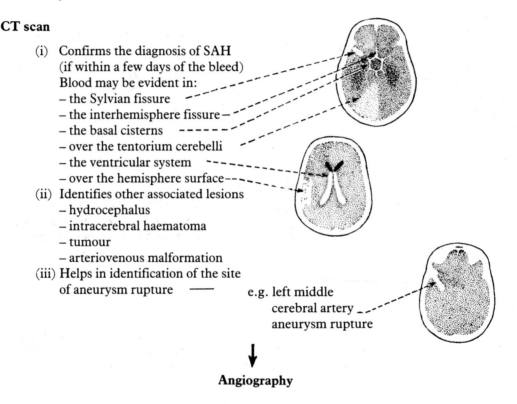

   (i) Confirms the diagnosis of SAH
      (if within a few days of the bleed)
      Blood may be evident in:
      – the Sylvian fissure
      – the interhemisphere fissure
      – the basal cisterns
      – over the tentorium cerebelli
      – the ventricular system
      – over the hemisphere surface
   (ii) Identifies other associated lesions
      – hydrocephalus
      – intracerebral haematoma
      – tumour
      – arteriovenous malformation
   (iii) Helps in identification of the site
      of aneurysm rupture ——— e.g. left middle
      cerebral artery
      aneurysm rupture

Angiography

MRI scan

In patients with multiple aneurysms, MRI may provide greater sensitivity than CT in detecting small areas of subarachnoid clot and help determine the lesion responsible for the bleed.

Angiography

Angiography is usually carried out at the earliest convenience, although in patients in poor clinical condition, the clinician may prefer to delay investigation until improvement has occurred. If a patient deteriorates from the mass effect of an intracranial haematoma, then emergency angiography is required prior to any decompressive operation.

SUBARACHNOID HAEMORRHAGE

Angiography *(contd)*
Four-vessel angiography is usually performed in all patients, although in older patients vertebral angiography may be omitted in view of the greater operative risks of posterior circulation aneurysms.

Antero-posterior, lateral and *oblique* views are required.

Carotid angiogram – lateral view

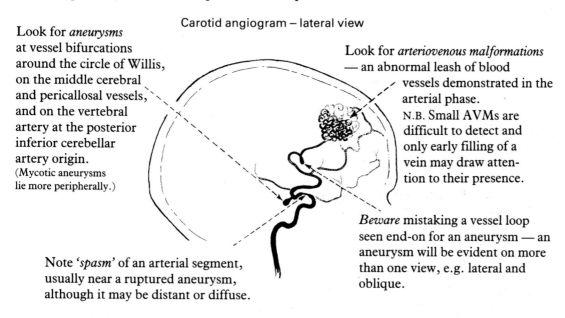

Look for *aneurysms* at vessel bifurcations around the circle of Willis, on the middle cerebral and pericallosal vessels, and on the vertebral artery at the posterior inferior cerebellar artery origin.
(Mycotic aneurysms lie more peripherally.)

Look for *arteriovenous malformations* — an abnormal leash of blood vessels demonstrated in the arterial phase.
N.B. Small AVMs are difficult to detect and only early filling of a vein may draw attention to their presence.

Note *'spasm'* of an arterial segment, usually near a ruptured aneurysm, although it may be distant or diffuse.

Beware mistaking a vessel loop seen end-on for an aneurysm — an aneurysm will be evident on more than one view, e.g. lateral and oblique.

DIGITAL SUBTRACTION ANGIOGRAPHY (DSA)

The resolution of intravenous DSA is as yet insufficient to detect small aneurysms. Some centres may use intra-arterial contrast injection DSA instead of standard angiographic techniques. This permits the use of smaller quantities of contrast medium and reduces the risk of contrast 'reactions'.

Negative angiography

Angiography fails to reveal a source of the subarachnoid haemorrhage in approximately 20% of patients. In the presence of arterial spasm, reduction in flow may prevent the demonstration of an aneurysm and repeat angiography may be required at a later date.

Prognosis: In patients with negative angiography the outlook is excellent and the risk of rebleeding extremely small.

N.B. Rupture of a spinal angioma also results in SAH — if the patient's pain begins in the back before spreading to the head, or if any features of cord compression are apparent, then myelography should be the preliminary investigation (see page 407).

CEREBRAL ANEURYSMS

INCIDENCE

At autopsy intracranial aneurysms are found in approximately 1% of the population.
Aneurysm rupture occurs in 6–12 per 100 000 per year.
Female:male = 3:2   <40 years, male > females.
        but this ratio varies with age —— >40 years, females ≫ males

Inheritance: familial occurrence is rare and is occasionally associated with connective tissue disease. e.g. Ehlers-Danlos syndrome.
Age: rupture is most common between 40 and 60 years but can occur in any age group, though rarely in children.

MORPHOLOGY

Intracranial aneurysms are usually *saccular,* – – – – – – – – – – – – – – –
occurring at vessel bifurcations.

    Size varies from a few millimetres to several centimetres.
Those over 2.5cm are termed 'giant' aneurysms.

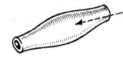

Fusiform dilatation and ectasia of the carotid and
the basilar artery may follow atherosclerotic
damage. These aneurysms seldom rupture.
Mycotic aneurysms, secondary to vessel wall infection, arise from
haematogenous spread, e.g. subacute bacterial endocarditis.

Aneurysm rupture: usually occurs at the fundus of the aneurysm and the risk appears related to size; rupture seldom occurs until the aneurysm is over 6 mm in diameter. In some, rupture occurs during exertion, straining or coitus, but in many there is no associated relationship. Giant aneurysms surprisingly are less likely to rupture, probably due to multiple layers of thrombus reinforcing the inner wall.

Sites of saccular aneurysm

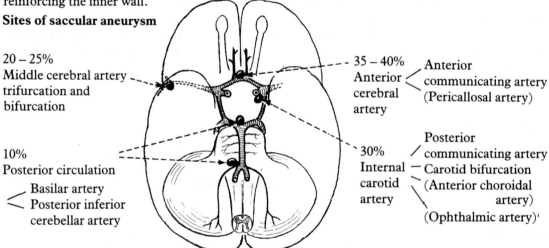

20 – 25%
Middle cerebral artery
trifurcation and
bifurcation

35 – 40%
Anterior
cerebral
artery

Anterior
communicating artery
(Pericallosal artery)

10%
Posterior circulation

Basilar artery
Posterior inferior
cerebellar artery

30%
Internal
carotid
artery

Posterior
communicating artery
Carotid bifurcation
(Anterior choroidal
artery)
(Ophthalmic artery)'

Multiple aneurysms: in approximately 30% of patients with aneurysmal SAH, more than one aneurysm is demonstrated on angiography.

CEREBRAL ANEURYSMS

PATHOGENESIS
The exact cause of aneurysm formation may be multifactorial.

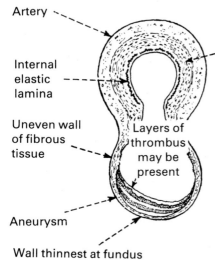

Artery

Internal
elastic
lamina

Uneven wall
of fibrous
tissue

Layers of
thrombus
may be
present

Aneurysm

Wall thinnest at fundus

Aneurysms were once thought to be 'congenital' due to the finding of *developmental defects in the tunica media.* These defects occur at the apex of vessel bifurcation as do aneurysms, but they are also found in many extracranial vessels as well as intracranial vessels; saccular aneurysms in contrast are seldom found outwith the skull. Tunica media defects are often evident in children, yet aneurysms are rare in this age group. It now appears that *defects of the internal elastic lamina* are more important in aneurysm formation and these are probably related to arteriosclerotic damage.

Hypertension may play a role; more than half the patients with ruptured aneurysm have pre-existing evidence of raised blood pressure. (Aneurysm formation is common in patients with hypertension from coarctation of the aorta.)

CLINICAL PRESENTATION
Of those patients with intracranial aneurysms, 90% presenting to neurosurgeons have SAH and 7% have symptoms or signs from compression of adjacent structures. The remainder are found incidentally.

1. Rupture (90%).
The features of SAH have already been described in detail (page 270); they include sudden onset of headache, vomiting, neck stiffness, loss of consciousness, focal signs and epilepsy.

Since the severity of the haemorrhage relates to the patient's clinical state and this in turn relates to outcome, much emphasis has been placed on categorising patients into 5 level grading systems, e.g. Hunt and Hess, Nishioka. Recently a new scale has been formed and approved by the World Federation of Neurosurgeons, incorporating the Glasgow Coma Scale (page 29):

WFNS Grade	Glasgow Coma Scale	Motor deficit
I	15	absent
II	14 – 13	absent
III	14 – 13	present
IV	12 – 7	present or absent
V	6 – 3	present or absent

Glasgow Coma Score

eye opening	1 – 4
verbal response	1 – 5
motor response	1 – 6
	3 – 15

e.g. no eye opening (1)
no verbal response (1)
flexing to pain (3) } = 5

This grading scale correlates well with final outcome and provides a prognostic index for the clinician. In addition, it enables matching of patient groups before comparing the effects of different management techniques.

275

CEREBRAL ANEURYSM

CLINICAL PRESENTATION (*contd*)
2. Compression from aneurysm sac (7%)
A large *internal carotid artery aneurysm (or anterior communicating artery aneurysm)* may compress —

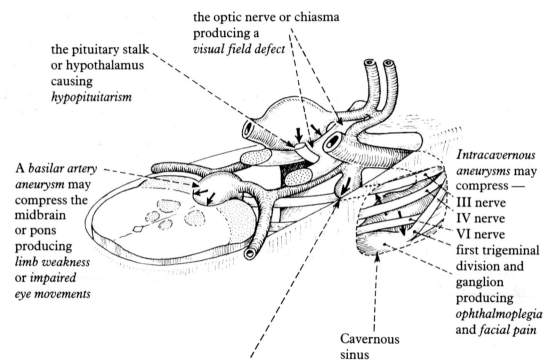

the optic nerve or chiasma producing a *visual field defect*

the pituitary stalk or hypothalamus causing *hypopituitarism*

A *basilar artery aneurysm* may compress the midbrain or pons producing *limb weakness* or *impaired eye movements*

Intracavernous aneurysms may compress —
III nerve
IV nerve
VI nerve
first trigeminal division and ganglion producing *ophthalmoplegia* and *facial pain*

Cavernous sinus

A *posterior communicating artery aneurysm* may produce a *III nerve palsy*. This indicates aneurysm expansion and the need for urgent treatment. Alternatively, it occurs concurrent with SAH.

3. Incidental finding (3%)
Angiography performed for reasons other than SAH, e.g. investigation of ischaemic or neoplastic disease, occasionally reveals previously undetected aneurysms.

CEREBRAL ANEURYSM

NATURAL HISTORY OF RUPTURED ANEURYSM

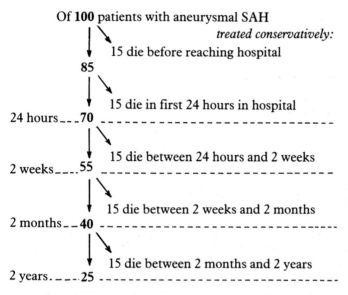

Of **100** patients with aneurysmal SAH

treated conservatively:

15 die before reaching hospital

85

15 die in first 24 hours in hospital

24 hours — 70

15 die between 24 hours and 2 weeks

2 weeks — 55

15 die between 2 weeks and 2 months

2 months — 40

15 die between 2 months and 2 years

2 years — 25

SAH from ruptured aneurysm carries a high initial mortality which gradually declines with time. Of those who survive the initial bleed, rebleeding and cerebral infarction (see below) are the major causes of death.

These figures are based on studies of conservative treatment carried out in the 1960s, at a time when the risks of operation were greater and benefits uncertain.

COMPLICATIONS OF ANEURYSMAL SAH

INTRACRANIAL

- Rebleeding
- Cerebral ischaemia/infarction
- Hydrocephalus
- 'Expanding' haematoma
- Epilepsy.

EXTRACRANIAL

- Myocardial infarction
- Cardiac arrhythmias
- Pulmonary oedema
- Gastric haemorrhage (stress ulcer).

277

CEREBRAL ANEURYSMS — COMPLICATIONS

REBLEEDING

Rebleeding is a major problem following aneurysmal SAH. In the first 28 days (in *untreated* patients), approximately 30% of patients would rebleed; of these 70% die. In the following few months the risk gradually falls off but it never drops below 3.5% per year.

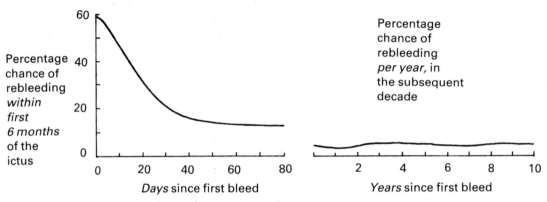

Percentage chance of rebleeding *within first 6 months* of the ictus

Days since first bleed

Percentage chance of rebleeding *per year,* in the subsequent decade

Years since first bleed

Adapted from Winn, Richardson, Jane 1977
Annals of Neurology

Thus, for example, if a patient survives the first 15 days after a bleed, there is a 40% chance of a rebleed occurring in the next 5½ months. Even if patients survive the 'high risk' period in the first 6 months, there is still a considerable chance of rebleeding and death in the subsequent years.

The clinical picture of rebleeding is that of SAH, but usually the effects are more severe than the initial bleed. Most patients lose consciousness; the risk of death from a rebleed is more than twice that from the initial bleed.

Investigation

All patients deteriorating suddenly require a CT scan. This helps in establishing the diagnosis of rebleeding and excludes a remediable cause of the deterioration, e.g. acute hydrocephalus.

CEREBRAL ANEURYSMS — COMPLICATIONS

CEREBRAL ISCHAEMIA/INFARCTION

Following subarachnoid haemorrhage, patients are at risk of developing cerebral ischaemia or infarction and this is an important contributory factor to mortality and morbidity. Approximately 25% of patients develop clinical evidence of ischaemia/infarction; of these 30% die as a result; permanent neurological deficit persists in 50% of survivors. Cerebral ischaemia/infarction most frequently develops from the 4th to the 12th day from the onset — hence the term 'delayed cerebral ischaemia', but it can occur at any time from within 24 hours to several weeks, either before or after operation.

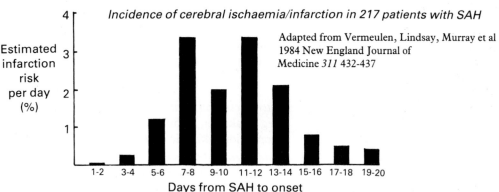

Incidence of cerebral ischaemia/infarction in 217 patients with SAH

Adapted from Vermeulen, Lindsay, Murray et al 1984 New England Journal of Medicine *311* 432-437

Estimated infarction risk per day (%)

Days from SAH to onset

Aetiology of cerebral ischaemia/infarction

Several factors probably contribute to the development of cerebral ischaemia or infarction:
'Vasospasm': arterial narrowing on angiography occurs in up to 60% of patients after SAH and is either focal or diffuse. The development of 'vasospasm' shows a similar pattern of delay to that of cerebral ischaemia.

The angiogram appearance was initially thought to result from arterial constriction; this may be so, but the pathogenesis of 'vasospasm' now seems more complex. Many vasoconstrictive substances either released from the vessel wall or from the blood clot appear in the CSF after SAH, e.g. serotonin, prostaglandin, oxyhaemoglobin, but all studies with vasoconstrictor antagonists have failed to reverse vessel narrowing or reduce the incidence of ischaemia. *Arteriopathic* changes have been observed in the vessel wall.

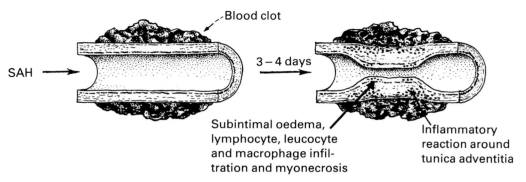

Blood clot

SAH →

3 – 4 days

Subintimal oedema, lymphocyte, leucocyte and macrophage infiltration and myonecrosis

Inflammatory reaction around tunica adventitia

The greater the amount of blood in the basal cisterns (as shown on CT scan), the higher the incidence of arterial narrowing and associated ischaemic deficits.

CEREBRAL ANEURYSMS — COMPLICATIONS

Hypovolaemia

Hyponatraemia develops after SAH in many patients due to excessive renal secretion of sodium rather than a dilutional effect from inappropriate antidiuretic hormone secretion. Fluid loss and a fall in plasma volume follow.

These patients are particularly at risk of developing cerebral ischaemic deficits, probably as a result of increased blood viscosity.

Reduced cerebral perfusion pressure

Following SAH, intracranial haematoma or hydrocephalus may cause a rise in intracranial pressure (ICP). Since cerebral perfusion pressure = mean BP – ICP, a subsequent reduction in cerebral perfusion may occur.

Clinical effects of cerebral ischaemia/infarction

This may affect one particular arterial territory producing characteristic signs:

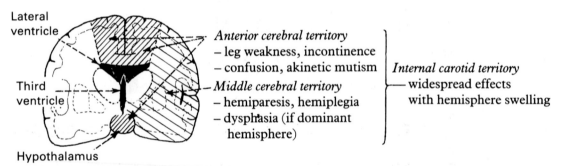

Lateral ventricle

Third ventricle

Hypothalamus

Anterior cerebral territory
– leg weakness, incontinence
– confusion, akinetic mutism

Middle cerebral territory
– hemiparesis, hemiplegia
– dysphasia (if dominant hemisphere)

Internal carotid territory
– widespread effects with hemisphere swelling

Commonly the ischaemia occurs in multiple areas, often in both hemispheres. This correlates with the pattern of arterial 'spasm'.

HYDROCEPHALUS

Following SAH, cerebrospinal fluid drainage may be impaired by:

– blood clot within the basal cisterns ⎫ 'communicating' hydrocephalus
– obstruction of the arachnoid villi ⎬ (see page 359)
– blood clot within the ventricular system — 'obstructive' hydrocephalus.

Hydrocephalus occurs in about 20% of patients, usually in the first few days after the ictus; occasionally this is a late complication. In only one-third are symptoms of headache, impaired conscious level, dementia, incontinence, or gait ataxia severe enough to warrant treatment.

CEREBRAL ANEURYSMS — COMPLICATIONS

'EXPANDING' INTRACEREBRAL HAEMATOMA
Brain swelling around an intracerebral haematoma may aggravate the mass effect of the haematoma; this may cause a progressive deterioration in conscious level or progression of focal signs.

EPILEPSY
Epilepsy may occur at any stage after SAH, especially if a haematoma has caused cortical damage.
   Seizures may be generalised or partial (focal).

EXTRACRANIAL COMPLICATIONS
Myocardial infarction/cardiac arrhythmias: electrocardiographic and pathological changes in the myocardium are occasionally evident after SAH, and ventricular fibrillation has been recorded. These problems are likely to occur secondarily to catecholamine release following ischaemic damage to the hypothalamus.

Pulmonary oedema: this occasionally occurs after SAH, probably as a result of massive sympathetic discharge; note the 'pink, frothy' sputum and typical auscultatory and chest X-ray findings.

Gastric haemorrhage: bleeding from gastric erosions occasionally occurs after SAH but rarely threatens life.

CEREBRAL ANEURYSMS — MANAGEMENT FOLLOWING SAH

Headache requires *analgesia* — codeine or dihydrocodeine. Stronger analgesics may depress conscious level and mask neurological deterioration. Management is otherwise aimed at preventing complications —

PREVENTION OF REBLEEDING
Bed rest: Usually enforced after SAH, although there is no evidence that this reduces the rebleed risk. If conservative treatment is planned, most restrict bed rest to 1 – 2 weeks.

Antifibrinolytic agents: tranexamic acid, epsilon aminocaproic acid.

   These agents have been used for many years with the aim of preventing rebleeding by delaying clot dissolution around the aneurysm fundus. A recent large multicentre trial showed that tranexamic acid does reduce rebleeding (by more than 50%) but at the expense of increasing the incidence of cerebral ischaemia. The overall results showed no improvement in mortality or morbidity.

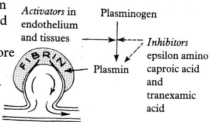

Fibrinolytic mechanism

Operation: Clipping of the aneurysm neck is the only certain way of preventing rebleeding, but this technique is not always possible and other methods are sometimes employed. The timing of operation is a controversial topic.

CEREBRAL ANEURYSMS — MANAGEMENT FOLLOWING SAH

OPERATIVE METHODS
Direct clipping of the aneurysm neck
is the optimal method of treatment and prevents further rupture; aneurysm clips rarely slip after application. The operating microscope and improved anaesthetic techniques have considerably lowered mortality and morbidity. Careful dissection of arachnoid tissue around the neck of the aneurysm enables accurate positioning of the clip.

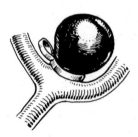

Wrapping: If the width of the aneurysm neck or its involvement with adjacent vessels prevents clipping then muslin gauze may be wrapped around the fundus. This provides some protection but rebleeding can still occur.

Trapping: clipping of proximal and distal vessels is the only possible treatment for some aneurysms, e.g. 'giant' and intracavernous aneurysms. This prevents rebleeding but carries a high risk of producing an ischaemic deficit. A bypass procedure — superficial temporal to middle cerebral anastomosis, prior to trapping — may help minimise the risk of this complication (see page 286).

Induced thrombosis: several methods have been employed to induce thrombosis within the aneurysm sac, ranging from insertion of yards of fine wire into the exposed sac to external electromagnetic induction. These methods, however, are not without risk; thrombus formation may be short-lived and rebleeding may occur.

Proximal occlusion — common carotid ligation: this technique is used for aneurysms arising directly from the carotid artery where clipping has failed or was not attempted, e.g. an intracavernous aneurysm or 'giant' ophthalmic artery aneurysm. Most patients tolerate common carotid occlusion; collateral circulation through the circle of Willis and perhaps from reverse flow in the external carotid artery usually provides sufficient hemispheric flow to prevent ischaemic complications.

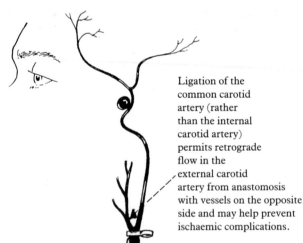

Ligation of the common carotid artery (rather than the internal carotid artery) permits retrograde flow in the external carotid artery from anastomosis with vessels on the opposite side and may help prevent ischaemic complications.

Efforts are made to predict patients who will not tolerate common carotid occlusion.
1. Compression of the carotid artery during angiography demonstrates the extent of cross circulation from the other side.
2. Cerebral blood flow studies performed preoperatively (xenon inhalation) and peroperatively (intra-arterial xenon) before and during temporary occlusion are of value in identifying those patients with an inadequate collateral circulation. Pressure from the internal carotid artery stump provides additional information.
3. Alternatively, the common carotid artery is temporarily occluded under local anaesthetic for a 30-minute period; if no neurological deficit develops, the vessel is permanently ligated.
   These methods are not infallible and late ischaemic deficits occasionally occur.

Carotid ligation prevents the patient from rebleeding in the 'high-risk' period. Beyond the first 6 months, the rebleed risk reverts to that of an untreated aneurysm, i.e. 3.5% per year.

CEREBRAL ANEURYSMS – MANAGEMENT FOLLOWING SAH

TIMING OF OPERATION

Pioneers of aneurysm surgery found that operation within a day or two of the haemorrhage carried an unacceptably high risk. Operative mortality rates dramatically fell when operation was delayed for several weeks. The longer the delay, the better the results; but the longer the delay, the greater the possibility of death from rebleeding. The clinical condition or 'grade' of the patient also played a major part; the worse the grade the worse the outcome. As a result, surgeons adopted an optimal delay period of *6–14 days from the haemorrhage, the exact time depending on the patient's clinical condition.*

In recent years, with improved operative and anaesthetic techniques, 'early' operation within a few days of the haemorrhage has become feasible. Most surgeons now advocate operation within 3 days if possible for patients in grade I or II. The additional risks appear small and are by far outweighed by the benefit of preventing rebleeding.

Once the aneurysm is clipped, aggressive methods of treating ischaemia with induced hypertension can be applied (see below). The optimal time for operation in poorer grade patients remains controversial and requires further study.

Operative mortality (i.e. mortality rate in patients undergoing operation) ranges from 5–50% depending on the patient's clinical condition and the timing of operation. *Management mortality* figures are of more value when comparing results of different management regimes.

Operative mortality (at 3 months).
No. of patients undergoing operation—187

		No.	Mortality
Preoperative	1	82	5%
grade (Hunt and Hess)	2	55	24%
	3	46	20%
	4	4	50%
	5	–	–

Management mortality (at 3 months).
No. of patients admitted to the neurological/neurosurgical unit within 3 days from the haemorrhage — 479

		No.	Mortality
Grade on	1	79	22%
admission	2	180	32%
(Hunt and Hess)	3	132	31%
	4	82	63%
	5	6	100%

Adapted from Vermeulen, Lindsay, Murray et al 1984 New England Journal of Medicine. *311*, 432-427.

CEREBRAL ANEURYSMS — MANAGEMENT FOLLOWING SAH

PREVENTION OF CEREBRAL ISCHAEMIA/INFARCTION
Despite considerable clinical and experimental research, cerebral ischaemia is still a major cause of morbidity and mortality after subarachnoid haemorrhage. In recent years some advances have proved beneficial.

Avoidance of antihypertensive therapy: antihypertensive therapy was widely used after SAH to reduce 'reactive' hypertension and to theoretically minimise the risk of rebleeding. In the normal subject a drop in BP results in cerebral vasodilatation to maintain cerebral flow (autoregulation, page 75). After SAH, autoregulation is often impaired; a drop in BP causes a reduction in cerebral blood flow with a subsequent risk of cerebral ischaemia. Accumulated evidence shows that patients with SAH on antihypertensive therapy have a significantly higher risk of cerebral infarction.

High fluid intake: maintenance of a high fluid input (3 litres per day) may help prevent a fall in plasma volume from sodium and fluid loss. If hyponatraemia develops do not restrict fluids (this significantly increases the risk of cerebral infarction). If sodium levels fall below 125 mmol/1, give fludrocortisone.

Plasma volume expansion: expanding the plasma volume with colloid, e.g. plasma proteins, dextran 70, Haemacel, increases blood pressure and improves cerebral blood flow. If clinical evidence of ischaemia develops despite this treatment, then combine with:

Hypertensive therapy: treatment with inotropic agents, e.g. dobutamine, increases cardiac output and blood pressure. Since cerebral autoregulation commonly fails after subarachnoid haemorrhage, increasing blood pressure increases cerebral blood flow. Up to 70% of ischaemic neurological deficits developing after aneurysm operations can be reversed by inducing hypertension; often a critical level of blood pressure is evident.
  Early recognition and treatment of a developing neurological deficit may prevent progression from ischaemia to infarction. Delayed treatment may merely aggravate vasogenic oedema in an ischaemic area. This technique of induced hypertension is now widely applied, with good results, but requires careful, intensive monitoring. In veiw of the risk of precipitating aneurysm rupture, it is reserved until after aneurysm clipping.

Brain protective agents: a recent large multicentre study has shown that the calcium antagonist Nimodipine (60 mg 4-hourly) reduces the incidence of cerebral ischaemia from 33% to 22%. The drug does not appear to prevent 'vasospasm' and presumably acts either by opening up collateral circulation or by reducing the harmful effect of calcium influx into brain cells (see page 238).

Steroids — Rheomacrodex/Mannitol: many clinicians use steroids, or a combination of Rheomacrodex and Mannitol infusion, either prophylactically or following the development of a neurological deficit, but since there are no adequate trials of their use in SAH, benefits remain unknown.

Antispasmodic agents: despite numerous studies in the last 10 – 20 years, antispasmodic drugs remain a dismal failure in the prophylaxis and treatment of 'vasospasm' and cerebral ischaemia. None appears to prevent or reverse arterial narrowing occurring after subarachnoid haemorrhage.

CEREBRAL ANEURYSMS — MANAGEMENT FOLLOWING SAH

Hydrocephalus

Hydrocephalus causing acute deterioration in conscious level requires urgent CSF drainage with a ventricular catheter (in 'communicating' hydrocephalus lumbar puncture may provide temporary benefit).

Gradual deterioration or failure to improve in the presence of enlarged ventricles indicates the need for permanent CSF drainage with either a ventriculoperitoneal or lumboperitoneal shunt.

Expanding intracerebral haematoma

Intracerebral haematomas from ruptured aneurysms do not require specific treatment unless 'mass' effect causes a deterioration of conscious level. This necessitates urgent angiography followed by evacuation of the haematoma with or without simultaneous clipping of the aneurysm; under these circumstances, operative mortality is high.

OUTCOME AFTER SUBARACHNOID HAEMORRHAGE

Of patients surviving the initial bleed and admitted within 3 days to the neurosurgical unit, approximately one-third die within the following 3 months. Almost half make a good recovery and regain former employment, although in a proportion, minor personality change and intellectual deficit persist.

Factors providing a prognostic guide are: age, quantity of subarachnoid blood on CT scan, loss of consciousness at the ictus, clinical condition on admission and the presence of pre-existing hypertension or arterial disease.

Comparing different operative or management policies: Comparison of different treatments for ruptured aneurysms is difficult, unless conducted under the confines of a randomised controlled trial. 'Operative mortality' provides little information unless patient groups are carefully matched for age, clinical condition and timing of operation. 'Management mortality' (e.g. outcome of all admitted patients up to 3 months from the ictus) is of more practical value, but even then, admission policies require careful scrutiny (see page 283).

CEREBRAL ANEURYSMS — MANAGEMENT

ANEURYSMS CAUSING COMPRESSIVE SYMPTOMS AND SIGNS

Aneurysms may present as a result of compression of adjacent neurological structures. An oculomotor (III) nerve palsy from a posterior communicating aneurysm often precedes rupture by a few days or weeks and indicates the need for urgent operative treatment.

A giant aneurysm (over 25 mm in diameter), causing compressive problems, seldom ruptures but the symptoms and signs are unlikely to resolve unless spontaneous thrombosis occurs.

Direct clipping and aspiration or excision of the sac provides the best treatment. In some patients the size of the aneurysm neck prevents clipping and either common carotid ligation (if a carotid aneurysm) or 'trapping' provide alternative methods. Prior to 'trapping', superficial temporal middle cerebral anastomosis may help prevent ischaemic complications.

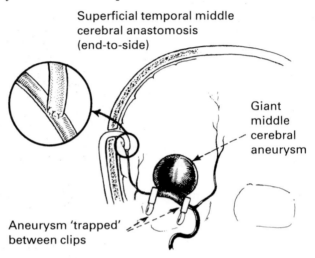

Superficial temporal middle cerebral anastomosis (end-to-side)

Giant middle cerebral aneurysm

Aneurysm 'trapped' between clips

INCIDENTAL ANEURYSMS

Opinions vary as to whether incidental aneurysms (i.e. aneurysms not causing symptoms or signs) require operation. Recent studies suggest that risk of bleeding from a previously unruptured aneurysm is approximately 1% per year, with aneurysms over 10 mm in diameter carrying the highest risk.

Operative mortality of aneurysm clipping in the absence of SAH lies well below 5%. Thus, younger patients (e.g. under 45 years) with an otherwise normal life expectancy may well benefit from operation.

When angiography after SAH reveals multiple aneurysms the neurosurgeon must decide whether to operate on the intact as well as the ruptured aneurysm. If accessible through the one craniotomy flap, many clip unruptured aneurysms at the initial operation, although delayed clipping at a second operation several weeks later minimises the risk of ischaemic complications.

ARTERIOVENOUS MALFORMATIONS

Arteriovenous malformations (AVMs) are developmental anomalies of the intracranial vasculature; they are not neoplastic despite their tendency to expand with time and the descriptive term 'angioma' occasionally applied.

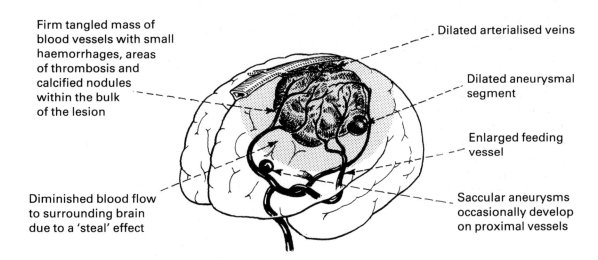

Firm tangled mass of blood vessels with small haemorrhages, areas of thrombosis and calcified nodules within the bulk of the lesion

Dilated arterialised veins

Dilated aneurysmal segment

Enlarged feeding vessel

Diminished blood flow to surrounding brain due to a 'steal' effect

Saccular aneurysms occasionally develop on proximal vessels

Dilated arteries feed directly into a tangled mass of blood vessels of varying calibre; they bypass the capillary network and shunt oxygenated blood directly into the venous system. As a result of raised intraluminal pressure, veins may adopt an 'aneurysmal' appearance. Arteriovenous malformations may occur at any site but are commonest in the middle cerebral artery territory.

Vascular malformations vary in size and different forms exist:

Capillary telangiectasis: an area of dilated capillaries, like a small petechial patch on the brain surface — especially in the pons. These lesions are often only revealed at autopsy.

Cavernous malformation/angioma: plum coloured sponge-like mass composed of a collection of blood filled spaces, but without enlargement of feeding or draining vessels.

CLINICAL PRESENTATION

Haemorrhage

About 40–60% of patients with an AVM present with haemorrhage — often with an intracerebral or intraventricular component. In comparison with saccular aneurysms, AVMs tend to bleed in younger patients, i.e. 20–40 years, and are less likely to have a fatal outcome. In addition, vasospasm and delayed ischaemic complications rarely develop. Small AVMs are at greater risk of bleeding than larger lesions.

Risk of initial and recurrent bleeding: the risk of haemorrhage over a 5-year period in patients with a previously unruptured AVM is approximately 15% (i.e. 2–3% per year); however, this risk increases to 50% over 5 years for lesions under 3 cm in size.

After a haemorrhage, the chance of a further bleed is slightly increased in the first year but beyond that the risk reverts to that of an unruptured AVM.

Mortality from haemorrhage: in contrast to the high mortality following aneurysm rupture, haemorrhage from an AVM carries the relatively low mortality rate of approximately 10%.

ARTERIOVENOUS MALFORMATIONS

CLINICAL PRESENTATION (*contd*)
Epilepsy
Generalised or partial seizures commonly occur in patients with arteriovenous malformation, especially if the lesion involves the cortical surface.

Neurological deficit
Large AVMs, especially those involving the basal ganglia, may present with a slowly progressive dementia, hemiparesis or visual field defect, probably as a result of a 'steal' effect. The infrequent brain stem AVM may also produce a motor or sensory deficit, with or without cranial nerve involvement.

Headache
Attacks of well localised headache — unilateral and throbbing — occur in a proportion of patients subsequently shown to have an AVM.

Cranial bruit
Auscultation, especially over the eyeball, occasionally reveals a bruit.

INVESTIGATIONS
CT scan
Most AVMs are evident on CT scan unless masked by the presence of an intracranial haematoma. A double dose of intravenous contrast may aid visualisation, especially with small 'cryptic' lesions.

Before i.v. contrast

Area of mixed density with high density patches (calcification) = AVM

High density area = intracerebral haematoma

After i.v. contrast

Lesion irregularly enhanced

Streaks of enhancement represent dilated feeding and draining vessels

Angiography
Four-vessel angiography confirms the presence of an AVM and delineates the feeding and draining vessels. Occasionally small AVMs are difficult to detect and only early venous filling may draw attention to their presence.

N.B. If angiography investigation of patients with intracranial haematoma is unexpectedly negative (e.g. in younger, normotensive patients with a lobar haematoma) repeat investigation with CT scan and double dose of contrast following haematoma resolution is advisable.

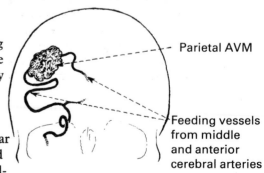

Parietal AVM

Feeding vessels from middle and anterior cerebral arteries

ARTERIOVENOUS MALFORMATIONS

MANAGEMENT

Various methods of treating arteriovenous malformations are available, but all risk further damage. The urgency of the patient's clinical condition and the risks of treatment must be weighed against the risk of a conservative approach.

Indications for intervention

– 'Expanding' haematoma associated with the AVM
– Risk of haemorrhage, especially in younger patients with many years 'at risk'
– Progressive neurological deficit.
N.B. Operative removal appears to have little effect on the control of epilepsy; epilepsy is therefore not a reason for intervention unless it causes 'intractable' problems.

Methods of treatment

Operation: *Excision* — complete excision of the AVM (confirmed by per- or postoperative angiography) is the most effective method of treatment, but some deeply situated lesions in the basal ganglia or brain stem are inoperable in view of the risk of neurological deficit.
Occlusion of feeding vessels — widely used in the past, this method is no longer acceptable since repeat investigation inevitably shows persistent filling of the AVM from dilated collateral vessels.

Embolisation: Skilled catheterisation techniques permit selective embolisation of feeding vessels with sponge, muscle, beads, pieces of lyophilised dura, isobutyl-cyanoacrylate or detachable balloons. Long-term benefits of this technique still require assessment; it is not without risk and recurrence rates may be high. Isobutyl-cyanoacrylate has been injected directly into the AVM at the time of operation to aid excision.

Radiotherapy: In the past, standard radiotherapy was employed in many patients with inoperable AVMs; although some workers claimed limited success, this approach has not been generally adopted. Recent developments include the use of a *focussed proton beam* (only available in centres with a cyclotron) and *focussed beams of irradiation from multiple sources sited on a stereotactic frame* (only available in a few centres). Preliminary results with these treatments look promising, especially for small lesions. The advantage of both techniques is the minimal damage to surrounding tissue; the disadvantage is a delay of up to two years before complete tissue destruction occurs. Despite this, these methods may prove ideal for some deeply situated lesions.

ARTERIOVENOUS MALFORMATIONS

ANEURYSM OF THE VEIN OF GALEN

This is a type of arteriovenous malformation in which arteries feed directly into the great vein of Galen causing massive aneurysmal dilatation. Patients present either in the neonatal period with severe high output cardiac failure due to the associated arteriovenous shunt, in infancy with cranial enlargement due to an obstructive hydrocephalus, or in childhood with subarachnoid haemorrhage. A cranial bruit is always evident. Cardiac failure usually develops in the neonatal period and is invariably fatal. In the other groups operation is feasible; ventricular drainage combined with clipping of feeding vessels from the carotid and basilar circulation may cure, but mortality and morbidity are high.

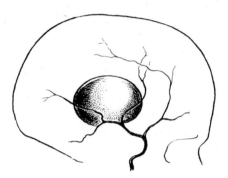

Presentation rarely occurs in later years when operative results are more favourable.

STURGE-WEBER SYNDROME

Angiomatosis affecting the facial skin, eyes and leptomeninges produces the characteristic features of the Sturge-Weber syndrome — a capillary naevus over the forehead and eye, epilepsy and intracranial calcification. (See page 540.)

ARTERIOVENOUS MALFORMATIONS

CAROTID-CAVERNOUS FISTULA

A fistulous communication between the internal carotid artery and the cavernous sinus may follow skull base trauma either immediately or after a delay of several days or weeks. Less often carotid-cavernous fistulae occur spontaneously when a saccular aneurysm ruptures.

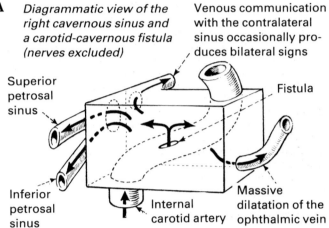

Diagrammatic view of the right cavernous sinus and a carotid-cavernous fistula (nerves excluded)

Venous communication with the contralateral sinus occasionally produces bilateral signs

Superior petrosal sinus

Fistula

Inferior petrosal sinus

Internal carotid artery

Massive dilatation of the ophthalmic vein

Clinical features

Symptoms develop *suddenly* (cf. cavernous sinus thrombosis) — the patient becomes aware of a 'noise' inside his head. Pain may follow. Examination reveals definitive signs:

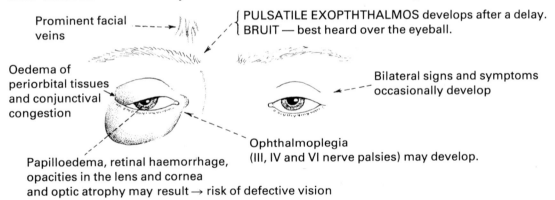

Prominent facial veins

{ PULSATILE EXOPHTHALMOS develops after a delay.
{ BRUIT — best heard over the eyeball.

Oedema of periorbital tissues and conjunctival congestion

Bilateral signs and symptoms occasionally develop

Ophthalmoplegia (III, IV and VI nerve palsies) may develop.

Papilloedema, retinal haemorrhage, opacities in the lens and cornea and optic atrophy may result → risk of defective vision

Methods of fistula repair

Trapping: ligation of the supraclinoid carotid and ophthalmic arteries intracranially, followed by ligation of the internal carotid artery in the neck.

Direct operative repair: repair of the fistula within the cavernous sinus with the aid of cardiopulmonary bypass.

Embolisation: – with muscle emboli or plastic beads introduced into the internal carotid artery
– with detachable balloon catheterisation.

The multiplicity of methods of fistula repair reflect the difficulties and limitations of each technique. None are without risk. The recently developed method — detachable balloon catheterisation — in expert hands may prove to be the most satisfactory.

N.B. In a proportion of patients in whom treatment failed or was postponed, symptoms and signs resolve, presumably due to spontaneous thrombosis.

291

INTRACRANIAL TUMOURS

INCIDENCE
Primary brain tumours occur in approximately 6 persons per 100 000 per year. Fewer patients with metastatic tumours reach a neurosurgical centre, although the actual incidence must equal, if not exceed that of primary tumours. About 1 in 12 primary brain tumours occur in children under 15 years.

SITE
In adults, the commonest tumours are gliomas, metastases and meningiomas; most lie in the supratentorial compartment.

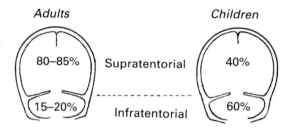

In children, medulloblastomas and cerebellar astrocytomas predominate.

PATHOLOGY
Intracranial tumours are often described as 'benign' or 'malignant', but these terms cannot be directly compared with their extracranial counterparts:

A *benign* intracranial tumour may have devastating effects if allowed to expand within the rigid confines of the skull cavity. A benign astrocytoma may infiltrate widely throughout brain tissue preventing complete removal, or may occupy a functionally critical site preventing even partial removal.

A *malignant* intracranial tumour implies rapid growth, poor differentiation, increased cellularity, mitosis, necrosis and vascular proliferation, but metastases to extracranial sites rarely occur.

Pathological classification
In 1979, the World Health Organisation drew up an internationally agreed classification of intracranial tumours based on the tissue of origin. This system avoids the term 'glioma' — previously encompassing astrocytoma, oligodendroglioma, ependymoma and glioblastoma multiforme. Since the cell origin of the highly malignant glioblastoma is unrecognisable, this is classified along with tumours of embryonic origin.

INTRACRANIAL TUMOURS — PATHOLOGICAL CLASSIFICATION

NEUROEPITHELIAL

— Astrocytes → **Astrocytoma:** The most common primary brain tumour. Histological features permit separation into four grades depending on the degree of malignancy. Grading is of limited accuracy and only reflects the features of the biopsy specimen and not necessarily those of the whole tumour. The most malignant type — anaplastic astrocytoma (grade IV) — occurs most frequently and widely infiltrates surrounding tissue. The less common low-grade astrocytomas include the pilocytic (juvenile) type, fibrillary, protoplasmic and gemistocytic types.

Composite diagram showing the characteristic features of a malignant astrocytoma.

Vascular proliferation

Mitosis

Poor cellular differentiation throughout

Palisading of cells around an area of necrosis

Multinucleate giant cell

— Oligodendrocytes → **Oligodendroglioma:** Usually a slowly growing, sharply defined tumour. Variants include an anaplastic (malignant) form and a 'mixed' astrocytoma oligodendroglioma.

— Ependymal cells and choroid plexus → **Ependymoma:** Occurs anywhere throughout the ventricular system or spinal canal, but is particularly common in the 4th ventricle and cauda equina. It infiltrates surrounding tissue and may spread throughout the CSF pathways. Variants include an anaplastic type and a subependymoma arising from subependymal astrocytes.

→ **Choroid plexus papilloma:** Rare tumours and an uncommon cause of hydrocephalus due to excessive CSF production. They are usually benign but occasionally occur in a malignant form.

— Neurons → **Ganglioglioma/gangliocytoma/neuroblastoma:** Rare tumours containing ganglion cells and abnormal neurons. Occur in varying degrees of malignancy.

— Pineal cells → **Pineocytoma/pineoblastoma:** Extremely rare tumours. The latter are less well differentiated and show more malignant features.

— Poorly differentiated and embryonic cells → **Glioblastoma multiforme:** A highly malignant tumour with no cell differentiation, preventing identification of its tissue origins.

→ **Medulloblastoma:** A malignant tumour of childhood arising from the cerebellar vermis. Small closely packed cells are often arranged in rosettes surrounding abortive axons. May seed through the CSF pathways.

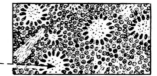

INTRACRANIAL TUMOURS — PATHOLOGICAL CLASSIFICATION

MENINGES → **Meningioma:** Arise from the arachnoid granulations, usually closely related to the venous sinuses but also found over the hemispheric convexity.

The tumours compress rather than invade adjacent brain. They also occur in the spinal canal and orbit. Most are benign (despite their tendency to invade adjacent bone) but some undergo sarcomatous change.

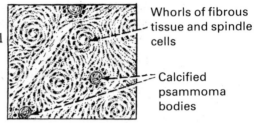

Whorls of fibrous tissue and spindle cells

Calcified psammoma bodies

Histological types — syncytial, transitional, fibroblastic and angioblastic.
Meningeal sarcoma and primary **Meningeal melanoma:** Exceedingly rare tumours.

NERVE SHEATH CELLS → **Neurilemmoma/schwannoma:** a non-invasive, slowly growing tumour of the Schwann cells, involving the VIII cranial nerve roots or the peripheral nerves. Different histological types exist:

Antoni type A
Antoni type B } see page 320.

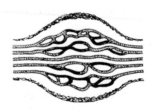

→ **Neurofibroma:** tumour of Schwann cells and fibroblasts producing a fusiform expansion through which nerve fibres run. It involves the spinal nerve roots or peripheral nerves but rarely affects cranial nerves and has a greater tendency to undergo malignant change than schwannoma. This tumour is the type associated with Von Recklinghausen's disease, although schwannomas and mixed tumours also occur (see page 538).

N.B. Many tumours have mixed characteristics in varying proportions.

BLOOD → **Haemangioblastoma:** Occurs **VESSELS** within the cerebellar parenchyma or spinal cord.
In 1926, Lindau described a syndrome relating cerebellar and/or spinal haemangioblastomas with similar tumours in the retina and cystic lesions in the pancreas and kidney (Von Hippel-Lindau disease).

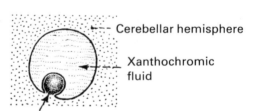

Cerebellar hemisphere

Xanthochromic fluid

Reddish brown tumour nodule lying in the wall of the cyst. Histology shows a mass of blood vessels separated by clear, foamy vacuolated cells

INTRACRANIAL TUMOURS — PATHOLOGICAL CLASSIFICATION

GERM CELLS

- **Germinoma:** Primitive spheroidal cell tumour comparable to seminoma of the testis.
- **Teratoma:** A tumour containing a mixture of well differentiated tissues — dermis, muscle, bone.

} uncommon tumours of the pineal region (not arising from pineal cells)

TUMOURS OF MAL-DEVELOP-MENTAL ORIGIN

- **Craniopharyngioma:** Arises from cell rests of buccal epithelium and lies in close relation to the pituitary stalk. Usually a nodular tumour with cystic areas containing greenish fluid and cholesteatomatous material.
- **Epidermoid/dermoid cysts:** Rare cystic tumours arising from cell rests predetermined to form epidermis or dermis.
- **Colloid cyst:** A cystic tumour arising from an embryological remnant in the roof of the 3rd ventricle.

ANTERIOR PITUITARY GLAND

- **Pituitary adenoma:** Benign tumour, usually secreting excessive quantities of prolactin, growth hormone or adrenocorticotrophic hormone.
- **Adenocarcinoma:** Malignant tumour occasionally arises in the pituitary.

LOCAL EXTENSION FROM ADJACENT TUMOURS

- **Chordoma:** Rare tumour arising from cell rests of the notochord. May occur anywhere from the sphenoid to the coccyx — but commonest in the basi-occipital and the sacrococcygeal region, invading and destroying bone at these sites.
- **Glomus jugulare tumour** (syn. chemodectoma): Vascular tumour arising from 'glomus jugulare' tissue lying either in the bulb of the internal jugular vein or in the mucosa of the middle ear. The tumour invades the petrous bone and may extend into the posterior fossa or neck.
- Other local tumours include **chondroma, chondrosarcoma** and **cylindroma**.

Primary malignant lymphoma (syn. microgliomatosis): Forms around parenchymal blood vessels. May be solitary or multifocal. It generally occurs in immuno-compromised patients, e.g. AIDS. Metastatic lymphoma (non-Hodgkin's) is less common, involves the meninges and is rarely intraparenchymal.

Metastatic tumours: May arise from any primary site but most commonly spread from the bronchus or breast.

INTRACRANIAL TUMOURS — CLASSIFICATION ACCORDING TO SITE

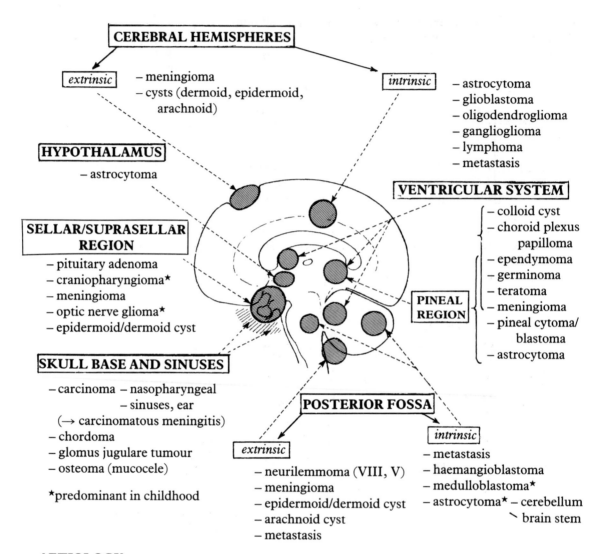

CEREBRAL HEMISPHERES

extrinsic
– meningioma
– cysts (dermoid, epidermoid, arachnoid)

intrinsic
– astrocytoma
– glioblastoma
– oligodendroglioma
– ganglioglioma
– lymphoma
– metastasis

HYPOTHALAMUS
– astrocytoma

VENTRICULAR SYSTEM
⎰ – colloid cyst
⎱ – choroid plexus papilloma

SELLAR/SUPRASELLAR REGION
– pituitary adenoma
– craniopharyngioma★
– meningioma
– optic nerve glioma★
– epidermoid/dermoid cyst

PINEAL REGION
– ependymoma
– germinoma
– teratoma
– meningioma
– pineal cytoma/blastoma
– astrocytoma

SKULL BASE AND SINUSES
– carcinoma – nasopharyngeal
        – sinuses, ear
  (→ carcinomatous meningitis)
– chordoma
– glomus jugulare tumour
– osteoma (mucocele)

★predominant in childhood

POSTERIOR FOSSA

extrinsic
– neurilemmoma (VIII, V)
– meningioma
– epidermoid/dermoid cyst
– arachnoid cyst
– metastasis

intrinsic
– metastasis
– haemangioblastoma
– medulloblastoma★
– astrocytoma★ – cerebellum
        ↘ brain stem

AETIOLOGY

The cause of most intracranial tumours remains unknown, but in some, predisposing factors are recognised:

Cranial irradiation: long term follow-up after whole head irradiation (e.g. for tinea capitis) shows an increased incidence of both benign and malignant tumours — astrocytoma, meningioma.

Immunosuppression: leads to an increased incidence of lymphoma and lymphoreticular tumours.

Neurofibromatosis: linked to an increased incidence of optic nerve glioma and meningioma (page 538).

Tuberose sclerosis: related to the formation of subependymal astrocytomas.

INTRACRANIAL TUMOURS — INCIDENCE

The table below details the incidence of intracranial tumours examined by the Neuropathology Department, Institute of Neurological Sciences, Glasgow (population 2.7 millions) over a 5-year period.

SUPRATENTORIAL	Adults		Children (< 15 years)	
Anaplastic astrocytoma (including glioblastoma multiforme)	347	(40%)	5	(7%)
Meningioma	134	(15%)	–	
Metastasis	105	(12%)	–	
Astrocytoma	73	(8%)	5	(7%)
Pituitary adenoma	31	(4%)	–	
Craniopharyngioma	13	(1%)	9	(13%)
Oligodendroglioma	9	(1%)	1	(1%)
Colloid cyst	4	(<1%)	–	
Lymphoma	2	(<1%)	–	
Others	11	(1%)	6	(9%)
INFRATENTORIAL				
Neurilemmoma	50	(6%)	–	
Metastasis	39	(4%)	–	
Haemangioblastoma	17	(2%)	–	
Astrocytoma	12	(1%)	19	(27%)
Meningioma	12	(1%)	–	
Medulloblastoma	6	(<1%)	17	(24%)
Dermoid/epidermoid	3	(<1%)	1	(1%)
Ependymoma			4	(6%)
Others	8	(1%)	3	(4%)
Total	876		70	

(Adapted from Adams, Graham and Doyle, 1981 Brain Biopsy)

297

INTRACRANIAL TUMOURS — CLINICAL FEATURES

Symptoms tend to develop insidiously, gradually progressing over a few weeks or years, depending on the degree of malignancy (cf. acute onset of a cerebrovascular accident followed by a gradual improvement if the patient survives). Occasionally tumours present acutely due to haemorrhage or the development of hydrocephalus.

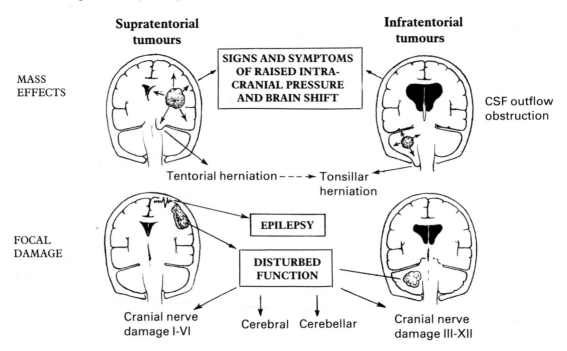

Supratentorial tumours

Infratentorial tumours

MASS EFFECTS

SIGNS AND SYMPTOMS OF RAISED INTRA-CRANIAL PRESSURE AND BRAIN SHIFT

CSF outflow obstruction

Tentorial herniation - - - ➤ Tonsillar herniation

FOCAL DAMAGE

EPILEPSY

DISTURBED FUNCTION

Cranial nerve damage I-VI

Cerebral   Cerebellar

Cranial nerve damage III-XII

CLINICAL EFFECTS:

RAISED INTRACRANIAL PRESSURE – headache, papilloedema

BRAIN SHIFT – vomiting, deterioration of conscious level, pupillary dilatation

} see pages 77 – 79

EPILEPSY (see page 87)

– generalised
– partial (focal)
– partial progressing to generalised

} occur in 30% of patients with brain tumours

Partial motor seizures arise in the motor cortex – tonic or clonic movements in the contralateral face or limbs.

Partial sensory seizures arise in the sensory cortex and cause numbness and tingling in the contra-lateral face, limbs.

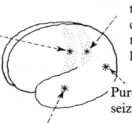

Pure visual (or auditory) seizures are rare

Partial seizures help localise the tumour site.

Complex partial (temporal lobe) seizures arise from the medial temporal lobe — formed visual or auditory hallucinations, awareness of abnormal taste, feelings of fear, déjà vu, unfamiliarity or depersonalisation and automatisms.

INTRACRANIAL TUMOURS — CLINICAL FEATURES

DISTURBED FUNCTION
Supratentorial — see higher cortial dysfunction, pages 105–113.

OCCIPITAL LOBE
Visual field defect
– homonymous hemianopia

CORPUS CALLOSUM — dysconnection
syndromes
(page 113)
Apraxia
Word blindness

FRONTAL LOBE
Contralateral face,
   arm or leg weakness
Expressive dysphasia
   (dominant hemisphere)
Personality change
– antisocial behaviour
– loss of inhibitions
– loss of initiative
– intellectual impairment
→ profound dementia
   especially if the corpus
   callosum is involved

PARIETAL LOBE
Disturbed sensation
– localisation of touch
– two point discrimination
– passive movement
– astereognosis
– sensory inattention
Visual field defect
– lower homonymous
   quadrantanopia

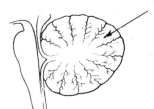

Right/left confusion
Finger agnosia
Acalculia
Agraphia
} dominant hemisphere

Apraxia
Agnosia
} non-dominant hemisphere

TEMPORAL LOBE
Receptive dysphasia (dominant hemisphere)
Visual field defect
– upper homonymous quadrantanopia

Supratentorial tumours may directly damage
the I and II cranial nerves. Cavernous sinus
compression or invasion may involve the III-VI
cranial nerves.

HYPOTHALAMUS/PITUITARY
Endocrine dysfunction.

Infratentorial

MIDBRAIN/BRAIN STEM
Cranial nerve lesions III–XII
Long tract signs
   – motor and sensory
Deterioration of conscious level
Tremor (red nucleus)
Impaired eye movements
Pupillary abnormalities
Vomiting, hiccough (medulla)

CEREBELLUM — see cerebellar
   dysfunction, pages 176–179
Ataxic gait
Intention tremor
Dysmetria
Dysarthria
Nystagmus

N.B. Intrinsic brain stem tumours in contrast to
extrinsic tumours are more likely to produce long
tract (motor and sensory) signs early in the
course of the disease.

INTRACRANIAL TUMOURS — INVESTIGATION

Chest X-ray
ESR: } The high incidence of metastatic tumour makes these tests mandatory in patients with suspected intracranial tumour.

Skull X-ray   Note:
Calcification
– oligodendroglioma
– meningioma (look for hyperostosis of adjacent bone)
– craniopharyngioma

Osteolytic lesion
– primary or secondary bone tumour
– dermoid/epidermoid
– chordoma
– nasopharyngeal carcinoma
– myeloma
– reticulosis

Signs of raised intracranial pressure
– Suture separation (diastasis) in infants.
– 'Beaten brass' appearance — of limited value since it may occur normally in children and in some adults.

– *erosion of the posterior clinoids* (may also occur from local pressure, e.g. craniopharyngioma.

Lateral view

Pineal shift — if gland is calcified (ensure 'shift' is not due to film rotation).

Towne's view

CT scanning   Note:
SITE
e.g. frontal, occipital
– *intrinsic: within brain* substance, e.g. meningioma.
– *intrinsic: within brain* parenchyma, e.g. astrocytoma.

MASS EFFECT
– midline shift.
– ventricular compression.
– hydrocephalus (secondary to 3rd ventricular or posterior fossa lesion).

Effect on adjacent bone
i.e. if meningioma ⟶ hyperostosis

Single or multiple lesions
i.e. if multiple ⟶ metastasis

Effect of contrast enhancement
e.g. none – low grade astrocytoma
irregular – malignant astrocytoma
homogeneous – meningioma

HIGH DEFINITION SCANS (1.5 mm slice width) — useful in the detection of pituitary, orbital and posterior fossa tumours.

CORONAL AND SAGITTAL RECONSTRUCTION DIRECT CORONAL SCANNING } – useful in demonstrating the vertical extent of a tumour and its relationship with other structures — especially when intraventricular or arising from the pituitary fossa or skull base.

INTRACRANIAL TUMOURS — INVESTIGATION

MRI scanning Of particular value in demonstrating tumours around the skull base and posterior fossa.

SITE
 – extrinsic:
 – intrinsic:
coronal and
sagittal views
provide most
information.

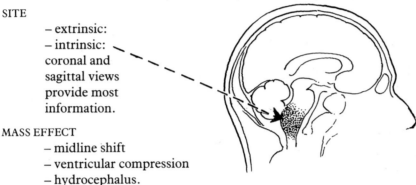

MASS EFFECT
 – midline shift
 – ventricular compression
 – hydrocephalus.

Single or multiple lesions: MRI appears more sensitive than CT scanning in detecting some tumours — improved detection of multiple lesions, e.g. metastases.

Paramagnetic enhancement: intravenous gadolinium may increase sensitivity of detection and clarify the site of origin, i.e. intrinsic or extrinsic, and may delineate the border between tumour and surrounding oedema.

Angiography: although angiography may reveal a tumour 'blush' or vessel displacement, it is only occasionally required to supplement CT scanning. In some patients, it provides useful preoperative information, e.g. identifies feeding vessels to a vascular tumour or tumour involvement and constriction of major vessels.

Isotope scanning: useful in the detection of supratentorial intracranial pathology if CT scanning is unavailable — but will not distinguish the nature of the lesion.

CSF examination: lumbar puncture is contraindicated if the clinician suspects intracranial tumour. If CSF is obtained by another source, e.g. ventricular drainage or during shunt insertion, then cytological examination may reveal tumour cells.

Tumour markers: as yet attempts to find a substance in blood or CSF which reflects growth of a specific tumour have been limited — only the link between elevated alpha fetoprotein and human chorionic gonadotrophins with germinomas of the third ventricle aids diagnosis. The development of monoclonal antibodies, with further improvements in their specificity may provide a useful approach to tumour localisation and identification in the future.

DIFFERENTIAL DIAGNOSIS OF INTRACRANIAL MASS LESIONS (other than tumour)

Vascular – haematoma
 – giant aneurysm
 – arteriovenous malformation
 – infarct with oedema
 – venous thrombosis.

Infection – abscess
 – tuberculoma
 – sarcoidosis
 – encephalitis.

Trauma – haematoma
 – contusion.

Cysts – arachnoid
 – parasitic (hydatid).

301

INTRACRANIAL TUMOURS — MANAGEMENT

STEROID THERAPY

Steroids dramatically reduce oedema surrounding intracranial tumours, but do not affect tumour growth.

A loading dose of 12 mg i.v. dexamethasone followed by 4 mg q.i.d. orally or by injection often reverses progressive clinical deterioration within a few hours. After several days treatment, gradual dose reduction minimises the risk of unwanted side effects.

Sellar/parasellar tumours occasionally present with steroid insufficiency. In these patients, steroid cover is an essential prerequisite of any anaesthetic or operative procedure.

OPERATIVE MANAGEMENT

Most patients with intracranial tumours require one or more of the following approaches:

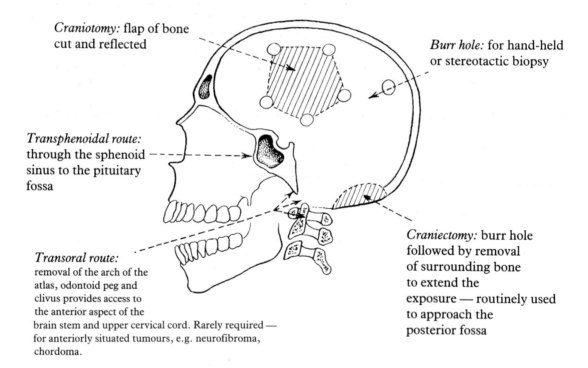

Craniotomy: flap of bone cut and reflected

Burr hole: for hand-held or stereotactic biopsy

Transphenoidal route: through the sphenoid sinus to the pituitary fossa

Transoral route: removal of the arch of the atlas, odontoid peg and clivus provides access to the anterior aspect of the brain stem and upper cervical cord. Rarely required — for anteriorly situated tumours, e.g. neurofibroma, chordoma.

Craniectomy: burr hole followed by removal of surrounding bone to extend the exposure — routinely used to approach the posterior fossa

The subsequent procedure — *biopsy, partial tumour removal/internal decompression* or *complete removal* — depends on the nature of the tumour and its site. The infiltrative nature of primary malignant tumours prevents complete removal and often operation is restricted to biopsy or tumour decompression. Prospects of complete removal improve with benign tumours such as meningioma or craniopharyngioma; if any tumour tissue is overlooked, or if fragments remain attached to deep structures, then recurrence will result.

INTRACRANIAL TUMOURS — MANAGEMENT

RADIOTHERAPY

Present-day treatment of intracranial tumours with radiotherapy utilises one of the following:
– *megavoltage X-rays.*
– γ rays from *cobalt-60*
– electron beam from a *linear accelerator.*
– *accelerated particles from a cyclotron,* e.g. neutrons, nuclei of helium, protons (awaits full evaluation).

Alternatively the tumour is treated from within (brachytherapy) by the implantation of a radioactive seed, e.g. iodine-125.

In contrast to older methods of 'deep X-ray therapy', these modern techniques produce greater tissue penetration and avoid radiation damage to the skin surface.

The effect of radiotherapy depends on the total dose — usually up to 60 Gy, and the treatment duration. This must be balanced against the risk to adjacent normal structures. In general, the more rapidly the tumour cells divide, the greater the sensitivity. Radiotherapy is of particular value in the management of malignant tumours — malignant astrocytoma, metastasis, medulloblastoma and germinoma, but also plays an important part in the management of some benign tumours — pituitary adenoma, craniopharyngioma. Since some tumours seed throughout the CSF pathways, e.g. medulloblastoma, *whole neural axis irradiation* minimises the risk of a distant recurrence.

Complications of radiotherapy: following treatment, deterioration in a patient's condition may occur for a variety of reasons:
during treatment — increased oedema — reversible.
after weeks, months — demyelination — usually reversible.
6 months–10 years — *radionecrosis* — irreversible
(usually 1–2 years).
Similar complications may involve the spinal cord after irradiation of spinal tumours.

Hypoxic cell sensitisers: during radiotherapy, part of the destructive process involves conversion of oxygen to hydroxyl ions. The presence of hypoxic areas within the tumour substance increases radioresistance. Recent use of hypoxic cell sensitisers aims to increase sensitivity within these regions. Benefits of these drugs await evaluation.

INTRACRANIAL TUMOURS — MANAGEMENT

CHEMOTHERAPY

Chemotherapeutic agents have been used for many years in the management of malignant brain tumours, but benefits remain uncertain.

Drugs most commonly employed include BCNU, CCNU, methyl-CCNU, procarbazine, vincristine and methotrexate.

In patients with malignant tumours, some studies demonstrate that individual or combined therapy produces a degree of tumour remission, but randomised controlled trials show disappointing results. In malignant astrocytoma, however, BCNU may produce a modest benefit. In medulloblastoma, combined therapy including CCNU and vincristine may delay recurrence. In patients with benign or 'low-grade' tumours, chemotherapy is of no benefit.

Problems of drug administration

Toxicity: The ideal cytotoxic drug selectively kills tumour cells; but tumour cell response relates directly to the dose. High drug dosage causes *bone marrow suppression*. Often marrow depression occurs before an adequate therapeutic dose is reached.

Drug access: 'Toxic' doses are usually required before sufficient amounts penetrate the blood-brain barrier and gain access to the tumour cells.

Intrinsic resistance: Some tumour cells appear to have an inbuilt resistance to certain drugs. The vast array of available cytotoxic drugs and the infinite permutations of combined therapy creates difficulties in drug selection.

New approaches

Cell targeting: Monoclonal antibodies have been used in the hope that they would serve as carriers, taking cytotoxic drugs, toxins or radionuclides directly to the tumour site. Initial studies on intrinsic tumours have not lived up to expectations due to problems with access and transfer across the blood-brain barrier. The use of monoclonal antibodies appears more beneficial in carcinomatous meningitis where direct intrathecal access is possible.

Improving access: Modifying the blood-brain barrier with mannitol or preliminary binding with *liposomes* may improve the passage of cytotoxic drugs and monoclonal antibodies to tumour tissue. Similarly direct *intracarotid injection* may improve access over conventional routes of administration. These methods await full evaluation.

In vitro chemosensitivity testing: This approach utilises cultured tumour cells from biopsy material. In vitro analysis of growth inhibition, or the rate of cell death following application of a specific drug, points to the tumour 'sensitivity' of the drug under test. In practice, this technique appears to be of limited value. Although successfully identifying drugs which have no effect on the tumour, the demonstration of cytotoxic activity in vitro does not always reflect its in vivo performance.

PROGNOSIS OF INTRACRANIAL TUMOURS

Patient prognosis depends on the specific tumour type; this is described for individual tumours in subsequent pages.

TUMOURS OF THE CEREBRAL HEMISPHERES — INTRINSIC

Intrinsic tumours arise within the brain substance.

ASTROCYTOMA (and glioblastoma multiforme)
Astrocytomas may occur in any age group, but are commonest between 40 and 60 years.
   Male:female = 2:1
Primary sites: Found in equal incidence throughout the frontal, temporal, parietal and thalamic regions, but less often in the occipital lobe. Microscopic classification defines 4 grades (Kernohan I–IV), but this is of limited accuracy. A more practical description for the clinician divides tumours into either 'malignant' or 'low grade'.

'Malignant' astrocytoma/glioblastoma multiforme

Malignant astrocytoma (grade III/IV) and glioblastoma multiforme (grade IV) constitute over 40% of all primary intracranial tumours. Peak age incidence is 55 years. These tumours widely infiltrate adjacent brain; growth is rapid. At autopsy, microscopic examination usually reveals spread to multiple distant sites.

Malignant astrocytoma

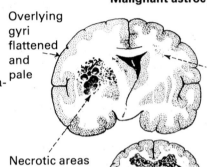

Overlying gyri flattened and pale

At autopsy 75% show microscopic spread to the contralateral hemisphere. Some patients may present with a bilateral corpus callosal tumour or 'butterfly' astrocytoma

Necrotic areas may coalesce and form cystic cavities

'Low grade' astrocytoma
Low grade astrocytomas (grade I/II) make up 14% of all primary intracranial tumours and occur on average at an earlier age than their malignant counterparts (about 40 years).

Fibrillary astrocytoma

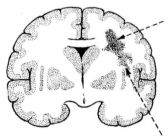

Firm, rubbery texture with or without cystic regions

Infiltrates surrounding brain with minimal mass effect and neuronal damage

These tumours are diffuse and slowly growing, and composed of well differentiated astrocytic cells subdivided into fibrillary, protoplasmic or gemistocytic types. Although 'benign' they widely infiltrate surrounding brain and lack a definitive edge or capsule. A further low grade type — the pilocytic (or 'juvenile') astrocytoma occurs in the hypothalamic region as well as in the optic nerve (page 335) and cerebellum (page 318). Since partial resection may result in a cure, some believe pilocytic astrocytomas are 'hamartomas' — mesodermal cell rests, rather than true tumours.

TUMOURS OF THE CEREBRAL HEMISPHERES — INTRINSIC

ASTROCYTOMA (*contd*)
CLINICAL FEATURES
Astrocytomas may present with:
   – epilepsy
   – signs and symptoms of focal brain damage — dysphasia, hemiparesis, personality change
   – signs and symptoms of raised intracranial pressure — headache, vomiting, depression of
     conscious level.
   Symptoms usually develop gradually, progressing over several weeks, months or years, the rate depending on the degree of malignancy. Sudden deterioration suggests haemorrhage into a necrotic area. In a patient with long standing epilepsy, the rapid development of further symptoms may result from malignant change within a previously 'low grade' lesion.

INVESTIGATIONS
Skull X-ray: of limited value; shift of a calcified pineal or erosion of the dorsum sella indicates the presence of an intracranial mass.
CT scan: appearances vary considerably; in general, malignant and low grade lesions show different characteristics:

Malignant astrocytoma/glioblastoma multiforme

The lesion,
site and
associated mass
effect
– ventricular compression
– midline shift
are clearly demonstrated

Areas of mixed density, *irregularly enhance with contrast*. No plane exists between tumour and brain indicating infiltration

Surrounding regions
of low density
indicate either
oedema or
infiltrative
tumour

Central, low density regions represent necrotic areas or cystic cavities; neither enhances with contrast

Low grade astrocytoma

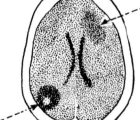

A low density region, *usually unenhancing with contrast* suggests a low grade infiltrative lesion; detection is often difficult in early stages.
Calcification occasionally occurs.

Some low grade tumours secrete
fluid which may encircle the lesion
— 'benign cystic astrocytoma'

TUMOURS OF THE CEREBRAL HEMISPHERES — INTRINSIC

ASTROCYTOMA *(contd)*

MANAGEMENT

Management varies for patients presenting with a mass lesion causing a rise in intracranial pressure or focal signs, and for those who present with epilepsy resulting from a small infiltrative tumour.

1. IN PATIENTS WITH RAISED INTRACRANIAL PRESSURE OR FOCAL SIGNS

Steroid therapy: A loading dose of dexamethasone 12 mg i.v. followed by 4 mg q.i.d., by injection or orally, reduces surrounding oedema and leads to rapid improvement in symptoms. After several days, a gradual reduction in dose avoids side effects.

Confirmation of diagnosis: In most patients the CT scan appearance is insufficient to diagnose a malignant tumour confidently. Lack of confirmation of the nature of the lesion risks omitting treatment of a benign condition such as abscess, tuberculoma or sarcoidosis. Identification of tumour type and grade by either burr hole or open biopsy provides a prognostic guide and aids further management.

Burr hole biopsy: A brain cannula inserted into the abnormal region permits aspiration of a small quantity of tissue for immediate (smear and frozen section) and later (paraffin section) examination. Provided patients receive preoperative steroid cover the risks are small, but occasionally biopsy produces or increases a focal deficit or causes a fatal haemorrhage.

Controlled suction

Dandy brain cannula — on introduction, a change in consistency may be detected on encountering tumour tissue

Aspiration of fluid from a cystic cavity may provide a temporary decompression

For small and/or deep inaccessible lesions (e.g. hypothalamus), a *stereotactic method*, guided by CT scan (see page 369), permits accurate placement of a fine cannula at a predetermined site. Although minimising tissue damage the minute specimen size makes histological examination more difficult.

N.B. The degree of malignancy may vary from region to region within a single lesion and this limits the accuracy of biopsy. If findings vary, then the region of greatest malignancy dictates the tumour grade.

TUMOURS OF THE CEREBRAL HEMISPHERES — INTRINSIC

ASTROCYTOMA *(contd)*

MANAGEMENT OF PATIENTS WITH RAISED INTRACRANIAL PRESSURE OR FOCAL SIGNS *(contd)*

Craniotomy – open biopsy
       – *internal tumour decompression*
       – *lobectomy*
	A bone flap turned over the appropriate region allows direct inspection of the cortical surface.

The surgeon may then perform an 'open' biopsy under direct vision, enter the tumour cavity and remove as much tissue as is feasible — internal decompression, or following histological confirmation perform a lobectomy (frontal, occipital or non-dominant temporal) in the hope that most tumour tissue is included. The difficulty with attempted resection lies in the absence of a plane of cleavage between tumour tissue and brain.

Radiotherapy: Most effective in rapidly growing malignant tumours – grade III and IV. Radiotherapy extends survival, but does not cure. Recent efforts to increase the local effect by implanting ^{125}I needles into the tumour requires further study.

Chemotherapy: Various combinations of chemotherapeutic agents (e.g. BCNU, 5-fluorouracil) have been used in the management of malignant astrocytoma and glioblastoma multiforme. Although a proportion of tumours undoubtedly respond to chemotherapy, studies have as yet failed to demonstrate any significant prolongation of survival. New methods of improving drug access await evaluation (see page 304).

Treatment selection and prognosis

After establishing the diagnosis, further treatment depends on the degree of malignancy, the tumour site, the extent of any presenting neurological deficit and the patient's age. The clinician must consider the quality of survival as well as the duration.

Malignant astrocytoma/glioblastoma multiforme: Despite modern techniques, these common primary tumours still carry an extremely grave prognosis, irrespective of the selected treatment.

Although there are many protagonists for aggressive operative treatment, benefits remain unconvincing. Extensive tumour resection extends average survival by only 1 or 2 months; at 1 year, the percentage of patients surviving varies little, irrespective of whether burr hole biopsy or tumour resection was performed. Complete removal is impossible; even the formidable 'hemispherectomy' fails due to interhemispheric spread.

	Median survival (months)
Burr hole biopsy	3–4
Tumour resection	6
Burr hole biopsy + radiotherapy	6–8
Tumour resection + radiotherapy	9–10

Radiotherapy appears to have the greatest effect, extending the mean survival period by 3–4 months.

Management policies vary widely. In Britain, most neurosurgeons adopt a relatively conservative policy, combining burr hole biopsy with radiotherapy. In general, *'partial' or 'complete' resection* (with radiotherapy) is only considered in:
   – younger patients
   – patients with 'accessible' lesions, e.g. frontal pole, non-dominant temporal lobe
   – patients with pressure symptoms, yet no disabling focal signs.

A *diagnostic burr hole biopsy* is appropriate in:
   – elderly patients, and patients with marked disability (e.g. severe dysphasia).

TUMOURS OF THE CEREBRAL HEMISPHERES — INTRINSIC

ASTROCYTOMA (contd)

Low grade astrocytoma: If biopsy reveals a low grade astrocytoma (grade I and II), then prognosis relatively improves but median survival is only 2 years for grade II and 4 years for grade I. In some instances, however, patients survive for more than 20 years. If the CT scan shows a well-defined tumour mass, then operative decompression is worthwhile; in some, the diffuse infiltrative nature of the tumour limits resection. Many clinicians advise radiotherapy, despite the expected limited sensitivity.

2. MANAGEMENT IN PATIENTS WITH EPILEPSY ALONE

A small poorly defined region of low density on the CT scan, without contrast enhancement, suggests a low grade astrocytoma. In these patients, the clinician may defer biopsy until follow-up CT scans or the development of focal signs indicate progression.

OLIGODENDROGLIOMA

Oligodendrogliomas are far less common than astrocytomas. They occur in a slightly younger age group — 30–50 years, and usually involve the frontal lobes. Occasionally involvement of the ventricular wall results in CSF seeding. Radiological calcification occurs in 40%.

In contrast to astrocytomas, the tumour margin often appears well defined. The rate of growth of oligodendrogliomas and the degree of malignancy are variable. Many tumours exhibit a 'mixed' histological picture with areas of astrocytic change scattered between the oligodendroglia. In these, grading is judged by the astrocytic component. Malignant change may result in a histological pattern resembling glioblastoma multiforme.

Oligodendroglioma

Tumour edge well demarcated

Radiological calcification present in 40%

Some tumours involve the ventricular wall — CSF seeding may occur

Management: matches that of astrocytomas. Low grade lesions may benefit from 'complete' or 'partial' excision. In malignant tumours, radiotherapy may have the greatest effect.

Prognosis: depends on the tumour grade. Long term survival (over 20 years) is occasionally recorded, but in tumours showing malignant change, expected survival compares closely with the depressing figures for malignant astrocytoma.

HYPOTHALAMIC ASTROCYTOMA

Hypothalamic tumours usually occur in children; they are usually astrocytomas of the pilocytic (juvenile) type.

Clinical presentation takes different forms. Initially the child *fails to thrive* and becomes *emaciated*. Signs of *panhypopituitarism* may be evident. Eventually an anabolic phase results in *obesity* accompanied by *diabetes insipidus* and *delayed puberty*.

Upward tumour extension may obstruct the foramen of Munro and cause *hydrocephalus*.

Involvement of the tuberal region may result in the rare presentation of *precocious puberty* with secondary sexual characteristics developing in children perhaps only a few years old.

Downward extension invades the optic chiasma and *impairs vision*.

Management: The site of the lesion prevents operative removal; a stereotactic biopsy may aid tumour identification. If hydrocephalus is present, a bilateral ventriculoperitoneal/atrial shunt relieves pressure symptoms. Radiotherapy is of doubtful value.

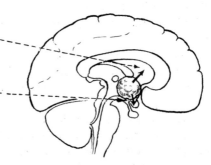

TUMOURS OF THE CEREBRAL HEMISPHERES — INTRINSIC

METASTATIC TUMOURS

Any malignant tumour may metastasise to the brain. Malignant melanomas show the highest frequency (66% of patients); this contrasts with tumours of the cervix and uterus where < 3% develop intracranial metastasis. The most commonly encountered metastatic intracranial tumours arise from the bronchus and the breast; of patients with carcinomas at these sites, 25% develop intracranial metastasis.

Common primary sites
– bronchus
– breast
– kidney
– thyroid
– stomach
– prostate
– testis
– melanoma

   In up to 50% of patients, metastases are multiple.

Spread usually haematogenous. Occasionally a metastasis to the skull vault may result in a nodule or plaque forming over the dural surface from direct spread.

Intracranial sites < *¾ cerebral hemispheres* / *¼ cerebellum*
      (see page 316)

Involvement of the ventricular wall or encroachment into the basal cisterns may result in tumour cells seeding through the CSF pathways.

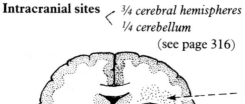

Surrounding oedema is often marked.

Tumour margin — well defined.

Necrotic areas may break down to form cystic cavities containing a pus-like fluid.

Clinical features

Patients with supratentorial metastatic tumours may present with epilepsy, or with signs and symptoms occurring from focal damage or raised intracranial pressure. Cerebellar metastases are discussed on page 316. Carcinomatous meningitis causes single or multiple cranial nerve palsies and may obstruct CSF drainage (see page 495).

Investigations

A CT scan shows single or multiple well demarcated lesions of variable size. Often an extensive low density area, representing oedema, surrounds the lesion.

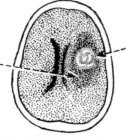

Metastatic lesions usually enhance with contrast. A ring-like appearance may resemble an abscess — but the wall is irregular and thickened.

   MRI scanning, with or without paramagnetic enhancement, is even more sensitive than CT in detecting small metastatic lesions.

   The search for a primary lesion must include a thorough clinical examination and a chest X-ray. Other investigations including barium studies, intravenous pyelogram (IVP), abdominal CT scans, ultrasound and sputum and urine cytology have questionable value, unless clinically indicated.

TUMOURS OF THE CEREBRAL HEMISPHERES — INTRINSIC

METASTATIC TUMOURS
Management and prognosis:
1. Solitary lesions: If the tumour lies in an accessible site, complete excision followed by radiotherapy provides good results — survival usually depends on the extent of extracranial disease and its ability to respond to treatment rather than on intracranial recurrences.

In general, in patients with no other evidence of systemic cancer, the median survival period approaches 2 years after the intracranial operation. In patients with other evidence of systemic disease, results are less good with a median survival of 8 months.

2. Multiple lesions: In these patients, operative removal is seldom practical or possible. Provided no doubt exists about the diagnosis (i.e. multiple abscesses or tuberculomata may resemble metastatic deposits) then whole brain irradiation is administered. This diminishes the need for prolonged steroid therapy.

PRIMARY LYMPHOMA (syn. MICROGLIOMATOSIS)
Single or multifocal tumours occurring at any hemispheric site. Some are discreet lesions, others extensively invade surrounding brain. They are prone to develop in immunosuppressed patients. Histology shows sleeves of primitive reticulum cells around and extending outwards from the blood vessels.

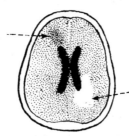

CT scan: shows either a poorly enhancing low density region or ...

Multiplicity also suggests lymphoma.

... a strongly enhancing homogeneous hyperdense region, often in a periventricular location.

Management: Biopsy confirms the nature of the lesion. Although radiotherapy may produce dramatic shrinkage, the mean survival period of about 1 year is little better than that of malignant glioma.

GANGLIOGLIOMA
This is a rare tumour occurring in the younger age group (< 30 years), composed of abnormal neuronal growth mixed with a glial component. The proportion of each component varies from patient to patient. Growth is slow and malignant change uncommon; when this occurs it probably develops in the glial component.

Management follows that of low grade astrocytomas.

NEUROBLASTOMA
Rarely occurs intracranially in children <10 years. Highly cellular, malignant lesion composed of small round cells, some showing neuronal differentiation.

TUMOURS OF THE CEREBRAL HEMISPHERES — EXTRINSIC

Extrinsic tumours arise outwith the brain substance.

MENINGIOMA

Meningiomas constitute about one-fifth of all primary intracranial tumours. They are slowly growing and arise from the arachnoid granulations. These lie in greatest concentration around the venous sinuses, but they also occur in relation to surface tributary veins. Meningiomas may therefore develop at any meningeal site. Occasionally they are multiple.

Meningiomas present primarily in the 40–60 age group and have a slight female preponderance. They are principally benign tumours, although a malignant form exists.

Pathology

Various histological types are described — syncytial, transitional, fibroblastic and angioblastic; different types may coexist within the same tumour. These distinctions serve little clinical value, although it is important to identify the haemangiopericytic variant of the angioblastic group as well as the malignant type, as these indicate the likelihood of rapid growth and a high rate of recurrence following removal.

Sites of intracranial meningioma

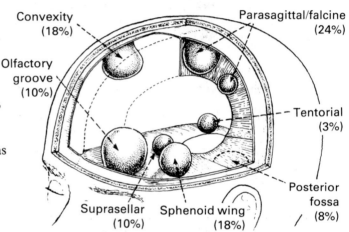

Convexity (18%)

Olfactory groove (10%)

Parasagittal/falcine (24%)

Tentorial (3%)

Posterior fossa (8%)

Suprasellar (10%)

Sphenoid wing (18%)

The remainder arise from the middle fossa, orbital roof and lateral ventricle

Macroscopic appearance
The dural origin usually incorporates the main arterial supply.
The tumour surface, although often lobulated, is well demarcated from the surrounding brain and attached only by small bridging vessels.
Marked *oedema* often develops in the surrounding brain.

A reactive *hyperostosis* develops in adjacent bone, forming a swelling on the inner table. Hyperostosis affecting the outer table may produce a palpable lump. Tumour tissue may infiltrate adjacent bone.

Parasagittal tumours may invade and obstruct the sagittal sinus.

Tumour texture and vascularity varies considerably from patient to patient — some are firm and fibrous, others soft. *Calcified deposits* (psammoma bodies) are often found.

En-plaque meningioma: In some patients, rather than developing a spherical form, the meningioma spreads 'en-plaque' over the dural surface. This type often arises from the outer aspect of the sphenoid wing.

TUMOURS OF THE CEREBRAL HEMISPHERES — EXTRINSIC

MENINGIOMA   Clinical features:

Approximately a quarter of patients with meningioma present with epilepsy — often with a focal component. In the remainder, the onset is insidious with pressure effects (headache, vomiting, papilloedema) often developing before focal neurological signs become evident.

Notable characteristic features occur, dependent on the tumour site — PARASAGITTAL/ PARAFALCINE tumours lying near the vertex affect the 'foot' and 'leg' area of the motor or sensory strip. *Partial seizures* or a *'pyramidal' weakness* may develop in the leg (i.e. primarily affecting foot dorsiflexion, then knee and hip flexion). Extension of the lesion through the falx can produce *bilateral leg weakness.* Posteriorly situated parasagittal tumours may present with a *homonymous hemianopia.* Tumours arising anteriorly may grow to extensive proportions before causing focal signs; eventually minor *impairment of memory, intellect* and *personality* may progress to a *profound dementia.*

INNER SPHENOIDAL WING tumours may compress the optic nerve and produce *visual impairment.* Examination may reveal a central *scotoma* or other *field defect* with *optic atrophy.*

N.B. The FOSTER KENNEDY syndrome denotes a tumour causing optic atrophy in one fundus from direct pressure and papilloedema in the other due to increased intracranial pressure.

Involvement of the cavernous sinus or the superior orbital fissure may produce *ptosis* and *impaired eye movements* (III, IV and VI nerve palsies) or *facial pain and anaesthesia* (V$_1$ nerve damage) — see diagram on page 149. *Proptosis* occasionally results from venous obstruction from tumour extension into the orbit.

OLFACTORY GROOVE tumours destroy the olfactory bulb or tract causing unilateral followed by bilateral *anosmia.* Often unilateral loss passes unnoticed by the patient; with tumour expansion, dementia may gradually ensue.

SUPRASELLAR tumours — see page 335.

Investigations:

SKULL X-RAY — note:
Associated signs of long-standing increased ICP, i.e. posterior clinoid erosion.

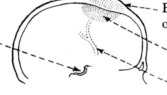

Bony hyperostosis — radiating spicules occasionally seen ('sunray' effect).

15% show calcification.

Dilated middle meningeal groove.

CT SCAN

Before i.v. contrast

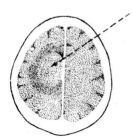

Meningioma — well circumscibed lesions of a density usually greater than, or equal to brain with a surrounding area of low attenuation (oedema). Calcification may be evident.

The lesion abuts the dura overlying the hemispheric cavity, the falx or the sagittal sinus or arises from the skull base.

After i.v. contrast

A dense, usually homogeneous enhancement occurs after contrast injection.

N.B. CT is more sensitive than MRI in meningioma detection.

TUMOURS OF THE CEREBRAL HEMISPHERES — EXTRINSIC

MENINGIOMA   Investigations *(contd)*
ANGIOGRAPHY: Characteristically shows a highly
vascular lesion with a typical tumour 'blush'. It provides useful preoperative information — identifying the
site of major feeding vessels, e.g. inner sphenoid wing
meningioma may encircle and constrict the internal
carotid artery.

   Selective catheterisation and embolisation of
external carotid feeding vessels can reduce tumour
vascularity and diminish operative risks from
excessive haemorrhage.

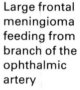

Large frontal
meningioma
feeding from
branch of the
ophthalmic
artery

Management
Management aims at complete removal of both the tumour and its origin without damaging
adjacent brain; but this depends on the tumour site and its nature. Even with 'convexity' tumours,
where complete excision of the dural origin is possible, overlooking a small piece of tumour
imbedded in adjacent brain will result in recurrence. This is particularly likely with malignant
meningiomas where the plane of cleavage is often obscured.

Parasagittal meningioma

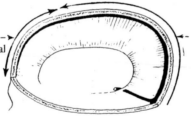

Involvement of the
anterior one-third of the sagittal
sinus permits total
resection of the tumour
and origin.

Resection of the posterior two-thirds of the sagittal sinus carries an unacceptably high
risk of bilateral venous infarction; in
this region every effort is made to spare
the sinus and its draining veins.

Tumours arising from the skull base seldom permit excision of the origin. Occasionally the
patient's age or the tumour site prevents operation or allows only a limited removal; in these
patients radiotherapy is often administered but its value remains unknown. Radiotherapy should
be administered in malignant tumours.

Operative results: With modern techniques, operative mortality has fallen to less than 5%, but
varies depending on the position and the size of the tumour.

Tumour recurrence: depends predominantly on the completeness of removal. Tumour type
seems less important although a higher rate of recurrence has been reported in the
haemangiopericytic variant of the angioblastic group as well as in tumours showing malignant
features.
   Meningiomas recur in up to one-third of patients followed up for more than 10 years.

TUMOURS OF THE CEREBRAL HEMISPHERES — EXTRINSIC

ARACHNOID CYSTS

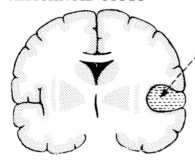

These cystic collections of CSF-like fluid lie in the Sylvian fissure, the chiasmatic cistern, the cisterna magna or over the hemisphere convexity. Some are related to a previous infective meningitis with subsequent adhesions but most are probably congenital in origin. Those occurring in the Sylvian fissure may be associated with temporal lobe agenesis.

Occasionally arachnoid cysts present as an intracranial mass, but more often they are found by chance on CT scan.

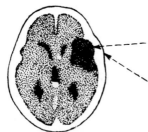

CT scan: shows a low density (CSF density well demarcated lesion, occasionally producing expansion of the overlying bone.

Treatment: only required if the mass effect becomes symptomatic — *marsupialisation* or *cystopertioneal shunt.*

EPIDERMOID/DERMOID CYSTS

These cysts, more commonly found in the posterior fossa (page 324), occasionally develop in the Sylvian or interhemispheric fissure. They may present with epilepsy, features of raised intracranial pressure or with focal neurological signs. Rupture into the subarachnoid space causes a chemical meningitis.

On CT scan, the extreme low attenuation of the cyst contents is characteristic. Symptoms may necessitate operative evacuation of the cyst contents. Removal of the cyst wall is often impossible and reaccumulation may occur.

TUMOURS OF THE POSTERIOR FOSSA — INTRINSIC

CEREBELLAR METASTASIS

In adults, metastasis is the commonest tumour of the cerebellar hemisphere. Primary tumour sites match those of supratentorial lesions (page 310).

Clinical features: may present acutely or progress over several months.

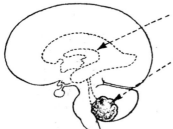

CSF obstruction *hydrocephalus* — signs and symptoms of raised intracranial pressure.
Cerebellar signs — ataxia, nystagmus, dysarthria, inco-ordination.

Extension into the cerebello-pontine angle may damage cranial nerves V-XII — especially if a *carcinomatous plaque* develops.

Investigations

CT scan shows a well-defined solid or cystic lesion lying within the cerebellar hemisphere and enhancing irregularly with contrast. Obstructive hydrocephalus is often evident on higher scan cuts.

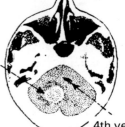

4th ventricle displaced

Management

Operative removal of a single metastasis through a suboccipital craniectomy is worthwhile, provided the patient has a reasonable prognosis from the primary tumour. Risks are small — extensive cerebellar hemisphere resection (on one side) seldom produces any significant permanent deficit. A course of *radiotherapy* should follow operation. Persistence of obstructive hydrocephalus requires a ventriculoperitoneal or atrial shunt.

HAEMANGIOBLASTOMA

This tumour of vascular origin occurs primarily in the middle-aged; it is slightly more prevalent in males. In some patients, haemangioblastomas occur at other sites, e.g. the spinal cord and retina and may be associated with other pathologies, e.g. polycythaemia and cysts in the pancreas and kidneys — *Von Hippel-Lindau disease* (page 540).

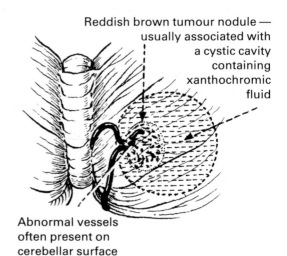

Reddish brown tumour nodule — usually associated with a cystic cavity containing xanthochromic fluid

Abnormal vessels often present on cerebellar surface

TUMOURS OF THE POSTERIOR FOSSA — INTRINSIC

HAEMANGIOBLASTOMA *(contd)*

Clinical features

Cerebellar signs and symptoms or the effects of CSF obstruction usually develop insidiously. Occasionally subarachnoid haemorrhage occurs. In female patients, symptoms often appear during pregnancy. Polycythaemia due to increased erythropoietin production is common.

Investigations

CT scan shows a well defined low density cystic region in the cerebellum with a strongly enhancing nodule in the wall. Occasionally, multiple lesions are evident.

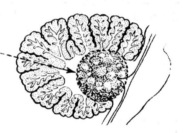

Management

In most patients *operative removal* of the tumour nodule is straightforward, but recurrences (or further tumours at other sites, e.g. spine) develop in 20%.

MEDULLOBLASTOMA

Medulloblastomas occur predominantly in childhood, with a peak age incidence of about 5 years. They arise in the cerebellar vermis and usually extend into the 4th ventricle. All are highly malignant and spread readily throughout the CSF pathways, often seeding to the lateral ventricles or the spinal theca.

Clinical features

Destruction of the cerebellar vermis causes truncal and gait ataxia often developing over a few weeks.

Alternatively, the patient presents with signs and symptoms of raised intracranial pressure due to blockage of CSF drainage. In the very young, failure to recognise these features has resulted in permanent visual loss from severe papilloedema.

Investigations

CT scan shows an isodense midline lesion in the cerebellar vermis, compressing and displacing the 4th ventricle and enhancing strongly with contrast.

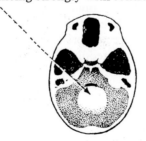 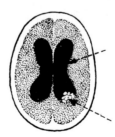

Higher cuts often show hydrocephalus

Look for evidence of CSF tumour seedings.

317

TUMOURS OF THE POSTERIOR FOSSA — INTRINSIC

MEDULLOBLASTOMA *(contd)*
Management
Operation: The aim is to remove as much tumour as possible, yet producing minimal damage to surrounding tissue, in particular crucial structures in the floor of the 4th ventricle. Some patients require a CSF shunt, although this provides a further potential route for tumour seeding.
Radiotherapy: Medulloblastomas are radiosensitive. Whole neural axis irradiation attempts to cover any undetected CSF seeding.
Chemotherapy: Appears to provide effective supplementary treatment, but initial encouraging results await full evaluation.

Prognosis
Studies in the last decade show a 5-year survival of approximately 40–60%. With present treatment methods, it is hoped this figure will approach 70%.

CEREBELLAR ASTROCYTOMA
In contrast to astrocytomas of the cerebral hemispheres, cerebellar astrocytomas are usually low grade tumours of the fibrillary or pilocytic types. They are particularly common in children and carry an excellent prognosis. Occasionally a more diffuse or anaplastic type occurs with a less favourable outcome. They usually lie in the cerebellar hemisphere or vermis but occasionally extend through a peduncle into the brain stem. Many have cystic components.

Clinical features
Cerebellar signs and symptoms tend to develop gradually over many months; if CSF obstruction occurs, the patient may present acutely with headache, papilloedema and deteriorating conscious level.

Investigations
CT scan — density changes and the degree of contrast enhancement are variable.

Often a low density cystic area abuts or encircles the tumour mass

Displaced 4th ventricle

Management
Ideally, complete *operative removal* is attempted provided the brain stem is not involved. With 'juvenile' pilocytic tumours, long-term survival is likely. Even after partial removal 'cures' have been reported; although histologically similar to some supratentorial lesions, growth characteristics clearly differ. Persistent hydrocephalus may require a ventriculoperitoneal/atrial shunt.

TUMOURS OF THE POSTERIOR FOSSA — INTRINSIC

BRAIN STEM ASTROCYTOMA
Rarely, astrocytomas arise within the brain stem. Most are of the fibrillary or pilocytic types and diffusely expand the pontine region although they can be malignant. They develop mainly in children or young adults.

Clinical features
Cranial nerve palsies and long tract signs gradually develop as the tumour progresses. Eventually conscious level is impaired. More malignant gliomas are associated with a rapidly progressing course, often with signs of raised intracranial pressure.

Investigations
CT scan shows:
– absence of the cisterns surrounding the brain stem
– posterior displacement of the 4th ventricle

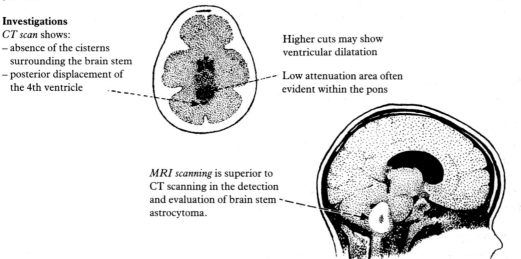

Higher cuts may show ventricular dilatation

Low attenuation area often evident within the pons

MRI scanning is superior to CT scanning in the detection and evaluation of brain stem astrocytoma.

Management
Operative exploration is rarely indicated. Usually radiotherapy is administered without histological confirmation of the diagnosis.

Prognosis
At best, the 5-year survival following radiotherapy is 35%. Rarely, patients may survive for up to 20 years with minimum disability.

TUMOURS OF THE POSTERIOR FOSSA — EXTRINSIC

ACOUSTIC NEURILEMMOMA/SCHWANNOMA
Nerve sheath tumours are the commonest infratentorial tumours, constituting 6% of all primary intracranial tumours and 80% of cerebellopontine angle lesions. They usually present in middle age (40–50 years) and occur more frequently in women. Bilateral neurilemmomas occur in 5% of patients and are characteristic of type 2 neurofibromatosis (page 538).

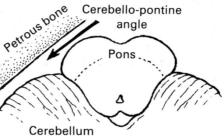

Petrous bone Cerebello-pontine angle

Pons

Cerebellum

They are benign, slowly growing tumours which arise primarily from the vestibular portion of the VIII cranial nerve and lie in the cerebellopontine angle — a wedge shaped area bounded by the petrous bone, the pons and the cerebellum. Rarely these tumours arise from the V cranial nerve.

TUMOURS OF THE POSTERIOR FOSSA — EXTRINSIC

ACOUSTIC NEURILEMMOMA/SCHWANNOMA *(contd)*

Pathology: The other type of nerve sheath tumour — neurofibroma (page 294) — does not occur intracranially.

Different histological types exist, often within the same tumour:

Antoni type A —
shoals and
whorls of
tightly packed
cells in groups
or palisades

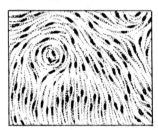

Antoni type B —
a meshwork of
interlinked
loosely packed
stellate cells.

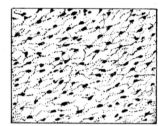

Clinical features

Patients with acoustic tumours often complain of *occipital pain* on the side of the tumour.
In addition:

VIII nerve damage causes a *gradually progressive sensorineural deafness* noted over many months or years. *Vertigo* is rarely troublesome since slow tumour growth readily permits compensation. Similarly *tinnitus* is usually minimal.

V nerve damage causes *facial pain, numbness* and *paraesthesia. Depression of the corneal reflex* is an important early sign.

Compression of the aqueduct and the 4th ventricle may result in hydrocephalus with *symptoms and signs of raised intracranial pressure.*

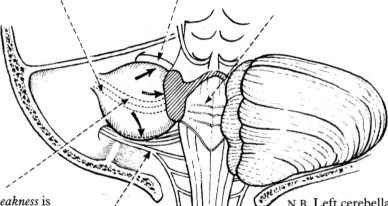

Facial weakness is surprisingly *uncommon* despite marked VII nerve compression

IX, X and XI nerve damage seldom occurs but occasionally large tumours cause *swallowing difficulty, voice change* and *palatal weakness.*

N.B. Left cerebellar hemisphere removed to expose the divided cerebellar peduncles.

Cerebellar and pontine damage — large tumours may compress the cerebellum causing *ataxia, ipsilateral inco-ordination* and *nystagmus.* Pontine damage may produce a *contralateral hemiparesis.*

320

TUMOURS OF THE POSTERIOR FOSSA — EXTRINSIC

ACOUSTIC NEURILEMMOMA/SCHWANNOMA *(contd)*
Investigations

Neuro-otological test (see pages 60–62)
— audiometry
— tone decay
— speech audiometry
— acoustic impedence
— brain stem auditory evoked potential

help differentiate deafness due to:
  conductive deficit
          cochlear deficit
  sensorineural
          retrocochlear deficit
          (e.g. acoustic tumour)

— caloric testing — invariably shows absence or impairment of the response on the affected side.

CT scan

Acoustic
neurilemmoma

Look for
dilatation of
the IAM

I.V. contrast is essential, since acoustic tumours are often isodense. After contrast the tumour, lying adjacent to the IAM enhances strongly. Low density cystic areas are occasionally seen. Patients with 4th ventricle compression may show associated dilatation of the 3rd and lateral ventricles.

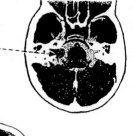

Metrizemide CT scan — the introduction of contrast into the *basal cisterns* (by lumbar or cisternal puncture) helps outline small acoustic tumours projecting from the internal auditory meatus. Alternatively, *air* insufflation may be used.

MRI scanning will also clearly demonstrate large tumours, but it is of particular value in identifying small intracanalicular lesions

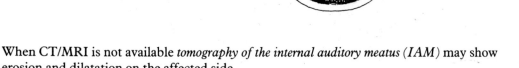

When CT/MRI is not available *tomography of the internal auditory meatus (IAM)* may show erosion and dilatation on the affected side.

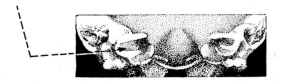

TUMOURS OF THE POSTERIOR FOSSA — EXTRINSIC

ACOUSTIC NEURILEMMOMA/SCHWANNOMA Management

The treatment of acoustic tumours is operative removal. A conservative approach gains nothing; operative risks relate directly to tumour size — the larger the tumour, the higher the operative mortality and the smaller the chance of preserving VII nerve function.

Technique

Middle fossa approach: temporal lobe retraction exposes the acoustic tumour and facial nerve from above. The tentorium cerebelli and the superior petrosal sinus are divided if necessary.

TRANSLABYRINTHINE APPROACH: approaching the tumour through the mastoid air cells and the labyrinth permits early identification of the facial nerve; tumour decompression and removal follows.

SUBOCCIPITAL APPROACH: the cerebellopontine angle is approached from below by removing occipital bone and retracting the cerebellum.

Tumour debulking aids dissection of the tumour capsule from the surrounding structures, including the facial nerve. Drilling away of the roof of the internal meatus exposes the tumour and facial nerve lying within the canal.

Some surgeons prefer a joint translabyrinthine/suboccipital approach.

All methods have their advocates. Limited visualisation of the brain stem structures through a translabyrinthine approach makes this inappropriate for large tumours. Inevitably this approach damages hearing. With very small tumours (which usually arise from the vestibular portion of the nerve), careful removal via the suboccipital route may preserve cochlear nerve as well as facial nerve function. Peroperative electrical monitoring may aid preservation of these structures.

Results

The mortality rate relates to tumour size and may approach 5% for very large tumours. Death usually results from damage to important vascular structures (e.g. anterior inferior cerebellar artery) or from postoperative cerebellar swelling. The incidence of facial nerve preservation also depends on tumour size. In most patients with small tumours (e.g. under 2 cm) facial nerve integrity is preserved compared to only 20% of patients with large tumours (e.g. over 4 cm), although recovery may take many months. Incomplete eyelid closure may require *tarsorrhaphy* to prevent corneal ulceration. When facial nerve palsy persists, *hypoglossal-facial anastomosis* may alleviate the final cosmetic result.

Swallowing difficulty from X cranial nerve damage seldom persists; intravenous or cautious oral fluid administration during this period should prevent aspiration.

Every effort should be made to remove all tumour tissue, with a two-stage operation if necessary. Incomplete removal results in late recurrence. Despite this, in some elderly patients, a subtotal intracapsular decompression may provide the safest approach.

TUMOURS OF THE POSTERIOR FOSSA — EXTRINSIC

TRIGEMINAL NEURILEMMOMA/SCHWANNOMA

Rarely neurilemmomas arise from the trigeminal ganglion or nerve root. These lie in the middle fossa or extend into the cerebellopontine angle, compress surrounding structures — cavernous sinus, midbrain and the pons — and erode the apex of the petrous bone.

Clinical features are usually long-standing — facial pain, paraesthesia and numbness. Compression of posterior fossa structures results in nystagmus, ataxia and hemiparesis.

Skull X-ray shows erosion of the petrous apex and CT scan demonstrates an enhancing lesion extending into the middle and/or posterior fossa.

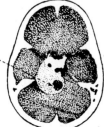

Management: Operative removal, even if subtotal, should provide long-lasting benefit. The tumour is approached through either the middle fossa or through a suboccipital craniectomy depending on the predominant site.

MENINGIOMA

Approximately 8% of all intracranial meningiomas arise in the posterior fossa.

Clinical features

These depend on the exact tumour site. Those arising over the *cerebellar convexity* may not present until the mass obstructs CSF drainage. Meningiomas arising in the *cerebellopontine angle* may involve any cranial nerve from V to XII. A *clivus* meningioma may cause bilateral VI nerve palsies before pontine pressure causes long tract signs.

Tumours growing at the *foramen magnum,* compressing the cervico-medullary junction, produce characteristic effects — pyramidal weakness initially affecting the ipsilateral arm, followed by the ipsilateral leg, spreading to the contralateral limbs with further tumour growth.

Investigations

CT scan identifies the exact tumour site.

Most meningiomas enhance homogeneously with contrast.

Management

As with supratentorial meningiomas, treatment aims at complete tumour removal. In the posterior fossa, cranial nerve involvement makes this difficult and exacting; excision of the tumour origin is seldom possible.

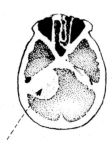

CT scan showing cerebellopontine angle meningioma. The absence of dilatation of the internal auditory meatus supports the diagnosis of meningioma rather than acoustic neurilemmoma.

323

TUMOURS OF THE POSTERIOR FOSSA — EXTRINSIC

EPIDERMOID/DERMOID CYSTS
These rare cysts of embryological origin develop from cells predestined to become either epidermis or dermis. They most commonly arise in the cerebellopontine angle but may also occur around the suprasellar cisterns, in the lateral ventricles and in the Sylvian fissures, often extending deeply into brain tissue.

Pathology: Depends on cell of origin:
Epidermoid (epidermis) — a thin transparent cyst wall often adheres firmly to surrounding tissues; the contents — keratinised debris and cholesterol crystals — produce a 'pearly' white appearance.
Dermoid (dermis) — as above, but thicker walled and, in addition, containing hair follicles and glandular tissue. Midline dermoid cysts lying in the posterior fossa often connect to the skin surface through a bony defect. This presents a potential route for infection.

Clinical features
When lying in the cerebellopontine angle, epidermoid/dermoid cysts often cause *trigeminal neuralgia* (see page 159). Neurological findings may range from a depressed corneal reflex to multiple cranial nerve palsies. Rupture and release of cholesterol into the subarachnoid space produces a severe and occasionally fatal *chemical meningitis*. The presence of a *suboccipital dimple* combined with an attack of infective meningitis should raise the possibility of a posterior fossa dermoid cyst with a cutaneous fistula.

Investigations
CT scan shows a characteristic low density (often 'fat' density) lesion, unchanged after contrast enhancement or showing only slight peripheral enhancement. Calcification may be evident.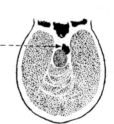

MRI scanning appears more sensitive than CT in detecting this tumour, with a T2 weighted scan demonstrating a high density lesion.

Treatment
Adherence of the cyst wall to important structures invariably prevents complete removal but evacuation of the contents provides symptomatic relief. Recollection of the keratinised debris usually takes many years.

SELLAR/SUPRASELLAR TUMOURS — PITUITARY ADENOMA

Tumours of the pituitary gland constitute about 5% of intracranial tumours. They arise from the anterior portion of the gland and are usually benign.

Previous classification
Previously based on the light microscopic appearance of the tumour cell type — ADENOMA EFFECT

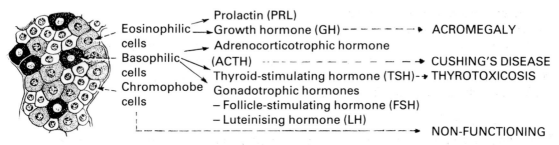

PRESENT classification
Recent immunoassay techniques permit a more practical classification based on the hormone type secreted. About half of the 'non-functioning' chromophobe adenomas secrete prolactin.

- **GH secreting tumour**
- **Prolactinoma**
- **ACTH secreting tumour**
- TSH secreting tumour
- FSH/LH secreting tumour
} rare

CLINICAL PRESENTATION

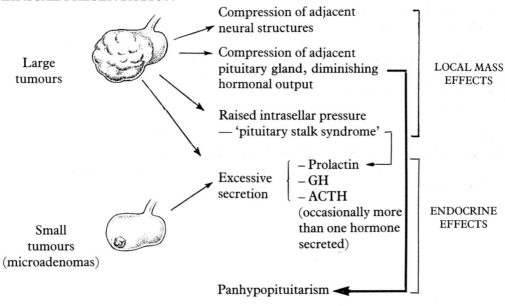

SELLAR/SUPRASELLAR TUMOURS — PITUITARY ADENOMA

LOCAL MASS EFFECT

Headache
Occurs in most patients with enlargement of the pituitary fossa. It is not specific in site or nature.

Visual field defects
Pressure on the inferior aspect of the optic chiasma causes *superior temporal quadrantanopia* initially, with progression to bitemporal hemianopia.

Cavernous sinus compression

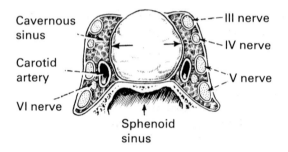

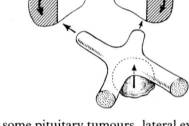

In some pituitary tumours, lateral expansion may compress nerves lying within the walls of the cavernous sinus. The III nerve is especially vulnerable.

ENDOCRINE EFFECT

1. Hypersecretion
The clinical syndrome produced is dependent on the hormone secreted.

GROWTH HORMONE (GH)
Stimulates growth and plays a part in control of protein, fat and carbohydrate metabolism. Excess GH in the adult causes ACROMEGALY.

In childhood, prior to fusion of bone epiphyses, GH excess causes GIGANTISM.

GH levels are usually increased to >10 ng/ml.

Hyperglycaemia normally suppresses GH secretion. GH samples are taken in conjunction with blood glucose during a glucose tolerance test. The lack of GH suppression after glucose administration confirms the presence of a tumour.

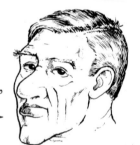

Enlargement of soft tissues, cartilage and bones in face, hands and feet

Coarse skin

'Soft, doughy' hands

Enlarged finger pulps and heel pads.

Enlarged viscera — heart, liver, thyroid

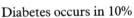

Diabetes occurs in 10%

SELLAR/SUPRASELLAR TUMOURS — PITUITARY ADENOMA

1. Hypersecretion (*contd*)
PROLACTIN

This hormone helps to promote lactation. The introduction of immunoassay techniques has shown prolactinaemias to be the commonest type of pituitary tumour and aided early detection of prolactin microadenomas.

This tumour may present with

- INFERTILITY
- AMENORRHOEA
- GALACTORRHOEA

In males, the tumour may present with IMPOTENCE or remain undetected until local pressure effects occur.

In most centres, a serum prolactin of 360 mU/l is considered abnormal, but before assuming the presence of a prolactin secreting tumour, other causes must be excluded.

Causes of hyperprolactinaemia
- Stress
- Pregnancy
- Drugs (phenothiazines, oestrogens)
- Hypothyroidism
- Renal disease
- Pituitary adenoma
- Hypothalamic lesion (e.g. sarcoid, craniopharyngioma) or pituitary stalk section
- Seizures

Since thyrotrophic hormone (TRH) stimulates prolactin release, prolactin levels are high in hypothyroidism.

Prolactin differs from other anterior pituitary hormones in that it is under tonic inhibitory control from the hypothalamus. Hypothalamic lesions or raised intrasellar pressure, compromising hypothalamic-pituitary perfusion (i.e. the 'pituitary stalk syndrome') produce a rise in serum prolactin, but levels seldom exceed 2000 mU/l. Prolactin levels above 4000 mU/l invariably indicate prolactinoma.

The following tests suggest the presence of a prolactin secreting tumour, but these are of limited reliability.
- Loss of the normal diurnal fluctuation in prolactin levels.
- Loss of reduction in response to TRH injection (normal increases $\times$ 500).
- Loss of response to metoclopramide (normal increases $\times$ 2000).

SELLAR/SUPRASELLAR TUMOURS — PITUITARY ADENOMA

ADRENOCORTICOTROPHIC HORMONE (ACTH)

ACTH stimulates secretion of cortisol and androgens. Hypersecretion from a pituitary adenoma or hyperplasia causes CUSHING'S DISEASE (bilateral adrenal hyperplasia) which presents with the characteristic features of CUSHING'S SYNDROME.

This syndrome may also be produced by an adrenal tumour or by ectopic secretion from a bronchial carcinoma, but steroid administration is the commonest cause.

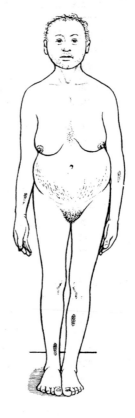

Features
– Moon face
– Acne
– Hirsutism and baldness
– Buffalo-type obesity
– Purple striae over flanks and abdomen
– Bruising
– Muscle weakness and wasting
– Osteoporosis
– Hypertension
– Increased susceptibility to infection
– Latent diabetes mellitus

The diagnosis of a pituitary disorder is established by finding normal or moderately raised ACTH levels which suppress with dexamethasone.

Ectopic ACTH production does not suppress with dexamethasone.

With adrenal tumours, ACTH levels are virtually undetectable.

Bilateral adrenalectomy for Cushing's syndrome is sometimes followed by the development of Nelson's syndrome — high ACTH levels, pituitary enlargement and marked skin pigmentation.

TSH — stimulates thyroid hormone secretion
FSH — controls growth of ovarian follicles/spermatogenesis
LH — induces ovulation/testosterone secretion
⎫
⎬ Hypersecreting
⎭ tumours
very rare.

SELLAR/SUPRASELLAR TUMOURS — PITUITARY ADENOMA

2. Hyposecretion

Many pituitary tumours are diagnosed before panhypopituitarism develops, but large tumours may cause gradual impairment of pituitary hormone secretion. Growth hormone and the gonadotrophins are first affected, followed by TSH and ACTH. Panhypopituitarism only occurs when more than 80% of the anterior pituitary is destroyed.

Impaired secretion	Adults	Children
GH	—	Pituitary dwarfism —
Gonadotrophins —	Amenorrhoea, sterility, loss of libido	diminished skeletal growth,
ACTH —	Glucocorticoid and androgen deficiency, muscle weakness and fatigue	retarded sexual development, hypoglycaemic episodes,
TSH —	Secondary hypothyroidism — sensitivity to cold, dry skin, physical and mental sluggishness, coarseness of hair	normal intelligence
Prolactin* —	Failure of lactation	

*Prolactin secretion is most resistant to pituitary damage. Deficiency is seldom evident, usually only presenting after postpartum haemorrhage (Sheehan's syndrome) as a failure of lactation associated with the other features of panhypopituitarism.

Pituitary hormone assay cannot distinguish low 'normal' levels from impaired secretion, *but low levels of pituitary hormone in the presence of low target gland hormones* confirm hyposecretion, e.g. low TSH levels despite a low serum thyroxine.

The lack of response to tests designed to increase specific pituitary hormones provides additional confirmation of hypofunction:

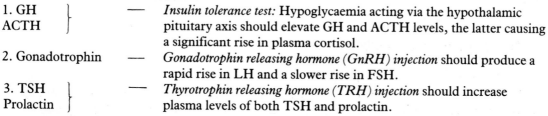

1. GH
   ACTH — *Insulin tolerance test:* Hypoglycaemia acting via the hypothalamic pituitary axis should elevate GH and ACTH levels, the latter causing a significant rise in plasma cortisol.

2. Gonadotrophin — *Gonadotrophin releasing hormone (GnRH) injection* should produce a rapid rise in LH and a slower rise in FSH.

3. TSH
   Prolactin — *Thyrotrophin releasing hormone (TRH) injection* should increase plasma levels of both TSH and prolactin.

The above tests can be carried out simultaneously as the *Combined pituitary stimulation test.* Insulin, GnRH and TRH are injected intravenously and all anterior pituitary hormones measured from repeated blood samples taken over a 2-hour period. Glucose levels are also checked to ensure adequacy of the hypoglycaemia.

PITUITARY APOPLEXY

This is an uncommon complication of pituitary tumours due to the occurrence of haemorrhage into the tumour substance. Severe headache of sudden onset simulating subarachnoid haemorrhage, rapidly progressive visual failure and extraocular nerve palsies accompany acute pituitary insufficiency. Death may follow unless urgent treatment is instituted.

SELLAR/SUPRASELLAR TUMOURS — PITUITARY ADENOMA

NEURORADIOLOGICAL INVESTIGATION

Skull X-ray

Large tumours
cause expansion or
'ballooning' of the
pituitary fossa
and may erode
the floor

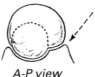

A-P view

Asymmetrical fossa expansion gives the
appearance of a 'double floor'
effect on the *lateral view*

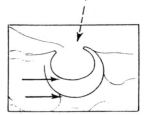

CT scan

CT scan with contrast enhancement clearly demonstrates
tumours filling the pituitary fossa and expanding into
the suprasellar compartment.

Suprasellar extension

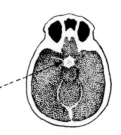

Large tumours: Coronal and axial views of the pituitary
region obtained either by reconstruction or direct scanning
demonstrate the exact extent of the suprasellar extension.

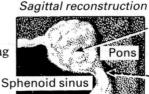

Sagittal reconstruction

Large tumour
with
suprasellar
extension

Pons

Sphenoid sinus   4th ventricle

Microadenomas: One- or two-millimetre slices may
demonstrate a low density region within the gland tissue
(or may show deviation of the pituitary stalk from the
midline. Tumours >5 mm diameter produce
these characteristic appearances. Tumours
under this size are difficult to detect.

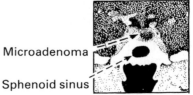

Coronal view

Microadenoma

Sphenoid sinus

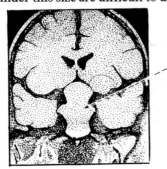

MRI provides most information on large tumours,
clearly delineating any suprasellar extension and
the effect on adjacent structures.

MRI is no better than CT scanning in the detection
of microadenomas; both have false positives and
false negatives.

Angiography or **MRI** may be required before
trans-sphenoidal operation to exclude the presence of
an incidental medially projecting aneurysm.

SELLAR/SUPRASELLAR TUMOURS — PITUITARY ADENOMA

MANAGEMENT
A variety of different forms of treatment are available:

Drug therapy
Bromocriptine: a dopamine agonist which lowers abnormal circulating hormone concentrations, especially prolactin. In two-thirds of patients with prolactinomas, the prolactin levels fall and the tumour shrinks. These patients require long-term therapy as the source of the hyperprolactinaemia persists. Cessation of treatment can result in rapid tumour re-expansion.

Somatostatin analogues: inhibit growth hormone production and cause tumour shrinkage in a proportion of patients. Some TSH secreting tumours may also respond to this therapy. Results of long-term therapy await evaluation.

Operative approach

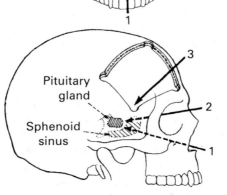

From BELOW:
1. *Trans-sphenoidal*
Through an incision in the upper gum the nasal mucosa is stripped from the septum and the pituitary fossa approached through the sphenoid sinus.

2. *Transethmoidal*
An incision is made on the medial orbital wall and the pituitary fossa approached through the ethmoid and sphenoid sinuses.
    With the transethmoidal and trans-sphenoidal routes the pituitary gland can be directly visualised and explored for microadenoma. Even large tumours with suprasellar extensions may be removed from below, avoiding the need for craniotomy.

From ABOVE
3. *Transfrontal*
Through a craniotomy flap the frontal lobe is retracted to provide direct access to the pituitary tumour. This approach is usually reserved for tumours with large frontal or lateral extensions.

N.B. All patients require steroid cover before any anaesthetic or operative procedure.

Radiotherapy
Pituitary adenomas are radiosensitive and external irradiation is commonly employed. Occasionally, radioactive seeds of yttrium or gold are implanted into the pituitary fossa, either via a trans-sphenoidal approach or stereotactically through a frontal burr hole.
    Several months elapse before hormone levels begin to fall. Pituitary function gradually declines over a 5 – 10 year period after treatment and most patients eventually require replacement hormone therapy to prevent symptoms of hypopituitarism developing.

SELLAR/SUPRASELLAR TUMOURS — PITUITARY ADENOMA

MANAGEMENT (*contd*)

Treatment selection

Treatment choice depends on:
- — presenting problems and patient's requirements, e.g. restoring fertility, halting visual deterioration.
- — patient's age.
- — preference and experience of the treatment centre.

Microadenomas

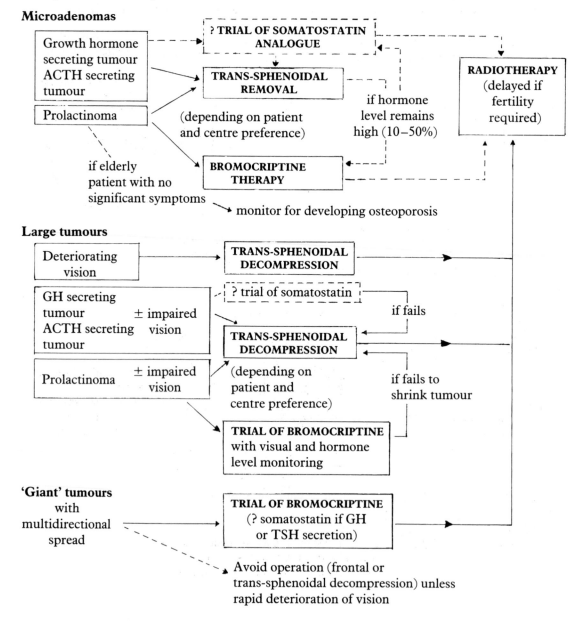

Large tumours

'Giant' tumours

SELLAR/SUPRASELLAR TUMOURS

CRANIOPHARYNGIOMA

These cystic tumours constitute about 3% of all primary intracranial tumours. They present predominantly in children and in young adults but symptoms may develop at any age. Although benign, their proximity to crucial structures poses complex problems of management. Most craniopharyngiomas have solid components of squamous epithelium with calcified debris and one or more cystic regions containing greenish cholesteatomatous fluid. In some, the tumour is solid throughout. Although the tumour capsule appears well defined, histological examination reveals finger-like projections extending into adjacent tissue with marked surrounding gliosis.

Sites: Growth usually begins near the pituitary stalk, but may extend in many directions.

Clinical features: depend on the exact site and size of the tumour. Growth is slow and most signs and symptoms develop insidiously.

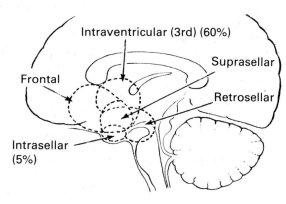

Intraventricular (3rd) (60%)

Suprasellar

Frontal

Retrosellar

Intrasellar (5%)

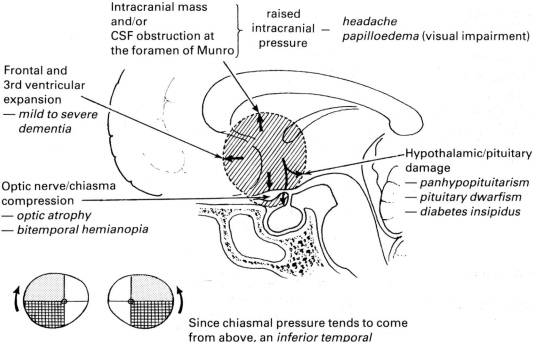

Intracranial mass and/or CSF obstruction at the foramen of Munro } raised intracranial — *headache* pressure *papilloedema* (visual impairment)

Frontal and 3rd ventricular expansion
— *mild to severe dementia*

Hypothalamic/pituitary damage
— *panhypopituitarism*
— *pituitary dwarfism*
— *diabetes insipidus*

Optic nerve/chiasma compression
— *optic atrophy*
— *bitemporal hemianopia*

Since chiasmal pressure tends to come from above, an *inferior temporal quadrantanopia* usually develops first

SELLAR/SUPRASELLAR TUMOURS

CRANIOPHARYNGIOMA *(contd)*
Investigations
Skull X-ray: shows calcification above or within the pituitary fossa in most children and in 25% of adults.

CT scan: shows a lesion of mixed density containing solid and cystic components lying in the suprasellar region.

In children, CT scan invariably shows calcification

Coronal or sagittal CT reconstruction or MRI helps by demonstrating the exact relationships of the tumour to the 3rd ventricle

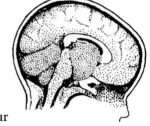

The cyst capsule often enhances with contrast.

Pituitary function studies (page 329): often demonstrate the need for hormone replacement.

Management
Several options exist; the more aggressive the treatment, the higher the risks, but the lower the recurrence rate.

All patients require steroid cover before any anaesthetic or operative procedure.

Operative removal usually involves a subfrontal or subtemporal craniotomy, perhaps combined with a transcallosal approach (i.e. splitting the anterior corpus callosum from above and approaching the tumour through the 3rd ventricle). The trans-sphenoidal route may permit removal of purely intrasellar tumours.

Methods
1. *Total tumour excision (+ radiotherapy if recurrence develops)*
2. *Subtotal tumour excision + radiotherapy*
3. *Cyst drainage +* ——————— *radiotherapy*
   (with an indwelling   *or*
   catheter and reservoir)   *implantation of yttrium-90*

Attempted total excision carries a risk of life-threatening hypothalamic damage, but if successful avoids the immediate need and associated risks of radiotherapy to a developing brain. Operative mortality lies between 0–10% and depends on the tumour site and the extent of the attempted removal. Some report a recurrence rate of 50% within 10 years of an apparent 'total' removal. This presumably results from residual tumour extensions lying beyond the capsule.

With subtotal removal the recurrence rate approaches 90%, but with radiotherapy this falls to 30–50%.

The decision to aim for total or subtotal removal requires careful judgement. Preoperative investigations help but the final decision often awaits direct exploration.

SELLAR/SUPRASELLAR TUMOURS

OPTIC NERVE (GLIOMA) ASTROCYTOMA

This rare tumour usually presents in children under 10 years. Up to two-thirds are associated with neurofibromatosis. Tumour growth expands the nerve in a fusiform manner. Some extend anteriorly into the orbit, others posteriorly to involve the optic chiasma. All are of the pilocytic type and growth is slow.

Optic nerve tumour may 'dumbbell' through the optic foramen.

Clinical features

Visual field scotomas gradually progress to *complete visual loss.*
   Orbital extension causes *proptosis.*
   In some patients posterior expansion beyond the chiasma causes *hypothalamic damage (precocious puberty and other endocrine disturbance)* and/or *hydrocephalus.*
   X-rays of the orbital foramen show dilatation and *CT scans* demonstrate an enhancing mixed attenuation mass within the orbit or lying in the suprasellar region.

Management

| Unilateral within orbit | — Complete excision with orbital enucleation if necessary |
| Lesion involving the optic chiasma | — Conservative approach (the value of radiotherapy is not known) |

Prognosis

— Long-term survival expected.

— Patients may retain vision for many years; survival is often long-term. Those with hypothalamic damage have a poor prognosis.

SUPRASELLAR MENINGIOMA

Meningiomas arising from the tuberculum sellae often present early as a result of chiasmal compression causing visual field defects — usually a *bitemporal hemianopia.*

Straight X-rays may show *hyperostosis* of the tuberculum sellae or planum sphenoidale.

Hyperostotic sphenoid

CT scan shows a rounded, often partly calcified suprasellar mass homogeneously enhancing with contrast.
   Unfortunately the visual defect often persists after operation, but attempted removal is essential to prevent further progression.

MENINGIOMA OF THE OPTIC NERVE SHEATH

Rarely, meningiomas arise from the optic nerve sheath, usually extending in dumbbell fashion through the optic foramen. Some penetrate the orbital dura and invade the orbital contents. Total excision is impossible without sacrificing the adjacent optic nerve.

SUPRASELLAR EPIDERMOID/DERMOID (see page 324).

Note: large aneurysms or granulomas (TB, sarcoid) may simulate a sellar/suprasellar tumour on CT scan. If in doubt, perform angiography prior to operative exploration.

PINEAL REGION TUMOURS

Pineal region tumours are relatively uncommon. They consist of a variety of different pathological types and as a result of the direct anatomical relationship with the third ventricle include tumours arising at this site. Less than 20% actually originate from 'pineal' cells.

PATHOLOGICAL TYPES

Teratoma: well differentiated tumour occurring predominantly in males, and formed from various cell types — muscle, bone, cartilage, dermis.

Tumour consistency depends on the predominant cell type. In most patients the tumour margin is well defined. Malignant, poorly differentiated forms occasionally occur.

Germinoma: a malignant tumour, resembling seminoma of the testis. The tumour adheres firmly to the surrounding tissues and cells readily spread to the floor or anterior wall of the third ventricle. Cells may also seed through the CSF pathways to the spinal cord or cauda equina.

Pineocytoma: well differentiated, slowly growing tumour } rare tumours of true
Pineoblastoma: poorly differentiated, highly malignant tumour } 'pineal' origin.

Glial cell tumours — astrocytoma — arising from cells within the pineal gland, or from adjacent brain.

ependymoma — arising from cells lining the third ventricle.

Meningioma
Dermoid } rarely occur in the pineal region.
Epidermoid

CLINICAL FEATURES   Develop due to:

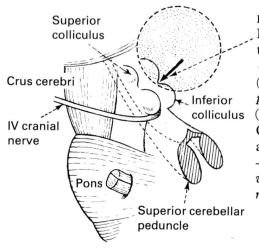

Superior colliculus
Crus cerebri
IV cranial nerve
Pons
Inferior colliculus
Superior cerebellar peduncle

LOCAL MASS EFFECT
Pressure on the tectal region (midbrain) — PARINAUD'S *syndrome (impaired upward gaze, pupillary abnormalities)* (page 153).
Compression of the aqueduct of Sylvius — *obstructive hydrocephalus with signs and symptoms of raised intracranial pressure.*

EFFECTS FROM SPREAD THROUGH THE THIRD VENTRICLE
e.g. germinoma
— *hypothalamic damage, diabetes insipidus, hypo/hyperphagia, precocious puberty, hypopituitarism.*
— *optic chiasmal involvement with visual field defects.*

336

PINEAL REGION TUMOURS

INVESTIGATIONS

CT scan shows a mass projecting into the posterior aspect of the third ventricle with associated dilatation of the third and lateral ventricles.

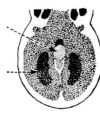

3rd ventricle   Pineal tumour

Pituitary fossa   Tentorium cerebelli

Sagittal CT reconstruction or *MRI scanning* clarifies the exact tumour relationship to the third ventricle.

Pineocytomas — may appear calcified.
Teratomas — may contain mixed densities from fat to calcification.

CSF cytology: occasionally reveals malignant cells and may indicate the tumour type.
Serum human chorionic gonadotrophin
Serum alpha fetoprotein } may rise in patients with germinoma.

MANAGEMENT

Hydrocephalus often requires urgent treatment with a *ventriculoperitoneal* or *ventriculo-atrial shunt*. Large tumours may obstruct the foramen of Munro, making *bilateral* ventricular drainage. necessary.

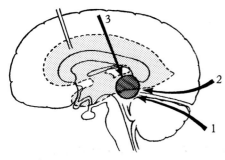

The site of pineal region tumours makes the operative approach difficult. Although modern techniques considerably diminish the risk of a direct operation, many neurosurgeons advocate initial treatment with *radiotherapy* (without tissue diagnosis). About 70% of tumours are radiosensitive and show a dramatic reduction in size. Failure to respond would indicate the need for tissue diagnosis, with a *stereotactic biopsy* or *direct operative exploration*.

Routes of direct approach
1 — Infratentorial
2 — Supratentorial
3 — Transventricular

Patients undergoing a CSF shunt followed by radiotherapy survive 4 years on average.

TUMOURS OF THE VENTRICULAR SYSTEM

EPENDYMOMA
Intracranial ependymomas originate from cells lining the ventricular cavities. Most arise in the 4th ventricle and in this site occur predominantly in children. Both low grade and malignant forms are found and tumour cells may seed throughout CSF pathways.

In the *4th ventricle*, ependymomas present with cerebellar signs or, more commonly, with signs and symptoms of raised intracranial pressure from CSF obstruction. *Vomiting* is often an early feature from direct brain stem involvement.

CT scanning shows an isodense mass, with or without calcification, lying within the 4th ventricle and usually enhancing with contrast.

Management
The aim is complete operative removal, although infiltration of the floor of the 4th ventricle may prevent this. Most clinicians advise radiotherapy postoperatively, but its value is limited in the low grade tumours.

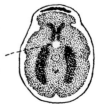

Prognosis
Despite relatively slow growth, results are often disappointing with 5-year survival ranging from 20–50%.

CHOROID PLEXUS PAPILLOMA
Rare, benign tumour with a granular surface and a gritty texture.

They develop from the choroid plexus — in the *4th ventricle* — *adults*,
— in the *lateral venticle* — *children*.

Malignant forms occasionally occur in children.
Most patients present with hydrocephalus, either due to obstruction or to excessive CSF secretion from the tumour.
CT scanning shows a hyperdense mass within the ventricular system.
Operative removal gives good results.

COLLOID CYST OF THE THIRD VENTRICLE
A benign cyst, containing a mucoid fluid may arise from embryological remnants in the roof of the third ventricle. When of sufficient size (about 2 cm) it occludes CSF drainage from both lateral ventricles through the foramen of Munro.

Clinical features: Symptoms may be intermittent, possibly due to a ball-valve effect, with episodes of loss of consciousness or sudden weakness of legs.

CT scan shows a small round mass of increased density, lying level with the foramen of Munro, causing lateral ventricular dilatation. Cyst drainage through a stereotactically placed needle is usually feasible and safe. If this fails operative removal through the right lateral ventricle carries little additional risk.

MENINGIOMA: rarely arises in the *lateral* ventricles. Often symptoms are mild and long standing. Operative removal only becomes necessary when symptoms and signs appear.

GERMINOMA }
TERATOMA } see Pineal region tumours, page 336

TUMOURS OF THE ORBIT

The orbital cavity is bounded —

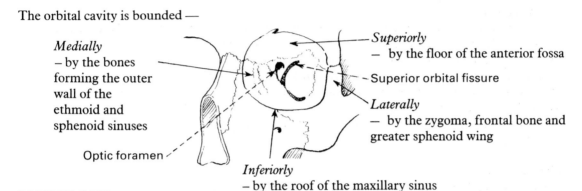

Medially
— by the bones forming the outer wall of the ethmoid and sphenoid sinuses

Optic foramen

Superiorly
— by the floor of the anterior fossa

Superior orbital fissure

Laterally
— by the zygoma, frontal bone and greater sphenoid wing

Inferiorly
— by the roof of the maxillary sinus

PATHOLOGY
Tumours may arise from any of the structures lying within or around the orbit.

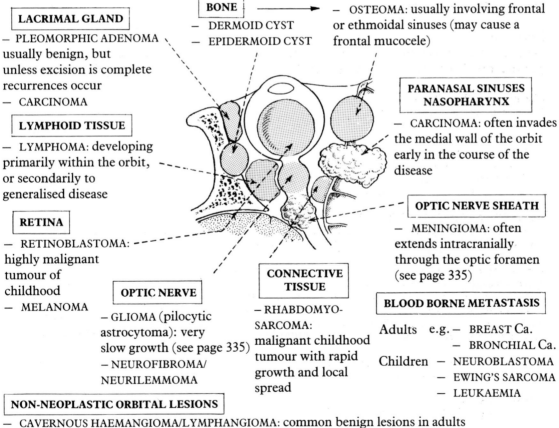

LACRIMAL GLAND

— PLEOMORPHIC ADENOMA usually benign, but unless excision is complete recurrences occur
— CARCINOMA

LYMPHOID TISSUE

— LYMPHOMA: developing primarily within the orbit, or secondarily to generalised disease

RETINA

— RETINOBLASTOMA: highly malignant tumour of childhood
— MELANOMA

BONE ⟶
— DERMOID CYST
— EPIDERMOID CYST

— OSTEOMA: usually involving frontal or ethmoidal sinuses (may cause a frontal mucocele)

PARANASAL SINUSES NASOPHARYNX

— CARCINOMA: often invades the medial wall of the orbit early in the course of the disease

OPTIC NERVE SHEATH

— MENINGIOMA: often extends intracranially through the optic foramen (see page 335)

OPTIC NERVE

— GLIOMA (pilocytic astrocytoma): very slow growth (see page 335)
— NEUROFIBROMA/ NEURILEMMOMA

CONNECTIVE TISSUE

— RHABDOMYO-SARCOMA: malignant childhood tumour with rapid growth and local spread

BLOOD BORNE METASTASIS

Adults e.g. — BREAST Ca.
        — BRONCHIAL Ca.
Children — NEUROBLASTOMA
        — EWING'S SARCOMA
        — LEUKAEMIA

NON-NEOPLASTIC ORBITAL LESIONS

— CAVERNOUS HAEMANGIOMA/LYMPHANGIOMA: common benign lesions in adults
— ORBITAL GRANULOMA (PSEUDOTUMOUR) ⎱ (see over)
— DYSTHYROID EXOPHTHALMOS ⎰
— WEGENER'S GRANULOMATOSIS
— SARCOIDOSIS   N.B. CAROTID-CAVERNOUS FISTULA presents
— HISTIOCYTOSIS X   with a pulsatile exophthalmos.   339

TUMOURS OF THE ORBIT

CLINICAL SYMPTOMS AND SIGNS

Orbital pain: prominent in rapidly growing malignant tumours, but also a characteristic feature of orbital granuloma and carotid-cavernous fistula.

Proptosis: forward displacement of the globe is a common feature, progressing gradually and painlessly over months or years (benign tumours) or rapidly (malignant lesions).

Lid swelling: may be pronounced in orbital granuloma, dysthyroid exophthalmos or carotid-cavernous fistula.

Palpation: may reveal a mass causing globe or lid distortion — especially with lacrimal gland tumours or with a mucocele. *Pulsation* indicates a vascular lesion — carotid-cavernous fistula or arteriovenous malformation — listen for a bruit.

Eye movements: often limited for mechanical reasons, but if marked, may result from a dysthyroid ophthalmoplegia or from III, IV or VI nerve lesions in the orbital fissure (e.g. Tolosa Hunt syndrome) or cavernous sinus.

Visual acuity: may diminish due to direct involvement of the optic nerve or retina, or indirectly from occlusion of vascular structures.

INVESTIGATIONS

X-ray of the orbit: may reveal local erosion (malignancy), dilatation of the optic foramen (meningioma, optic nerve glioma) and occasionally calcification (retinoblastoma, lacrimal gland tumours). A meningioma often causes local sclerosis.

CT scan of the orbits demonstrates the precise site of intraorbital pathology and shows the presence of any intracranial extension.

Axial view showing an optic nerve glioma. Coronal views are of value in assessing the size of the optic nerve and extraocular muscles and the floor and roof of the orbit

MRI may provide more information in certain conditions, e.g. meningioma of the optic nerve sheath.

MANAGEMENT

BENIGN tumours: require excision, but if visual loss would inevitably result, the clinician may adopt a conservative approach.

MALIGNANT tumours: require biopsy plus radiotherapy. Lymphomas may also benefit from chemotherapy. Occasionally localised lesions (e.g. carcinoma of the lacrimal gland) require radical resection.

Operative approach

Frontal-transcranial: for tumours with intracranial extension or lying posterior and medial to the optic nerve

Ethmoidal: for anterior tumours, lying medial to the optic nerve

Lateral: for tumours lying superior, lateral or inferior to the optic nerve

340

NON-NEOPLASTIC ORBITAL LESIONS

ORBITAL GRANULOMA (pseudotumour)

Sudden onset of *orbital pain* with *lid oedema, proptosis* and *chemosis* due to a diffuse granulomatous infiltrate of lymphocytes and plasma cells involving multiple structures within the orbit.

This condition usually occurs in middle age and seldom occurs bilaterally. CT scanning shows a diffuse orbital lesion, although one structure may be predominantly involved, e.g. optic nerve, extraocular muscles or the lacrimal gland. If diagnostic doubt remains, a biopsy is required. Most patients show a dramatic response to high dose *steroid therapy*. If symptoms persist, the lesion should respond well to radiotherapy.

DYSTHYROID EXOPHTHALMOS

The thyrotoxic patient with bilateral exophthalmos presents no diagnostic difficulty, but dysthyroid exophthalmos, with marked lid oedema, lid retraction and ophthalmoplegia *may occur unilaterally* without evidence of thyroid disease.

Coronal CT scanning establishes the diagnosis by demonstrating enlargement of the extraocular muscles — primarily the medial and inferior recti.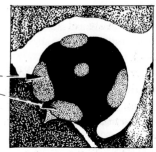

Circulating thyroid hormone levels are often normal. Thyroid releasing hormone stimulation or thyroid suppression tests may support the diagnosis.

Management

Steroids should help. A few patients require orbital decompression in an attempt to prevent corneal ulceration, papilloedema and blindness.

TUMOURS OF THE SKULL BASE

MALIGNANT
CARCINOMA
Carcinoma of the nasopharynx, paranasal sinuses or ear may extend intracranially either by direct erosion or through the skull foramina. It frequently penetrates the dura (in contrast to metastatic carcinoma of the spinal cord) and may involve almost any cranial nerve. Symptoms of nasopharyngeal or sinus disease are often associated with facial pain and numbness. Spread to the CSF pathways leads to *carcinomatous meningitis* and may cause multiple cranial nerve palsies.
Skull X-ray, CT scan and *MRI scan* will demonstrate a lesion involving the skull base.
Treatment is usually restricted to retropharyngeal biopsy plus radiotherapy.

Chordoma —
sites of
intracranial
origin

CHORDOMA
Rare tumours of notochordal cell rests arising predominantly in the sphenoido-occipital (clivus) and sacrococcyeal regions. Although growth begins in the midline, they often expand asymmetrically into the intracranial cavity. Chordomas may present at any age, but the incidence peaks in the 4th decade. They are locally invasive and rarely metastasise.
Clinical: most patients develop nasal obstruction. Cranial nerve palsies usually follow and depend on the exact tumour site.
Skull X-ray shows a soft tissue mass with an osteolytic lesion of the sphenoid, basi-occiput or petrous apex.
CT scan confirms the presence of a partly calcified mass causing marked bone destruction and extending into the nasopharyngeal space.
MRI scan more clearly demonstrates the structural relationships.
Management: the tumour site prevents complete removal. Usually extensive debulking (sometimes through the transoral route) is combined with radiotherapy. Most patients die within 10 years of the initial presentation.

BENIGN
GLOMUS JUGULARE TUMOUR (syn: chemodectoma, paraganglioma)
Rare tumour arising from chemoreceptor cells in the jugular bulb or from similar cells in the middle ear mucosa. This tumour extensively erodes the jugular foramen and petrous bone; many patients present with cranial nerve palsies, especially IX-XII. Chemodectomas occasionally arise at other sites and metastasis may occur.
X-ray and *CT scan* demonstrate an osteolytic lesion expanding the jugular foramen.
Angiography reveals a vascular tumour, usually only filling from the external carotid artery, but occasionally from vertebral branches.
Management: tumour vascularity makes excision difficult. Selective embolisation may considerably reduce the operative risks or provide an alternative treatment. The value of radiotherapy is uncertain.

OSTEOMA
Rare tumours, usually occurring in the frontal sinus and eroding into the orbit, nasal cavity or anterior fossa. If sinus drainage becomes obstructed, a *mucocele* develops, often with infected contents. These lesions require excision, either through an ethmoidal approach or through a frontal craniotomy.

INTRACRANIAL ABSCESS

The advent of antibiotics and improved treatment of ear and sinus infection has led to a reduction in intracranial abscess formation but the incidence still lies at 2–3 patients per million per year.

Pus may accumulate in:
- the extradural space — — — — —
  EXTRADURAL ABSCESS
- the subdural space — — — —
  SUBDURAL EMPYEMA
- the brain parenchyma — — —
  CEREBRAL ABSCESS

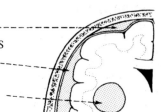

CEREBRAL ABSCESS
Source of infection

HAEMATOGENOUS SPREAD
- Subacute bacterial endocarditis
- Congenital heart disease (especially right to left shunt)
- Bronchiectasis or pulmonary abscess

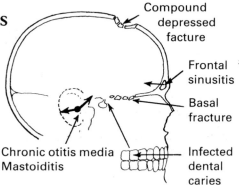

Compound depressed facture

Frontal sinusitis

Basal fracture

Chronic otitis media
Mastoiditis

Infected dental caries

Local spread

direct penetration of the dura

indirect —— extension of an infected thrombus. embolic spread along a vein

Abscess *site* depends on the source, e.g. frontal sinusitis
→ frontal lobes
mastoiditis → temporal lobe
↘ or cerebellum

Organisms: *Streptococcus* (especially *Strep. viridans*)

Anaerobic streptococci ⎫
Bacteroides ⎬ Improved anaerobic culture techniques have demonstrated the
E. coli ⎭ frequent occurrence of these organisms in intracranial abscesses.
Proteus Prior to this, 50% of cultures appeared 'sterile'.
Staphylococcus aureus
Toxoplasma, Aspergillus — in immunocompromised
and Candida patients (see page 492)

Pathogenesis

Infection source

Local ← → Haematogenous

Small vessel occlusion or surface thrombophlebitis may precede parenchymal involvement (bacteria appear to favour damaged brain)

↓

Parenchymal bacterial invasion

↓

Polymorphonuclear infiltrate and impaired vascular permeability

Risk of rupture into adjacent ventricle

'Mass' + surrounding oedema → *raised ICP*

Extension to cortical surface → *purulent meningitis*

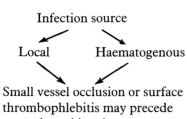

'Daughter' loculi may form

ABSCESS

Mature capsule forms with central zone of necrotic tissue, inflammatory cells and necrotic debris.

↑

Zone of granulation → Thin capsule of fibroblasts
tissue 'CEREBRITIS' and reticular fibres forms

343

INTRACRANIAL ABSCESS

CEREBRAL ABSCESS (contd)
Clinical effects
Symptoms and signs usually develop over 2–3 weeks. Occasionally the onset is more gradual, but features may develop acutely in the immunocompromised patient. Clinical features arise from:
— Toxicity — *pyrexia, malaise* (although systemic signs often absent).
— Raised intracranial pressure — *headache, vomiting → deterioration of conscious level.*
— Focal damage — *hemiparesis, dysphasia, ataxia, nystagmus.*
             ⟍ *epilepsy* — partial or generalised, occurring in over 30%.
— Infection source — *tenderness over mastoid* or *sinuses, discharging ear.*
                bacterial endocarditis — *cardiac murmurs, petechiae, splenomegaly.*
— Neck stiffness due to coexistent meningitis or tonsillar herniation occurs in 25%.

N.B. Beware attributing patient's deteriorating clinical state to the primary condition, e.g. otitis media, thus delaying essential investigations.

Investigations
X-ray of the sinuses and mastoids: opacities indicate infection.
CT scan: in the stage of 'cerebritis' the CT scan may appear normal or only show an area of low density. As the abscess progresses, a characteristic appearance emerges:

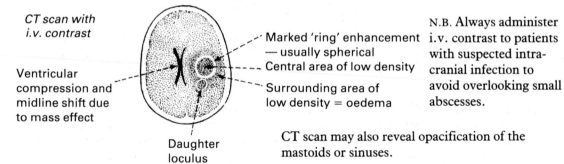

CT scan with i.v. contrast

Ventricular compression and midline shift due to mass effect

Daughter loculus

Marked 'ring' enhancement — usually spherical
Central area of low density
Surrounding area of low density = oedema

N.B. Always administer i.v. contrast to patients with suspected intra-cranial infection to avoid overlooking small abscesses.

CT scan may also reveal opacification of the mastoids or sinuses.

Prior to the availability of CT scanning, *isotope scans* accurately identified the lesion site, but did not confirm its nature. Lumbar puncture was occasionally performed showing ↑ protein, e.g. 1 g/l, ↑ white cell count (several hundred/ml) — polymorphs or lymphocytes.

Peripheral blood — may show ↑ ESR, leucocytosis, or positive blood culture.

N.B. Do not perform lumbar puncture in the presence of a suspected mass lesion.

INTRACRANIAL ABSCESS

CEREBRAL ABSCESS *(contd)*
Management:
1. Antibiotics
Commence i.v. antibiotics on establishing the diagnosis (prior to determining the responsible organism or its sensitivities). Antibiotics are selected for their ability to cross the blood–brain barrier. The ease with which they penetrate the abscess capsule remains uncertain.
Use combined
therapy:

—PENICILLIN 4 megaunits q.i.d. ⎫ Penicillin covers streptococcus,
— CHLORAMPHENICOL 1 g q.i.d. ⎬ metronidazole covers anaerobic
— METRONIDAZOLE 500 mg q.i.d. ⎭ organisms.

In immunocompromised patients — see page 492.

Later determination of the organism and its sensitivities permits alteration to more specific drugs. Antibiotic medication should continue for 4–6 weeks.

2. Abscess drainage
Various methods exist:

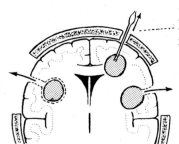

Burr hole aspiration of pus, with repeated aspirations as required.

Primary excision of the whole abscess including the capsule (standard treatment of cerebellar abscess)

Evacuation of the abscess contents under direct vision, leaving the capsule remnants.

Burr hole aspiration is simple and relatively safe. Persistent reaccumulation of pus despite repeated aspiration requires secondary excision. Primary excision removes the abscess in a single procedure, but carries the risk of damage to surrounding brain tissue. Open evacuation of the abscess contents requires a craniotomy, but avoids damaging surrounding brain.

3. Treatment of the infection site
Mastoiditis or sinusitis requires prompt operative treatment, otherwise this acts as a persistent source of infection.

Steroids help reduce associated oedema but they may also reduce antibiotic penetration. Their value in management remains controversial.
Conservative management: In some situations the risks of operative intervention outweigh its benefits. In those patients, treatment depends on i.v. antibiotics.
Indications: — small deep abscesses, e.g. thalamic (although stereotactic aspiration may help).
— multiple abscesses.
— early 'cerebritic' stage.

Prognosis
The use of CT scanning in the diagnosis and management of intracranial abscesses and the recognition and treatment of pathogenic anaerobic organisms have led to a reduction in the mortality rate from 40% to 10%. In survivors, focal deficits usually improve dramatically with time. Persistent seizures occur in 50%.

345

INTRACRANIAL ABSCESS

SUBDURAL EMPYEMA

Subdural empyema occurs far less frequently than intracerebral abscess formation. Infection usually spreads from infected sinuses or mastoids, but may arise from any of the aforementioned sources. Similarly organisms and clinical features match those of intracerebral abscess but since rapid extension occurs across the subdural space, overwhelming symptoms often develop suddenly. Seizures occur in 70% at onset.

CT scan shows a low density extracerebral collection with mass effect, often with enhancement on the cortical surface; occasionally isodense lesions make identification difficult.

Management: Intravenous antibiotic treatment is combined with evacuation of pus either through multiple burr holes or a craniotomy flap. Despite active treatment, the mortality rate still runs at approximately 20%.

GRANULOMA

TUBERCULOMA

Although tuberculomas still constitute an important cause of mass lesions in underdeveloped countries (20% in India), they are now rare in Britain. The lesions may be single or multiple. They often lie in the cerebellum, especially in children.

Clinical features are those of any intracranial mass; alternatively tuberculoma may present in conjunction with tuberculous meningitis.

CT scan clearly demonstrates an enhancing lesion — but this often resembles astrocytoma or metastasis; tuberculomas have no distinguishing features.
Other investigations: ESR, chest X-ray and Mantoux often fail to confirm the diagnosis.

Management: When tuberculoma is suspected, a trial of antituberculous therapy is worthwhile. Follow up CT scans should show a reduction in the lesion size. Other patients require an exploratory operation and biopsy followed by long-term drug treatment.

SARCOIDOSIS

Sarcoidosis is a systemic disease of unknown aetiology characterised by noncaseating epithelioid cell tubercles. Nervous system involvement occurs in 8%.

When sarcoid infiltrates the central nervous system it usually involves the meninges. In some patients mass lesions may arise from the dura, but more commonly signs and symptoms relate to an adhesive arachnoiditis involving the skull base, cranial nerves and pituitary stalk. Mass lesions may occasionally arise within the brain without obvious meningeal involvement.

Investigation: The CT appearances are not diagnostic. A definitive diagnosis is based on clinical and radiological evidence of multisystem disease confirmed by characteristic histology.

The diagnosis is often elusive and suggested by clinical presentation supported by
— elevated serum and CSF angiotensin converting enzyme (ACE),
— elevated serum immunoglobulins,
— elevated serum calcium,
— elevated CSF cell count (monocytes) and immunoglobulins.
The Kveim test is not specific and is rarely used.

Management: Long-term steroids.

MOVEMENT DISORDERS — EXTRAPYRAMIDAL SYSTEM

The control of voluntary movement is effected by the interaction of the pyramidal, cerebellar and extrapyramidal systems interconnecting with each other as well as projecting to the anterior horn region or cranial nerve motor nuclei.

The extrapyramidal system consists of paired subcortical masses or nuclei of grey matter.

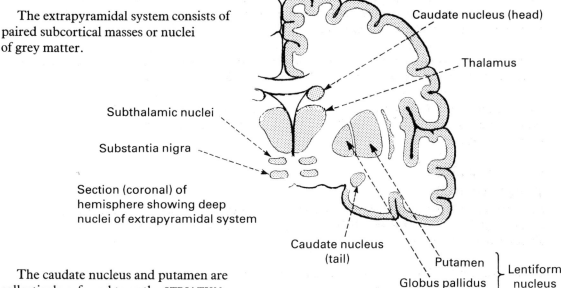

Caudate nucleus (head)

Thalamus

Subthalamic nuclei

Substantia nigra

Section (coronal) of hemisphere showing deep nuclei of extrapyramidal system

Caudate nucleus (tail)

Putamen

Globus pallidus

Lentiform nucleus

The caudate nucleus and putamen are collectively referred to as the STRIATUM.

Interconnections of the deep nuclei
The connections between components of the extrapyramidal system and other parts of the brain are complex. (See BRODAL — *Neurological Anatomay.*) However, certain simple observations can be made:

a — The thalamus plays a vital rôle in projecting information from the basal nuclei and cerebellum to the motor cortex via *thalamocortical pathways* and exerts an influence on the *corticospinal pathway* at its origin.
b — The cortical neurons project to the thalamus thus providing a feedback loop between these structures.
c — Outflow is solely through the corticobulbar and corticospinal (pyramidal) pathways.

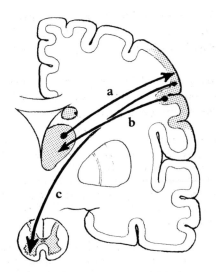

MOVEMENT DISORDERS — EXTRAPYRAMIDAL SYSTEM

NEUROPHARMACOLOGY

The observation that drugs such as reserpine and phenothiazines regularly produce extrapyramidal syndromes has clarified the neurochemical basis of movement disorders and delineated the role of neurotransmitters.

Neurotransmitter substances are synthesised and stored presynaptically. When released by an appropriate stimulus they cross the synaptic gap and combine with specific receptors on the postsynaptic cell,

Neuromodulator substances diminish or enhance the effects of neurotransmitters in the basal ganglia,

e.g.   — acetylcholine
          — dopamine
          — γ-aminobutyric acid
          — serotonin
          — glutamate

e.g.   — substance P
          — encephalin
          — cholecystokinin
          — somatostatin.

ACETYLCHOLINE

— Synthesised by small striatal cells
— Greatest concentration in striatum
— Excitatory effect.

DOPAMINE

— Synthesised by cells of substantia nigra (pars compacta) and nigral projections in striatum.
— Greatest concentration in substantia nigra.
— Inhibiting effect.

These two transmitters normally are 'in balance.'

Imbalance —

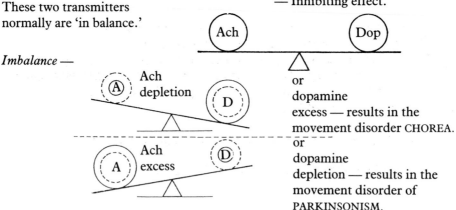

Ach depletion

or dopamine excess — results in the movement disorder CHOREA.

Ach excess

or dopamine depletion — results in the movement disorder of PARKINSONISM.

γ-Aminobutyric acid (GABA) is synthesised in the striatum and globus pallidus. It has inhibitory actions and deficiency is associated with Huntington's chorea.

Drugs may produce movement disorders by interfering with neurotransmission in the following ways:

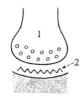

1. — By reducing transmitter at nerve terminal, e.g. tetrabenazine reduces dopamine.
2 — By blocking the receptor site postsynaptically — as phenothiazines do to dopamine receptors.

Both reduce effective dopamine and create a relative excess of acetylcholine
↓
Parkinsonism

MOVEMENT DISORDERS — EXTRAPYRAMIDAL DISEASES

CLINICAL FEATURES
The effects of disease of the extrapyramidal system on movement can be regarded as *negative* (primary functional deficit) and *positive* (secondary effect due to release or disinhibition in undamaged regions).

Negative features
1. *Bradykinesia:* — a loss or slowness of voluntary movement.
   This is a major feature of Parkinson's disease and produces:
   – reduced facial expression (mask-like)
   – reduced blinking
   – reduced adjustments of posture when seated.
   When agitated the patient will move swiftly — 'kinesia paradoxica'.

2. *Postural disturbance:* — most commonly seen in Parkinson's disease.
Flexion of limbs and trunk is associated with a failure to make quick postural or 'righting' adjustments to correct imbalance. The patient falls whilst turning or if pushed.

Positive features
1. *Involuntary movements:* — tremor — athetosis
                            — chorea — dystonia
                            — hemiballismus
Chorea and athetosis may merge into one another — choreoathetosis.

2. *Rigidity*

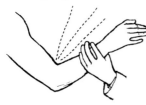 Stiffness felt by the examiner when passively moving a limb. This 'resistance' is present to the same degree throughout the full range of movement, affecting flexor and extensor muscle groups equally and is described as PLASTIC or LEAD PIPE rigidity. When tremor is superimposed upon rigidity it produces a COGWHEELING quality.

In Parkinson's disease both positive features, e.g. tremor, and negative features, e.g. bradykinesia, occur.
In Huntington's chorea positive features, e.g. chorea, predominate.

PARKINSON'S DISEASE

Described by James Parkinson (1817) in 'An essay on the shaking palsy'.
Recognised as an extrapyramidal disorder by Kinnier Wilson (1912).
Annual incidence: 20 per 100 000.
Prevalence: 190 per 100 000.
Sex incidence: male:female — 3:2
Age of onset: 50 years upwards. Incidence peaks in mid-70s then declines.
Familial incidence occurs in 5%.

AETIOLOGY

The cause of Parkinson's disease is unknown. Discordance in identical twins suggests that genetic factors are not important and environmental mechanisms appear to play a role.

Increased interest in the role of exogenous toxins has arisen through the recent observation that, in drug abusers, 1-methyl-4-phenyl 1236 tetrahydropyridine (MPTP) produces parkinsonism by selectively destroying nigral cells and their striatal projections.

Virus infection seems an unlikely explanation in view of the worldwide distribution, lack of viral antibodies in the brain and inability to transmit the disease to primates.

In view of the unclear aetiology of Parkinson's disease it is referred to as *Idiopathic Parkinson's Disease* as opposed to *Secondary Parkinsonism* where the causation is clear, e.g.

Drugs — phenothiazines
          reserpine
          haloperidol
Trauma — single or repetitive head injury.

PATHOLOGY of idiopathic Parkinson's disease

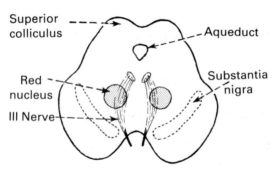

MIDBRAIN

The substantia nigra contains pigmented cells (neuromelanin) which give it a characteristic 'black' appearance (macroscopic). These cells are lost in Parkinson's disease and the substantia nigra becomes pale. Remaining cells contain atypical eosinophilic inclusions in the cytoplasm — *Lewy bodies* — although these are not specific to Parkinson's disease. The presence of 'cortical' inclusions is linked with dementia.

Minor changes are seen in other basal nuclei — striatum and globus pallidus.

Radiolabelled ligand studies have identified two dopamine receptors on striatal cell membranes — D1 and D2 receptors.

The D2 receptor correlates with Parkinson's disease. When blocked by phenothiazines it produces symptoms; when activated by dopamine or dopamine agonists it reduces symptoms.

PARKINSON'S DISEASE

CLINICAL FEATURES
Initial symptoms are vague, the patient often complains of aches and pains.

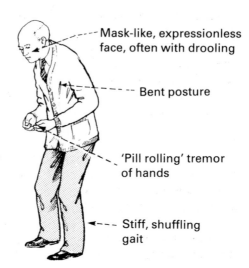

Mask-like, expressionless face, often with drooling

Bent posture

'Pill rolling' tremor of hands

Stiff, shuffling gait

1. A coarse TREMOR at a rate of 4 per second usually develops early in the disease. It begins unilaterally in the upper limbs and eventually spreads to all four limbs. The tremor is often *'pill rolling'*, the thumb moving rhythmically backwards and forwards on the palm of the hand. It occurs at rest, improves with movement and disappears during sleep.

2. RIGIDITY is detected by examination. It predominates in the flexor muscles of the neck, trunk and limbs and results in the typical *'flexed posture'*.

3. BRADYKINESIA: This slowness or paucity of movement affects facial muscles of expression (mask-like appearance) as well as muscles of mastication, speech, voluntary swallowing and muscles of the trunk and limbs.

   Dysarthria, dysphagia and a slow deliberate gait with little associated movement (e.g. arm swinging) result.

Tremor, rigidity and bradykinesia deteriorate simultaneously, affecting every aspect of the patient's life:
Handwriting reduces in size.
The gait becomes shuffling and festinant (small rapid steps to 'keep up with' the centre of gravity) and the posture more flexed.
Rising from a chair becomes laborious with progressive difficulty in initiating lower limb movement from a stationary position.
Eye movements may be affected with loss of ocular convergence and upward gaze.
Excessive sweating and greasy skin (seborrhoea) can be troublesome.

Depression, drug-induced confusional states and even dementia occur in a proportion of patients.
Occasionally autonomic features occur — postural hypotension. Postencephalitic Parkinson's disease (encephalitis lethargica), now rarely encountered, is characterised by an earlier age of onset and oculogyric crises (acute ocular deviation).

351

PARKINSON'S DISEASE

DIAGNOSIS

When tremor, rigidity and bradykinesia coexist, distinguish Parkinson's disease from secondary parkinsonism by the absence of a relevant drug history.

Distinguish TREMOR from

senile tremor
essential tremor } all are absent at rest and more pronounced on voluntary movement.
metabolic tremor

Distinguish RIGIDITY from spasticity — with passive limb movement, spasticity is felt towards the end rather than through the full range of movement.

Distinguish BRADYKINESIA from — gait disturbance of normal pressure hydrocephalus.

TREATMENT is symptomatic and does not halt the pathological process.

It aims at restoring the dopamine/acetylcholine balance (dopamine deficiency) by:

1. reducing acetylcholine
2. increasing dopamine.

1. Anticholinergic drugs

Synthetic anticholinergics, e.g. benzhexol — useful in control of tremor, but effect on rigidity and bradykinesia is often minimal.

Side effects:

Central { confusions, hallucinations, chorea }   *Peripheral* { dry mouth, blurred vision, urinary retention }

2. Increase dopamine

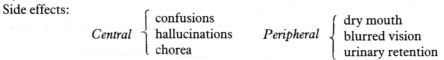

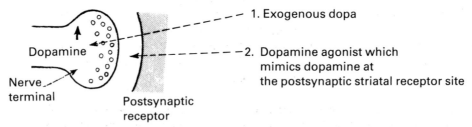

1. Exogenous dopa

2. Dopamine agonist which mimics dopamine at the postsynaptic striatal receptor site

Dopamine

Nerve terminal

Postsynaptic receptor

Exogenous dopa

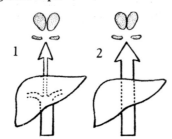

Given as 1 — levodopa, or 2 — levodopa + decarboxylase inhibitor, which prevents peripheral breakdown in the liver allowing a higher concentration of dopa to reach the blood–brain barrier; also the peripheral side effects (nausea, vomiting, hypotension) are diminished.

Central side effects: confusion, depression, choreatic movements and following long-term treatment — *'On/Off'* phenomenon (see later).

Exogenous dopa improves bradykinesia, rigidity and, to a lesser extent, tremor, but in 20% the response is poor. 'Good' responders often develop central side effects later — especially the 'on/off' phenomenon.

PARKINSON'S DISEASE

TREATMENT (*contd*)

Dopamine agonists: the ergot alkaloid bromocriptine acts directly on the postsynaptic dopamine receptor. It also increases dopamine at the synaptic gap by enhancing its release and blocking reuptake. Bromocriptine 'smooths' the response when used with levodopa. Side effects are similar to levodopa. Benefits of its usage as a single treatment in the early stages of the disease are under assessment.

Selegiline: the enzymes monoamine oxidase (MAO) A and B play a key role in the breakdown of dopamine. This drug is an MAO-B inhibitor. Its usage results in increased dopamine levels. The 'selective' action on only one enzyme ensures that the complication of hypertensive crises does not occur. The protective effect that this drug has upon the MPTP animal model suggests that selegiline may influence the rate of disease progression in man. Preliminary studies support this hypothesis and results of a large multicentre study are awaited.

Amantidine, an antiviral drug, may help rigidity. The mode of action is not known.

Advances in drug treatment in recent years have reduced the need for *stereotactic surgery* (see page 369), but in patients with intractable tremor this is still of benefit. A stereotactic lesion in the globus pallidus or ventrolateral nucleus of the thalamus (contralateral to the tremor) may produce dramatic results.

Human fetal and medullary transplantation: experimental evidence shows that transplantation to the striatum of tissue capable of synthesising and releasing dopamine reverses the motor symptoms of Parkinson's disease. Despite much publicity, this treatment remains experimental. As yet results appear disappointing.

Regime of treatment

Early Parkinson's disease	— Anticholinergics (and selegiline ?).
Established moderate disease	— Levodopa + decarboxylase inhibitor, selegiline and/or anticholinergics.
Established severe disease with central side effects	— Small, frequent doses of levodopa + decarboxylase inhibitor selegiline with consideration of low dose bromocriptine.

'On/off' phenomenon — a consequence of prolonged levodopa treatment in which signs of Parkinson's disease (undertreatment) and drug overdosage — choreatic or dystonic movements — (overtreatment) alternate rapidly as though being turned on and off. These changes may bear no relationship to the time of drug medication. *Treatment* is difficult. Reduce exogenous levodopa and consider bromocriptine.

CHOREA

Definition: (From the Greek — *dance*)
An involuntary, irregular, jerking movement affecting limb and axial muscle groups. These movements are suppressed with difficulty and are incorporated into voluntary gestures resulting in a 'semipurposeful' appearance, e.g. crossing and uncrossing of legs.

Dopamine agonists, levodopa and amphetamine, produce chorea. Dopamine antagonists, haloperidol and chlorpromazine, reduce it.

Chorea is a characteristic of several disorders:

HUNTINGTON'S CHOREA

Huntington's chorea is an autosomal dominant inherited disorder with onset in middle life and progression to death within 10 – 12 years.

It may occur in young persons (juvenile form); here chorea is less apparent and negative symptoms (rigidity) predominate.

Pathology

Neuronal loss in the striatum is associated with a reduction in projections to other basal ganglia structures. In addition, cells of the deep layers of the frontal and parietal cortex are lost (corticostriatal projections). The neurochemical basis of this disorder involves deficiency of GABA and acetylcholine as well as the neuromodulators enkephalin and substance P.

Symptoms

Chorea — may be the inital symptom. This progresses from mere fidgetiness to gross involuntary movements which interrupt voluntary movement and make feeding and walking impossible.

Dementia — this is of a subcortical type with impaired performance but preserved verbal skills (see page 122).

Behavioural disturbance — personality change, affective disorders and frank psychosis are common. Schizophrenia occurs in 10%.

Hypotonicity often accompanies fidgety, choreiform movements. Primitive reflexes — grasp, pout and palmomental — are usually elicited.

Diagnosis

On clinical grounds with a family history (although true parents may be unknown, or knowledge of illness suppressed). Distinguish from benign hereditary chorea in which intellect is preserved. Exclude senile chorea by older age of onset and absence of dementia. Exclude other causes of chorea (see over page).

Prediction of disease

The gene for Huntingdon's chorea is located at the tip of the short arm of chromosome 4. The identification of this locus provides a reliable method of predicting the disease. Presymptomatic testing is now available in many centres. Most individuals do not have sufficient affected relatives to make a definitive prediction. A positive test suggests a 95% risk of the disease and a negative test a 5% risk.

Treatment

Phenothiazines, haloperidol or tetrabenazine, may control the chorea in the preliminary stages.

CHOREA

SYDENHAM'S CHOREA
Acute onset. Associated with streptococcal infection. Remits in weeks.
Pathology: Necrotising arteritis in thalamus, caudate nucleus and putamen.
Diagnosis is confirmed by elevated ESR and ASO (antistreptolysin) titre.
Treatment: Sedation, phenothiazines.
   The condition may become recurrent — during pregnancy, intercurrent infection.

CHOREA GRAVIDARUM
Acute onset in pregnancy, usually the first trimester.
Restricted to face or generalised. Perhaps caused by reactivation of Sydenham's chorea.
Pathology: Unknown.
Treatment: Haloperidol.

OTHER CAUSES OF CHOREA
Drug induced — levodopa	Tricyclic antidepressants
Polycythaemia rubra vera	Alcohol abuse
Lupus erythematosus	Senile chorea
Wilson's disease	Oral contraceptive

DYSTONIA

DYSTONIA manifests as a prolonged
abnormal posture produced by spasms
of large trunk and limb muscles, e.g.
sustained head retraction .....

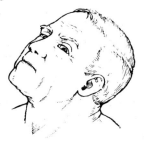

.... or sustained
inversion of
the foot.

Dystonias may be:
   generalised — dystonia musculorum deformans,
   or *partial* (focal), e.g. spasmodic torticollis.
   The precise neuropathological basis of dystonia is uncertain. Vascular and traumatic lesions of
the putamen occasionally produce this movement disorder. PET scan studies of blood flow and
metabolism may accurately localise the lesion site.

DYSTONIA MUSCULORUM DEFORMANS
Onset in childhood usually with autosomal recessive inheritance.
   Initially, a flexion deformity of leg develops when walking.
   Movements then become generalised with abnormal posturing of the head,
trunk and limbs. They are initially intermittent but ultimately constant. Despite
eventual gross contortion the postures disappear during sleep.
Diagnosis is made on clinical grounds and by exclusion
— Normal perinatal history
— No laboratory evidence of Wilson's disease.
Pathology: unknown
Treatment: levodopa or carbamezapine are of benefit in some patients;
anticholinergics help in others.
   Stereotactic surgery — a lesion in the region of the ventrolateral nucleus of
the thalamus may reduce the dystonia in the contralateral limb.

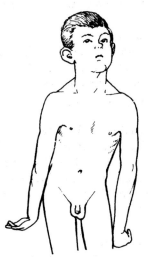

DYSTONIAS — PARTIAL

SPASMODIC TORTICOLLIS (Wry neck)

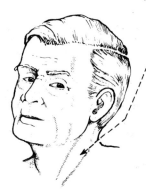

Unilateral deviation of the head.

Aetiology is unknown. Vestibular abnormalities occur on testing, but it is uncertain whether these cause torticollis or result from the abnormal head posture. Dystonic contraction of the *left* sternomastoid produces head turning to the *right*. Pressure of the index finger on the *right* side of the chin may turn the head back to the neutral position.

Turning of the head is specially noticeable when the patient is walking. Eventually hypertrophy of the sternomastoid occurs.

Pathology: unknown. **Diagnosis** is based on clinical findings.

Treatment: anticholinergics and phenothiazines produce some benefit in 50% of patients. Injection of *Botulinum* toxin into the sternomastoid muscle gives variable symptomatic relief though requires regular repetition.

Operative techniques: – Myotomy
– Section of spinal accessory and upper cervical anterior roots. (Results from these procedures are unpredictable and varied.)

Prognosis: Remission occurs in 20% of patients. Dystonia may spread into other muscle groups. In the long term, psychological disturbance often occurs.

WRITER'S CRAMP Variable age of onset.

Muscles of the hand and forearm tighten on attempting to write and pain may occur in the forearm muscles. Previously regarded as an 'occupational neurosis' but now classified as a partial dystonia.

May be a precursor of Parkinson's disease.

Treatment: Benzodiazepines and anticholinergics are of limited value.

OROMANDIBULAR DYSTONIA

Constant involuntary prolonged tight eye closure (blepharospasm) is associated with dystonia of mouth, tongue or jaw muscles. Response to treatment is poor though phenothiazines should be tried. Section of the nerves to orbicularis oculi muscles will relieve blepharospasm. Botulinum toxin injection is also effective.

DRUG INDUCED DYSTONIA

Acute adoption of abnormal dystonic posture — usually head and neck or oculogyric crisis (upward deviation of eyes) — caused by phenothiazines, butyrophenones, e.g. haloperidol, metoclopramide.

Anticholinergics, e.g. benztropine for 24–48 hours helps symptoms settle.

PROGRESSIVE SUPRANUCLEAR PALSY

A condition characterised by gaze palsies, extrapyramidal features, *axial dystonia* (truncal dystonia) and progressive pseudobulbar palsy. Onset in the 5th to 6th decade.

Aetiology: unknown.

Pathology: Neuronal loss is evident in periaqueductal grey matter, brain stem, nuclei, subthalamic nuclei and the superior colliculi.

Neurofibrillary tangles as seen in Alzheimer's disease are also found.

Signs: Downward eye movement is initially impaired followed by all other voluntary eye movement. Lid retraction is common. Pseudobulbar signs develop (see page 534).

The head then hyperextends (dystonia) and rigidity ensues in the limbs.

Treatment: Levodopa and anticholinergics give disappointing results.

The course is relentless with progression and death in 2–5 years.

OTHER EXTRAPYRAMIDAL MOVEMENT DISORDERS

HEMIBALLISMUS

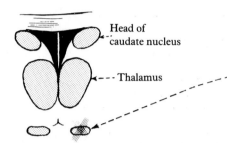

Head of
caudate nucleus

Thalamus

This is a movement disorder characterised by unilateral, violent flinging of the limbs. This involuntary movement is occasionally severe enough to throw the patient off balance or even from his bed.

The anatomical basis is a lesion of the *subthalamic nuclei* or its connections contralateral to the abnomal movement. It usually results from vascular disease (posterior cerebral artery territory), buy occasionally occurs in multiple sclerosis.

Drug treatment is ineffective. The condition often settles spontaneously.

ATHETOSIS

Athetosis presents in childhood and appears as a slow writhing movement disorder with a rate of movement between that of chorea and dystonia. It usually involves the digits, hands and face on each side.

These abnormal movements may result from:
– Hypoxic neonatal brain damage,
– Kernicterus,
– Lipid storage diseases.

Response to anticholinergics is variable and occasionally dramatic.

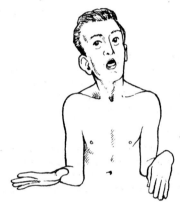

TARDIVE DYSKINESIA

This is a consequence of long-term treatment with neuroleptic drugs — phenothiazines, butyrophenones — and results from the development of drug-induced supersensitive dopamine receptors.

Involuntary movements in the face, mouth and tongue (orofacial dyskinesia) as well as limb movements of a *choreathetoid nature* occur.

This movement disorder may commence even after stopping the responsible drug and can persist indefinitely.

Prevention

Incidence may be reduced by:
   1. Drug 'holidays' (periods of rest from causal drug).
   2. Early recognition and drug withdrawal.

The practice of increasing the dose of the offending drug when movements occur should be avoided. This will improve movements initially, but they will 'break through' later.

Treatment

Discontinue neuroleptic. If not possible, continue on lowest possible dose. Drugs which increase acetylcholine (Deanol), reduce catecholamine release (lithium), or deplete dopamine (reserpine) are variably effective.

357

OTHER EXTRAPYRAMIDAL MOVEMENT DISORDERS

WILSON'S DISEASE (hepatolenticular degeneration)
A rare autosomal recessive disorder of copper metabolism in which extrapyramidal features are evident. The primary genetic defect is unknown.

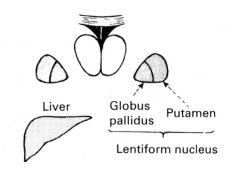

Liver Globus pallidus Putamen

Lentiform nucleus

Pathology
Cavitation and neuronal loss occurs within the putamen and the globus pallidus.
   The liver shows the appearance of coarse cirrhosis.
Copper accumulates in all organs, especially in Descemet's membrane in the eye, nail beds and kidney.

Biochemistry
There is deficiency of α_2 globulin — Ceruloplasmin — which normally binds 98% of copper in the plasma. This results in an increase in loosely bound copper/albumin, and deposition occurs in all organs. Urinary copper is increased.

Clinical features
There are two clinical forms:

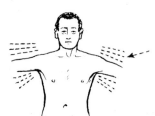

1. *Acute* (Children)
Bradykinesia
Behavioural change
Involuntary movements
Liver involvement common

Untreated: death in 2 years

2. *Chronic* (Young adults)
Marked proximal 'wing beating' tremor
Dysarthria
Choreoathetoid movements
Liver involvement less severe

Untreated: death in 10 years

   The deposition of copper in Descemet's membrane produces the golden brown *Kayser-Fleischer* ring, which is seen by the naked eye and is diagnostic.

Diagnosis
Clinical findings supported by biochemical evidence:
   1. Low ceruloplasmin (less than 20 mg/dl)
   2. Elevated unbound serum copper
   3. High urinary copper excretion
   4. Liver biopsy and copper metabolism tests with radioactive [64]Cu.
   In families, biochemical tests will identify low ceruloplasmin in carriers and in presymptomatic patients. These relatives require appropriate genetic counselling and treatment when indicated.

Treatment
Low copper diet and a chelating agent, e.g. penicillamine 1–2 g daily. Zinc sulphate was initially used in patients who could not tolerate toxic effects of chelating agents; now it is regarded as an effective and well tolerated first-line treatment.
   Therapy is necessary for the rest of the patient's life. Adequate treatment is compatible with normal life expectancy. Kayser-Fleischer rings will disappear with time.

HYDROCEPHALUS

DEFINITION

Hydrocephalus is an increase in cerebrospinal fluid (CSF) volume, usually resulting from impaired absorption, rarely from excessive secretion.

This definition excludes ventricular expansion secondary to brain shrinkage from a diffuse atrophic process (hydrocephalus ex vacuo).

CSF FORMATION AND ABSORPTION

CSF forms at a rate of 500 ml/day (0.35 ml/min), secreted predominantly by the choroid plexus of the lateral, third and fourth ventricles. CSF flows in a caudal direction through the ventricular system and exits through the foramina of Luschka and Magendie into the subarachnoid space. After passing through the tentorial hiatus and over the hemispheric convexity, absorption occurs through the arachnoid granulations into the venous system.

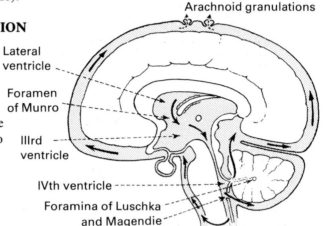

CLASSIFICATION

'Obstructive' hydrocephalus — obstruction of CSF flow *within* the ventricular system.
'Communicating' hydrocephalus — obstruction to CSF flow *outwith* the ventricular system i.e. ventricular CSF 'communicates' with the subarachoid space.

CAUSES OF HYDROCEPHALUS

Obstructive

Congenital – Aqueduct stenosis or forking
– Dandy-Walker syndrome (atresia of foramina of Magendie and Luschka)
– Arnold-Chiari malformation
– Vein of Galen aneurysm

Acquired – Acquired aqueduct stenosis (adhesions following infection or haemorrhage)
– Supratentorial masses causing tentorial herniation
– Intraventricular haematoma
– Tumours – ventricular, e.g. colloid cyst
– pineal region
– posterior fossa
– Abscesses/granuloma
– Arachnoid cysts

Communicating

Thickening of the leptomeninges and/or involvement of the arachnoid granulations
– infection (pyogenic, TB, fungal)
– subarachnoid haemorrhage
– spontaneous
– trauma
– postoperative
– carcinomatous meningitis
Increased CSF viscosity, e.g. high protein content
Excessive CSF production — choroid plexus papilloma (rare)

359

HYDROCEPHALUS

PATHOLOGICAL EFFECTS

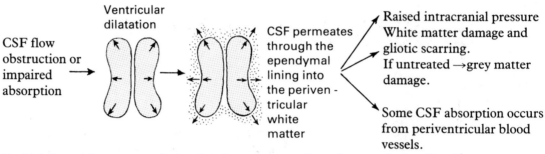

CSF flow obstruction or impaired absorption → Ventricular dilatation → CSF permeates through the ependymal lining into the periventricular white matter →

Raised intracranial pressure
White matter damage and gliotic scarring.
If untreated →grey matter damage.

Some CSF absorption occurs from periventricular blood vessels.

In the infant, prior to suture fusion, head expansion and massive ventricular dilatation may occur, often leaving only a thin rim of cerebral 'mantle'. Untreated, death usually results, but in many cases the hydrocephalus *'arrests';* although the ventricles remain dilated, intracranial pressure (ICP) returns to normal and CSF absorption appears to balance production. When hydrocephalus arrests, normal developmental patterns resume, although pre-existing mental or physical damage may leave a permanent handicap. In these patients, the rapid return of further pressure symptoms following a minor injury or infection suggests that the CSF dynamics remain in an unstable state.

CLINICAL FEATURES
Infants and young children

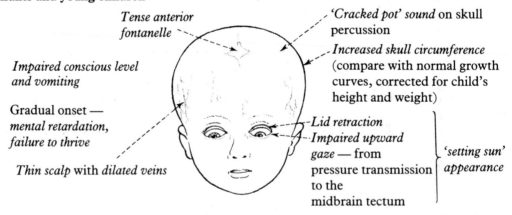

Tense anterior fontanelle

'Cracked pot' sound on skull percussion

Increased skull circumference (compare with normal growth curves, corrected for child's height and weight)

Impaired conscious level and vomiting

Gradual onset — *mental retardation, failure to thrive*

Thin scalp with *dilated veins*

Lid retraction
Impaired upward gaze — from pressure transmission to the midbrain tectum

'setting sun' appearance

Juvenile/adult type hydrocephalus

Acute onset — signs and symptoms of ↑ ICP ⟨ *headache, vomiting, papilloedema.*
— *impaired upward gaze*   *deterioration of conscious level.*

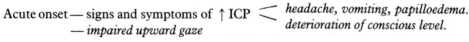

Gradual onset — *dementia*
— *gait ataxia*
— *incontinence*

This triad of symptoms may occur despite an apparently 'normal' CSF pressure, i.e. NORMAL PRESSURE HYDROCEPHALUS (see page 125).
The condition often relates to previous trauma, meningitis or subarachnoid haemorrhage.

HYDROCEPHALUS

INVESTIGATIONS
Skull X-ray
Note: — skull size and suture width.
  — evidence of chronic raised pressure — erosion of the posterior clinoids.
  — associated defects — platybasia, basilar invagination.

CT scan
The *pattern of
ventricular enlargement*
helps determine the cause, i.e.

The presence of *periventricular
lucency* (and absent sulci) suggests
raised CSF pressure.

*lateral
+
3rd ventricular
dilatation*

*normal 4th
ventricle* — suggests
aqueduct
stenosis.

*deviated or
absent 4th
ventricle* — suggests a
posterior
fossa mass.

The absence of periventricular
lucency and prominent sulci suggests
appearances resulting from an
atrophic process.

-Dilated 3rd ventricle
-Dilated lateral ventricle (temporal horns)
-Normal 4th ventricle

*generalised
dilatation* — suggests a communicating
hydrocephalus.

Ultrasonography through the anterior fontanelle, usefully demonstrates ventricular enlargement
in infants but provides less precise information than CT scanning.

Isotope cisternography/CSF infusion studies/ICP monitoring: investigations in patients with
suspected normal pressure hydrocephalus designed to predict the likelihood of a beneficial
response to shunting.

Developmental assessment and psychometric analysis detect impaired cerebral function and
provide a baseline for future comparison.

MANAGEMENT

*Acute
deterioration*

ventricular drainage or
ventricular-peritoneal (VP) or ventriculoatrial (VA) shunt
lumbar puncture — if communicating hydrocephalus, e.g. following
subarachnoid haemorrhage.

*Gradual
deterioration*

VP or VA shunt (lumboperitoneal shunts are occasionally used for
communicating hydrocephalus).
removal of a mass lesion if present — this may obviate the need for a shunt.

'Arrested hydrocephalus' — symptomless ventricular dilatation requires no treatment, but
regular development or psychometric assessment ensures no ill
effects develop from this potentially unstable state.

361

HYDROCEPHALUS

Shunt techniques

A *reservoir* permits CSF aspiration for analysis.

A *valve* is incorporated in the system, either proximally — ball or diaphragm type (Hakim, Pudenz, Spitz-Holter), or distally — slit valve at distal tip (Pudenz).

Valve opening pressures range from 5–150 mm H$_2$O.

A *ventricular catheter* is inserted through the occipital (or frontal) horn. The tip lies at the level of the foramen of Munro.

Ventriculoatrial shunt — distal catheter inserted through the internal jugular vein to the right atrium (T6/7 level on chest X-ray).

Silastic tubing tunnelled subcutaneously.

[*Lumboperitoneal shunt* — catheter inserted into the lumbar theca either directly at open operation or percutaneously through a Tuohy needle. The distal end is sited in the peritoneal cavity.]

Ventriculoperitoneal shunt — distal catheter inserted into the peritoneal cavity. In children, redundant coils permit growth without revision.

Complications of shunting

Infection: results in meningitis, peritonitis or inflammation extending along the subcutaneous channel. In patients with a V-A shunt, bacteraemia may lead to shunt 'nephritis'. *Staphylococcus epidermidis* or *aureus* are usually involved, with infants at particular risk. Prophylactic antibiotics may minimise the risk of infection, but, when established, eradication usually requires shunt removal.

Subdural haematoma: ventricular collapse pulls the cortical surface from the dura and leaves a subdural CSF collection or tears bridging veins causing subdural haemorrhage. Lying the patient supine for 24–48 hours after shunting helps reduce this risk.

Shunt obstruction: blockage of the shunt system with choroid plexus, debris, high CSF protein, omentum or blood clot results in intermittent or persistent recurrence of symptoms and indicates the need for shunt revision. Demonstration of an increase in ventricular size compared to a previous baseline CT scan confirms shunt malfunction. In children, growth pulls the distal tip of a ventriculoatrial shunt out of the right atrium, resulting in thrombus formation and occlusion. Ventriculoperitoneal shunting avoids this complication.

Low pressure state: following shunting, some patients develop headache and vomiting on sitting or standing. This low pressure state usually resolves with a high fluid intake and gradual mobilisation. If not, conversion to a high pressure valve is required.

Prognosis: Provided treatment precedes irreversible brain damage, results are good with most children attaining normal IQs. Repeated complications, however, particularly prevalent in infancy and in young children carry a significant morbidity.

BENIGN INTRACRANIAL HYPERTENSION

Benign intracranial hypertension (pseudotumour cerebri) is a term applied to patients with raised intracranial pressure and no evidence of any 'mass' lesion or of hydrocephalus.

AETIOLOGY: This condition is related to a variety of clinical problems:

Some clearly demonstrate a direct causal link —
VENOUS OUTFLOW OBSTRUCTION TO CSF ABSORPTION

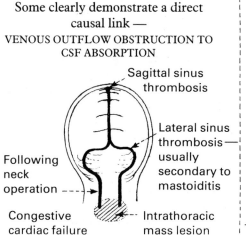

Sagittal sinus thrombosis

Lateral sinus thrombosis — usually secondary to mastoiditis

Following neck operation

Congestive cardiac failure

Intrathoracic mass lesion

In the majority, the causal link remains obscure, but a variety of factors are associated —
DIET — obesity.
     — hyper/hypovitaminosis A.
ENDOCRINE — pregnancy, menarche, menstrual irregularities, Addison's disease.
HAEMATOLOGICAL — iron deficiency anaemia.
     — polycythaemia vera.
DRUGS — oral contraceptives.
     — steroid withdrawal.
     — tetracycline.
     — nalidixic acid.
Various mechanisms have been postulated.

— BRAIN SWELLING
— ↓ CSF ABSORPTION
— ↑ CSF SECRETION

Different studies support different mechanisms. The link with obesity suggests an underlying endocrine basis, but, except in Addison's disease, endocrine assessment has failed to reveal abnormalities.

CLINICAL FEATURES

Age: any age, but usually in 3rd and 4th decades.
Sex: female > male—especially in the idiopathic group.

Symptoms
Headache
Visual obscurations
Impaired visual acuity } ← Papilloedema
Diplopia ← VI nerve palsy
In women the condition is often associated with — recent weight gain, fluid retention, menstrual dysfunction, the first trimester of pregnancy and the postpartum period.

Signs
Obesity
Papilloedema
VI nerve palsy

Investigations
CT scan negative — ventricles usually small.
Visual field charting —
Enlarged blind spot (often used to monitor
Peripheral field constriction.   progress).
Lumbar puncture and pressure measurement.
ICP monitoring — if diagnostic doubt persists.

PROGNOSIS
Most patients respond rapidly to short-term treatment, but up to one-third develop recurrent attacks. In 10% visual impairment persists.

TREATMENT
Treat the underlying cause if known.
Weight reduction diet.
Drugs — acetazolamide (reduces CSF production).
     — *thiazide diuretics.*
     — *steroid therapy.*
If above fail → *lumboperitoneal shunt* (subtemporal decompression, now rarely required).
Optic nerve decompression — if progressive impairment of visual acuity despite treatment.

ARNOLD-CHIARI MALFORMATION

Although the names of two authors are linked to the description of malformations at the medullary-spinal junction, Chiari must take most credit for providing a detailed description of this condition.

TYPE I	TYPE II	TYPE III

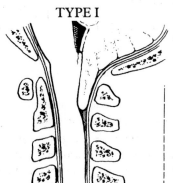 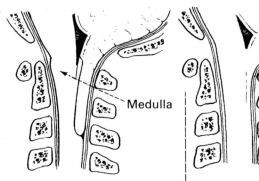

Medulla

Meningo-myelocele

TYPE I

The cerebellar *tonsils* lie below the level of the foramen magnum (cerebellar ectopia). This may not produce symptoms.

Associated conditions
(in symptomatic patients):

SPINAL

Syringomyelia
Hydromyelia } (50%)

CRANIAL

Hydrocephalus (10%) (occurs less often than Chiari originally described)

OTHERS

TYPE II

Part of the cerebellar *vermis*, medulla and 4th ventricle extend through the foramen magnum, often to the midcervical region. The lower cranial nerves are stretched and the cervical nerve roots run horizontally or in an upward direction.

Syringomyelia
Hydromyelia } (90%)
Spina bifida — meningomyelocele, diastomatomyelia
Cervical fusion (Klippel-Feil)

Hydrocephalus (85%)
Aqueduct stenosis and forking
Small posterior fossa
Basilar impression
Fusion of both thalami
Fusion of the superior and inferior colliculi
Microgyria
Hypoplastic tentorium cerebelli and falx
Skull lacunia — vault thinned or defective

Developmental anomalies of the cardiovascular, gastrointestinal and genitourinary systems in 10%

TYPE III

Part of the cerebellum and medulla lie within a cervico-occipital meningomyelocele.
[TYPE IV
Cerebellar hypoplasia — best considered as a separate entity.]

ARNOLD-CHIARI MALFORMATION

PATHOGENESIS

Several hypotheses have been proposed to explain the pathological findings of these malformations. Gardner suggested that downward pressure from *hydrocephalus* played an important role in displacing the posterior fossa structures and, when associated with a patent central canal, explained the high incidence of syringomyelia (page 385). Others supposed that *traction* from a tethered spinal cord (dysraphism), or a *CSF leak* through a myelocele into the amniotic sac in fetal life resulted in caudal displacement of the posterior fossa structures. Of these theories, none provides an entirely satisfactory explanation; a more realistic view attributes the hindbrain deformity to *maldevelopment* during early fetal life. This would explain the presence of other developmental anomalies.

CLINICAL PRESENTATION

Depends on age

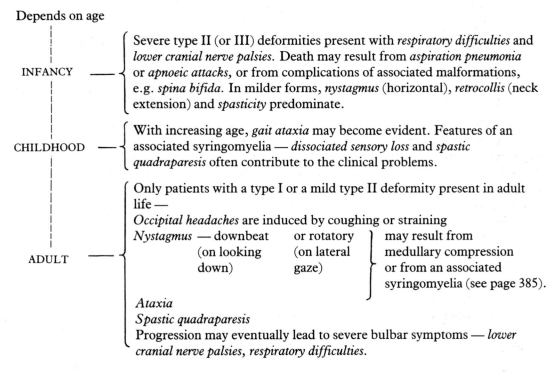

INFANCY — Severe type II (or III) deformities present with *respiratory difficulties* and *lower cranial nerve palsies*. Death may result from *aspiration pneumonia* or *apnoeic attacks*, or from complications of associated malformations, e.g. *spina bifida*. In milder forms, *nystagmus* (horizontal), *retrocollis* (neck extension) and *spasticity* predominate.

CHILDHOOD — With increasing age, *gait ataxia* may become evident. Features of an associated syringomyelia — *dissociated sensory loss* and *spastic quadraparesis* often contribute to the clinical problems.

ADULT — Only patients with a type I or a mild type II deformity present in adult life —
Occipital headaches are induced by coughing or straining
Nystagmus — downbeat (on looking down) or rotatory (on lateral gaze) may result from medullary compression or from an associated syringomyelia (see page 385).
Ataxia
Spastic quadraparesis
Progression may eventually lead to severe bulbar symptoms — *lower cranial nerve palsies, respiratory difficulties.*

INVESTIGATIONS

Magnetic resonance imaging (MRI) is the investigation of choice. This will clearly demonstrate cerebellar ectopia; in addition it will identify the presence or absence of an associated syringomyelia.

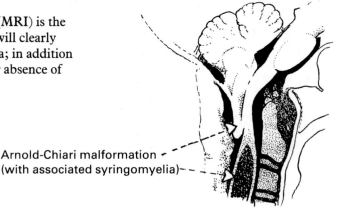

Arnold-Chiari malformation
(with associated syringomyelia)

365

ARNOLD-CHIARI MALFORMATION

Investigation (*contd*)

Straight X-rays

Skull: note the presence of platybasia, basilar impression or lacuniae (vault defects).

Cervical spine: note increased canal width or fusion of vertebrae (especially C2,3) — Klippel Feil syndrome.

Lumbosacral spine: note spina bifida.

Myelography (if MRI unavailable)

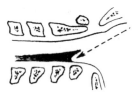

Contrast run up to the foramen magnum with the patient in the supine position outlines a posteriorly situated filling defect.

CT scan: preferably with contrast in the theca demonstrates cerebellar tissue lying within the cervical canal.

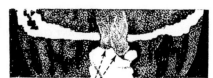

MANAGEMENT (see also syringomyelia, page 385)

In patients with hydrocephalus and signs and symptoms of raised intracranial pressure. → *Ventriculoperitoneal* or *atrial shunt* may significantly improve signs and symptoms attributed to the Chiari malformation.

In patients with other symptoms and signs → *Posterior fossa decompression* — by removing the posterior rim of the foramen magnum and the arch of the atlas. The dura is opened and a dural graft inserted. Attempts at freeing tonsilar adhesions should be resisted. An apnoea monitor in the initial postoperative period helps detect potentially fatal apnoea, especially during sleep. In some instances, patients with minimal symptoms or with no evidence of progression may warrant a conservative approach.

PROGNOSIS

Patients with mild symptoms and signs often respond well to operation, but those with long-standing neurological deficits rarely improve. Treatment should aim at preventing further progression.

Further deterioration eventually occurs in one-third, despite operative measures.

SYRINGOBULBIA

Extension of a syringomyelic cavity upwards into the medulla may produce signs and symptoms which are difficult to distinguish from those of medullary compression in the Arnold-Chiari syndrome:

— difficulty in swallowing, dysphonia, dysarthria, vertigo, facial pain

— nystagmus, palatal and vocal cord weakness, occasional facial and tongue weakness.

DANDY-WALKER SYNDROME

This rare developmental anomaly comprises:

1. Dilatation of the lateral and third ventricles (but to a lesser extent than the fourth ventricle)

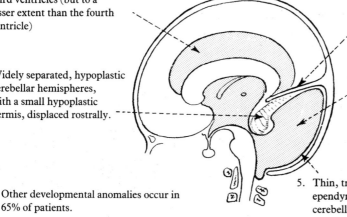

3. Enlarged posterior fossa with high tentorium cerebelli and transverse sinuses.

2. Widely separated, hypoplastic cerebellar hemispheres, with a small hypoplastic vermis, displaced rostrally.

4. Cystic dilatation of the 4th ventricle — *usually* related to congenital absence of the foramina of Luschka and Magendie.

Other developmental anomalies occur in 65% of patients.

5. Thin, transparent membrane containing ependymal cells and occasionally cerebellar tissue.

CLINICAL PRESENTATION

Infancy: Symptoms and signs of hydrocephalus (page 360) combined with a prominent occiput.
Childhood: Signs of cerebellar dysfunction with or without signs of hydrocephalus.

INVESTIGATIONS

Skull X-ray: Usually shows elevation of the transverse sinuses and occipital bulging, confirming the presence of an enlarged posterior fossa.

CT scan:

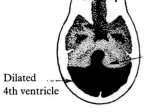

Dilated 4th ventricle

Confirms dilatation of the 4th ventricle with lateral displacement of hypoplastic cerebellar tissue.

Differentiate from:
— Midline arachnoid cyst
— Enlarged cisterna magna

distinguish from Dandy-Walker by identifying cerebellar tissue or septum between the cyst and the 4th ventricle

MANAGEMENT

Excision of the cyst membrane, 'marsupialising' the 4th ventricle.
Alternatively, and more simply, cystoperitoneal shunt.

PROGNOSIS

Marked neurological impairment prior to treatment carries a poor outlook. In less impaired patients, the prognosis relates more to the presence of other developmental anomalies.

CRANIOSYNOSTOSIS

In normal childhood development, the cranial sutures allow passive skull enlargement as the brain grows. *Premature fusion of one or more sutures* results in restricted growth of bone alongside the suture and excessive compensatory growth at the non-united joints. The effect depends on the site and number of sutures involved. Sagittal synostosis is the most frequently occurring deformity (80%).

SAGITTAL SYNOSTOSIS
Lateral growth is restricted, resulting in a long narrow head with a pronounced sagittal suture (scaphocephaly).
Treatment: by excision of the sagittal suture. Lining the bone edges with a silicon film helps prevent reossification.

CORONAL SYNOSTOSIS
Bilateral or unilateral.

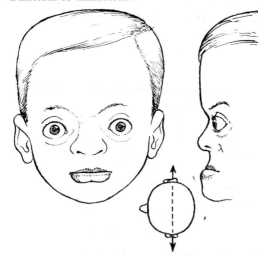

Expansion occurs in a superior and lateral direction (brachiocephaly). This produces a short anterior fossa, shallow orbits and hypertelorism (widening of the interocular distance). Exophthalmos, elevated ICP and visual impairment from papilloedema may result. Bilateral coronal synostosis commonly occurs as one of several congenital defects incorporated in *Crouzon's* and *Apert's syndromes*.

Involvement of several sutures (oxycephaly) results in skull expansion towards the vertex, the line of least resistance.

PANSYNOSTOSIS (all sutures affected) results in failure of skull growth with a symmetrical abnormally small head and raised intracranial pressure. It is important to distinguish this from microcephaly due to inadequate primary brain development.

Treatment of coronal, metopic and pansynostosis involves extensive craniofacial surgery correcting both cranial and orbital deformities.

Indication for operative treatment is primarily cosmetic when only one suture is involved, but with involvement of two or more sutures operation is also aimed at prevention of visual and cerebral damage during growth.

STEREOTACTIC SURGERY

Stereotactic techniques developed initially for lesion making, enable accurate placement of a cannula or electrode at a predetermined target site within the brain with the least risk.

Many different stereotactic frames have been developed, e.g. Leksell, Todd-Wells, Guiot. These, combined with radiological landmarks (usually ventriculography) and a brain atlas, provide anatomical localisation to within ± 1 mm. Since some functional variability occurs at each anatomical site, electrode localisation is also based on the recorded neuronal activity and on the effects of electrical stimulation.

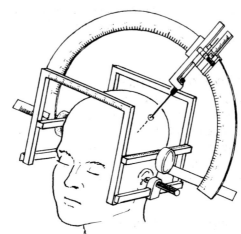

CT/MRI STEREOTACTIC SYSTEM

Several CT and MRI compatible stereotactic systems are now available which allow cannula insertion to any point selected on the image. They are all based on the concept of identifiable external reference (fiducial) markers,

e.g. Brown-Robert-Wells (BRW) system:

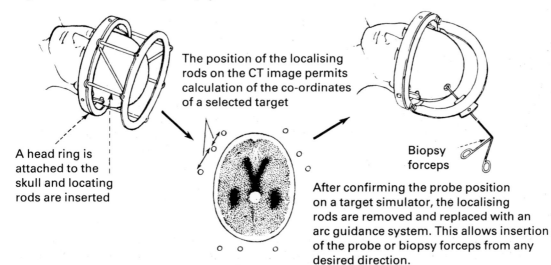

The position of the localising rods on the CT image permits calculation of the co-ordinates of a selected target

A head ring is attached to the skull and locating rods are inserted

Biopsy forceps

After confirming the probe position on a target simulator, the localising rods are removed and replaced with an arc guidance system. This allows insertion of the probe or biopsy forceps from any desired direction.

CT/MRI stereosurgery provides the optimal method for the biopsy or aspiration of *small, deeply situated tumours* or *abscesses*.

When combined with craniotomy it permits direct endoscopic examination of a lesion and may aid localisation, e.g. a small arteriovenous malformation. The improved resolution now available with CT/MRI scanning has led to sufficient anatomical localisation for accurate lesion making, obviating the need for ventriculography.

369

STEREOTACTIC SURGERY

METHODS OF LESION MAKING

Heat — radiofrequency current delivered through a fine electrode ⎫ lesion size
Cooling — with a cryogenic probe   ⎪ determined by
Radiation — implantation of radioactive seed, e.g. yttrium-90.   ⎬ temperature
— focussed beam from cobalt-60 rods (sited on a specially   ⎪ change and
adapted Leksell frame) or from a linear accelerator.   ⎭ duration.

USES OF STEREOTACTIC SURGERY

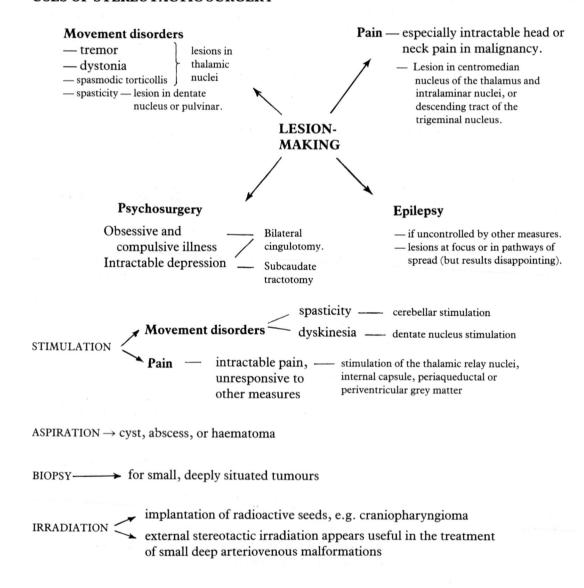

Movement disorders
— tremor   ⎫ lesions in
— dystonia   ⎬ thalamic
— spasmodic torticollis ⎭ nuclei
— spasticity — lesion in dentate
nucleus or pulvinar.

Pain — especially intractable head or
neck pain in malignancy.
— Lesion in centromedian
nucleus of the thalamus and
intralaminar nuclei, or
descending tract of the
trigeminal nucleus.

LESION-MAKING

Psychosurgery
Obsessive and
compulsive illness —— Bilateral
cingulotomy.
Intractable depression —— Subcaudate
tractotomy

Epilepsy
— if uncontrolled by other measures.
— lesions at focus or in pathways of
spread (but results disappointing).

spasticity —— cerebellar stimulation
Movement disorders — dyskinesia —— dentate nucleus stimulation

STIMULATION
Pain — intractable pain, —— stimulation of the thalamic relay nuclei,
unresponsive to   internal capsule, periaqueductal or
other measures   periventricular grey matter

ASPIRATION → cyst, abscess, or haematoma

BIOPSY ——— for small, deeply situated tumours

IRRADIATION
implantation of radioactive seeds, e.g. craniopharyngioma
external stereotactic irradiation appears useful in the treatment
of small deep arteriovenous malformations

PSYCHOSURGERY

In 1935, observation of behavioural changes in chimpanzees following bilateral ablation of the frontal association area, led to the introduction of lesion-making for psychiatric disease (Moniz). The operation of *prefrontal leucotomy* was perfected and used on patients with a wide variety of problems. In Britain, between 1940 – 1955, neurosurgeons performed over 10 000 operations. It became evident that patients with affective problems — depression, anxiety and obsessional neurosis — showed better results than those with schizophrenia.

As a consequence of the introduction of *chlorpromazine* in the 1950s, and the operative complications and results — perhaps limited by poor case selection, prefrontal leucotomy fell into disrepute. The need for a surgical procedure persisted, however, in those patients where drugs had little effect. Despite pharmacological improvements, some patients developed chronically disabling conditions requiring continual hospital care; in others with acute depressive illness, the suicide rate was high.

Stereotactic surgery provided a method of lesion-making which was virtually risk free and this is now generally accepted as a suitable treatment in *selected patients where drug treatment has failed.*

INDICATIONS FOR STEREOTACTIC SURGERY AND LESION SITE

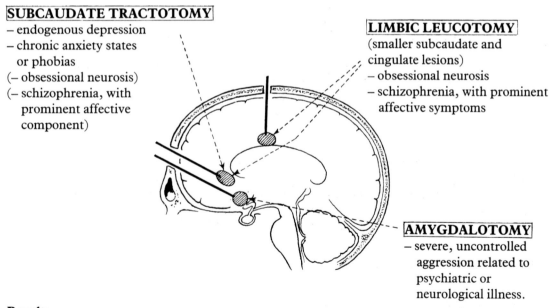

SUBCAUDATE TRACTOTOMY
– endogenous depression
– chronic anxiety states
  or phobias
(– obsessional neurosis)
(– schizophrenia, with
  prominent affective
  component)

LIMBIC LEUCOTOMY
(smaller subcaudate and
cingulate lesions)
– obsessional neurosis
– schizophrenia, with prominent
  affective symptoms

AMYGDALOTOMY
– severe, uncontrolled
  aggression related to
  psychiatric or
  neurological illness.

Results

Depression/anxiety states — up to two-thirds benefit from subcaudate tractotomy.

Obsessional neurosis — 80% improve following limbic leucotomy.

Schizophrenia — poor results, unless operation is restricted to those patients with concurrent depression, anxiety or obsession, where some benefit may occur.

LOCALISED NEUROLOGICAL DISEASE AND ITS MANAGEMENT
B. SPINAL CORD AND ROOTS

SPINAL CORD AND ROOTS

Disorders localised to the spinal cord or nerve roots are detailed below, but note that many diffuse neurological disease processes also affect the cord (see Section V, e.g. multiple sclerosis, Friedreich's ataxia).

SPINAL CORD AND ROOT COMPRESSION

As the spinal canal is a rigidly enclosed cavity, an expanding disease process will eventually cause cord and/or root compression.

Causes

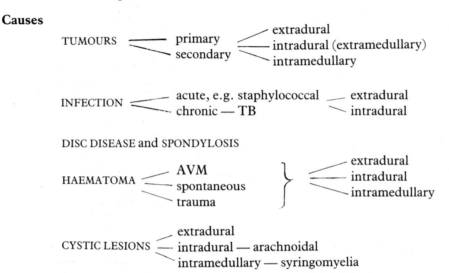

Manifestations of cord or root compression depend upon the following:

Site of lesion within the spinal canal: an expanding lesion outside the cord produces signs and symptoms from root and segmental damage.

ROOT — lower motor neuron (l.m.n.) and sensory impairment appropriate to the distribution of the damaged root.

SEGMENTAL — l.m.n. and sensory impairment appropriate to segmental level.

Interruption of ascending sensory and descending motor tracts produces sensory impairment and an upper motor neuron (u.m.n.) deficit below the level of the lesion.

Lesions within the cord (intramedullary) only produce segmental signs and symptoms.

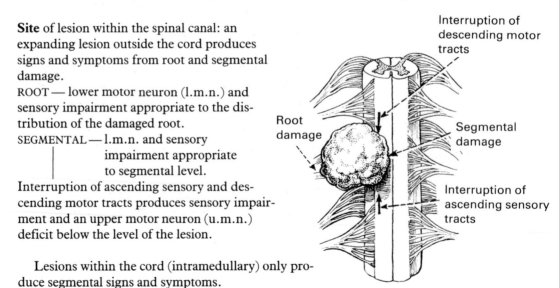

Interruption of descending motor tracts

Root damage

Segmental damage

Interruption of ascending sensory tracts

SPINAL CORD AND ROOT COMPRESSION

Level of the lesion: a lesion above the L1 vertebral body may damage both the cord and its roots. Below this, only roots are damaged.

Vascular involvement: whether neuronal damage results from mechanical stretching or is secondary to ischaemia remains uncertain. On occasions, clinical findings indicate cord damage well beyond the level of the compressive lesion; this implies a distant ischaemic effect due to blood vessel compression at the lesion site.

Speed of onset: speed of compression affects the clinical picture. Despite producing upper motor neuron damage, a rapidly progressive cord lesion often produces a 'flaccid paralysis' with loss of reflexes and absent plantar responses. This state is akin to 'spinal shock' seen following trauma. Several days or weeks may elapse before tone returns accompanied by the expected 'upper motor neuron' signs.

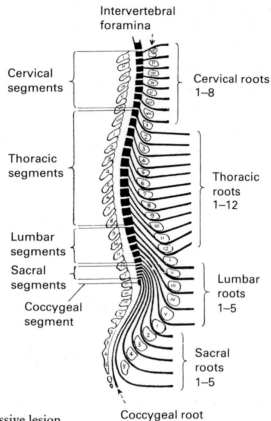

Intervertebral foramina

Cervical segments — Cervical roots 1–8

Thoracic segments — Thoracic roots 1–12

Lumbar segments

Sacral segments — Lumbar roots 1–5

Coccygeal segment

Sacral roots 1–5

Coccygeal root

(After BING A. Local Diagnosis in Neurological Disease 15 ed.)

Clinical features

These depend on the site and level of the compressive lesion.

PAIN

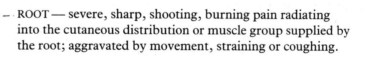

ROOT — severe, sharp, shooting, burning pain radiating into the cutaneous distribution or muscle group supplied by the root; aggravated by movement, straining or coughing.

SEGMENTAL — continuous, deep aching pain radiating into whole leg or one half of body; not affected by movement.

BONE — continuous, dull pain and tenderness over the affected area; may or may not be aggravated by movement.

375

SPINAL CORD AND ROOT COMPRESSION — NEUROLOGICAL EFFECTS

LATERAL COMPRESSIVE LESION

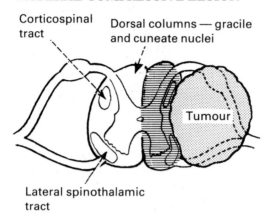

Corticospinal tract

Dorsal columns — gracile and cuneate nuclei

Tumour

Lateral spinothalamic tract

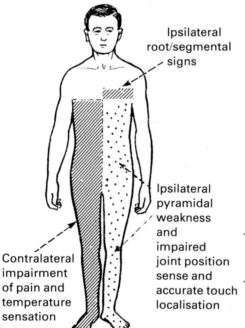

Ipsilateral root/segmental signs

Ipsilateral pyramidal weakness and impaired joint position sense and accurate touch localisation

Contralateral impairment of pain and temperature sensation

Root/segmental damage
MUSCLE WEAKNESS in groups supplied by the involved root and segment with
LOWER MOTOR NEURON (l.m.n.) signs:
— wasting; — loss of tone; — fasciculation;
— diminished or absent reflexes.
N.B. motor deficit is seldom detected
with root lesions above C5 and from T2 to L1.

SENSORY DEFECT of all modalities or hyperaesthesia in area supplied by the root, but overlap from adjacent roots may prevent detection.

Long tract — signs and symptoms
Partial cord lesion (Brown-Séquard syndrome)
MOTOR DEFICIT — dragging of the leg. In high cervical lesions weakness of finger movements is noted on the side of the lesion.
Upper motor neuron (u.m.n.) signs
(maximal on side of lesion):
— weakness in a 'pyramidal' distribution,
    i.e. arms — extensors predominantly
    affected; legs — flexors predominantly affected.
— increased tone, clonus; — increased reflexes;
— extensor plantar response.

SENSORY DEFICIT — numbness may occur on the same side as the lesion and a burning dysaesthesia on the opposite side.
— joint position sense and accurate touch localisation (two point discrimination) impaired on side of lesion.
— pinprick and temperature sensation impaired on opposite side.

In practice, cord damage is seldom restricted to one side. Usually a mixed picture occurs, with an asymmetric distribution of signs and symptoms.

Damage to sympathetic pathways in the T1 root or cervical cord causes an ipsilateral *Horner's syndrome* (page 141).

BLADDER symptoms are infrequent and only occur when cord damage is bilateral. Precipitancy or difficulty in starting micturition may precede retention.

SPINAL CORD AND ROOT COMPRESSION — NEUROLOGICAL EFFECTS

LATERAL COMPRESSIVE LESION *(contd)*
Long tract damage — complete cord lesion

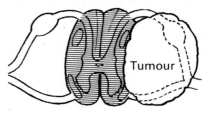

MOTOR DEFICIT: the speed of cord compression
affects the clinical picture. Slowly growing lesions
present with difficulty in walking;
the legs may 'jump' at night. Examination
reveals u.m.n. signs often with an
asymmetric distribution. Rapidly progressive
lesions produce 'spinal shock' — the limbs are flaccid, power
and reflexes diminished or absent and plantar responses are
absent or extensor.

SENSORY DEFICIT: involves all modalities and occurs
up to the level of the lesion.

BLADDER: patient first notices difficulty in initiating
micturition. Retention follows, associated with
incontinence as automatic emptying occurs.
Constipation is only noticed after a few days. Some
patient develop *priapism* (painful erection).

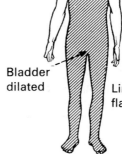

Impairment of all
sensory modalities
up to the level of
the lesion.

Power and reflexes
diminished or
absent

Bladder
dilated

Limbs
flaccid

CENTRAL CORD LESION

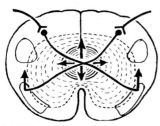

'CAPE' sensory
deficit

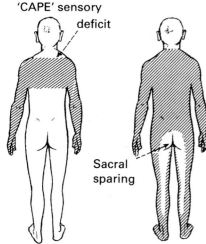

Sacral
sparing

Segmental damage
A central lesion initially damages the second sensory neuron
crossing to the lateral spinothalamic tract; pain and
temperature sensations are impaired in the distribution of
the involved segment. As the lesion expands, anterior horn
cells are also involved and a l.m.n. weakness occurs.

Long tract effects: further lesion expansion damages
the spinothalamic tract and corticospinal tracts, the most
medially situated fibres being involved first. With lesion in
the cervical region, the sensory deficit to pain and
temperature extends downwards in a 'CAPE'-like distribution. As the sacral fibres lie peripherally in the lateral
spinothalamic tract, SACRAL SPARING can occur, even
with a large lesion. Involvement of the corticospinal tracts
produces u.m.n. signs and symptoms in the limbs below the
level of the lesion. The bladder is usually involved late.
  In the cervical cord, sympathetic involvement may
produce a unilateral or bilateral *Horner's syndrome.*

377

SPINAL CORD AND ROOT COMPRESSION — NEUROLOGICAL EFFECTS

LOWER CORD/CAUDA EQUINA LESIONS

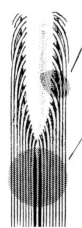

Root or segmental lesions may involve the upper part of the cauda equina and produce root/segmental and long tract signs as described on the previous page, e.g. an expanding L4 root lesion causes weakness and wasting of the foot dorsiflexors, sensory deficit over the inner calf, an increased ankle jerk and an extensor plantar response. Bladder involvement tends to occur late.

The lower sacral roots are involved early, producing loss of motor and sensory bladder control with detrusor paralysis. Overflow incontinence ensues. Impotence and faecal incontinence may be noted. A l.m.n. weakness is found in the muscles supplied by the sacral roots (foot plantarflexors and evertors), the ankle jerks are absent or impaired and a sensory deficit occurs over the 'saddle' area.

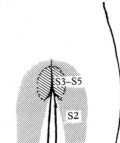

'Saddle' area

VERTEBRAL COLUMN

If a spinal cord or root lesion is suspected look for:

— *Scoliosis, loss of lordosis* or
    limitation of straight leg raising } — suggests root irritation

— *Paravertebral swelling*
— *Tenderness* on bone percussion } — suggests malignant disease or infection

— *Restricted spinal mobility*   — suggests bone, disc or root involvement
— Sacral *dimple or tuft of hair*   — suggests spina bifida oculta /dermoid.

SPINAL CORD AND ROOT COMPRESSION — INVESTIGATIONS

STRAIGHT X-RAY

On the ANTERO-POSTERIOR views look for:

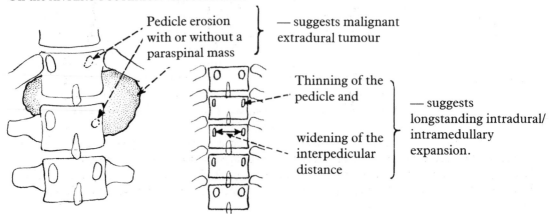

Pedicle erosion with or without a paraspinal mass } — suggests malignant extradural tumour

Thinning of the pedicle and

widening of the interpedicular distance } — suggests longstanding intradural/intramedullary expansion.

378

SPINAL CORD AND ROOT COMPRESSION — INVESTIGATIONS

STRAIGHT X-RAY (*contd*)
On the LATERAL view

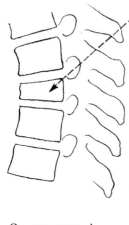

Collapse of the vertebral body suggests malignant infiltration or osteoporosis
(If the disc space is destroyed, infection is more likely)

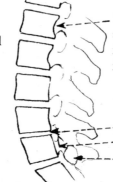

'Scalloping' of the posterior surface of the vertebral body indicates a longstanding intradural lesion

Narrow disc space, narrow canal and hypertrophic facet joints support a diagnosis of disc disease or lumbar spinal stenosis
(but not diagnostic)

Expansion of the intervertebral foramina suggests neurofibroma

On OBLIQUE views

Narrowing from osteophytic encroachment indicates possible root compression
(but often seen in asymptomatic elderly patients)

MYELOGRAPHY
Myelography identifies the level of the compressive lesion and its site, e.g. intradural, extradural.

Extradural		Intradural	
PARTIAL BLOCK	COMPLETE BLOCK	EXTRAMEDULLARY BLOCK	INTRAMEDULLARY BLOCK

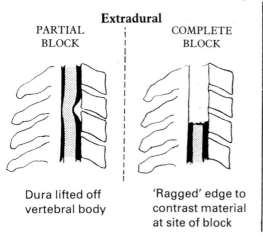
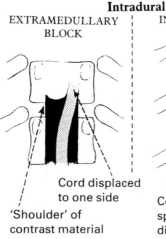
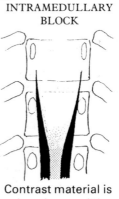

Dura lifted off vertebral body

'Ragged' edge to contrast material at site of block

Cord displaced to one side

'Shoulder' of contrast material

Contrast material is splayed around the dilated cord

Even with an apparent 'complete' block, sufficient contrast medium may be 'coaxed' beyond the lesion to determine its upper extent. If not, a cervical puncture may be necessary.

Radio-opaque markers on the skin surface at the site of the block are a useful operative guide.

Lesions in the lumbar and sacral regions require a '*radiculogram*', outlining the lumbosacral roots.

SPINAL CORD AND ROOT COMPRESSION — INVESTIGATIONS

CSF ANALYSIS

This is of limited value in cord compression. Abnormalities frequently occur, but *lumbar puncture may precipitate neurological deterioration,* presumably due to the creation of a pressure gradient. *If cord compression is suspect then lumbar puncture and CSF analysis should await myelography.*

CSF protein: often increased, especially below a complete block.

CSF cell count: a marked leucocyte count suggests an infective cause — abscess or tuberculosis.

Queckenstedt's Test: absence of pressure transmission to the CSF during lumbar puncture when the neck veins are compressed indicates a complete block.

CT SCAN

It is impracticable to use this as a screening investigation for cord compression, but if the level is known, CT scanning can provide useful information. *Plain CT* clearly identifies disc disease of the lumbar and sacral spine and demonstrates narrowing of the bony canal and thickening of the facet joints. *Intrathecal contrast,* however, is required to show cord compression; scanning is best performed about 6–12 hours after myelography. This will demonstrate the degree of compression and identifies the extraspinal extent of an intraspinal lesion, e.g. neurofibroma.

Neurofibroma

Vertebral body eroded by tumour

Displaced thecal sac containing contrast medium

Facet joint

Dilated intravertebral foramen

MRI

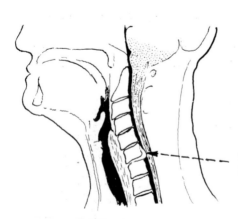

Cord compression by a cervical disc

Sagittal views are of particular value in outlining the spinal cord and the cervicomedullary junction. In contrast, axial views (as obtained in CT scanning) are seldom of sufficient clarity to be of value. MRI will demonstrate cord swelling and differentiate a syrinx (page 385) from an intramedullary tumour (page 384).

SPINAL CORD AND ROOT COMPRESSION

TUMOURS

Incidence: The table shows the number of patients with histologically confirmed tumours admitted to the Institute of Neurological Sciences, Glasgow, over a 5-year period (population 2.7 millions). Tumour types differ in adults and children and are considered separately.

Adults		Children	
EXTRADURAL (**78%**)		EXTRADURAL (**18%**)	
Metastasis	118	Metastasis	1
Myeloma	19	Lymphoma	1
Neurofibroma	15		
Lymphoma	14		
Others	7		
INTRADURAL (**18%**)		INTRADURAL (**64%**)	
Meningioma	22	Dermoid/	
Schwannoma	13	epidermoid	6
Others	4	Others	1
INTRAMEDULLARY (**4%**)		INTRAMEDULLARY (**18%**)	
Astrocytoma	8	Astrocytoma	2
Others	1		

(Table adapted from Adams, Graham and Doyle: Brain Biopsy, 1982)

Pathology: The pathological features of spinal tumours match those of their intracranial counterparts (see page 293).

METASTATIC TUMOUR

Primary site: Usually breast, lung, prostate or kidney.

Metastatic site: Thoracic vertebrae most often involved, but metastasis may occur at any site and may be multiple.

Clinical features: Bone pain and tenderness are common features usually preceding limb and autonomic dysfunction.

Investigations: Plain radiology may be diagnostic as osteolytic lesions or vertebral collapse are often present. Myelography or MRI will identify extradural compression and help exclude multiple lesions.

Management

Until the last few years most patients with cord compression from metastatic tumour underwent a decompressive *laminectomy*, i.e. removal of the laminae and spinous processes.

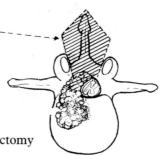

This procedure was usually combined with *radiotherapy*.

Literature reviews, however, suggest that laminectomy does *not* increase the chance of regaining useful limb function when compared to radiotherapy administered alone and, if anything, adds to the risk of neurological deterioration.

— In *ambulant* patients, one-third were unable to walk after laminectomy and radiotherapy.

— In *paraparetic* patients, one-third became ambulant, but a quarter progressed to complete paraplegia, irrespective of treatment.

— Virtually no patients with *paraplegia* of >24 hours duration regained useful leg or bladder function.

SPINAL CORD AND ROOT COMPRESSION

Management *(contd)*

Metastatic tumour often involves the vertebral body. Laminectomy removes the posterior support. The poor operative results in these patients may result from instability.

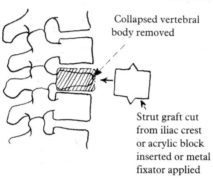

Collapsed vertebral body removed

Strut graft cut from iliac crest or acrylic block inserted or metal fixator applied

ANTERIOR VERTEBRAL DECOMPRESSION WITH FUSION/FIXATION overcomes this problem. Inevitably this involves a major procedure — usually TRANSTHORACIC and it is inappropriate in the elderly, in patients with paraplegia of >24 hours duration and in patients with a dismal prognosis from their primary tumour (e.g. small cell bronchial carcinoma). As yet, results appear far superior to laminectomy, but comparison is difficult in view of the more stringent patient selection.

SUGGESTED SCHEME OF MANAGEMENT

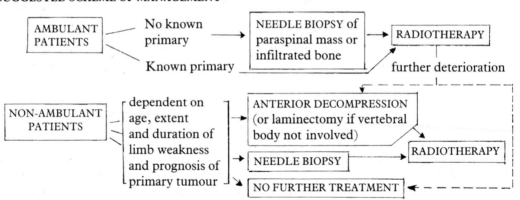

With this approach fewer patients are submitted to the demands of operation, yet overall results appear as good as, if not better than by more traditional methods.

MYELOMA

This malignant condition usually affects older age groups. It is often multifocal, involving the vertebral bodies, pelvis, ribs and skull, but solitary tumours may occur ('plasmacytoma'). Spinal cord compression occurs in 15% of patients with myeloma and rarely without vertebral body involvement due to intradural deposits. If suspect, look for characteristic changes in the plasma immunoglobulins and for Bence-Jones protein in the urine. An isotope bone scan may be less informative than a radiological skeletal survey. Bone marrow shows infiltration of plasma cells. Serum calcium levels may be high.

Management is as for metastatic tumour with additional chemotherapy. The prognosis is variable.

SPINAL CORD AND ROOT COMPRESSION

MENINGIOMA

Spinal meningiomas tend to occur in elderly patients and are more common in females than in males. They usually arise in the thoracic region and are almost always intradural. Slow growth often permits considerable cord flattening to occur before symptoms become evident.

The operative aim is complete removal. Results are usually good, but if the tumour arises anteriorly to the cord, excision of the dural origin is difficult, if not impossible, and recurrence may result.

SCHWANNOMA/NEUROFIBROMA

Schwannomas are slowly growing benign tumours occurring at any level and arising from the posterior nerve roots. They lie either entirely within the spinal canal or 'dumbbell' through the intervertebral foramen, on occasions presenting as a mass in the thorax or posterior abdominal wall.

Neurofibromas are identical apart from their microscopic appearance (page 294) and their association with multiple neurofibromatosis (Von Recklinghausen's disease) — look for café au lait patches in the skin.

Schwannomas tend to occur in the 30–60 age group. Typically they present with root pain, but in contrast to the pain from disc disease, this is often worse at night. Root signs and/or signs of cord compression may follow.

Myelography identifies an intradural/extramedullary lesion. Oblique X-rays may show foraminal enlargement;

Nerve root entering tumour

Neurofibroma 'dumbbelling' through intervertebral foramen

CT scan will delineate any extraspinal extension (see page 380). Complete operative removal is feasible but the nerve root of origin is inevitably sacrificed. Overlap from adjacent nerve roots usually minimises any resultant neurological deficit.

INTRAMEDULLARY TUMOURS

Intrinsic tumours of the spinal cord occur infrequently. In the Glasgow series (Table, page 381) almost all were slowly growing *astrocytomas* (grades I and II) although other series report an equal incidence of *ependymomas*. Cystic cavities may lie within the tumour or at the upper or lower pole.

Clinical features

The onset is usually gradual. Segmental pain is common. Interruption of the decussating fibres to the lateral spinothalamic tract causes loss of pain and temperature sensation at the level of the involved segments.

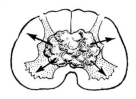

Tumour expansion and involvement of the anterior horn cells produces a lower motor neuron weakness of the corresponding muscle groups; corticospinal track involvement produces an upper motor neuron weakness below the level of the lesion. The sensory deficit spreads downwards bilaterally, the sacral region being the last to become involved.

SPINAL CORD AND ROOT COMPRESSION

INTRAMEDULLARY TUMOURS (*contd*)

Investigations
Straight X-rays occasionally show widening of the
interpedicular distance or 'scalloping' of the vertebral bodies.
Myelography confirms the presence of an intramedullary lesion,
but MRI provides most information, differentiating
tumour from syringomyelia, and identifying the
extent of the lesion and the presence of any
associated cysts.

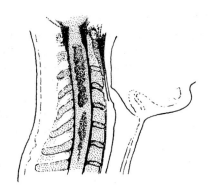

Management
When an intrinsic cord tumour is suspect, an exploratory laminectomy is required. An attempt is made to obtain a diagnosis
either through a longitudinal midline cord incision or by needle biopsy. Cystic cavities within a tumour or an associated
syringomyelia may benefit from aspiration. Rarely benign lesions (e.g. tuberculoma, epidermoid, haemangioblastoma,
lipoma) are found. With some tumours, particularly ependymomas, a plane of cleavage is evident and partial or even total
removal is possible. After tumour biopsy or removal, radiotherapy is often administered, but its value is uncertain.

EPENDYMOMA OF THE CAUDA EQUINA
Over 50% of spinal ependymomas occur around the cauda equina and present with a central cauda equina syndrome (page
378). Operative removal combined with radiotherapy usually gives good long-term results, although metastatic seeding
occasionally occurs through the CSF.

SPINAL CYSTIC LESIONS

Enterogenous cysts: cysts with a
mucoid content are occasionally
found lying ventral or dorsal to the
cord. They are often associated
with vertebral malformation or
other congenital abnormality, and
are thought to arise from remnants
of the neuroenteric canal.

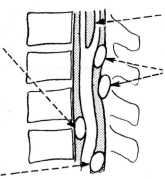

Intramedullary cystic lesion:
syringomyelia (see over) or cystic
cavitation within a glioma.

Arachnoid cysts: arachnoid pouches
filled with contrast medium are
occasionally found incidentally during
myelography. These may seal off,
producing CSF filled cysts. They
occur predominantly in the
thoracic region and sometimes cause
cord compression. Children with
extradural arachnoid cysts
frequently develop kyphosis; the
causal relationship remains
unknown.

Epidermoid/dermoid cysts:
may be of developmental origin or
may follow implantation from a
preceding lumbar puncture
procedure.

SPINAL CORD AND ROOT COMPRESSION

SYRINGOMYELIA

Syringomyelia is the acquired development of a cavity (syrinx) within the spinal cord substance. The lower cervical segments are usually affected, but extension may occur upwards into the brain stem (syringobulbia, see page 366) or downwards as far as the filum terminale.

The cavitation appears to develop in association with obstruction:
– usually around the foramen magnum in conjunction with the *Arnold-Chiari malformation*.
– also secondarily to *trauma* or *arachnoiditis*.

The syrinx may obliterate the central canal leaving clumps of ependymal cells in the wall. In contrast HYDROMYELIA is the congenital persistence and widening of the central canal.

Syringomyelia should be distinguished from cystic intramedullary tumours, although both pathologies may coexist.

Pathogenesis

The exact cause of this condition remains unknown but theories abound. In 1965, Gardner proposed the *'hydrodynamic theory'*, suggesting that the craniovertebral anomaly may impair CSF outflow from the 4th ventricle to the cisterna magna. This in turn was believed to result in transmission of a CSF arterial pulse wave through a patent central canal, dilating the canal below the level of compression. This theory, however, does not explain the occurrence of syringomyelia in patients with non-patent central canals. Most now attribute the formation of the syrinx to pressure changes transmitted through the epidural veins to the spinal canal during coughing or straining. In the presence of an obstructive element these pressure changes appear to force CSF into the cord substance. This develops into a cystic cavity which progressively extends.

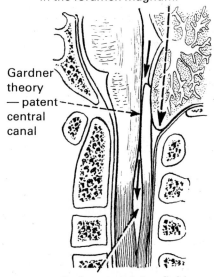

Arnold-Chiari malformation with cerebellar tonsils impacted in the foramen magnum.

Gardner theory — patent central canal

Syrinx containing fluid identical to CSF

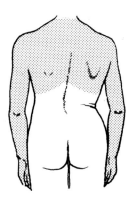

Clinical features
– *Dissociated sensory loss* (i.e. loss of pain and temperature sensation with retention of other senses) occurring in a cape-like distribution. Painless burns are a classical sign.
– *Wasting and weakness of the small muscles of the hand* and *winging of the scapula* from anterior horn cell involvement. *Scoliosis* often results.
– *Long tract signs* follow.
– *Brain stem signs* may appear, either from syringobulbia or an associated Arnold-Chiari malformation.
– *Hydrocephalus* occurs in 25% but is usually asymptomatic.

385

SPINAL CORD AND ROOT COMPRESSION

SYRINGOMYELIA *(contd)*
Investigations
MRI is the investigation of choice (see page 365). This will demonstrate the syrinx and any associated Arnold-Chiari malformation and exclude intramedullary tumour. If MRI is unavailable — MYELOGRAPHY demonstrates dilatation of the spinal cord. With coexisting Arnold-Chiari malformations, screening in the *supine* position will show the cerebellar tonsils descending below the foramen magnum.

The introduction of air into the CSF space — AIR MYELOGRAPHY — may cause 'collapse' of the dilated segment thereby excluding an intrinsic cord tumour. A CT scan, six hours after injection of intrathecal contrast, may show uptake within the syrinx, but beware of misinterpreting normal contrast uptake within spinal cord tissue. Puncture of the syrinx is occasionally possible and subsequent injection of contrast shows its exact extent.

Management
Operative techniques are only of limited benefit. The approach depends on the presence or absence of an associated Arnold-Chiari malformation.

1. If Arnold-Chiari malformation is present — *decompression* by removing the posterior rim of the foramen magnum and posterior arch of the atlas results in improvement of long tract and brain stem signs in approximately 30%. Progression is halted in a further 40%. These benefits are probably due to relief of hind brain pressure, rather than an alteration of the hydrodynamics of the syrinx.

   If deterioration in the above patients continues, or if no associated Arnold-Chiari malformation exists, attempt either:

2. Syringostomy: or   3. Filum terminale division:

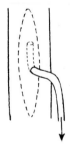 The syrinx is drained via a silastic tube into the surrounding CSF space.
    Alternatively, a syringoperitoneal shunt is performed. Some patients benefit from this procedure but in one-third, progressive deterioration continues.

To CSF space or peritoneum

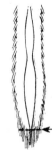 In some patients the syrinx or a patent central canal extends down to the conus medullaris; in these, division of the filum terminale permits syrinx drainage. Although a relatively safe technique, benefits require confirmation.

Syringomyelia remains a difficult condition to treat. Draining the syrinx into the CSF space by syringostomy or filum terminale division may not significantly alter the haemodynamics. Syringoperitoneal shunt may seem to be the most logical approach. Despite all efforts, at least one-third of patients suffer progressive deterioration.

SPINAL CORD AND ROOT COMPRESSION

SPINAL INFECTION

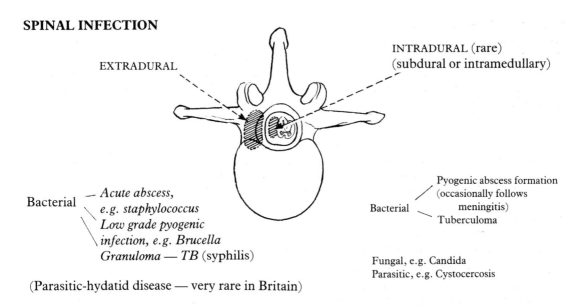

EXTRADURAL

INTRADURAL (rare)
(subdural or intramedullary)

Bacterial — Acute abscess,
e.g. staphylococcus
Low grade pyogenic
infection, e.g. Brucella
Granuloma — TB (syphilis)

Bacterial — Pyogenic abscess formation
(occasionally follows
meningitis)
Tuberculoma

Fungal, e.g. Candida
Parasitic, e.g. Cystocercosis

(Parasitic-hydatid disease — very rare in Britain)

ACUTE EXTRADURAL ABSCESS

Organism: Invariably *Staphylococcus aureus*.

Spread: Haematogenous, e.g. from a boil or furuncle, or direct from vertebral osteomyelitis.

Site: Usually thoracic, but may affect any level. Cord damage occurs either from direct compression or secondary to a thrombophlebitis and venous infarction.

Clinical features: May mimic a rapidly progressive extradural tumour or haematoma with bilateral leg weakness, a sensory level and urinary retention, but distinguishing features are:
– very severe pain and tenderness over the involved site.
– toxaemia: pyrexia, malaise, increased pulse rate.
– rigidity of neck and spinal column, with marked resistance to flexion.
As the abscess extends upwards, the sensory level may rise.

Investigations: *Straight X-ray* may or may not show an associated osteitis.
An *MRI* or *myelogram* confirms the site of the extradural lesion.
CSF examination, if performed shows an increased white cell count, usually polymorphonuclear, but may be normal.
A *leucocytosis* is usually present in the peripheral blood and the *ESR* raised.

Management: Urgent decompressive laminectomy and abscess drainage combined with intravenous antibiotic therapy provides the best chance of recovery of function.

SPINAL CORD AND ROOT COMPRESSION

SPINAL TUBERCULOSIS (Pott's disease of the spine)
In developing countries, spinal TB is mostly a disease of childhood or adolescence. In Britain it usually affects the middle aged and is particularly prevalent in immigrant populations.

The lower thoracic spine is commonly involved and the disease initially affects two adjacent vertebral bodies.

Clinical features:
The classical systemic features of weight loss, night fever and cachexia are often absent.

Pain occurs over the affected area and is only relieved by rest.

Symptoms and signs of cord compression occur in approximately 20% of cases.

The onset may be gradual as pus, caseous material or granulation tissue accumulate, or sudden as vertebral bodies collapse and a kyphosis develops.

STRAIGHT X-RAYS are characteristic.

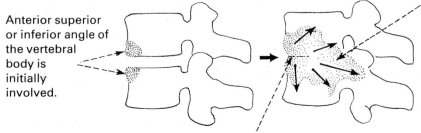

Anterior superior or inferior angle of the vertebral body is initially involved.

Infective process spreads throughout the vertebral body and may involve the pedicles or facet joints.

The disc space collapses as the vertebral plate is destroyed.

Management:
Every effort is made to establish the diagnosis. A *needle biopsy* is often sufficient, but occasionally an exploratory operation (costotransversectomy) is required. Long-term *antituberculous therapy* is commenced.

If signs of cord compression develop, decompression is required.

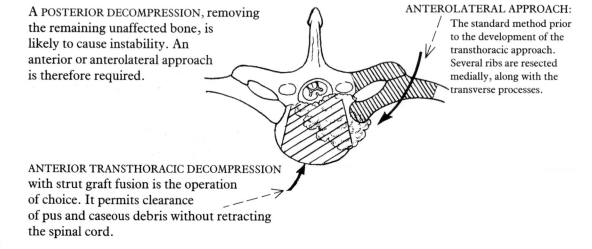

A POSTERIOR DECOMPRESSION, removing the remaining unaffected bone, is likely to cause instability. An anterior or anterolateral approach is therefore required.

ANTEROLATERAL APPROACH: The standard method prior to the development of the transthoracic approach. Several ribs are resected medially, along with the transverse processes.

ANTERIOR TRANSTHORACIC DECOMPRESSION with strut graft fusion is the operation of choice. It permits clearance of pus and caseous debris without retracting the spinal cord.

388

DISC PROLAPSE AND SPONDYLOSIS

Intervertebral discs act as shock absorbers for the bony spine.

A tough outer layer — the annulus fibrosis surrounds a softer central nucleus pulposus.

Discs degenerate with age, the fluid within the nucleus pulposus gradually drying out. Disc collapse produces excessive strain on the facet joints, i.e. the superior and inferior articulatory processes of each vertebral body, and leads to degeneration and hypertrophy.

LUMBAR DISC PROLAPSE

An *acute disc prolapse* occurs when the soft nucleus herniates through a tear in the annulus and may result from a single or repeated traumatic incidents. Herniation usually occurs laterally and compresses adjacent nerve roots, but may occasionally occur centrally, compressing the cauda equina.

A 'free fragment' of the nucleus pulposus may extrude and lie above or below the level of the disc space.

Associated hypertrophy of degenerated facet joints is often a further source of back and leg pain and is an important cause of root compression.

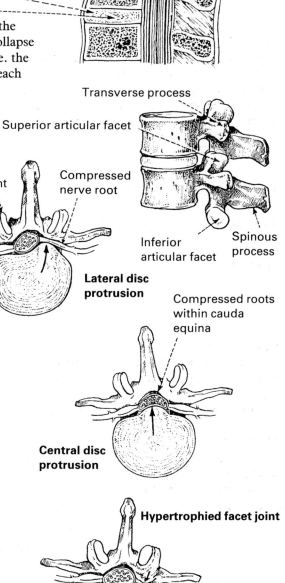

Transverse process

Superior articular facet

Facet joint

Compressed nerve root

Inferior articular facet

Spinous process

Lateral disc protrusion

Compressed roots within cauda equina

Central disc protrusion

Hypertrophied facet joint

Compressed nerve root

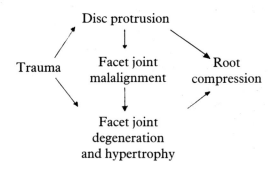

Trauma → Disc protrusion → Root compression

Disc protrusion → Facet joint malalignment → Facet joint degeneration and hypertrophy → Root compression

LUMBAR DISC PROLAPSE

A *congenitally narrowed spinal canal* increases susceptibility to the development of nerve root compression. Here the spinal canal diameter is considerably diminished and minor disc protrusion or mild joint hypertrophy may more readily compress the nerve root.

Lateral disc herniations usually compress the nerve root exiting through the foramen below the affected level, e.g. an L3/4 disc lesion will compress the L4 nerve root, but large disc protrusions or a free fragment may compress any adjacent root.

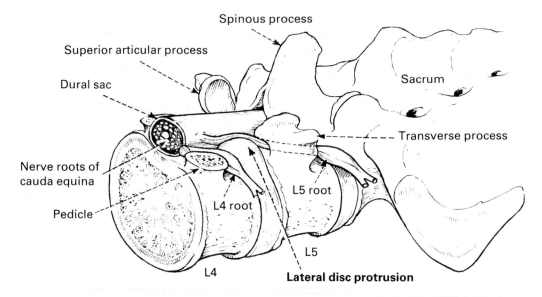

Lumbar disc lesions may occur at any level but L4/5 and L5/S1 are the commonest sites (95%).

LUMBAR DISC PROLAPSE

CLINICAL FEATURES
Lateral disc protrusion

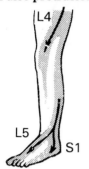

Injury: A history of falling, or lifting heavy weights often precedes the onset of symptoms.

Leg pain: Root irritation or compression produces pain in the distribution of the affected root and this should extend below the mid-calf. Coughing, sneezing or straining aggravates the leg pain which is usually more severe than any associated backache. If compression causes severe root damage the leg pain may disappear as neurological signs develop.

Paraesthesia: Numbness or tingling occurs in the distribution of the affected root.

'MECHANICAL' SIGNS: Spinal movements are restricted, scoliosis is often present and is related to spasm of the erector spinae muscles, and the normal lumbar lordosis is lost.

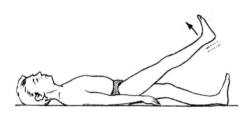

Straight leg raising: L5 and S1 root compression causes limitation to less than 60° from the horizontal and produces pain down the back of the leg. Dorsiflexion of the foot while the leg is elevated aggravates the pain. Elevation of the 'good' leg may produce pain in the other leg.

(If in doubt about the veracity of a restricted straight leg raising deficit, sit the patient up on the examination couch with the legs straight. This is equivalent to 90° straight leg raising.)

Reverse leg raising (femoral stretch)
Tests for irritation of
higher nerve roots
(L4 and above)

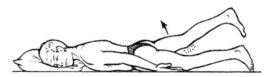

NEUROLOGICAL DEFICIT: Depends on the root involved:

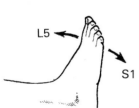

L4 — Quadriceps wasting and weakness; sensory impairment over medial calf; impaired knee jerk.

L5 — Wasting and weakness of dorsiflexors of foot, extensor digitorum longus and extensor hallucis longus; wasting of extensor digitorum brevis; sensory impairment over lateral calf and dorsum of foot.

S1 — Wasting and weakness of plantar flexors; sensory impairment over lateral aspect of foot and sole; impaired ankle jerk.

Root signs cannot reliably localise the level of disc protrusion due to variability of the anatomical distribution.

LUMBAR DISC PROLAPSE

CLINICAL FEATURES (*contd*)
Central disc protrusion
Symptoms and signs of central disc protrusion are usually bilateral, although one side is often worse than the other.

Leg pain: Extends bilaterally down the back of the thighs. Pain may disappear with the onset of paralysis.

Paraesthesia: Occurs in the same distribution.

Sphincter paralysis: Loss of bladder and urethral sensation with intermittent or complete retention of urine occurs in most patients. Anal sensation is usually impaired and accompanies constipation.

Severe pain associated with lateral disc protrusion may inhibit micturition. In this instance, strong analgesia should allow normal micturition; the presence of normal perineal sensation excludes root compression as the cause of the retention.

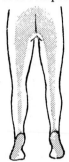

Sensory loss: Extends over all or part of the sacral area ('saddle' anaesthesia) and confirms a neurogenic cause for the sphincter disturbance.

Motor loss: Usually presents as foot drop with complete loss of power in the dorsiflexors and plantarflexors of both feet.

Reflex loss: The ankle jerks are usually absent on each side.

INVESTIGATION
Straight X-ray of lumbosacral spine is of limited benefit in the investigation of lumbar disc disease — it may show loss of a disc space or an associated spondylolisthesis (see page 394). Straight X-rays are *important in excluding other pathology* such as metastatic carcinoma.

Radiculography outlines the thecal sac and nerve roots.
Disc protrusion may cause:
1. A filling defect in the theca on the AP or lateral view at the appropriate disc level.
2. Obliteration or displacement of the nerve root sleeve.

Oblique view:

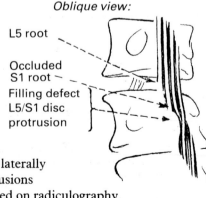

L5 root

Occluded S1 root

Filling defect L5/S1 disc protrusion

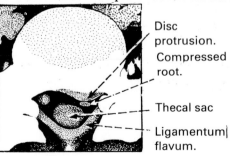

Disc protrusion.
Compressed root.

Thecal sac

Ligamentum flavum.

Spinal CT scan may detect small laterally placed disc protrusions occasionally missed on radiculography.

In addition, it clearly shows hypertrophied facet joints and the diameter of the spinal canal.

LUMBAR DISC PROLAPSE

MANAGEMENT

(a) Lateral disc protrusion

CONSERVATIVE: Most bouts of leg pain settle spontaneously by taking simple measures:
- *Bed rest* for 2–3 weeks on an orthopaedic mattress or with a hard board under mattress;
- *Traction* may help, but pain may return when traction is removed;
- *Plaster jacket* or *spinal brace* is of benefit in some patients and provides rest yet retains mobility.
When the pain settles, the patient is advised to *avoid heavy lifting*. Even picking up objects from the floor should be accompanied by bending the knees and keeping the back straight.

INDICATIONS FOR OPERATION
- Severe *unremitting leg pain* despite conservative measures.
- *Recurrent attacks* of leg pain, especially when causing repeated time loss from work.
- The development of a *neurological deficit*.

TECHNIQUE: Fenestration usually provides good access. Retraction of the root and dural sac exposes the disc protrusion and allows removal with rongeurs. Any protuberance from the facet joint causing root pressure or narrowing of the root canal is also removed. 'Microdiscectomy' with an operating microscope allows disc removal through a smaller skin and muscle incision and may reduce the period of hospital care.

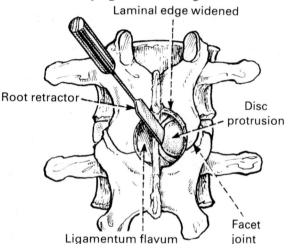

RESULTS: Approximately 80% of patients obtain good results after operation. The remainder m ty have recurrent problems due to a further disc protrusion at the same or another level. Occasionally bony instability complicates the operation. Now that a water-soluble contrast medium is used for investigation (instead of oil-based Myodil), arachnoiditis rarely occurs.

After disc operation, patients are advised to avoid heavy lifting, preferably for an indefinite period. Persistance in a heavy manual job may lead to further trouble.

In general, patients with clear-cut indications for operation do well, whereas those with dubious clinical or radiographic signs tend to have a high incidence of recurrent problems.

(b) Central disc protrusion

In contrast to lateral disc protrusion, *compression of the cauda equina from a central disc constitutes a neurosurgical emergency.* Delay in root decompression results in a reduced chance of motor and sphincter recovery.

A full laminectomy at the appropriate level rather than fenestration is usually required to obtain adequate exposure.

Motor, sensory and sphincter function should gradually recover over a two year period but results are often disappointing. Although most regain bladder control, few have completely normal function and in many, sexual difficulties persist.

LUMBAR SPINAL STENOSIS

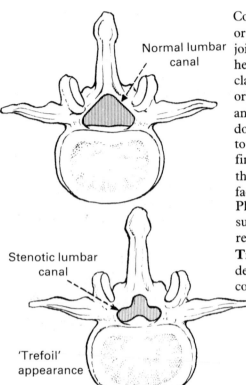

Normal lumbar canal

Stenotic lumbar canal

'Trefoil' appearance

Congenital narrowing of the lumbar spinal cord, or secondary narrowing due to hypertrophic facet joints, may predispose to root compression from a herniated disc, but in addition may produce 'neurogenic claudication'. Symptoms of root pain, paraesthesia or weakness develop after standing or walking and may be relieved by sitting, bending over or lying down. Straight leg raising is seldom impaired, in contrast to patients with disc protrusion. Objective neurological findings may only appear after exercise. In some patients this condition only affects one side — the 'unilateral facet syndrome'.

Plain X-rays and radiculography may suggest lumbar spinal stenosis but CT scanning is required to establish the diagnosis.

Treatment: A wide laminectomy with root decompression usually produces good results with complete relief of symptoms.

SPONDYLOLISTHESIS

Spondylolisthesis is a forward shift of one vertebral body on another. Slip occurs due to degenerative disease of the facet joints (always at L4/L5) or

to a developmental break or elongation of the L5 lamina causing an L5/S1 spondylolisthesis.

Spondylolisthesis is often symptomless but the resultant narrowing in canal width may accentuate symptoms of root compression from disc protrusion or joint hypertrophy.

L4

L5

Treatment: usually conservative, but if signs of root compression are present, then decompression of the root canal is necessary. Occasionally fusion is required, especially if back pain predominates.

THORACIC DISC PROLAPSE

This occurs rarely (0.2% of all disc lesions) due to the relative rigidity of the thoracic spine.

PRESENTATION
– Root pain and/or
– Progressive of fluctuating paraparesis (may lead to mistaken diagnosis).
As vascular involvement may produce damage above the level of compression, sensory findings may be misleading.

INVESTIGATION
Myelography, although difficult in the thoracic spine, demonstrates an anterior filling defect at the level of the disc space.
An *axial CT* scan (within 6–12 hours) at the appropriate level with or without sagittal reconstruction, should clearly demonstrate the lesion (see illustration on page 37). *MRI* will also demonstrate a midline thoracic disc protrusion, although a lateral disc may be harder to identify.

MANAGEMENT
Root pain — may settle with bed rest.

In the presence of cord compression or unremitting root pain, *anterior transthoracic decompression* provides the safest approach. (A posteror approach — laminectomy — carries an unacceptably high risk of paraplegia.)

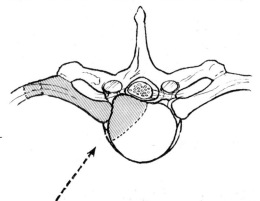

The head of the rib is removed and the vertebral body adjacent to the disc space is drilled away permitting clearance of herniated disc material.

CERVICAL SPONDYLOSIS

The mobile cervical spine is particularly subject to osteoarthritic change and this occurs in more than half the population over 50 years of age; of these approximately 20% develop symptoms. Relatively few require operative treatment.

PATHOGENESIS

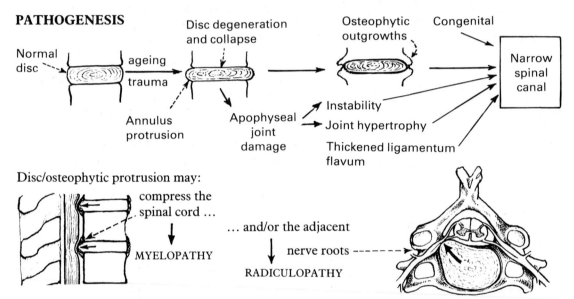

Disc/osteophytic protrusion may:

compress the spinal cord ...

↓

MYELOPATHY

... and/or the adjacent

↓

nerve roots - - - - - - →

RADICULOPATHY

Resultant damage to the spinal cord may arise from direct pressure or may follow vascular impairment. The onset is usually gradual. Trauma may or may not predispose to the development of symptoms.

CLINICAL FEATURES
Radiculopathy
Pain: A sharp stabbing pain, worse on coughing, may be superimposed on a more constant deep ache radiating over the shoulders and down the arm.
Paraesthesia: Numbness or tingling follows a nerve root distribution.
Root signs:
– *Sensory loss,* i.e. pin prick deficit in the appropriate dermatomal distribution.
– *Muscle (l.m.n.) weakness* and wasting in appropriate muscle groups, e.g. C5, C6...biceps, deltoid: C7...triceps.
– *Reflex impairment/loss,* e.g. C5,6...biceps, supinator jerk: C7...triceps jerk.
– *Trophic change:* In long-standing root compression, skin becomes dry, scaly, inelastic, blue and cold.

CERVICAL SPONDYLOSIS

CLINICAL FEATURES *(contd)*
Myelopathy

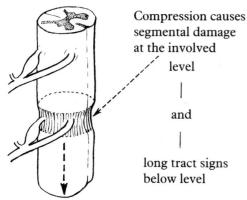

Compression causes segmental damage at the involved

level

|

and

|

long tract signs below level

Arms: l.m.n. signs and symptoms, as above, at the level of the lesion
and/or
u.m.n. signs and symptoms below the level of the lesion

e.g. C5 lesion { biceps weakness, wasting: diminished biceps jerk: increased finger jerks.

Legs: u.m.n. signs and symptoms, i.e. difficulty in walking due to stiffness; 'pyramidal' weakness, increased tone, clonus and extensor plantar responses; sensory symptoms and signs are variable and less prominent.

Sphincter disturbance is seldom a prominent early feature.

N.B. Involved segments may extend above or below the level of compression if the vascular supply is also impaired.

INVESTIGATION
Plain X-ray of cervical spine
Look for:
- – congenital narrowing of canal, loss of lordosis.
- – disc space narrowing and osteophyte protrusion (foraminal encroachment is best seen in oblique views).
- – subluxation. Flexion/extension views may be required.

Cervical myelogram
Lateral view: Identifies anterior disc bars compressing the cord.
Antero-posterior view: Shows root obliteration/filling defect due to disc or osteophyte protrusion.
If doubt persist, an **axial CT** within 6 – 12 hours of contrast administration should clearly demonstrate the degree and site of root compression.

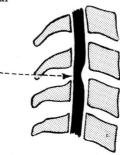

MRI: provides a non-invasive method of identifying cord compression (see page 380) but this technique is at present of limited value in patients with radiculopathy.

MANAGEMENT
Conservative
– Analgesics
– Cervical collar
– Traction

Symptoms of radiculopathy, whether acute or chronic, usually respond to these conservative measures plus reassurance. Progression of a disabling neurological deficit however demands surgical intervention. The clinician may adopt a conservative approach when a myelopathy is mild, but undue delay in operation may reduce the chance of recovery.

CERVICAL SPONDYLOSIS

MANAGEMENT (*contd*)
Indications for operation
1. Progressive neurological deficit — myelopathy or radiculopathy.
2. Intractable pain, when this fails to respond to conservative measures. This is rarely the sole indication for operation and usually applies to acute disc protrusions (see below) rather than chronic radiculopathy.

Operative techniques

1. *Anterior approach*
   Cloward's anterior fusion
   A core of bone and disc is
   drilled out allowing removal
   of the osteophytic projection.
   Although not essential, most
   combine this with fusion using
   a dowel from the iliac crest or
   bovine xenograft.

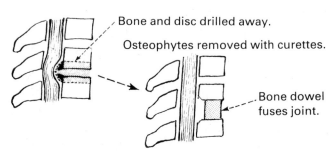

Bone and disc drilled away.

Osteophytes removed with curettes.

Bone dowel fuses joint.

Suitable for root or cord compression from an anterior protrusion at one level, although two and even three levels may be fused.

2. *Posterior approach*

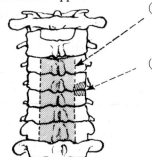

    (a) *Laminectomy:* a wide decompression, usually from C3–C7, is carried out. Suitable for multilevel cord compression especially when superimposed on a congenitally narrow spinal canal.

    (b) *Foraminotomy:* the nerve root at one or more levels may be decompressed by drilling away overlying bone.

Results
Operative results vary widely in different series and probably depend on patient selection. Some improvement occurs in 50–80% of patients. Operation should be aimed at preventing progression rather than curing all symptoms.

Cervical disc prolapse
In contrast to cervical spondylosis, cervical 'soft disc' protrusion is uncommon. This tends to occur acutely in younger patients and may be related to a specific incident such as a sudden twist or injury to the neck. The protrusion usually occurs posterolaterally at the C5/C6 or C6/C7 level causing a radiculopathy rather than a myelopathy. *CT scan with intrathecal contrast* clearly outlines the disc protrusion.
Sagittal T1 weighted *MRI* will demonstrate soft tissue spinal cord impingement.
    Operative removal through an anterior approach may be required for intractable pain or neurological deficit and gives good results.

SPINAL TRAUMA

Approximately 2 per 100 000 of the population per year sustain a spinal injury. Of these, 50% involve the cervical region.

At impact, *spinal cord damage* may or may not accompany the *bony or ligamentous damage*. After impact, stability at the level of injury plays a crucial part in further management. Injudicious movement of a patient with an unstable lesion may precipitate spinal cord injury or aggravate any pre-existing damage.

MECHANISMS OF INJURY
The mechanism of injury helps determine the degree of stability:

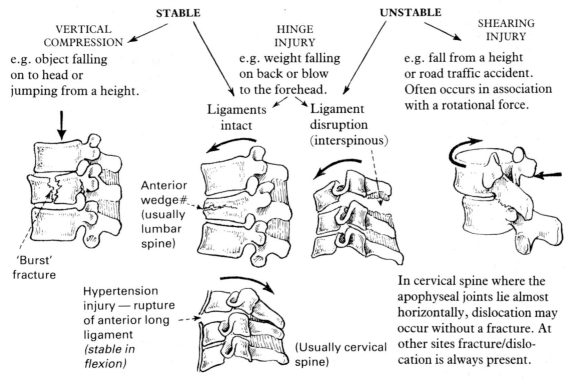

STABLE

VERTICAL COMPRESSION
e.g. object falling on to head or jumping from a height.

HINGE INJURY
e.g. weight falling on back or blow to the forehead.

UNSTABLE

SHEARING INJURY
e.g. fall from a height or road traffic accident. Often occurs in association with a rotational force.

Ligaments intact

Ligament disruption (interspinous)

'Burst' fracture

Anterior wedge# (usually lumbar spine)

Hypertension injury — rupture of anterior long ligament *(stable in flexion)*

(Usually cervical spine)

In cervical spine where the apophyseal joints lie almost horizontally, dislocation may occur without a fracture. At other sites fracture/dislocation is always present.

Initial assessment
The possibility of spinal injury must be considered at the scene of the accident and all movements and transportation of the patient undertaken with extreme caution especially when comatose. Most spinal injuries occur in conscious patients who complain of *pain, numbness or difficulty with limb movements.*

Examination may reveal *tenderness over the spinous processes, paraspinal swelling* or *a gap between the spinous processes*, indicating rupture of an interspinous ligament.
Neurogenic paradoxical ventilation (indrawing of the chest on inspiration due to absent intercostal function) may occur with cervical cord damage.
Bilateral absence of limb reflexes in flaccid limbs, unresponsive to painful stimuli, indicates spinal cord damage (unless death is imminent from severe head injury.)
Painless urinary retention or *priapism* may also occur.

399

SPINAL TRAUMA — INVESTIGATIONS

STRAIGHT X-RAYS
LATERAL VIEW
In the *cervical spine:*
– note evidence of
soft tissue swelling
between the pharynx
and the vertebrae.

– ensure *C6 and C7*
are included in the film.
If not, repeat with gentle
downward arm traction.

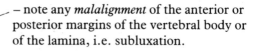

– note any *malalignment* of the anterior or posterior margins of the vertebral body or of the lamina, i.e. subluxation.

– note any undue *widening of the interspinous distance or of the disc space.*

– note *damage to the vertebral body, apophyseal joints, lamina or spinous process,* e.g. anterior wedge collapse, 'burst' fracture.

In the upper thoracic spine only **Tomography** may satisfactorily demonstrate the lateral view.

ANTERO-POSTERIOR VIEW
– note the
alignment and
the *width of
the apophyseal
joints* and look
for *vertical*
fracture lines.

ANTERO-POSTERIOR 'OPEN MOUTH' VIEW
– required to
demonstrate a
*fracture of
the odontoid
peg.*

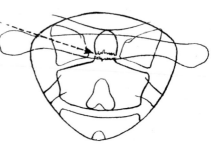

If doubt remains —
take **OBLIQUE VIEWS** to demonstrate the intervertebral foramina.

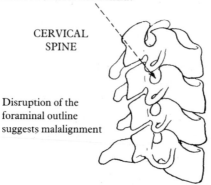

CERVICAL
SPINE

Disruption of the
foraminal outline
suggests malalignment

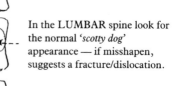

In the LUMBAR spine look for the normal *'scotty dog'* appearance — if misshapen, suggests a fracture/dislocation.

If in doubt about cervical stability, take **FLEXION/EXTENSION VIEWS**, but only with expert supervision.

Myelography and **CT scanning** show the extent to which bone fragments indent the spinal cord, but these investigations only help if operative decompression and/or stabilisation is considered.

SPINAL TRAUMA — MANAGEMENT

Management depends on the site and stability of the lesion, but basic principles apply.
1. An *unstable* lesion risks further damage to the spinal cord and roots and requires either —
   – *operative fixation* or
   – *immobilisation*, e.g. skull traction, Halo or plaster jacket.
2. There is no evidence that 'decompressing' the cord lesion (either anteriorly or posteriorly) improves the neurological outcome, but —
3. If a patient with normal cord function or with an incomplete cord lesion (i.e. with some residual function) *progressively deteriorates*, then *operative decompression* is required.

Many additional therapies and techniques (e.g. steroids, cord cooling, hyperbaric oxygen) are employed with the aim of improving neurological outcome; as yet none have been shown to produce any significant benefit.

Management of injury at specific sites

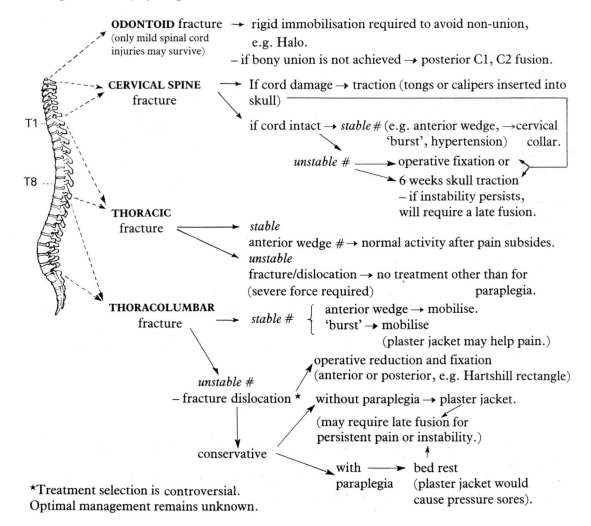

ODONTOID fracture → rigid immobilisation required to avoid non-union,
(only mild spinal cord injuries may survive)   e.g. Halo.
– if bony union is not achieved → posterior C1, C2 fusion.

CERVICAL SPINE fracture → If cord damage → traction (tongs or calipers inserted into skull)

if cord intact → *stable #* (e.g. anterior wedge, →cervical 'burst', hypertension)   collar.

unstable # ——→ operative fixation or
6 weeks skull traction
– if instability persists, will require a late fusion.

THORACIC fracture → *stable*
anterior wedge # → normal activity after pain subsides.
unstable
fracture/dislocation → no treatment other than for
(severe force required)   paraplegia.

THORACOLUMBAR fracture → *stable #* { anterior wedge → mobilise.
'burst' → mobilise
(plaster jacket may help pain.)

unstable #
– fracture dislocation *
operative reduction and fixation
(anterior or posterior, e.g. Hartshill rectangle)
without paraplegia → plaster jacket.
(may require late fusion for persistent pain or instability.)

conservative

with ——→ bed rest
paraplegia   (plaster jacket would cause pressure sores).

*Treatment selection is controversial.
Optimal management remains unknown.

401

SPINAL TRAUMA — MANAGEMENT

Management of the paraplegic patient

After spinal cord injury, transfer to a spinal injury centre with medical and nursing staff skilled in the management of the paraplegic patient provides optimal daily care and rehabilitation.
Important features include:

1. *Skin care* — requires meticulous attention. Two-hourly turning should prevent pressure sores. Attempt to avoid contact with bony prominences or creases in the bed sheets. Air or water beds or a sheepskin may help.
2. *Urinary tract*—long-term catheter drainage or intermittent self-catheterisation is required. Infection requires prompt treatment. Eventually, training may permit automatic reflex function (in cord lesions) or micturition by abdominal compression (in root lesions). In some, urodynamic studies may indicate possible benefit from bladder neck resection.
3. *Limbs* — intensive physiotherapy helps prevent flexion contractures (in cord injury) and plays an essential rôle in rehabilitation.

OUTCOME FOLLOWING SPINAL CORD OR ROOT INJURY

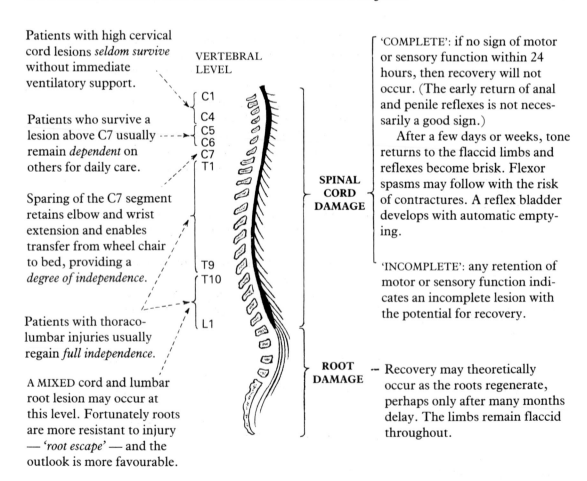

Patients with high cervical cord lesions *seldom survive* without immediate ventilatory support.

Patients who survive a lesion above C7 usually remain *dependent* on others for daily care.

Sparing of the C7 segment retains elbow and wrist extension and enables transfer from wheel chair to bed, providing a *degree of independence.*

Patients with thoraco-lumbar injuries usually regain *full independence.*

A MIXED cord and lumbar root lesion may occur at this level. Fortunately roots are more resistant to injury — *'root escape'* — and the outlook is more favourable.

VERTEBRAL LEVEL

C1
C4
C5
C6
C7
T1

T9
T10

L1

SPINAL CORD DAMAGE

ROOT DAMAGE

'COMPLETE': if no sign of motor or sensory function within 24 hours, then recovery will not occur. (The early return of anal and penile reflexes is not necessarily a good sign.)
After a few days or weeks, tone returns to the flaccid limbs and reflexes become brisk. Flexor spasms may follow with the risk of contractures. A reflex bladder develops with automatic emptying.

'INCOMPLETE': any retention of motor or sensory function indicates an incomplete lesion with the potential for recovery.

Recovery may theoretically occur as the roots regenerate, perhaps only after many months delay. The limbs remain flaccid throughout.

VASCULAR DISEASES OF THE SPINAL CORD

Blood supply to the spinal cord is complex; the main vessels are the anterior and posterior spinal arteries.

The posterior spinal arteries: - — ⌐
usually arise from the posterior inferior cerebellar arteries and form a plexus on the posterior surface of the spinal cord.

The anterior spinal artery: _ _ _
branches from each vertebral artery unite to form a single vessel lying in the median fissure of the spinal cord.

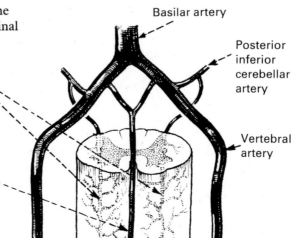

Basilar artery

Posterior inferior cerebellar artery

Vertebral artery

Vertebral artery

Both anterior and posterior spinal arteries run the length of the spinal cord and receive anastomotic vessels.

The plexus of the posterior spinal artery is joined by approximately 12 *unpaired* radicular feeding arteries. This rich collateral circulation protects the posterior part of the spinal cord from vascular disease.

The anterior spinal artery has a much less efficient collateral supply and is thus more vulnerable to the effects of vascular disease. It is joined by 7–10 *unpaired* radicular branches, usually from the left side.

Cervical arteries arise from vertebral and subclavian vessels, form plexuses and supply the cervical and upper thoracic cord.

Intercostal artery branches supply the midthoracic cord.

Anterior spinal artery is at its narrowest at T8. This level of the spinal cord is liable to damage during hypertension — watershed area.

Artery of Adamkiewicz, the largest radicular artery, supplies the low thoracic and lumbar cord. It usually enters at T9–T11 level and is on the left side in 70% of the population.

Sacral artery arises from the hypogastric artery and supplies the sacral cord and cauda equina.

Anterior radicular
branches joining anterior spinal artery

403

VASCULAR DISEASES OF THE SPINAL CORD

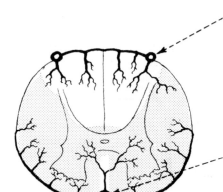

Posterior spinal artery territory
– Posterior one-third of spinal cord.
– Dorsal column.

Virtually no anastomotic communication.

Anterior spinal artery territory
Penetrating branches — anterior and part of posterior grey matter.
Circumferential branches — anterior white matter.
– Anterior two-thirds of spinal cord.

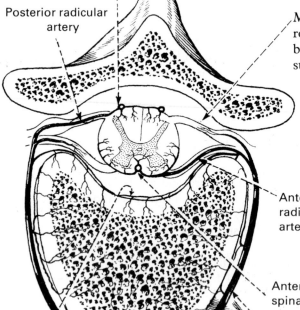

Posterior spinal artery

Posterior radicular artery

Most radicular vessels only supply the root. On average 12 posterior radicular branches and 8 anterior radicular branches supply the spinal cord.

Atherosclerosis of spinal arteries is rare. When infarction occurs in the anterior spinal artery territory it is often a consequence of disease in the vessels of origin of the segmental arteries, i.e. atheroma or dissection of the aorta.

Anterior radicular artery

Anterior spinal artery

Segmental artery

Aorta

Section through spinal cord in thoracic region.

Rich anastomotic network occurs between each segmental artery through the vertebral body and across the extradural space

VASCULAR DISEASES OF THE SPINAL CORD

SPINAL CORD INFARCTION
Anterior spinal artery syndrome

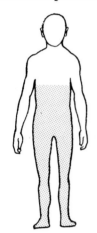

The level at which infarction occurs determines symptoms and signs. Characteristic features include:
– Radicular pain at onset
– Sudden para/quadraplegia
– Flaccid limbs $\xrightarrow{\text{days}}$ spastic
– Areflexia $\xrightarrow{\text{days}}$ hyper-reflexia and extensor plantar responses
– Sensory loss to pain and temperature up to the level of cord damage
– Preserved vibration and joint position sensation (dorsal columns supplied by the posterior spinal arteries)
– Urinary and faecal incontinence

When only penetrating branches are involved, long tract damage may be selective and sensory loss may not occur.

The spinal cord symptoms due to aortic atheroma may slowly be progressive and need not be acute.

Investigation: Exclude other causes of acute paraplegia — cord compression (page 379), transverse myelitis (page 489) and Guillain-Barré syndrome (page 422). A specific explanation for infarction should be sought, e.g.

– *Small blood vessel disease*	– diabetes
	– polyarteritis nodosa
	– systemic lupus erythematosus
	– neurosyphilis
	– endarteritis secondary to local infection (tuberculous meningitis, pneumococcal meningitis)
– *Arterial compression or occlusion*	– *spinal artery* – disc fragments, extradural mass (abscess or tumour)
	– *segmental artery* – posterior spinal mass, abdominal paravertebral mass
	– dissecting aneurysm
	– aortic surgery
– *Embolic occlusion*	– decompression sickness (Caisson's disease)
	– aortic arteriography
– *Hypotension*	– myocardial infarction/cardiac arrest.

Treatment is symptomatic and the outcome variable.

Posterior spinal artery syndrome
This is rare as white matter structures are less vulnerable to ischaemia. The dorsal columns are damaged and ischaemia may extend into the posterior horns.

Clinical features : – Loss of tendon reflexes
– Loss of joint position sense.

Transient ischaemic attack
These rarely affect the spinal cord. Spinal AVM is the commonest cause though mechanism is unclear. TIAs also result from emboli (calcific aortic disease) and vascular 'steal' (aortic coarctation).

405

VASCULAR DISEASES OF THE SPINAL CORD

SPINAL ARTERIOVENOUS MALFORMATION (Angiomatous malformation)

Arterio-venous malformations (AVMs) are congenital abnormalities of blood vessels rather than neoplastic growths. Arteries communicating directly with veins bypass the capillary network which has failed to develop, creating a 'shunt'. The AVM appears as a mass of convoluted dilated vessels.

Site

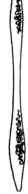

Cervical: uncommon site (~15%)
Arises from the anterior spinal artery and usually lies within the cord substance (intrameduallary).

Upper thoracic: (20%)

Thoracolumbar: this is the commonest site (~65%). It may be extra- or intradural or within both compartments. Intramedullary lesions at this site are less common.

Spinal AVMs may present clinically at any age in either sex, but are most common in males.

Clinical features

SUDDEN ONSET (10–15%)

Due to – subarachnoid haemorrhage: headache, neck stiffness, back and leg pain
    – extradural haematoma
    – subdural haematoma   } signs of acute cord compression.
    – intramedullary haematoma (haematomyelia)

GRADUAL ONSET (85–90%)
Probably due to ↑ *venous pressure* but other factors may play a part:
    – venous thrombosis
    – 'steal' phenomenon
    – venous bulk
    – arachnoiditis (if previous bleed).

Progressive deterioration of all spinal modalities simulating cord compression. Pain is common. With thoracolumbar lesions a mixed u.m.n./l.m.n. weakness in the legs is typical.
    Intramedullary AVMs may cause fluctuating signs and symptoms and may mimic intermittent claudication.

A bruit may be heard overlying a spinal AVM and occasionally midline cutaneous lesions — haemangiomas, naevi or angiolipomas — are found. (Note that cutaneous angiomas are not uncommon and do not necessarily imply an underlying lesion.)

VASCULAR DISEASES OF THE SPINAL CORD

SPINAL ARTERIOVENOUS MALFORMATION (*contd*)

Investigation

Myelography: Contrast material outlines
'serpent-like' vessels on the cord surface.

If the myelogram is positive, *spinal angiography* is required to delineate the extent of the AVM and the exact site of the shunt and feeding vessel.

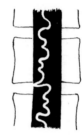

MRI may show flow voids at the appropriate site.

Management

Untreated, 50% of patients with gradual onset of symptoms would be unable to walk within 3 years.

Operation should prevent progression and may well improve a gait or bladder disturbance. Operative delay may result in irreversible cord damage.

Techniques: It is important to identify and divide the feeding vessel and excise the shunt. Total excision of all the dilated veins is probably unnecessary and would increase the operative hazards. A decompressive laminectomy alone is of no benefit. Intramedullary AVMs and/or AVMs lying ventral to the cord cannot be excised and embolisation of the feeding vessel may be tried. The long-term benefits of this procedure are unknown.

Intraspinal haematoma: If the patient presents with signs of a rapid onset of spinal cord compression, and myelogram confirms an extra- or intradural block, then urgent laminectomy and decompression is required (without waiting for angiography). Examination of the haematoma whether extra- or intradural may reveal angiomatous tissue. In some patients there is no evident cause and the bleed is designated as 'spontaneous'.

SPINAL DYSRAPHISM

SPINAL DYSRAPHISM: This term encompasses all defects (open or closed) associated with a failure of closure of the posterior neural arch.

Embryology

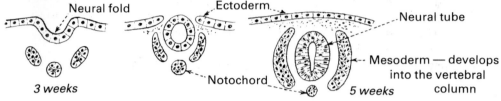

Developmental errors may occur early in fetal life and lead to a variety of spinal defects:

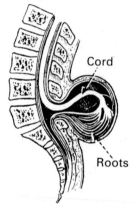
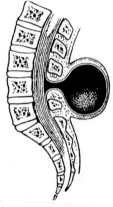
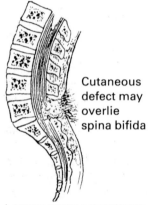

MYELOMENINGOCELE
The spinal cord and roots protrude through the bony defect and lie within a cystic cavity, lined with meninges and/or skin. In most patients, the meningeal covering ruptures and the spinal cord and roots lie exposed to the air — myelodysplasia. CSF may leak from the open lesion.

Site: 80% occur in the lumbosacral region.

MENINGOCELE
Cystic CSF filled cavity — lined with meninges but devoid of neural tissue. The cavity communicates with the spinal canal through the bone defect (usually lumbosacral). Meningoceles occur far less frequently than myelomeningocele; they are rarely associated with other congenital anomalies.

SPINA BIFIDA OCCULTA
A bony deficit — present in 5–10% of the population and not clinically significant. Those who also have a lumbosacral cutaneous abnormality however (*tuft of hair, dimple, sinus or 'port wine' stain*) have a high incidence of related underlying defects:
– *diastomatomyelia*
– *lipoma*
– *dermoid cyst.*
These defects may cause symptoms of pain or neurological impairment after many years.

Incidence: 2/1000 births in Britain, but there is a geographical variation (0.2/1000 in Japan). A familial incidence increases the risk (5% if a sibling is affected). This suggests a genetic factor, but teratogens, e.g. sodium valproate, also have a role.

Associated abnormalities: *Hydrocephalus*
Arnold-Chiari, type II,
aqueduct forking.

SPINAL DYSRAPHISM

Clinical assessment

Myelomeningocele: This lesion should be carefully examined for the presence of neural elements. Transillumination of the sac may help. Observation of movement in the limbs and in specific muscle groups, occurring spontaneously and in response to pain applied both above and below the level of the lesion, helps determine the degree and level of neurological damage. Also note the presence of a dilated bladder and a patulous anal sphincter. Look for any associated congenital anomalies, e.g. hydrocephalus, scoliosis, foot deformities.

Meningocele: Patients with this lesion seldom show any neurological deficit.

Investigations

Not required at the initial stage.

Management

Myelomeningocele: Advances in both orthopaedic and urological procedures have considerably improved the long-term management of the associated disabilities in most patients. Active treatment, however, in patients with gross hydrocephalus, complete paraplegia and other multiple anomalies as well as the spinal dysraphism, may merely prolong a painful existence. In these patients, many adopt a thoughtful conservative approach.

Immediate treatment requires closure and replacement of the neural tissues into the spinal canal to prevent infection. If necessary, this initial step provides more time to consider the wisdom of embarking on further active management.

Meningocele: In the presence of a CSF leak, urgent excision is performed; otherwise this is deferred, perhaps indefinitely if the lesion is small.

Spina bifida occulta: No treatment is required, although in patients with a cutaneous abnormality (and a higher incidence of an intraspinal anomaly), some recommend investigation with a view to prophylactic treatment.

Antenatal diagnosis

Screening the maternal serum and amniotic fluid for alpha-fetoprotein and acetylcholinesterase, fetal ultrasonography and contrast enhanced amniography in high risk patients (e.g. with an affected sibling) provides an effective method of detecting neural tube defects. This gives the parents the possibility of therapeutic abortion and in the long term may reduce the incidence of this condition.

SPINAL DYSRAPHISM

DIASTOMATOMYELIA: a congenital splitting of part of the spinal cord usually at the upper lumbar vertebral level.

A *bony, fibrous* or *cartilagenous spur* often extends directly across the spinal canal in an antero-posterior direction. The split cord does not always reunite distal to the spur (diplomyelia). In most patients, the conus medullaris lies well below its normal level, '*tethered*' by the filum terminale. Since vertebral growth proceeds more rapidly than growth of the spinal cord, tethering may produce progressive back pain or neurological impairment as the spinal cord is stretched.

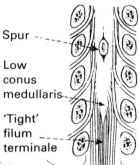

Spur

Low conus medullaris

'Tight' filum terminale

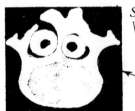

Straight X-ray
  may reveal associated congenital anomalies:
    spina bifida occulta, fused or hemivertebrae.
    tomography may demonstrate a bony spur.
  Myelography combined with CT scan: provides more definitive evidence of diastomatomyelia and clearly demonstrates the presence of a bony spur and the level of the conus medullaris.

Management: Although some recommend prophylactic exploration— despite the absence of neurological impairment, most reserve operative treatment for those who present with a neurological deficit, especially if there is evidence of progression, or prior to the correction of any spinal deformity. At operation, any spur is removed and if tethering exists, the filum terminale and any fibrous bands are divided.

LIPOMENINGOCELE
Lipomas may occur in association with spinal dysraphism and range from purely intraspinal lesions to very large masses extending along with neural tissues through the bony defect. All are adherent to the conus and closely related to the lumbosacral roots, preventing complete removal and increasing operative hazards.

CONGENITAL DERMAL SINUS TRACT/DERMOID CYST
This congenital defect results from a failure of separation of neuronal from epithelial ectoderm and may occur with other midline fusion defects, e.g. diastomatomyelia and a tethered cord. A tiny sinus in the lumbosacral region may represent the opening of a blind ending duct or may extend into the spinal canal. Dermoid cysts arise at any point along the sinus tract and often lie adjacent to the conus.

Clinical presentation varies from repeated attacks of unexplained meningitis to neurological deficits arising from the presence of an intraspinal mass. Treatment involves excision of the whole tract and any associated cyst (after treating any meningitic infection).

LOCALISED NEUROLOGICAL DISEASE AND ITS MANAGEMENT
C. PERIPHERAL NERVE AND MUSCLE

THE POLYNEUROPATHIES – FUNCTIONAL ANATOMY

The function of the peripheral nervous system is to carry impulses to and from the central nervous system. These impulses regulate motor, sensory and autonomic activities.

The peripheral nervous system is comprised of structures which lie outside the pial membrane of the brainstem and spinal cord and can be divided into cranial, spinal and autonomic components.

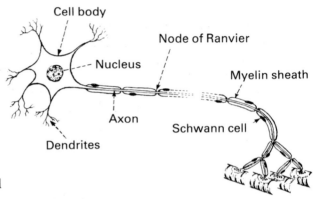

STRUCTURE OF THE NERVE CELL AND AXON

Each axon represents an elongation of the nerve cell — this lying within the central nervous system, e.g. anterior horn cell, or in an outlying ganglion, e.g. dorsal root ganglion. The cell body maintains the viability of the axon, being the centre of all cellular metabolic activity.

Many axons are surrounded by an insulation of myelin, which is enveloped by the Schwann cell membrane. Myelin is a protein-lipid complex. The membrane of the Schwann cell 'spirals' around the axon resulting in the formation of a multilayered myelin sheath.

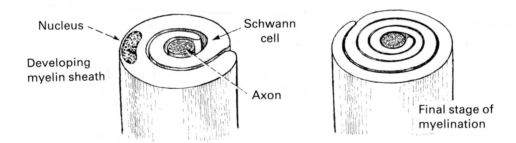

All axons have a cellular sheath — Schwann cell — but not all axons are myelinated.

Schwann cells with associated myelin are 250–1000 μm in length and separated from each other by the node of Ranvier. The axon is bare at this node and, during conduction, impulses jump from one node to the next — *saltatory* conduction. The rate of conduction is markedly increased in comparison with unmyelinated fibres. Myelin thus facilitates fast conduction. In unmyelinated fibres conduction depends upon the diameter of the nerve fibre, this determining the rate of longitudinal current flow.

THE POLYNEUROPATHIES — FUNCTIONAL ANATOMY

SPINAL PERIPHERAL NERVOUS SYSTEM

Entry to and exit from the central
nervous system is achieved by paired
spinal nerve roots (30 in all).

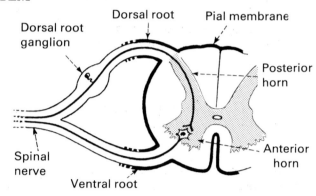

These dorsal and ventral roots lie in the
spinal subarachnoid space and come together at the intervertebral foramen to
form the spinal nerve.

The dorsal root contains sensory fibres,
arising from specialised sensory receptors
in the periphery.

The dorsal root ganglia are collections of sensory cell bodies with axons extending peripherally
as well as a central process which passes into the spinal cord in the region of the posterior horn of
grey matter and makes appropriate central connections.

Sensation can be divided into:
- *Pain and temperature*
- *Simple touch*
- *Discriminatory sensation* – proprioception, vibration.

These different forms of sensation are carried from the periphery by axons with specific
characteristics. The central connections and pathways vary also (see page 196).

The anterior horns of the spinal cord contain cell bodies whose axons pass to the periphery to
innervate skeletal muscle — the alpha motor neurons. Smaller cell bodies also project into the
anterior root and innervate the intrafusal muscle fibres of muscle spindles — the gamma motor
neurons.

Each alpha motor neuron through its peripheral ramifications will innervate a number of muscle
fibres. The number of fibres innervated from a single cell varies from less than 20 in the eye
muscles to more than 1000 in the large limb muscles (innervation ratio). The alpha motor neuron
with its complement of muscle fibres is termed the *motor unit*.

PERIPHERAL NERVES

Peripheral nerves are composed of many axons bound together by connective tissue. A 'mixed' nerve contains
motor, sensory and autonomic axons.

The blood supply to these bundles is by means of small
nutrient vessels within the epineurium — the *vasa nervorum*.

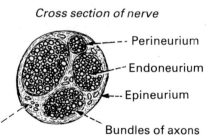

Cross section of nerve

413

THE POLYNEUROPATHIES — FUNCTIONAL ANATOMY

PERIPHERAL NERVES (*contd*)

Nerve fibre type

Axons within the peripheral nerve vary structurally. This is related to function.

Three distinct fibre types can be distinguished:

TYPE A   2–20 μm in diameter.
             Myelinated.
  Function: Motor and sensory (vibration, proprioception).
             Conduction velocity: 10–70 metres/second.

TYPE B   3 μm diameter.
             Thinly myelinated.
  Function: Mainly preganglionic autonomic, some pain and temperature.
             Conduction velocity: 7–5 metres/second.

TYPE C   < 1μm diameter.
             Unmyelinated.
  Function: Sensory — pain and temperature.
             Conduction velocity: <2 metres/second.

   The structure of the spinal peripheral nervous system has been considered but the arrangement is also important. Spinal nerves, after emerging from the intervertebral foramen pass into the brachial plexus to supply the upper limbs and the lumbosacral plexus to supply the lower limbs.

   The thoracic nerves supply skeletal muscles and subserve sensation of the thorax and abdomen.

   The Autonomic Nervous System is described on page 439.

PATTERNS OF INJURY

Damage may occur to: axon, myelin sheath, cell body, supporting connective tissue, nutrient blood supply to nerves.

Three basic pathological processes occur:

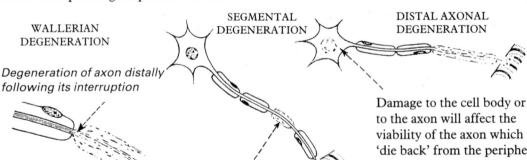

WALLERIAN DEGENERATION

Degeneration of axon distally following its interruption

The axon disintegrates and the myelin breaks up into globules.

   Regeneration of nerve is possible because the basement membrane of the Schwann cell survives and acts as a skeleton along which the axon regrows.

SEGMENTAL DEGENERATION

Scattered destruction of the myelin sheath occurs without axonal damage.

   The primary lesion affects the Schwann cell.

DISTAL AXONAL DEGENERATION

Damage to the cell body or to the axon will affect the viability of the axon which will 'die back' from the periphery. Loss of the myelin sheath occurs as a secondary event.

   Recovery is slow here because the axon must regenerate. When the cell body is destroyed no regrowth will occur.

THE POLYNEUROPATHIES — SYMPTOMS

Sensory

Negative phenomena — loss of sensation.
Disease of large myelinated fibres produces loss of touch and joint position perception.
Patients complain of difficulty in discriminating textures. Their hands and feet feel like cotton
wool. Gait is unsteady, especially when in darkness where vision cannot compensate for loss of
joint position sensation (proprioception).

Disease of small unmyelinated fibres produces loss of pain and temperature appreciation as a
consequence of which painless burns/trauma result. Damage to joints without pain results in a
'neuropathic' joint (Charcot's joint) in which traumatic deformity is totally painless.

Positive phenomena

Disease of large myelinated fibres produces paraesthesia — a 'pins and needles' sensation with a
peripheral distal distribution.

Disease of small unmyelinated fibres produces painful positive phenomena:
– Burning extremities
– Dysaesthesia — when touching is painful
– Hyperalgesia — when threshold to pain appears lowered
– Hyperpathia — when threshold to pain appears elevated but, once reached, the painful
           stimulus is excessively felt.

Lightning pains take the form of sudden, very severe shooting pains and are virtually
pathognomonic for tabes dorsalis.

Causalgia results from nerve trauma. A spontaneous burning sensation in the distribution of the
injured nerve is associated with an increased sensitivity to painful stimulation.

Motor

The patient notices weakness:
– When distal, e.g. difficulty in clearing the kerb when walking
– When proximal, e.g. difficulty in climbing stairs or combing hair
– Cramps may be troublesome
– Twitching of muscles (fasciculation) may be felt.

415

THE POLYNEUROPATHIES — SIGNS

SENSORY EXAMINATION

All modalities are tested
Light touch ⎫
Two point discrimination ⎬ Functions of large
Vibration sensation ⎪ myelinated sensory
Joint position perception ⎭ fibres.
Temperature perception ⎫ Functions of small unmyelinated
Pain perception ⎭ and thinly myelinated sensory fibres.

Initially the area of total sensory loss is defined. The test object, e.g. a pin, should be moved from anaesthetic to normal area; it is more accurate to state when an object is felt rather than when it disappears.

In polyneuropathies, sensory loss is symmetrical and follows a characteristic stocking and glove distribution.

Examination of gait is important; with joint position impairment, sensory ataxia is evident. Romberg's test is positive (see page 187). Neuropathic burns/ulcers or joints may be present.

Trophic changes
— Cold blue extremities.
— Cutaneous hair loss.
— Brittle finger/toe nails occasionally occur.

The AXON REFLEX can be used to 'place' lesions in the sensory pathway.
Normally:
the skin is scratched — local vasoconstriction (white reaction) ⎫ due to local
next — local oedema (red reaction) ⎭ histamine release.
and finally — surrounding vasodilatation or flare, dependent on antidromic impulses from the dorsal root ganglion along an intact sensory neuron.

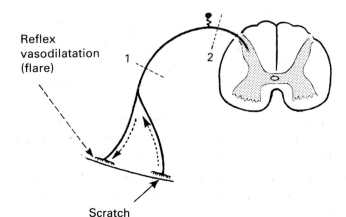

Reflex
vasodilatation
(flare)

1

2

Scratch

1. A distal sensory lesion will result in an absent flare response.

2. A proximal root lesion will not impair the response.

THE POLYNEUROPATHIES — SIGNS

MOTOR EXAMINATION

Muscle wasting is evident in subacute or chronic mixed or motor neuropathies. Oedema of immobile limbs may mask such a change. All muscle groups should be examined. The 1st dorsal interosseous muscle in the upper limbs and extensor digitorum brevis in the lower limbs are muscles which commonly show wasting in the neuropathies. The muscles should be examined for *fasciculations* — irregular twitches of groups of muscle fibres; this may be induced by exercise or muscle percussion and suggests anterior horn cell disease.

Muscle power is tested next. The pattern of weakness — proximal or distal, symmetrical or asymmetrical, flexors or extensors — must be properly analysed in order to locate the site of the cause of weakness (see Muscle weakness, page 189). In the neuropathies, weakness is generally symmetrical and either distal or proximal in distribution.

The degree of weakness is 'scored' using the MRC (Medical Research Council) scale:

Score 0 – No contraction
Score 1 – Flicker
Score 2 – Active movement/gravity eliminated
Score 3 – Active movement against gravity
Score 4 – Active movement against gravity and resistance
Score 5 – Normal power.

Weakness is proportional to the number of motor neurons acutely involved. It may develop suddenly or very slowly and, usually symmetrical, it is noticed at the extremities — usually lower limbs first — and gradually spreads or ascends into more proximal muscles.

The reason for the onset of symptoms distally is supposedly due to the 'dying back' of the axons towards their nerve cells — the longest ones being the most vulnerable.

Some neuropathies may affect proximal muscle groups preferentially — Guillain-Barré and diabetic neuropathy — whereas others (especially axonal neuropathies) affect the longest axons initially and present with distal weakness.

In severe neuropathies, truncal and respiratory muscle involvement occurs. Respiratory muscle weakness may result in death.

Tendon reflexes

The tendon reflex depends on:
– stretch of the muscle spindle (1),
– activation of spindle afferent fibres (2),
– monosynaptic projections to the alpha motoneurons (3)

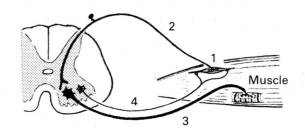

The gamma motoneuron fibres, projecting to the spindle (4) 'modulate' activity in the reflex loop.

Reflexes commonly tested:

Deltoid	— C5, 6 – Circumflex nerve	Triceps	—	C6,7,8 – Radial nerve
Biceps	— C5, 6 – Musculocutaneous nerve	Knee	—	L2,3,4 – Femoral nerve
Brachioradialis	— C5,6 – Radial nerve	Ankle	—	S1,2– Sciatic nerve

The tendon reflexes are lost when any component of the reflex response is affected by disease. Reflexes are lost early in peripheral neuropathies when power and muscle bulk appear normal. Distal reflexes are generally lost before proximal ones.

THE POLYNEUROPATHIES — CLASSIFICATION

There are several approaches to classification:

    by MODE of ONSET — acute, subacute, chronic

    by FUNCTIONAL DISTURBANCE — motor, sensory, autonomic, mixed

    by PATHOLOGICAL PROCESS — axonal, demyelinating

    by CAUSATION — e.g. infections; carcinomatous, diabetic, inflammatory, vascular

    by DISTRIBUTION — e.g. symmetrical, asymmetrical
                             proximal, distal.

Clinically it is of most value to classify the neuropathies according to mode of onset.

The following table is for reference. Certain neuropathies will be dealt with separately (see pages 422–426).

	CAUSE	FUNCTIONAL DISTURBANCE	PATHOLOGY
ACUTE A few days-4 weeks	**Inflammatory** (Postinfectious Guillain-Barré)	Predominantly motor Distal or proximal Autonomic disturbance	Demyelination with perivascular lymphocytic infiltration
	Diphtheria	Cranial nerve onset Mixed motor/sensory	Demyelinative. No inflammatory infiltration
	Porphyria	Motor (may begin in arm). Autonomic disturbance Minimal sensory loss.	Axonal
SUBACUTE Develop over weeks	**Drug-induced** Isoniazid Metronidazole Dapsone Disulfiram Nitrofurantoin Vincristine etc.	Vincristine — severe Usually mild sensory, motor disturbance Dapsone — pure motor involvement	Axonal degeneration
	Environmental toxins Solvents Lead Acrylamide Carbon disulphide Hexocarbons Organophosphates	Occasionally acute Usually sensory, motor disturbance; severity related to dose Lead — severe, predominantly motor with arms involved first	Lead-axonal degeneration with segmental demyelination. Other heavy metals and solvents produce axonal degeneration
	Nutritional Deficiency B complex (includes alcoholic neuropathy)	Sensory disturbance with 'burning feet' and other painful dysaesthesiae Motor component may be present and severe Autonomic disturbance is common but mild	Axonal degeneration with segmental demyelination. (Demyelination is minimal in alcoholic neuropathy)
	Substance abuse Solvents Heroin	Occasionally acute. Sensory, motor disturbance, Peripheral nerve lesion and plexopathies	Axonal degeneration

THE POLYNEUROPATHIES — CLASSIFICATION

CHRONIC

	CAUSE	FUNCTIONAL DISTURBANCE	PATHOLOGY
Develop over months, years	**Malignant disease**———— Carcinoma Lymphoma myeloma	Sensory or sensory/motor disturbance May predate recognition of malignancy by some years	– Axonal degeneration
	Paraproteinaemias———— Hypergamma- globulinaemia	Sensory/motor disturbance	– Axonal or demyelinative degeneration
	Collagenosis ———— (Connective tissue disorders) Rheumatoid arthritis Polyarteritis nodosa Scleroderma Systemic lupus erythematosis	In rheumatoid arthritis multiple mononeuropathy is common Motor/sensory disturbance is rare Systemic lupus erythematosis — mild motor/sensory disturbance Polyarteritis nodosa usually produces multiple mononeuropathy	– Occlusion of nutrient blood vessels to nerves (vasa nervorum)
	Amyloid disease ———— Primary, familial or secondary	Motor/sensory disturbance with autonomic involvement Also may develop 'entrapment' neuropathies	– Thickened nerves with amyloid deposition as well as small fibre axonal degeneration
	Metabolic disorders Diabetes, uraemia Hypothyrodism	– Uraemic neuropathy is sensory/motor in type. Hypothyroidism produces mild sensory/motor disturbance. Diabetic neuropathy takes many forms	– Axonal degeneration
	Inflammatory ————	Sensory, motor disturbance	– Demyelination
	Hereditary neuropathies — e.g. Peroneal muscular atrophy (Charcot-Marie-Tooth disease)	Onset in childhood or adolescence. Mainly motor with some sensory features. Wasting is distal, peroneal muscles first Dominant inheritance	– Demyelinative, axonal or neuronal types (Classification — see later).
	Hypertrophic ———— polyneuropathy (Dejerine-Sottas disease)	Onset in childhood with sensory symptoms followed by progressive distal weakness and wasting Claw hand and foot deformity common Autosomal recessive inheritance	– Recurrent demyelination and remyelination with Schwann cell hypertrophy
	Refsum's disease ————	A phytanic acid storage disorder. Onset in first decade and slowly progressive. A severe sensorimotor neuropathy with associated cerebellar ataxia, ichthyosis, pigmentory retinal degeneration, deafness and cardiac abnormalities. Elevated serum phytanate	– Schwann cell hyperplasia — hypertrophic neuropathy

419

INVESTIGATION OF NEUROPATHY

Despite extensive investigation, the cause of chronic neuropathy cannot be identified in 30% of such cases.

The following conditions require exclusion before a chronic neuropathy is classified as idiopathic or of unknown aetiology: diabetes, uraemia, deficiency states, connective tissue disorders, underlying malignancy, drugs and toxins. Hereditary disease can only be excluded by examining relatives.

The cause of acute or subacute neuropathy can usually be defined. Here, CSF examination may prove a useful diagnostic investigation, e.g. postinfectious polyneuropathy.

SPECIAL INVESTIGATIONS

1. Nerve conduction studies

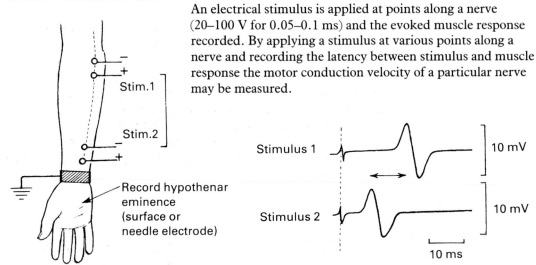

An electrical stimulus is applied at points along a nerve (20–100 V for 0.05–0.1 ms) and the evoked muscle response recorded. By applying a stimulus at various points along a nerve and recording the latency between stimulus and muscle response the motor conduction velocity of a particular nerve may be measured.

$$\text{Conduction velocity} = \frac{\text{Distance between two stimuli}}{\text{Difference in conduction time between the two sites}}$$

Motor conduction velocity can be measured in most motor peripheral nerves from the brachial plexus in the upper limbs and sciatic and femoral outlets in the lower limbs.

These studies not only aid in the diagnosis of generalised neuropathies but also in entrapments, e.g. ulnar nerve at elbow or median nerve at wrist (carpal tunnel syndrome).

INVESTIGATION OF NEUROPATHY

Sensory conduction can also be measured:

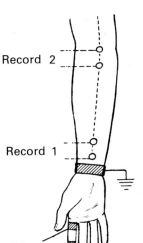

Record 2

Record 1

Stim.

The index finger is stimulated and the evoked sensory potential recorded at wrist and elbow. Measurements enable calculation to be made of the latencies and conduction velocity. Note the considerable difference in amplitude between sensory and motor evoked potentials.

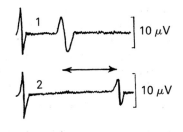

$$\text{Conduction velocity} = \frac{\text{Distance between two recording sites}}{\text{Difference in latency between the two evoked responses.}}$$

GENERAL OBSERVATIONS

Amplitude of response — a function of the number of axons which respond to stimulation.

Latency of response — a function of the speed at which the largest fibres in a nerve will conduct.

Axonal degeneration → *reduced amplitude or absence of response* to stimulation with mild slowing of conduction velocity.

Demyelinative disorders → marked *slowing of conduction velocity (30% at least reduced) with progressive reduction of amplitude.*

Localised compression of nerve → slowing of conduction in region of block, e.g. over the elbow when ulnar nerve is compressed at that site.

2. Electromyography

A fine needle is inserted into the muscle and the recorded activity displayed on an oscilloscope.

Electromyography is primarily of value in muscle disease but can also give indirect evidence of a neuropathic process. The presence of denervation in paraspinal muscles indicates proximal nerve root disease.

If chronic denervation has occurred, reinnervation may be present with long duration high amplitude motor unit potentials.

Also, with voluntary efforts, poor recruitment of motor units is seen on the oscilloscope screen.

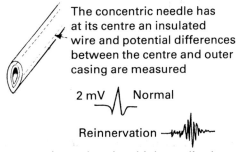

The concentric needle has at its centre an insulated wire and potential differences between the centre and outer casing are measured

2 mV Normal

Reinnervation

Long duration, high amplitude, polyphasia

3. Nerve biopsy

In neuropathies of uncertain cause, light and electron microscopy examination occasionally help diagnosis. The sural nerve is usually chosen for biopsy, provided its sensory conduction is abnormal.

421

THE POLYNEUROPATHIES — SPECIFIC TYPES

ACUTE INFLAMMATORY POSTINFECTIOUS POLYNEUROPATHY (syn. GUILLAIN-BARRÉ Syndrome)

Clinical features

Incidence: 2 per 100 000 population per year. Characteristically it occurs 1–3 weeks after a viral or other infection or immunisation.

Sensory symptoms predominate at the beginning with paraesthesia of the feet, then hands. Pain, especially back pain, is an occasional initial symptom. Weakness next develops — this may be generalised, proximal in distribution or commence distally and ascend. In severe cases, repiratory and bulbar involvement occurs. Weakness is maximal three weeks after the onset of neurological symptoms. Tracheostomy/ventilation is required in 20% of cases. Facial weakness is present to some extent in 50% of cases. Papilloedema may occur when CSF protein is markedly elevated (blocked arachnoid villi?). Autonomic involvement — tachycardia, fluctuating blood pressure, retention of urine — develops in some cases.

Sensory signs occur infrequently.

Aetiology/pathology

The condition may follow viral infection, especially cytomegalovirus. It is also associated with *Mycoplasma, Salmonella, Campylobacter* infections, immunisations with both live and dead vaccines, antitoxins, trauma, surgery and, rarely, malignant disease.

The finding of decreased suppressor T cell response suggests a cell mediated immunological reaction directed at peripheral nerves. Serum antibodies to myelin components are occasionally detected.

Segmental demyelination results with axonal damage if the process is severe. Perivascular infiltration with lymphocytes occurs within nerve roots. Lymphocytes probably release cytotoxic substances which damage Schwann cell/myelin. Macrophage infiltration then occurs with removal of myelin.

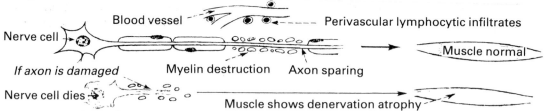

When axon damage and nerve cell death occur, regeneration cannot take place.

Investigations

CSF protein is elevated in most patients but often not until the second or third week of illness. The γ– globulin fraction is usually raised. Cells are often absent but in 20% up to 40 cells/mm^3 may be found.

Nerve conduction studies

When carried out early in the illness, these may be normal; this reflects the tendency initially for nerve root involvement with lesser distal damage. Later conduction velocities become prolonged.

Virological investigation

Viral studies occasionally reveal rising titres to specific viruses such as Epstein Barr, cytomegalovirus, mumps, rubella and enteroviruses.

THE POLYNEUROPATHIES — SPECIFIC TYPES

ACUTE INFLAMMATORY POSTINFECTIOUS POLYNEUROPATHY *(contd)*
Treatment
Treatment is mainly supportive, with management of the paralysed patient and occasionally management of respiratory failure by ventilation.

The effectiveness of specific immunosuppressive therapy — steroids and cytotoxic drugs — is disappointing; indeed, steroids have been found ineffective in a controlled trial. Reports of success with plasmapheresis have led to multi-centre prospective studies. The results are encouraging, showing significant improvement in the course of the illness. This treatment should be reserved for patients with deteriorating respiratory function.

Outcome
Mortality is 10%.
Of those in respiratory failure, 20% are left severely disabled and 10% moderately disabled.
In milder cases the outcome is excellent.
Physical signs, e.g. areflexia, may persist despite return to normal function.
Of all patients, 5% develop a chronic relapsing course.

Variant of Guillain-Barré
The Miller Fisher variant consists of ophthalmoplegia, areflexia and ataxia. Whether these features result from coexisting central nervous system involvement or wholly from peripheral disease remains controversial.

CHRONIC RELAPSING AND CHRONIC INFLAMMATORY POLYNEUROPATHY
These neuropathies represent chronic forms of the Guillain-Barré syndrome.

Segmental demyelination with lymphocytic infiltration occurs. Eventually the nerves show hypertrophy with concentric Schwann cell proliferation reminiscent of an 'onion bulb'.

This condition is sometimes remarkably steroid-responsive, with relapse often on reduction of dosage. In some patients, immunosuppressive drugs are necessary, in others plasmapheresis may be effective.

THE POLYNEUROPATHIES — SPECIFIC TYPES

DIABETIC NEUROPATHY

This condition is uncommon in childhood and increases with age.

Peripheral nerve damage is related to poor control of diabetes. This damage results from either metabolic disturbance with sorbitol accumulation in axons and Schwann cells or an occlusion of the nutrient vessels supplying nerves (vasa vasorum). The frequent occurrence of neuropathy with other vascular complications — retinopathy and nephropathy – suggests that the latter is the more usual mechanism.

Classification

Asymmetrical neuropathy

Polyneuropathy

Present in 5% of all diabetics. Distal weakness and sensory loss is usual. Two forms of sensory neuropathy occur — large fibre, causing ataxia and small fibre causing a painful anaesthesia.

Diabetic amyotrophy — Much less common than polyneuropathy. Pain and weakness rapidly develop. The anterior thigh is preferentially affected with wasting of the quadriceps, loss of the knee jerk and minimal sensory loss. The condition is due to anterior spinal root or plexus disease. Functional recovery is good.

Autonomic neuropathy

In most patients with peripheral neuropathy, some degree of autonomic disturbance is present. Occasionally this predominates:
- pupil abnormalities
- loss of sweating
- orthostatic hypotension
- gastroparesis and diarrhoea
- hypotonic dilated bladder
- impotence.

Cranial nerve palsy

An oculomotor palsy, usually without pain, may occur with pupillary sparing, which helps to differentiate from an aneurysmal cause. The 6th and 7th cranial nerves may also be involved in diabetes.

Treatment

Improved control of diabetes is essential.

Carbamazepine, antidepressants or α-adrenergic blockers, e.g. phenoxybenzene help control pain.

Drugs which reduce aldose reductase and halt accumulation of sorbitol are being evaluated.

Asymmetrical neuropathies usually spontaneously recover, whereas prognosis for symmetric neuropathies is less certain.

THE POLYNEUROPATHIES — SPECIFIC TYPES

CARCINOMATOUS POLYNEUROPATHY

Sensory or mixed 'sensorimotor' neuropathy is often associated with malignant disease, particularly small cell carcinoma of the bronchus. Of patients with bronchial carcinoma, 2–5% have symptomatic peripheral nerve involvement.

Pathology

The sensory type is characterised by degeneration and inflammatory changes in the dorsal root ganglion. The ventral roots and peripheral nerve motor fibres are spared. In the sensorimotor type, degeneration of the dorsal root ganglion is less marked and axonal and demyelinative changes affect motor and sensory fibres equally.

Clinical features

Symptoms and signs may predate the appearance of causal malignant disease by months or even years.

Sensory neuropathy: Progressive sensory loss is associated with paraesthesia, unpleasant 'burning' dysaesthesia and sensory ataxia.

Sensorimotor neuropathy: The onset is gradual with distal sensory loss and mild motor weakness. Occasionally a more acute, severe neuropathy resembling Guillain-Barré syndrome occurs.

Although there are anecdotal reports of improvement in symptoms after detecting and removing the underlying neoplasm, conclusive evidence is lacking.

PORPHYRIA

Acute intermittent porphyria is an autosomal dominant disorder in which symptoms of abdnominal pain, psychosis, convulsions and peripheral neuropathy occur.

The metabolic fault occurs in the liver. An increased production of porphobilinogen is reflected by its increased urinary excretion. δ-amino laevulic acid, a porphyrin precursor, is also increased.

Clinical features

The onset is acute and predominantly motor with upper limb and occasional cranial nerve involvement. Respiratory failure occurs in severe cases. Autonomic involvement with tachycardia, blood pressure changes, abdominal pain and vomiting often develop. The neuropathy must be distinguished from Guillain-Barré.

Clinical course is variable. Spontaneous recovery occurs over several weeks. Respiratory failure will require ventilation and carries a poor prognosis. During an attack, a high carbohydrate diet and prevention and treatment of electrolyte disturbances are essential. Recurrent attacks may be anticipated. Certain drugs may precipitate these attacks and must be avoided, e.g. sulphonamides, barbiturates, phenytoin, griseofulvin.

THE POLYNEUROPATHIES — SPECIFIC TYPES

HEREDITARY MOTOR AND SENSORY NEUROPATHY (HMSN)

PERONEAL MUSCULAR ATROPHY: CHARCOT-MARIE-TOOTH DISEASE

Characterised by distal wasting of lower limbs which usually stops at low thigh level, spreading to upper limbs. The legs resemble an inverted wine bottle. Pes cavus deformity of the foot develops. When the hands become involved, claw-like deformity is seen. Sensory signs are usually mild.

> Age of onset varies from childhood to middle age.
> Inheritance is usually autosomal dominant.
> Progression is slow with periods of stability.

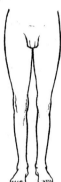

Pathology

Various forms of this disorder are recognised:

– *Hypertrophic type* – Segmental demyelination and hypertrophy with 'onion bulb' formation (HMSN type I).

– *Neuronal type* – Anterior horn cell/motor axon damage. No segmental demyelination (HMSN type II)

– *Spinal muscular atrophy type* – Anterior horn cell/motor axon damage. Usually autosomal dominant but occasionally recessive.

Clinically, these types differ and separation is aided by nerve conduction studies which reveal velocities in the arms lower than 38 m/s in the hypertrophic type.

Treatment

Correction of foot deformities may be helpful.

PROGRESSIVE HYPERTROPHIC NEUROPATHY: DEJERINE-SOTTAS DISEASE (HMSN TYPE III)

Commences in early childhood and progresses slowly. Sensory symptoms are more prominent, otherwise the picture resembles peroneal muscular atrophy.

> Inheritance is autosomal recessive. Kyphosis is often found.
> The nerves can be seen or palpated with ease, e.g. sural nerve or ulnar nerve.
> Enlarged spinal roots may even result in spinal compression.
> Nerve conduction velocity may be greatly reduced (5–10 m/s).

Pathology

Enlargement seems due to connective tissue as well as Schwann cell whorling — 'onion bulb' formation.

ROUSSY-LEVY SYNDROME

The features of distal limb wasting/weakness are associated with sensory ataxia, tremor and pes cavus.

The condition is separated from Friedreich's ataxia by the slow progression, lack of cerebellar signs and slow conduction velocities.

REFSUM's DISEASE

A rare autosomal recessive disorder in which neuropathy is associated with ataxia, retinal degeneration, deafness, cardiomyopathy and dry skin (ichthyosis). The disorder is due to an inability to metabolise phytanic acid — a long-chain fatty acid which accumulates in blood and tissues. It can be treated by a low phytol (precursor) diet.

HEREDITARY SENSORY NEUROPATHY

A rare autosomal dominant or recessive disorder present at birth and progressive, characterised by sensory loss, joint disruption and trophic skin lesions with resultant mutilation.

PLEXUS SYNDROMES AND MONONEUROPATHIES

Disease of a single peripheral or cranial nerve is termed *mononeuropathy*. When many single nerves are damaged one by one, this is described as *mononeuritis multiplex*. Damage to the brachial or lumbosacral plexus may produce widespread limb weakness which does not conform to the distribution of any one peripheral nerve. A knowledge of the anatomy and muscle innervation of the plexuses and peripheral nerves is essential to localise the site of the lesion and thus deduce the possible causes.

Certain systemic illnesses are associated with the development of mononeuropathy or mononeuritis multiplex:

– diabetes mellitus
– sarcoidosis
– rheumatoid arthritis
– polyarteritis nodosa.

Entrapment mononeuropathies result from damage to a nerve where it passes through a tight space such as the median nerve under the flexor retinaculum of the wrist. These are often related to conditions such as acromegaly, myxoedema and pregnancy, in which soft tissue swelling occurs. A familial tendency to entrapment neuropathy occasionally exists.

Cranial nerve mononeuropathies have been dealt with separately.

BRACHIAL PLEXUS

The plexus lies in the posterior triangle of the neck between the muscles scalenius anterior and scalenius medius.

At the root of the neck the plexus lies behind the clavicle.

The plexus itself gives off several important motor branches:
1. Nerve to rhomboids
2. Long thoracic nerve
   – to serratus ant.
3. Pectoral nerves
   – to pectoralis major
4. Suprascapular nerve
   – to supraspinatus
     and infraspinatus

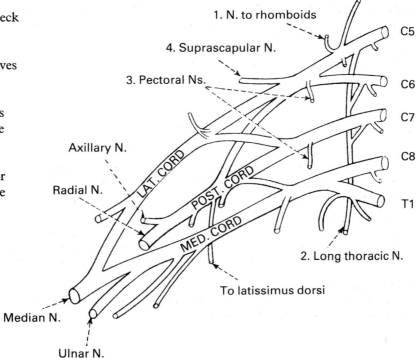

1. N. to rhomboids
4. Suprascapular N.
3. Pectoral Ns.
Axillary N.
Radial N.
LAT. CORD
POST. CORD
MED. CORD
C5
C6
C7
C8
T1
2. Long thoracic N.
To latissimus dorsi
Median N.
Ulnar N.

BRACHIAL PLEXUS SYNDROMES

UPPER PLEXUS LESION (C_5C_6)

Traction on the arm at birth (Erb–Duchenne paralysis) or falling on the shoulder may damage the upper part (C_5C_6) of the plexus.

Deltoid
Supraspinatus ⎱ paralysed.
Infraspinatus ⎰

Biceps ⎱ elbow flexors — also paralysed.
Brachialis ⎰

Adductors of shoulder — mildly affected.

When damage to C_5C_6 is more proximal, nerve to rhomboid and long thoracic nerve may be affected.

POSTERIOR CORD LESION ($C_5C_6C_7C_8$)

Deltoid
Extensors of elbow (triceps)
Extensors of wrist (extensor carpi radialis longus
   and brevis, extensor carpi ulnaris) ⎬ paralysed
Extensors of fingers (extensor digitorum)

LOWER PLEXUS LESION (C_8T_1)

Forced abduction of the arm at birth (Klumpke's paralysis) or trauma may produce damage to the lower plexus. This results in paralysis of the intrinsic hand muscles producing a claw hand, C_8T_1 sensory loss and a Horner's syndrome (page 141) if the T_1 root is involved.

N.B. A combined ulnar and median nerve lesion will produce a similar picture in the hand but with involvement also of flexor carpi ulnaris and pronator teres.

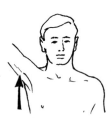

TOTAL BRACHIAL LESION

This results in complete flaccid paralysis and anaesthesia of the arm.
The presence of a Horner's syndrome indicates proximal T_1 nerve root involvement.

N.B. When trauma is the cause of brachial paralysis, early referral to a specialist unit with experience in the surgical repair of plexus injuries is advised.

BRACHIAL PLEXUS SYNDROMES

THORACIC OUTLET SYNDROME

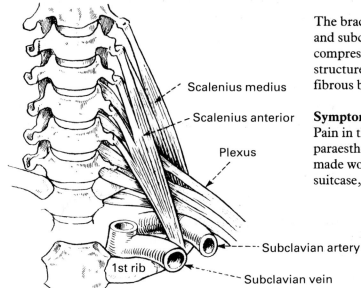

Scalenius medius

Scalenius anterior

Plexus

Subclavian artery

1st rib

Subclavian vein

The brachial plexus, subclavian artery and subclavian vein may be compressed in the neck by contiguous structures such as a cervical rib or tight fibrous band.

Symptoms
Pain in the neck and shoulder with paraesthesia in the forearm, made worse by carrying a suitcase, shopping bag, etc.

Signs
Sensory loss in a T_1 distribution.
Wasting and weakness of thenar and occasionally interosseous muscles.
Signs of vascular compression:
  – Unilateral Raynaud's phenomenon.
  – Pallor of limb on elevation.
  – Brittle trophic finger nails.
  – Loss of radial pulse in arm on abduction and external rotation at the shoulder or
    on bracing the shoulders — ADSON's sign.
  – Subclavian venous thrombosis may occur, especially after excessive usage of arm.

Investigation
Plain radiology of the thoracic outlet may reveal a cervical rib or prolonged transverse process.
Nerve conduction/electromyography will distinguish this from other peripheral nerve lesions.
Arteriography or venography is occasionally necessary if there are obvious vascular problems.

Treatment
In middle-aged people with poor posture and no evidence of abnormality on plain radiology, neck and postural exercises are helpful.
   In younger patients with clinical and electrophysiological changes supporting the radiological abnormalities, exploration and removal of a fibrous band or rib may afford relief.

BRACHIAL PLEXUS SYNDROMES

BRACHIAL NEURITIS (Neuralgic amyotrophy)
Brachial neuritis is a relatively common disorder sometimes associated with:
- Viral infection (infectious mononucleosis, cytomegalovirus).
- Vaccination (tetanus toxoid, influenza)
- Strenuous exercise.
- Intravenous heroin abuse (mainlining).
    In most cases it develops without any evident precipitating cause.

Clinical features
- Acute onset with preceding shoulder pain.
- Weakness is usually proximal, though the whole arm may be affected.
- Occasionally both arms are affected simultaneously.
- Sensory findings are minor (loss over the outer aspect of the shoulder) and occur in 50%.
- Reflex loss occurs.
- Wasting is apparent after 3–6 weeks.
- Recovery may be gradual over weeks or months and is not always complete.
- Recurrent episodes can occur, especially in the presence of a family history.

Differential diagnosis
A painful weak arm.
Consider:
- Cervical spondylosis.
- Cervical disc lesion.
- Brachialgia due to local bursitis.
- Polymyalgia rheumatica.

Investigation
Viral titres may be positive, e.g. Coxsackie.

CSF may show a mild protein rise and a pleocytosis.

Nerve conduction studies will show slowing in affected nerves after 7–10 days.

Familial brachial neuritis is associated with abnormalities of peripheral nerves (thickened myelin sheath) and evidence on nerve conduction studies of a diffuse neuropathy.

PANCOAST's TUMOUR
Involvement of the plexus by an apical lung tumour (usually squamous cell carcinoma). The lower cervical and upper thoracic roots are involved.

Clinical features
- Severe pain.
- Weak wasted hand muscles.
- Sensory loss (C_8T_1).
- Horner's syndrome.

BRACHIAL NEUROPATHY FOLLOWING RADIOTHERAPY
Irradiation of the axilla for breast carcinoma may damage the lower brachial plexus.
    Onset may be delayed from 5–30 months.
    Entrapment of the plexus by resultant fibrosis seems the probable cause.
    Distinguish from direct metastatic spread, in which plexus involvement is more widespread, pain more severe and Horner's syndrome often present.

UPPER LIMB MONONEUROPATHIES

LONG THORACIC NERVE ($C_5C_6C_7$)
Supplies: Serratus anterior muscle

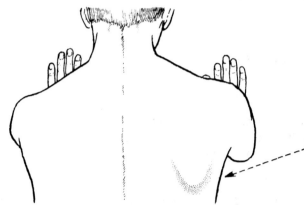

Damaged by:
– Carrying heavy objects
– Strapping the shoulder
– Limited brachial neuritis
– Diabetes mellitus

Results in:
Winging of the scapula
when arms are
stretched in front

SUPRASCAPULAR NERVE (C_5C_6)
Supplies: Supraspinatus and
infraspinatus muscles.

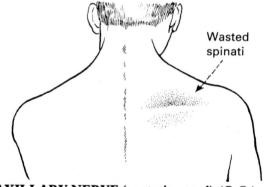

Wasted
spinati

Damaged by:
– [as for Long thoracic nerve (above)]

Results in:
– Weakness of abduction of arm
  (supraspinatus)
– Weakness of external rotation of arm
  (infraspinatus).

AXILLARY NERVE (posterior cord) (C_5C_6)
Supplies: Deltoid and teres minor muscles.

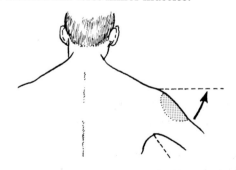

Damaged by:
– Shoulder dislocation.
– Limited brachial neuritis.

Results in:
– Weakness of abduction of shoulder
  between 15–90° and sensory loss
  over the outer aspect of the shoulder.

431

UPPER LIMB MONONEUROPATHIES

MUSCULOCUTANEOUS NERVE (Lateral cord) (5_5C_6)

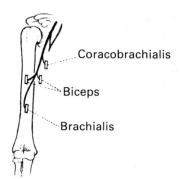

Sensory supply: Lateral border of the arm.

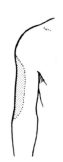

Coracobrachialis

Biceps

Brachialis

Damaged by:
– Fracture of the humerus.
– Systemic causes.

Reuslts in:
– Weakness of elbow flexion and
  forearm supination with characteristic
  sensory loss and absent biceps reflex.

RADIAL NERVE (Posterior cord) ($C_6C_7C_8$)

Sensory supply: Dorsum of hand.
The nerve descends from the axilla,
winding posteriorly around the humerus.
The deep branch — the posterior interosseous nerve — lies in the posterior
compartment of the forearm behind the
interosseous membrane.

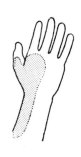

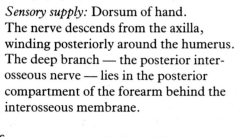

Triceps

Brachioradialis
Extensor carpi radialis longus
Extensor carpi radialis brevis
Supinator
Anconeus
Extensor digitorum
Extensor digiti minimi
Extensor carpi ulnaris

Radius
Ulna

Abductor pollicis longus
Extensor pollicis longus
Extensor pollicis brevis
Extensor indicis

Damaged by:
– Fractures of the humerus.
– Prolonged pressure (Saturday night palsy).
– Intramuscular injection.
– Lipoma, fibroma or neuroma.
– Systemic causes.

Results in:
– Weakness and wasting of muscles
  supplied, characterised by wrist drop
  with flexed fingers (weak extensors).
  Sensory loss on dorsum of hand and
  forearm. Loss of triceps reflex (when
  lesion lies in the axilla) and supinator
  reflex.

The *posterior interosseous branch* of the radial nerve can be compressed at
its point of entry into the supinator muscle. The clinical picture is similar
to a radial nerve palsy, only brachioradialis and wrist extensors are spared.
Examination shows weakness of finger extension with little or no wrist
drop.

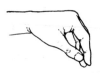

UPPER LIMB MONONEUROPATHIES

MEDIAN NERVE (Lateral and medial cords) (C_7C_8)

Sensory supply:
Palmar surfaces of the radial border of the hand.

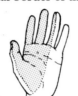

The nerve lies close to the brachial artery in the upper arm. It passes under the transverse carpal ligament as it approaches the palm of the hand.

Pronator teres
Flexor carpi radialis
Palmaris longus
Flexor digitorum sublimis
Flexor digitorum profundus
Flexor pollicis longus
Anterior interosseous nerve

Abductor pollicis brevis
Flexor pollicis brevis
Opponens pollicis

First lumbrical
Second lumbrical

Damaged by:
– Injury in axilla,
 e.g. dislocation of shoulder, compression in the forearm — anterior interosseous branch, compression at the wrist (carpal tunnel syndrome).

Results in:
– Weakness of abduction and apposition of thumb.
– Weakness of pronation of the forearm.
– Deviation of wrist to ulnar side on wrist flexion.
– Weakness of flexion of distal phalanx of thumb and index finger.
– Wasting of thenar muscles is evident.
– Sensory loss is variable but most marked on index and middle fingers

Carpal tunnel syndrome

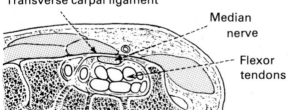

Transverse carpal ligament
Median nerve
Flexor tendons

This common disorder, more frequent in women, results from median nerve entrapment under the transverse carpal ligament at the wrist.
Causes: Connective tissue thickening, e.g.
 – Rheumatoid arthritis
 – Acromegaly
 – Hypothyroidism.
Infiltration of ligament, e.g. Amyloid disease.
Fluid retention, e.g. in pregnancy.
Weight gain.

Symptoms:
Pain, especially at night, and paraesthesia, eased by shaking the hand or dangling it out of the bed.

Objective findings may follow with cutaneous sensory loss and wasting and weakness of thenar muscles (abductor and opponens pollicis).

Nerve conduction studies are helpful in confirming diagnosis by showing slowing of conduction over the wrist.

Treatment: of the cause, weight loss and diuretics. Surgical division of the transverse ligament if symptoms fail to improve.

433

UPPER LIMB MONONEUROPATHIES

ULNAR NERVE (Medial cord) (C_7C_8)

Sensory supply:
Both palmar and dorsal surfaces of the ulnar border of the hand.

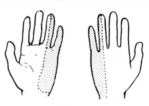

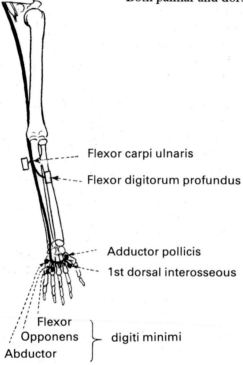

Flexor carpi ulnaris

Flexor digitorum profundus

Adductor pollicis

1st dorsal interosseous

Flexor
Opponens } digiti minimi
Abductor }

In the upper arm the nerve is closely related to the brachial artery and the median nerve, and passes behind the medial epicondyle of the humerus into the forearm.

In the hand, close to the hamate bone, it divides into deep and superficial branches.

Damaged by:
– Injury at elbow either 'acute', e.g. dislocation, or 'delayed'.
– Distal to the medial epicondyle, the ulnar nerve may be damaged by compression.
– Pressure on the nerve in the palm of the hand damages the deep branch resulting in wasting and weakness without sensory loss.

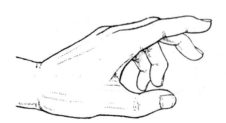

Results in:
– Weakness and wasting of muscles supplied, with a characteristic posture of the hand — *ulnar claw hand* — as well as sensory loss. The level of the lesion dictates the extent of the motor paralysis. Nerve conduction studies are helpful in confirming entrapment at the elbow.

Surgical transposition may be necessary in such cases.

LUMBOSACRAL PLEXUS

LUMBAR PLEXUS

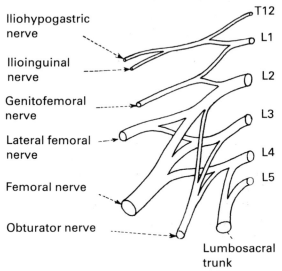

Iliohypogastric nerve

Ilioinguinal nerve

Genitofemoral nerve

Lateral femoral nerve

Femoral nerve

Obturator nerve

T12
L1
L2
L3
L4
L5

Lumbosacral trunk

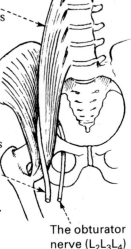

The plexus is located in the psoas muscle. The important branches are the femoral and obturator nerves.

The femoral nerve $(L_2L_3L_4)$ emerges from the lateral border of the psoas muscle and leaves the abdomen laterally below the inguinal ligament with the femoral artery.

The obturator nerve $(L_2L_3L_4)$

SACRAL PLEXUS

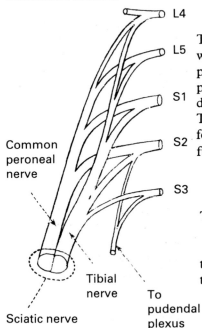

L4
L5
S1
S2
S3

Common peroneal nerve

Tibial nerve

Sciatic nerve

To pudendal plexus

Greater sciatic foramen

Sciatic nerve $L_4L_5S_1S_2S_3$

The plexus is located on the posterior wall of the pelvis. The five roots of the plexus divide into anterior and posterior divisions. The $L_4L_5S_1S_2$ divisions form the common peroneal nerve. The $L_4L_5S_1S_2S_3$ anterior divisions form the tibial nerve. Both these nerves fuse to form the sciatic nerve.

The posterior divisions S_2S_3 pass to the pudendal plexus.

The common peroneal and tibial nerves (sciatic nerve) leave the pelvis by the greater sciatic foramen. In the popliteal fossa the sciatic nerve splits into its constituent nerves.

LUMBOSACRAL PLEXUS SYNDROMES

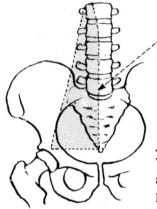

The proximity of the plexus to important abdominal and pelvic structures renders it liable to damage from diseases of these structures.

Trauma following abdominal or pelvic surgery, e.g. hysterectomy, lumbar sympathectomy. Compression from an abdominal mass, e.g. aortic aneurysm. Infiltration from tumour, e.g. cervical carcinoma.

Symptoms may be unilateral or bilateral, depending upon causation. Weakness, sensory loss and reflex changes are dictated by the location and extent of plexus damage. Pain of a severe burning quality may be present; it may be worsened by coughing, sneezing, etc.

In general:

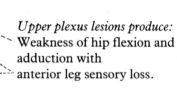

Lower plexus lesions produce: Weakness of posterior thigh (hamstring) and foot muscles with posterior leg sensory loss.

Upper plexus lesions produce: Weakness of hip flexion and adduction with anterior leg sensory loss.

The lumbosacral plexus may be affected in the same way as the brachial plexus in brachial neuritis — lumbosacral neuritis — the association with infection, etc., being similar. Recovery is usually good. Recurrent episodes may occur. Plexus lesions also occur in *diabetes mellitus* and *polyarteritis nodosa.* In both, the symptoms and signs may be bilateral.

LOWER LIMB MONONEUROPATHIES

FEMORAL NERVE (L$_1$L$_2$L$_3$)

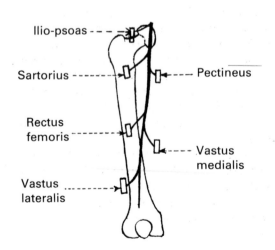

Ilio-psoas

Sartorius

Pectineus

Rectus femoris

Vastus medialis

Vastus lateralis

Damaged by:
– Fractures of the upper femur
– Congenital dislocation of the hip
– Neoplastic infiltration
– Psoas muscle abscess
– Haematoma in the iliacus muscle (haemophilia, anticoagulants)
– Systemic → causes of mononeuropathy, e.g. diabetes.

Results in:
– Weakness of hip flexion
– Weakness of knee extension with wasting of thigh muscles
– Sensory loss over the anterior and medial aspects of the thigh
– The knee jerk is lost.

LOWER LIMB MONONEUROPATHIES

OBTURATOR NERVE (L₂L₃L₄)

Damaged by: – Same process as the femoral nerve.
– During labour and occasionally as a consequence
   of compression by hernia in the obturator canal.
Results in: – Weakness of hip external rotation and adduction.
– The patient may complain of inability to cross the
   affected leg on the other.
– Sensory loss is confined to the innermost aspect
   of the thigh.
– The adductor reflex is absent (adductor response
   to striking the medial epicondyle).

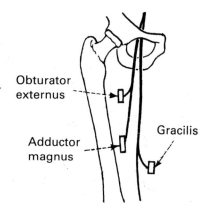

SCIATIC NERVE (L₄L₅S₁S₂)

The nerve descends between the ischial
tuberosity and the greater trochanter of the femur.
   In the thigh it innervates the hamstring muscles
(semitendinosus, semimembranosus and biceps).
Damaged by: Congenital or traumatic hip dislocation.
— Penetrating injuries.
— Accidental damage from 'misplaced'
      intramuscular injection.
— Systemic → causes of mononeuropathy
Results in: — Weakness of hamstring muscles with loss of knee flexion.
— Distal foot and leg muscles are also affected.
— Sensory loss involves the outer aspect of the leg.
— The ankle reflex is absent.

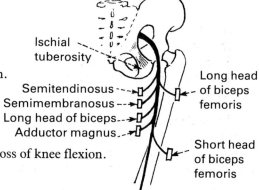

COMMON PERONEAL NERVE (L₄L₅)

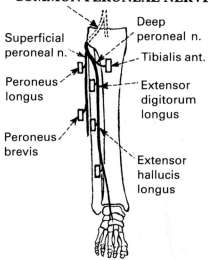

The nerve arises from the division of the sciatic nerve in
the popliteal fossa. It bears a close relationship with the
head of the fibula as it winds anteriorly. It divides into
superficial and deep branches as well as giving off a purely
sensory branch which, with sensory twigs from the tibial
nerve, forms the *sural nerve*, mediating sensation from the
dorsum and lateral aspect of the foot.
Damaged by: — Trauma to the head of the fibula; pressure
here from kneeling, crossing legs.
— Systemic → causes of mononeuropathy, e.g. diabetes.
Results in: Weakness of dorsiflexion and eversion of the foot.
The patient walks with a 'foot drop'. Sensory loss involves
the dorsum and outer aspect of the foot. Partial common
peroneal nerve palsies are common with very selective
muscle weakness.

437

LOWER LIMB MONONEUROPATHIES

POSTERIOR TIBIAL NERVE (S_1S_2)

This nerve also arises from the division of the sciatic nerve in the popliteal fossa and descends behind the tibia, terminating in the medial and lateral plantar nerves which innervate the small muscles of the foot.

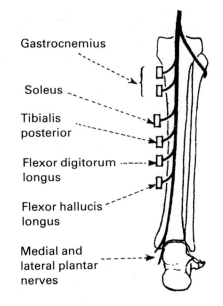

The sensory branch forms the *sural nerve*.

Damaged by:
– Trauma in the popliteal fossa.
– Fracture of the tibia.
– Systemic causes of mononeuropathy.

Results in:
– Weakness of plantar flexion and inversion of the foot.
– The patient cannot stand on toes.
– Sensory loss involves the sole of the foot.
– The ankle reflex is lost.

Tarsal tunnel syndrome

The posterior tibial nerve may be entrapped below the medial malleolus. This produces a burning pain in the sole of the foot. A prolonged sensory conduction velocity confirms the diagnosis. Surgical decompression is often required.

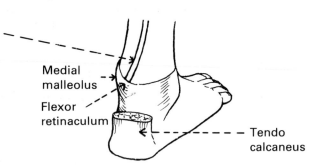

PLANTAR AND SMALL INTERDIGITAL NERVES

Compression of these nerves at the sole of the foot produces localised burning pain. Involvement of inter-digital nerves produces pain and analgesia in adjacent halves of neighbouring toes.

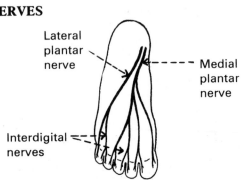

AUTONOMIC NERVOUS SYSTEM

The autonomic nervous sytem maintains the visceral and homeostatic functions essential to life. It is divided into SYMPATHETIC and PARASYMPATHETIC components and contains both motor (efferent) and sensory (afferent) pathways.

Both sympathetic and parasympathetic systems are regulated by the *limbic system, hypothalamus* and *reticular formation*. Fibres from these structures descend to synapse with preganglionic neurons in the intermediolateral column T1–L2 (sympathetic) and in the III, VII, IX and X cranial nerve nuclei and S2–S4 segments of the cord (parasympathetic).

PARASYMPATHETIC OUTFLOW

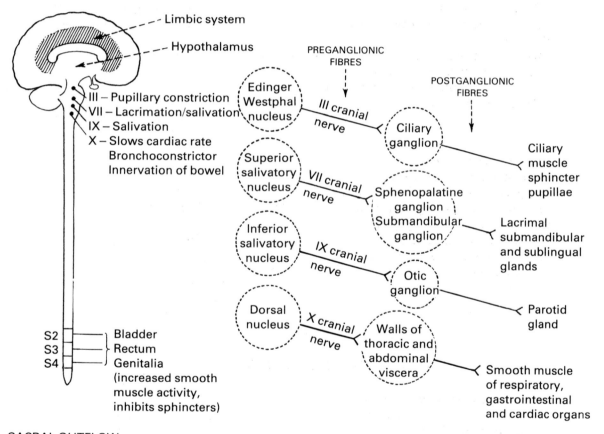

SACRAL OUTFLOW

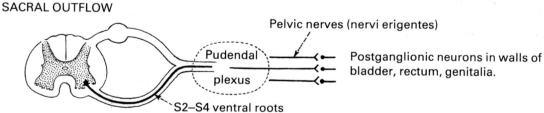

AUTONOMIC NERVOUS SYSTEM

SYMPATHETIC OUTFLOW

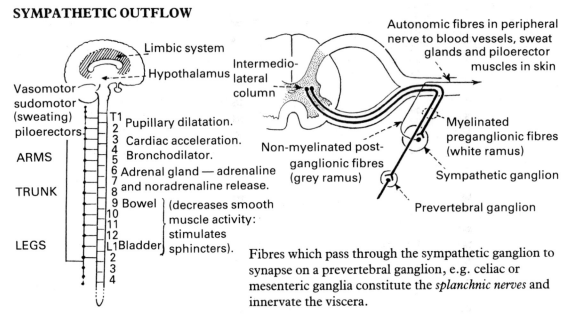

Fibres which pass through the sympathetic ganglion to synapse on a prevertebral ganglion, e.g. celiac or mesenteric ganglia constitute the *splanchnic nerves* and innervate the viscera.

AFFERENT AUTONOMIC NERVOUS SYSTEM

Sympathetic

Terminate in spinal cord in intermediate zone of grey matter — in relation to preganglionic neurons.

Function: Important in the appreciation of visceral pain.

Parasympathetic

Afferent fibres from the mouth and pharynx, and respiratory, cardiac and gastrointestinal systems, travelling in the VII, IX and X cranial nerves, terminate in the nucleus of tractus solitarius.

Function: Important in maintaining visceral reflexes.

The sacral afferents end in the S2–S4 region in relation to preganglionic neurons.

NEUROTRANSMITTER SUBSTANCES

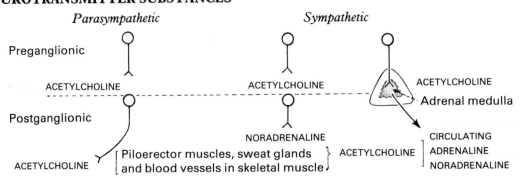

TESTS OF AUTONOMIC FUNCTION

BLOOD PRESSURE CONTROL
1. Maintenance of blood pressure with alteration in posture — dependent upon baroreceptor reflex function. A fall in BP occurs with efferent or afferent lesions — *postural hypotension.*
2. Exposure to cold induces vasoconstriction and a rise in BP — cold pressor test. Stress will produce a similar pressor response, e.g. ask patient to do mental arithmetic.
   Both central and peripheral lesions affect these tests.
3. Valsalva manoeuvre:
   The patient exhales against a closed glottis, increases intrathoracic pressure and thus reduces venous return and systemic BP. The heart rate accelerates to maintain BP. On opening the glottis, venous return increases and an overshoot of BP with cardiac slowing occurs. An impaired response occurs with afferent or efferent autonomic lesions.
4. Noradrenaline infusion test:
   A postganglionic sympathetic lesion results in 'supersensitivity' of denervated smooth muscle to adrenaline, with a marked rise in BP following infusion.

HEART RATE
1. Massage of the carotid sinus should stimulate the baroreceptors, increase vagal parasympathetic discharge and slow the heart rate. Either efferent or afferent lesions abolish this response.
2. Atropine test:
   Intravenous atropine 'blocks' vagal action and with intact sympathetic innervation results in an increase in heart rate.

SWEATING
A rise in body temperature causes increased sweating, detectable on the skin surface with starch-iodide paper. Any lesion from the central to the postganglionic sympathetic system impairs sweating.

SKIN TEMPERATURE
Skin temperature is a function of the sympathetic supply to blood vessels. With pre- or postganglionic lesions the skin becomes warm and red. With chronic postganglionic lesions the skin may become cold and blue (denervation hypersensitivity.) Compare the temperature of various regions.

PUPILLARY FUNCTION
Check the response to light and accommodation.
Pharmacological tests are important:
1. Atropine — blocks parasympathetic system — dilates pupil.
2. Cocaine — stimulates adrenergic receptors — dilates pupil.

441

AUTONOMIC NERVOUS SYSTEM — SPECIFIC DISEASES

IDIOPATHIC ORTHOSTATIC HYPOTENSION
Two types of this condition are recognised:
1. Due to degeneration of sympathetic postganglionic neurons.
2. Due to degeneration of sympathetic preganglionic neurons of the intermediolateral column T1–L2 — the SHY-DRAGER
SYNDROME.
In the latter disorder, features of extrapyramidal system involvement are also found.
Both disorders are characterised by: postural hypotension: anhidrosis (absent sweating):   impotence:
sphincter disturbance: pupillary abnormalities.
    The disorders may be separated pharmacologically; the postganglionic disorder shows hypersensitivity (denervation
hypersensitivity) to noradrenaline infusion.
Treatment
Drugs such as fludrocortisone increase blood volume and may prevent postural hypotension.

DIABETIC AUTONOMIC NEUROPATHY
Symptoms of autonomic dysfunction are common in long-standing insulin-dependent diabetics:
    Impotence/retrograde ejaculation.
    Bladder dysfunction — decreased detrusor muscle action — resulting in increased residual volume.
    Nocturnal diarrhoea.
    Gl dysfunction — vomiting from gastroparesis.
    Despite impairment of the cardiovascular reflexes (e.g. Valsalva manoeuvre), postural hypotension is never significant.
    These problems arise from damage to both sympathetic and parasympathetic postganglionic neurons.
Treatment
There is no specific treatment, although improved diabetic control may help..

POST-INFECTIOUS POLYNEUROPATHY — Guillain-Barré syndrome (see previous chapter).
Autonomic involvement occurs commonly in this disorder and may present major problems in patient management. The
lesion may involve the afferent or efferent limbs of the cardiovascular reflexes (baroreceptor reflexes) resulting in postural
hypotension, episodes of hypertension and cardiac dysrhythmias.
    Occasionally the postinfectious neuropathy is purely autonomic.

FAMILIAL DYSAUTONOMIA — RILEY-DAY SYNDROME.
This autosomal recessive disorder occurs in persons of Jewish descent.
    Features of autonomic dysfunction: postural hypotension, pain insensitivity, hyperpyrexia — present from birth.
Pathology
There is an absence of small unmyelinated sensory and sympathetic (postganglionic) axons.

PRIMARY AMYLOIDOSIS
Autonomic involvement with orthostatic hypotension, impotence, diarrhoea and bladder involvement may accompany
sensimotor neuropathy in the hereditary type of primary amyloidosis. Amyloid infiltration affects autonomic ganglia.

TOXIC DISORDERS
Drugs may damage the autonomic nervous system, e.g. cytotoxic agents, alcohol.

ADIE'S SYNDROME
A tonic pupil (page 140) associated with areflexia and occasionally widespread autonomic dysfunction, e.g. segmental
hypohidrosis (absent sweating) and diarrhoea.

AUTONOMIC DYSFUNCTION IN QUADRIPLEGIA (autonomic dysreflexia)
A high cervical lesion which completely severs the spinal cord, e.g. traumatic cervical fracture/dislocation will isolate all
but the cranial parasympathetic outflow. As a result, disturbed autonomic function is inevitable but variable.
    Autonomic reflexes are retained — Passive movement or tactile stimulation of limbs may result in blood pres-
sure rise, bradycardia, sweating, reflex penile erection (priapism).

AUTONOMIC NERVOUS SYSTEM — BLADDER INNERVATION

Efferent innervation

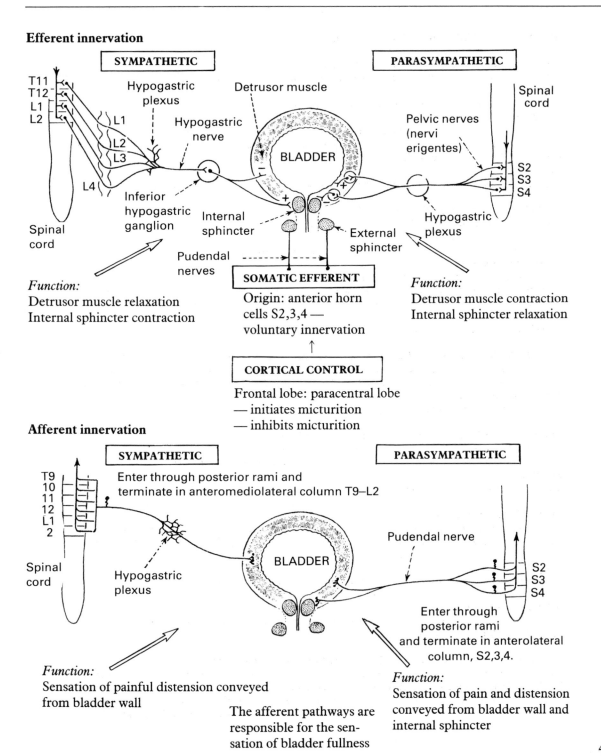

SYMPATHETIC

T11
T12
L1
L2

Hypogastric plexus

L1
L2
L3

L4

Hypogastric nerve

Detrusor muscle

BLADDER

Spinal cord

Inferior hypogastric ganglion

Internal sphincter

External sphincter

Spinal cord

Pudendal nerves

PARASYMPATHETIC

Spinal cord

Pelvic nerves (nervi erigentes)

S2
S3
S4

Hypogastric plexus

Function:
Detrusor muscle relaxation
Internal sphincter contraction

SOMATIC EFFERENT

Origin: anterior horn cells S2,3,4 — voluntary innervation

Function:
Detrusor muscle contraction
Internal sphincter relaxation

CORTICAL CONTROL

Frontal lobe: paracentral lobe
— initiates micturition
— inhibits micturition

Afferent innervation

SYMPATHETIC

T9
10
11
12
L1
2

Enter through posterior rami and terminate in anteromediolateral column T9–L2

Spinal cord

Hypogastric plexus

BLADDER

PARASYMPATHETIC

Pudendal nerve

S2
S3
S4

Enter through posterior rami and terminate in anterolateral column, S2,3,4.

Function:
Sensation of painful distension conveyed from bladder wall

The afferent pathways are responsible for the sensation of bladder fullness

Function:
Sensation of pain and distension conveyed from bladder wall and internal sphincter

443

MICTURITION

PROCESS OF MICTURITION
1. Cortical centre — removal of conscious inhibition of micturition.
2. Voiding — wave-like detrusor muscle contractions with relaxation of internal and external sphincters.
3. Voiding completed — detrusor muscle relaxation
   contraction of internal sphincter
   contraction of external sphincter.
4. Voiding may be voluntarily interrupted before complete bladder emptying by forced voluntary contraction of the external sphincter.

DISORDERS OF MICTURITION
Complete spinal cord lesion

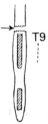 T9
isolates segmental innervation from cortical control.

Retention develops

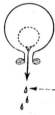

Increase in the intravesical pressure eventually overcomes internal sphincter integrity and 'dribbling overflow incontinence' results.

After some days or weeks a REFLEX BLADDER develops — *automatic emptying may be induced by abdominal tapping*. This voiding is often inadequate due to reflex contractions of the external sphincter before bladder emptying (autonomic dysynergia). High residual volumes result.

Lesions of the cauda equina

result in a parasympathetic denervated bladder which enlarges — flaccid neurogenic bladder — again with 'overflow incontinence'

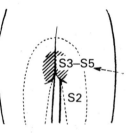

Sensation is lost in the sacral dermatomes. Anal tone is diminished and the anal reflex absent.

After weeks or months, abdominal compression combined with a Valsalva manoeuvre can induce efficient bladder emptying.

Urinary and, less commonly, associated faecal incontinence occurs in women following traumatic childbirth with injury to the innervation of striated pelvic floor musculature.

BOWEL AND SEXUAL FUNCTION

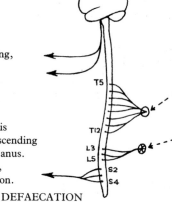

PARASYMPATHETIC

Vagus — gastric emptying, intestinal peristalsis.

Sacral nerve roots S2,3,4 — peristalsis from descending colon to anus.
— erection, ejaculation.

Paracentral lobule of frontal lobe
— voluntary initiation or inhibition of defaecation.

SYMPATHETIC
Celiac ganglion
— gastric and intestinal relaxation.
— contraction of internal anal sphincter.

Hypogastric plexus
— anti-erectile function.
? also erectile.

DEFAECATION

NORMAL PROCESS

1. Faeces arrive at rectosigmoid junction:
   — cortical awareness of urge to defaecate
   — release of sympathetic tone.
2. Relaxation of pelvic floor muscles and internal anal sphincter. Lowering of anorectum.
3. Voluntary opening of external anal sphincter.
4. Parasympathetic peristalsis and Valsalva manoeuvre empty the rectum.

SEXUAL FUNCTION
Parasympathetic:
— penile/clitoral erection.
Reflex — in response to tactile stimulation of erogenous zones.
Psychogenic — sexual thoughts or visual erotic stimulation.
— orgasm, ejaculation

Sympathetic:
— mainly anti-erectile action.

COMPLETE CORD LESION

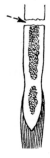

Bowel atony for up to 1 week.
→ Faecal retention with impaction and faecal fluid overflow (spurious diarrhoea). Impaired/absent external sphincter tone initially becomes spastic after days or weeks.
→ *Regular bowel emptying reflexly in response to digital stimulation or suppositories achieves continence.*

♂ Prolonged reflex erection (priapism) may occur for 2 – 3 days, then:
— Erections and ejaculation lost for weeks or months, then:
— Reflex actions (only tactile) appear but reflex ejaculation seldom returns.
Fertility is impaired or lost.

♀ Vaginal sensation and lubrication are lost. Fertility is retained.

CONUS LESION

MIXED PATTERN

Flaccid external sphincter.

Loss of genital sensation. Loss of reflex erections and ejaculation (psychogenic erection may be retained). Male infertile; female fertility retained. Male erections may be achieved by cavernosal blockade using intracavernosal injection of papaverine HCl.

CAUDA EQUINA LESION

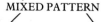

Faecal retention with impaction and faecal fluid overflow.
Regular clearance of constipated stool by manual evacuation or Valsalva maneouvre achieves continence.

445

DISEASES OF SKELETAL (VOLUNTARY) MUSCLE

Normal skeletal muscle morphology

A skeletal muscle is composed of a large number of muscle fibres separated by connective tissue (endomysium) and arranged in bundles (fasciculi) in which the individual fibres are parallel to each other. Each fasciculus has a connective tissue sheath (perimysium) and the muscle itself is composed of a number of fasciculi bound together and surrounded by a connective tissue sheath (epimysium).

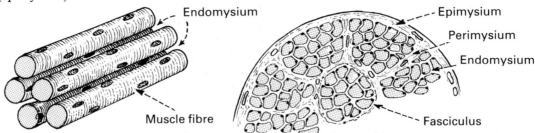

The three envelopes (sheaths) are made up of connective tissue richly endowed with blood vessels and fat cells (lipocytes).

The muscle fibre

This is a large multinucleated cell
with an outer membrane — SARCOLEMMA
       and a cytoplasm — SARCOPLASM
       within which lie the MYOFIBRILS

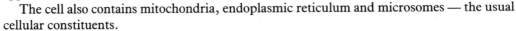

Each muscle fibre has its own endplate approximately half way along its length.

The cell also contains mitochondria, endoplasmic reticulum and microsomes — the usual cellular constituents.

Fats, glycogen, enzymes and myoglobin lie within the sarcoplasm and related structures.

The **MYOFIBRILS** are the contractile components of muscle.

Each myofibril is 1μ in diameter and contains filaments of *myosin* and *actin* interdigitating with each other between each Z line. When muscle contracts or relaxes these filaments slide over each other producing shortening and lengthening of the muscle fibre. The striated appearance of skeletal muscle is a consequence of differing concentrations of actin and myosin. These resultant bands are designated as shown.

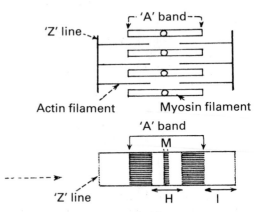

MUSCLE MORPHOLOGY

Fibre type
Muscle fibres vary with function. Two main types are recognised:
Type I: Slow continuous contractions — TONIC.
Type II: Sudden strong contractions — PHASIC.

Characteristics:

Type I	Type II
Red (rich in myoglobin)	White (little myoglobin)
Lower O_2 consumption	High O_2 consumption
Lower metabolism	High metabolism
Rich in sarcoplasm	Little sarcoplasm
AEROBIC.	May function ANAEROBICALLY.

Innervation
Type I — small alpha motor neuron. Type II — large alpha motor neuron.

Individual muscles contain a mixture of type I and type II fibres with a tendency for one type to predominate depending upon the specific muscle.

Neuromuscular junction
Muscle contraction is achieved by a nerve impulse. Each muscle fibre receives a nerve branch from the motor cell body in the anterior horn of the spinal cord or cranial nerve motor nuclei.
When a nerve fibre reaches the muscle it loses its myelin sheath and its neurilemma then merges with the sarcolemma under which the axon spreads out to form the motor endplate.

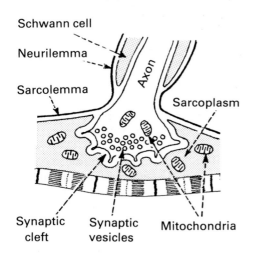

Schwann cell
Neurilemma
Axon
Sarcolemma
Sarcoplasm
Synaptic cleft
Synaptic vesicles
Mitochondria

The axon fibre with its endings and muscle fibres it supplies is called the MOTOR UNIT. The number of muscle fibres in a motor unit varies: in the eye muscles it is small (5 – 10), whereas in the limb muscles the number is large (in the gastrocnemius about 1800). Each motor unit contains only one type of muscle fibre, i.e. type I or type II. The neuromuscular junction is the point at which neuromusclar transmission is effected. The motor endplate is separated from the sarcoplasm by the synaptic cleft. Acetylcholine is found in the synaptic vesicles and released into the synaptic cleft when an electrical impulse passes down the axon. The endplate potential is produced by such a release and when a certain threshold is reached a muscle action potential results which causes contraction.

The enzyme cholinesterase, found in high concentration at motor endplates, destroys acetylcholine so that normally a single nerve impulse only gives rise to a single muscle contraction.

447

CLINICAL EXAMINATION

No muscle dystrophy affects all muscle groups.

Topography (distribution) of weakness, wasting or hypertrophy aids diagnosis and classification of muscle disorders.

Certain points should be elicited from history
— Whether muscles fatigue with exercise and recover with rest
      — non-specific in muscle disease but may suggest defective neuromuscular transmission.
— Tasks which are specifically difficult:
      proximal weakness — difficulty in climbing stairs
                            lifting hands above head
                            combing hair.
      distal weakness – 'scuffing' toes when walking
                      weak hands, e.g. cannot turn door handle, change gear in car.
— Speed of onset of weakness (whether acute, subacute, chronic).
— Muscle pains present at rest.
— Muscle pains and cramps during or after exercise.
— Whether contraction, e.g. hand grip, is slow to relax (myotonia).
— The presence of a family history of muscle disease or related disorders.

Examination should
— Note the presence of hypertrophy and the distribution of wasting and weakness, and grade weakness according to the MRC (Medical Research Council) scale:
      5 — Full strength.
      4 — Below normal.
      3 — Lift against gravity.
      2 — Movement with gravity eliminated.
      1 — Muscle twitch with no movement about the joint.
      0 — No muscle contraction.

— Palpate muscles for tenderness.
— Percussion to determine presence or absence of myotonia (see later).
— Reflex examination, initially normal, may change with marked wasting and weakness — hyporeflexia becoming apparent.
— General examination is essential. Muscle disease may be a reflection of an underlying metabolic, endocrine, neoplastic or connective tissue disorder, e.g. increased pigmentation in Addison's disease, malar rash in systemic lupus erythematosus, hepatosplenectomy in alcoholic liver disease.

MUSCULAR DYSTROPHIES

Muscular dystrophies are genetically determined myopathies in which progressive degeneration and wasting of muscles occur.

The pathogenesis of the dystrophies is unknown.

Classification is based upon the mode of inheritance and the clinical picture.

X-linked recessive
— Duchenne
— Becker
— Emery-Dreifuss.

Autosomal dominant
— facioscapulohumeral
— scapuloperoneal
— myotonic
— oculopharyngeal.

Autosomal recessive
— limb girdle.

DUCHENNE DYSTROPHY

Duchenne dystrophy is the commonest form of muscular dystrophy. The disorder is generally X-linked recessive in mode of inheritance. This means that 50% of females are carriers (XX) and 50% of the male offspring may be affected (XY). In Turner's syndrome (XO) females may develop Duchenne dystrophy and infrequent female involvement can also be explained by rare autosomal recessive (non-sex-linked) inheritance. The mutation rate is higher than in any other X-linked hereditary disease. This accounts for the high number (50%) of sporadic cases.

Estimated incidence
1 in 4000 live male births.

Clinical features:
Delayed motor development is common; at 18 months only 50% of subsequent sufferers can walk. Clinical presentation occurs before the age of 5 years.

Proximal muscle involvement initially:
— glutei/quadriceps → WADDLING GAIT.
— shoulder girdle and upper forearm.
— axial muscles → SWAY BACK POSTURE.

MUSCULAR DYSTROPHIES

Clinical features (*contd*)

The child, at the initial stage of the illness, cannot climb stairs or rise from a low chair, and when attempting to rise from the ground will 'climb up himself' — Gower's sign (not diagnostic of the condition, but indicative of pelvic muscle weakness).

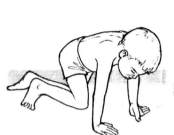
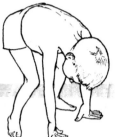
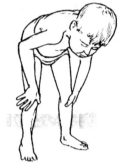
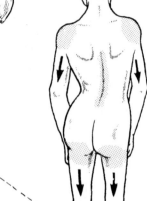

Pseudohypertrophy occurs in 80% of cases.

The gastrocnemius commonly is enlarged and rubbery hard. Quadriceps/deltoid and tongue likewise may be affected.

Mean IQ is 15-20 points lower than in the normal population; occasionally severe mental handicap may occur.

Progression

Between 7–12 years — child is no longer able to walk and weakness spreads distally in the limbs.

Kyphoscoliosis with respiratory distress and cardiac muscle involvement.

Aged 20 years — chest infection, cardiac failure and arrhythmias occur with severe muscle contractures. The patient by now is bedbound. Survival is rare beyond mid-20s.

Investigation

Muscle enzyme — creatine phosphokinase — is substantially elevated especially in early stages. The enzyme is raised at birth and is significantly elevated in the female carrier aiding detection of this state and genetic counselling.

Electromyographic (EMG) studies will support the diagnosis and may be important in doubtful early cases with no family history, i.e. spontaneous mutation. EMG studies do not detect carrier states.

Muscle biopsy will not always be necessary but will establish the diagnosis beyond doubt.

Treatment

There is no effective treatment. Orthopaedic procedures such as tenotomy may prolong mobility. Steroids are of no value. Detection of the carrier state and advice are essential as preventive treatment. Prenatal diagnosis is not yet possible. Fetal sexing indicates the risk, i.e. if male, 50% affected; if female, 50% carrier.

MUSCULAR DYSTROPHIES

BECKER'S DYSTROPHY
Becker's dystrophy is similar to Duchenne but less common (1/20 000 live male births).
Clinical features
Onset is later than Duchenne — aged 10 years.
Cardiac muscle is spared.
Most patients remain ambulant until 3rd and 4th decades.
Mental retardation is rare.

EMERY-DREIFUSS DYSTROPHY
This dystrophy is relatively benign, with survival well into middle age. Progressive proximal weakness is associated with facial weakness and flexion contractures.

FASCIOSCAPULOHUMERAL DYSTROPHY
This is inherited as an autosomal dominant trait. Described by Dejerine (1885) it is referred to as Dejerine's dystrophy.

Abortive forms of this condition in which selective muscle involvement occurs (e.g. unilateral shoulder muscle) may 'mask' the dominant mode of inheritance.
Incidence: 1–2 per 100 000.
Clinical features

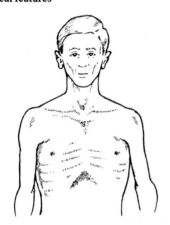

The expression of disease is variable and often mild.
Onset in first or second decade.
Initially the lower half of the face is involved — cannot purse lips or whistle — then spread into trapezius and pectorals occurs.
Lumbar lordosis develops from spinal muscle weakness. Pelvic musculature and quadriceps may eventually become involved. DROMEDARY or CAMEL-BACKED gait with protrusion of the buttocks is characteristic. Calf and deltoid muscles may be hypertrophic.

Unlike Duchenne dystrophy the clinical course is slow and arrest of progression may occur.

In some cases weakness of facial muscles is noted in childhood without spread to other muscles until middle age. Cardiac muscle is not involved. Sensorineural deafness and retinal vascular changes (telangiectasis and detachment) may occur. Life expectancy in this condition is normal.

Investigations
EMG studies show myopathic changes.
Muscle enzymes may be normal or slightly elevated.
Muscle biopsy shows increased fibre diameter; a cellular response of lymphocytes and plasma cells may be present between muscle fascicles.
Treatment
There is no specific treatment other than supportive with genetic guidance.

SCAPULOPERONEAL MUSCULAR DYSTROPHY

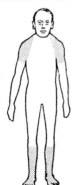

This is an autosomal dominant disorder with involvement of proximal upper limb and distal lower limb muscles. Onset is in adult life with foot drop (anterior tibial and peroneal muscle groups). Weakness next affects the upper limbs with spread from scapular muscles into deltoid, biceps and triceps. The disease runs a benign non-disabling course. Cardiac muscle involvement may occur in later life. A more aggressive X-linked form of this dystrophy has been described.

The *creatine phosphokinase (CPK)* enzyme is elevated.
The *electrocardiogram* may be abnormal with atrial arrhythmias.
EMG studies show myopathic changes.
Muscle biopsy will show non-specific myopathic features.
Differentiation from spinal muscular atrophy with the same distribution of muscle involvement may require EMG and biopsy.

451

MUSCULAR DYSTROPHIES

MYOTONIC DYSTROPHY

Myotonic dystrophy is a disorder characterised by the presence of MYOTONIA — failure of immediate muscle relaxation after voluntary contraction has stopped.

It can be demonstrated by:

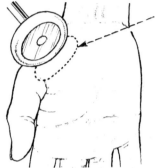

1. Striking a muscle with the tendon hammer and watching the resultant 'dimple' persist for a while before filling up.

2. Asking the patient to grip an object then suddenly release it. The slow relaxation and opening of the hand grip will make the object appear 'stuck' to the fingers.

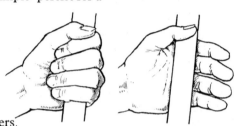

Physiologically, myotonia is due to instability of the muscle membrane with repetitive discharges following a short period of contraction. Although suggestive of myotonic dystrophy, myotonia may occur in other muscle disorders.

Clinical features

Myotonic dystrophy is an autosomal dominant inherited multisystem disorder with the causal gene located on chromosome 19.

The incidence is 5 per 100 000 with the onset occurring between 15 and 40 years.

The facial appearance is typical:

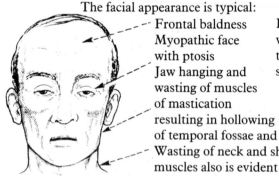

Frontal baldness
Myopathic face
with ptosis
Jaw hanging and
wasting of muscles
of mastication
resulting in hollowing
of temporal fossae and cheeks
Wasting of neck and shoulder girdle
muscles also is evident

In the limbs —
weakness and wasting are distal
though the hands are
spared until late.

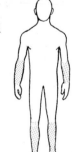

As the disease progresses, myotonia becomes less apparent and may disappear.
The disorder is progressive over 15–25 years.
Cataracts occur in 80% of cases.
Testicular atrophy occurs in males.
Infertility, habitual abortion and menstrual abnormalities in females.
Cardiac dysrhythmias occur in 70% occasionally resulting in sudden death.
Abnormalities of glucose/insulin metabolism with diabetes mellitus is present in some patients.
Mental deficiency is noted in 30% of patients.
Non-neurological manifestation — cataracts, frontal baldness, infertility — may predate the development of muscle weakness and myotonia.
In affected mothers, the disease may appear in the neonate.

MUSCULAR DYSTROPHIES

MYOTONIC DYSTROPHY (contd)

Investigation

The *creatine phosphokinase (CPK)* is elevated slightly.

The *ECG* may show conduction abnormalities.

The *EMG* shows classic features of myotonia, with waxing and waning in the amplitude and frequency of motor unit potentials, as well as myopathic changes.

Muscle biopsy may be normal or show a variety of changes.

Other investigations:

— Slit lamp examination of the eyes is essential to exclude cataract.

— Plain radiology may show certain bony abnormalities, e.g. hyperostosis frontalis interna, small pituitary fossa.

— Elevated blood insulin levels may be found as may a diabetic glucose tolerance curve.

Myotonic dystrophy must be distinguished from other disorders in which myotonia occurs.

Treatment

Drugs which act as membrane stabilisers, e.g. procainamide, phenytoin, quinine, quinidine, acetazolamide, may reduce myotonia.

Identification and treatment of diabetes mellitus and cataract is important.

Genetic counselling should be given.

Sedative drugs are to be avoided as patients show an excessive sensitivity.

General anaesthesia when necessary should be given cautiously — there is risk of malignant hyperthermia.

N.B. Although a Mendelian disorder, in some generations cataract or diabetes mellitus may be the sole manifestation.

OCULOPHARYNGEAL DYSTROPHY

This is an autosomal dominant disorder presenting in early middle age. Ptosis is the initial finding with progressive involvement of extraocular muscles until paralysis of all eye movements results. The pupillary reactions are spared. Dysphagia, facial weakness and proximal limb weakness develop later.

Laboratory findings demonstrate a high CPK (5 × normal). Muscle biopsy is characteristic with 'rimmed' vacuoles in a proportion of muscle fibres. Treatment is supportive, with death eventually from intercurrent infection. Swallowing difficulties may necessitate nasogastric feeding.

Distinction must be made from myasthenia gravis and mitochondrial myopathy (see later) in which ptosis is a distinctive feature.

LIMB-GIRDLE MUSCULAR DYSTROPHY

This is an autosomal recessive disorder with onset in second or third decade which may be delayed to middle age.

Often muscle involvement is asymmetrical and onset is usually in the pelvic girdle muscles. Progression is slow. The disease may arrest in some patients. Muscle enlargement (calves) occurs in a proportion of cases.

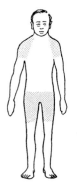

Attempts have been made to subdivide on the basis of pelvic or shoulder girdle onset — this has not been convincing.

The *creatine phosphokinase (CPK)* is moderately elevated.

Cardiac involvement does not occur (ECG normal).

EMG studies show non-specific myopathic features.

Muscle biopsy confirms myopathy with connective tissue proliferation.

Differentiation: This distribution of weakness in proximal muscles may be a feature of chronic spinal muscular atrophy, certain metabolic myopathies and polymyositis.

Investigation is essential to classify correctly as EMG and muscle biopsy will distinguish these disorders.

Treatment: Treatment is symptomatic. Genetic counselling is difficult because of the high frequency of sporadic cases, the recessive nature, and absence of CPK elevation in the carrier state.

453

INFLAMMATORY MYOPATHY

Inflammatory myopathy is a disorder of muscle in which there is clinical and laboratory evidence of an inflammatory process:

It is an acquired muscle disorder as opposed to the *inherited* dystrophies and may be classified as follows:

Polymyositis
Dermatomyositis — Childhood form
Adult form

Inflammatory myopathy associated with malignant disease (polymyositis or dermatomyositis forms)
Inflammatory myopathy associated with collagen vascular disorders, e.g. lupus erythematosus, systemic sclerosis, rheumatoid arthritis (polymyositis or dermatomyositis forms)
Infective — viral, bacterial and parasitic
Drug-induced — cimetidine, penicillamine.

POLYMYOSITIS/DERMATOMYOSITIS

There are two principal forms of inflammatory myopathy — polymyositis and dermatomyositis which are separated clinically by the dermatological findings in the latter. All age groups are affected. Annual incidence is 5 cases per 1 000 000 of the population.

An autoimmune basis for these disorders is supported by:
— response to immunosuppressive therapy.
— association with other known immunological disorders, e.g. collagen vascular disorders.
— elevated IgG in blood and presence of circulating autoantibodies, e.g. antinuclear antibody in some cases.
— an increased incidence of certain histocompatibility antigens (HLA antigens) B_8, DR3.
— the reproduction of a similar disorder in laboratory animals by injection of muscle extract with Freund's adjuvant.

Humoral and cell mediated immune mechanisms seem responsible for these disorders but the trigger factor(s) remain unknown.

INFLAMMATORY MYOPATHY

Clinical presentation

Onset is acute or subacute over a period of several weeks and may follow systemic infection.
(? Sensitisation to patient's own muscle.)

Systemic symptoms prevail at onset, e.g. lassitude, and are then followed by muscle weakness.
Extensive oedema of skin and subcutaneous tissues is common (especially in the periorbital
region).

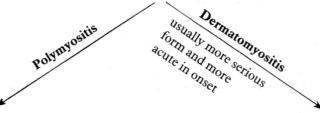

Polymyositis

Dermatomyositis usually more serious form and more acute in onset

Muscles may be painful and tender in 60%
of cases though onset is often painless.

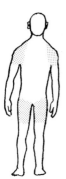

Proximal muscles are first
involved and initially weakness
may be asymmetrical, e.g.
one quadriceps only.

Weakness of
posterior neck
muscles will
result in
the head 'lolling'
forwards.

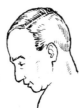

Occasionally weakness may spread into
distal limb muscle groups.

Pharyngeal and laryngeal involvement
results in dysphagia and dysphonia. Cardiac
muscle may also be involved.

The eye muscles are *not* involved unless
there is coexistent myasthenia gravis.

Reflexes are retained (if absent, consider
underlying carcinoma with added
neuropathy).

Characterised by skin rash.
Violet discoloration of light exposed skin.

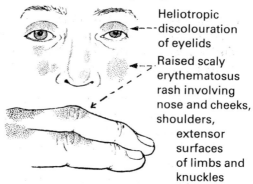

Heliotropic
discolouration
of eyelids

Raised scaly
erythematosus
rash involving
nose and cheeks,
shoulders,
extensor
surfaces
of limbs and
knuckles

Telangiectasia and tightening
of skin are common and small
ulcerated vasculitic lesions develop
over bony prominences.

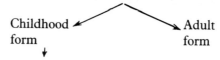

Childhood
form

Adult
form

Multisystem involvement.
Calcification develops in skin and muscle with
extrusion through skin.
Muscle contractures develop — tip-toe gait.
Gastrointestinal ulceration occurs.

The muscle weakness is as in polymyositis
but in childhood dermatomyositis may be
very severe, involving chewing, swallowing
and breathing.

INFLAMMATORY MYOPATHY

POLYMYOSITIS AND DERMATOMYOSITIS ASSOCIATED WITH MALIGNANT DISEASES

Approximately 10% of adults with inflammatory myopathy have underlying neoplasia. In dermatomyositis, of those over 40 years of age as many as 60% harbour neoplasia. Neoplasia may present before or after the development of inflammatory myopathy. The most frequently associated tumours are of lung, breast, ovary and gastrointestinal tract.

POLYMYOSITIS AND DERMATOMYOSITIS ASSOCIATED WITH COLLAGEN VASCULAR DISEASES

Approximately 25% of adults with inflammatory myopathy have symptoms and signs of an associated collagen vascular disorder.

In 5–10% of persons with these disorders (systemic lupus erythematosus etc), inflammatory myopathy develops at some stage in their illness.

In the 'overlap' syndromes (mixed collagen vascular diseases) muscle involvement is more common.

Diagnosis

The clinical picture is suggestive and diagnosis is supported by the following investigations:

Muscle enzymes
Creatine phosphokinase elevated in most patients along with other muscle enzymes.

Circulating antibodies
e.g. rheumatoid factor, antinuclear factor. Present in 40%.

Electromyogram
Shows a typical myopathic pattern with fibrillations.

Erythrocyte sedimentation rate (ESR)
Elevated in most patients.

Muscle biopsy shows necrosis of muscle fibres with inflammatory cells — lymphocytes, plasma cells, leucocytes — in the endomysium.

Prior to the availability of treatment the outcome in inflammatory myopathy was variable and obviously influenced by the presence of associated neoplasia or collagenosis. Periods of relative improvement could occur but generally progression prevailed. Death occurred as a result of chest infection, gastrointestinal haemorrhage, perforation and cardiac arrest in 20–30% of all patients.

Treatment

Steroids — Prednisolone 40–80 mg daily in divided doses with gradual reduction to maintenace dose once improved. If stopped too early, relapse may occur.

Cimetidine protects against the risk of gastrointestinal haemorrhage or perforation.

In refractory cases immunosuppressive drugs — methotrexate, azothiaprine or cyclophosphamide — may be used.

Plasmapheresis, thymectomy and low dose nodal or total body irradiation are 'last-line' treatments and while not fully evaluated should be considered in life-threatening disease.

Outcome

Mortality is now low though only 10% recover completely. In the rest, the disease becomes inactive after 2 years and patients are left with varying degrees of disability. When associated with collagen disease, eventual outcome will depend on the nature of that disease. When associated with neoplasm, steroids may cause temporary improvement. Removal of an associated tumour can result in remission.

ENDOCRINE/METABOLIC MYOPATHIES

Unlike inflammatory myopathy the weakness in these conditions is more chronic and is unassociated pathologically with inflammation. Correction of the underlying endocrine disturbance results in recovery. Usually the other features of endocrine dysfunction are more problematical and myopathy is of secondary importance.

Pituitary

Acromegaly

Proximal weakness with fatigue. Entrapment neuropathies, e.g. carpal tunnel syndrome may complicate the clinical picture of myopathy. Other features of growth hormone excess are evident.

Parathyroid

Hyperparathyroidism and osteomalacia.
Weakness of a proximal distribution with muscle tenderness occurs in 50% of patients with osteomalacia but is less common in primary hyperparathyroidism. The legs are mainly affected and a waddling gait results.

Adrenal

Hyperadrenalism and hypoadrenalism
These may both be associated with proximal myopathy. In patients treated with steroids, a similar picture may develop rapidly when drug induced. Reduction of steroid dosage results in improvement.

Thyroid

Hyperthyroidism

Weakness occurs in 20% of thyrotoxic patients. Shoulder girdle weakness is more marked than pelvic. Reflexes are brisk, fasciculation and atrophy may be present. *Distinction must be made from motor neuron disease.* There is always clinical evidence of thyrotoxicosis in these patients. Diagnosis is confirmed by thyroid function studies.

Hypothyroidism

Proximal weakness involves pelvic girdle more than shoulder. Painful cramps and muscle stiffness are common. Muscle enlargement in limbs and tongue often occur. There is always clinical evidence of hypothyroidism in these patients. Diagnosis is confirmed by thyroid function tests and response to thyroid hormone therapy is excellent.

In chronic proximal weakness, careful clinical history taking, examination and appropriate investigation will separate the various endocrine causes.

METABOLIC MYOPATHIES: THE PERIODIC PARALYSES

Acute episodes of weakness may result from alterations in serum potassium levels. Three separate forms exist:

Hypokalaemic periodic paralysis

Autosomal dominant.
Onset in second decade.
Precipitated by: exercise, carbohydrate load.
Commences in proximal lower limb muscles and rapidly becomes generalised. Onset usually in morning on wakening.
Bulbar muscles/respiration unaffected.
K^+ falls as low as 1.5 meq/l.
Treatment:
Acute — oral KCl.
Prophylactic – acetazolamide; low carbohydrate, high K^+ diet.
With age, attacks become progressively less frequent.

Non-familial hypokalaemic periodic paralysis may occur in patients suffering from hyperthyroidism.

Hyperkalaemic periodic paralysis

Autosomal dominant or recessive.
Onset in infancy/childhood.
Precipitated by: rest after activity or by cold.
Commences in the lower limbs and evolves rapidly.
Attacks are of short duration (less than 60 min).
Myotonia is evident in some patients.
K^+ rises only slightly.
Treatment:
Acute — intravenous calcium gluconate or sodium chloride.
Prophylactic — acetazolamide.

Paramyotonia congenita
A rare related disorder.
Periodic paralysis + myotonia — induced by exercise/cold.

Normokalaemic periodic paralysis

Autosomal dominant.
Onset variable.
Precipitated by: ingestion of K^+-containing substances.
Attacks appear more severe and prolonged.
Myotonia is absent.
Treatment:
Acute — supportive.
Prophylactic — acetazolamide or 9α fluorohydrocortisone.

NON-PROGRESSIVE CONGENITAL POLYMYOPATHIES

These are disorders which result from an abnormality in basic muscle morphology and usually have a familial incidence. No treatment exists, but they do not lead to progressive disability. Muscle biopsy with histochemical staining and electron microscopy should achieve the diagnosis.

Central core disease

Pathology: Hyaline changes in myofibrils lying centrally within the muscle fibres.
Clinically: Variable age of onset. Proximal muscle involvement (may resemble limb girdle dystrophy). Dominant inheritance.

Nemaline myopathy

Pathology: Presence of rod-like structures below the muscle sarcolemma.
Clinically: Onset in infancy. Bulbar muscles may be involved. Dominant or recessive inheritance.

Mitochondrial myopathy

Pathology: Large and excessive mitochondria within the muscle fibres.
Clinically: Onset in infancy/childhood.
Initial hypotonia and delayed motor development.
Several variations are recognised with variable inheritance.

METABOLIC MYOPATHIES

Disorders of glycogen or lipid metabolism may result in muscle weakness and diminished exercise tolerance.

McARDLE'S DISEASE — due to phosphorylase deficiency.

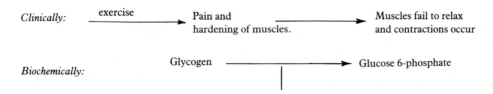

Clinically: exercise → Pain and hardening of muscles. → Muscles fail to relax and contractions occur

Biochemically: Glycogen ——————→ Glucose 6-phosphate

Absence of phosphorylase enzyme
blocks conversion

Myoglobin appears in the urine

Diagnosis: Failure of serum lactate to rise following exercise.
Muscle biopsy — absence of phosphorylase activity with appropriate histochemical staining.

McArdle's disease should be suspected in a patient who develops painful contracted muscles following exercise. Treatment with oral fructose may help, but persistent weakness often results.

ACID MALTASE DEFICIENCY
The development in adult life of limb girdle weakness characterises this disorder. In some, selective involvement of the respiratory muscles causes respiratory failure.
    Acid maltase deficiency occasionally presents in infancy with a floppy hypotonic weakness associated with an enlarged tongue.
Diagnosis: Confirmed by muscle biopsy.

CARNITINE DEFICIENCY
This results in disordered fatty acid transport.
    Clinically, muscle weakness and contractures occur with exercise in children or adults. A failure to produce ketones following prolonged fast and a normal elevation in serum lactate following exercise differentiates this condition from McArdle's disease.

MYASTHENIA GRAVIS

Myasthenia gravis is a disorder of neuromuscular transmission characterised by:
— Weakness and fatiguing of some or all muscle groups.
— Weakness worsening on sustained or repeated exertion, or towards the end of the day, relieved by rest.

This condition is a consequence of an autoimmune destruction of the NICOTINIC POSTSYNAPTIC RECEPTORS FOR ACETYLCHOLINE.

Myasthenia gravis is rare, with a prevalence of 40 per million. The increased incidence of autoimmune disorders in patients and first degree relatives and the association of the disease with certain histocompatibility antigens (HLA) — B_7, B_8 and DR_2 — suggests an IMMUNOLOGICAL BASIS.

AETIOLOGY

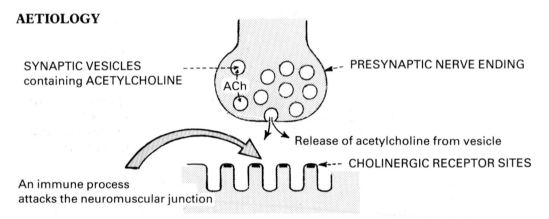

SYNAPTIC VESICLES containing ACETYLCHOLINE

ACh

PRESYNAPTIC NERVE ENDING

Release of acetylcholine from vesicle

CHOLINERGIC RECEPTOR SITES

An immune process attacks the neuromuscular junction

Antibodies bind to the receptor sites resulting in their destruction (complement mediated). These antibodies are referred to as ACETYLCHOLINE RECEPTOR ANTIBODIES (ACh R antibodies) and are demonstrated by radioimmunoassay in the serum of 90% of patients.

Human purified IgG (containing AChR antibodies) injected into mice induces myasthenia-like disease in these recipient animals.

In human myasthenia gravis a reduction of acetylcholine receptor sites has been demonstrated in the postsynaptic folds. Reduced receptor synthesis and increased receptor destruction, as well as the blocking of receptor response to acetylcholine, all seem responsible for the disorder.

The rôle of the thymus: Thymic abnormalities occur in 80% of patients. The main function of the thymus is to effect the production of T-cell lymphocytes, which participate in immune responses. Thymus dysfunction is noted in a large number of disorders which may be associated with myasthenia gravis, e.g. systemic lupus erythematosus.

MYASTHENIA GRAVIS — PATHOLOGY

Changes are found in the THYMUS gland and in muscle.

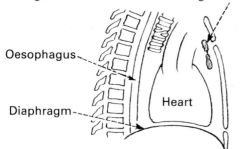

Oesophagus

Diaphragm

Heart

The gland is most active during the induction of normal immune responses in the neonatal period and attains its largest size at puberty after which it involutes.

Foci of lymphocytes

Epithelial cell (Hassall's corpuscle)

Normal structure

In myasthenia gravis:
20%: involuted gland

70%: show hyperplasia

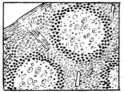

with lymphoid follicles demonstrating germinal centres

10%: thymoma, an encapsulate tumour of lymphoid and epithelial cells which may be locally invasive but rarely metastasises.

Muscle biopsy may show abnormalities:
— Lymphocytic infiltration associated with small necrotic foci of muscle fibre damage.
— Muscle fibre atrophy (type I and II or type II alone).
— Diffuse muscle necrosis with inflammatory infiltration (when associated with thymoma) producing anti striated muscle antibody.

Motor point biopsy may show abnormal motor endplates. Supravital methylene blue staining reveals abnormally long and irregular terminal nerve branching.
    Light and electron microscopy show destruction of ACh receptors with simplification of the secondary folds of the postsynaptic surface.

CLINICAL FEATURES

Up to 90% of patients present in early adult life (<40 years of age).
The disorder may be selective, involving specific groups of muscles.
Several clinical subdivisions are recognised:

        Grade I   — ocular muscles only ⁻20%
        Grade IIA — mild generalised weakness ⁻30%
        Grade IIB — moderate generalised weakness ⁻30%
        Grade III   — acute fulminating
        Grade IV   — severe upon mild or moderate at onset ⎭ ⁻ 20%

    Approximately 40% of grade I will eventually become grade II. The rest remain purely ocular throughout the illness.
Grades IIB, III and IV develop respiratory muscle involvement.

461

MYASTHENIA GRAVIS — CLINICAL FEATURES *(contd)*

Cranial nerve signs and symptoms

— Ocular involvement produces ptosis and muscle paresis.
— Weakness of jaw muscles allows the mouth to hang open.
— Weakness of facial muscles results in expressionless appearance.

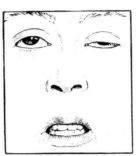
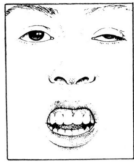

— On smiling, buccinator weakness produces a characteristic smile (myasthenic snarl).

Bulbar involvement may result in:
— dysarthric dysphonic speech and dysphagia.
— nasal regurgitation of fluids — nasal quality to speech.

Weakness of eye opening....  (ptosis) ...and closing... 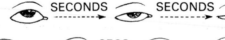 ...in the same patient is characteristic. (failure to 'bury' eyelashes)

The demonstration of *fatiguing* is important in reaching diagnosis and in monitoring the response to treatment:

'Look upwards' 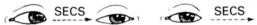 SECONDS ⟶ SECONDS ⟶ Ptosis becomes apparent and the eye drifts to neutral position

'Look left' SECS ⟶ SECS ⟶

Fatiguing of other bulbar muscles may be demonstrated by:
— blowing out cheeks against pressure.
— counting as far as possible in one breath, etc.

Ptosis becomes apparent and a dysconjugate drift develops

The tongue occasionally shows the characteristic triple grooved appearance with two lateral and one central furrow.

Limb and trunk signs and symptoms

Weakness of neck muscles may result in lolling of the head. Proximal limb muscles are preferentially affected. Fatigue may be demonstrated by movement against a constant resistance.
   Limb reflexes are often hyperactive and fatigue on repeated testing.
   Muscle wasting occurs in 15% of cases.
   Stress, infection and pregnancy all exacerbate the weakness.

Natural history:
(Before treatment became available)

10% of patients entered a period of remission of long duration.
20% experienced short periods of remission (1 to several months).
30% progressed to death.
The remainder showed varying degrees of disability accentuated by exercise.

MYASTHENIA GRAVIS — DIFFERENTIAL DIAGNOSIS

Distinguish from:
— The patient who complains of fatiguing easily — neurotic, hysterical or depressed individual.
— The patient with progressive ophthalmoplegia, e.g. ocular myopathy.
— The patient with multiple sclerosis — diplopia, dysarthria and fatigue with a relapsing and remitting course.
— The patient with the Eaton-Lambert myasthenic syndrome (see page 527).

INVESTIGATION

PHARMACOLOGICAL

Anticholinesterase drugs are used to confirm diagnosis.

Tensilon (edrophonium) — short action, 2–4 minutes, given i.v. 2–10 mg *slowly,* with atropine available to counter muscarinic side effects. This is positive when noticeable improvement in weakness occurs on objective testing.

SEROLOGICAL

Acetylcholine receptor antibodies are detected in 90% of patients and are specific to this disease.

Other antibodies — microsomal, colloid, rheumatoid factor, gastric parietal cell antibody — are occasionally found. These reflect the overlap between myasthenia gravis and other auto-immune disorders.

Anti striated muscle antibodies are found in 30% of all patients and in 90% of those with thymoma.

ELECTROPHYSIOLOGICAL

Reduction of the amplitude of the compound muscle action potential evoked by repetitive supramaximal nerve stimulation — 'the decrementing response'.

Various rates of stimulation; even as low as 3/second may produce a decrementing response.

Measure of 'Jitter' — the time interval variability of action potentials from two single muscle fibres of the same motor unit — is a more sensitive index of neuromuscular function and is increased.

ADDITIONAL

Patients with suspected thymoma, especially those over 40 years, require computerised tomography of the anterior mediastinum.

MYASTHENIA GRAVIS — TREATMENT

In the severely ill patients, the first priority is to protect respiration by intubation if necessary, and ventilation.

Anticholinesterase drugs
This is the longest established form of treatment (1934).

Anticholinesterase drugs interfere with **cholinesterase,** the enzyme responsible for the breakdown of acetylcholine, allowing enhanced receptor stimulation. As a result, more acetylcholine is available to effect neuromuscular transmission.

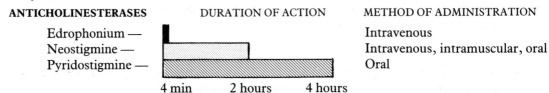

ANTICHOLINESTERASES	DURATION OF ACTION	METHOD OF ADMINISTRATION
Edrophonium —		Intravenous
Neostigmine —		Intravenous, intramuscular, oral
Pyridostigmine —		Oral
	4 min 2 hours 4 hours	

A muscarinic inhibitor, atropine, may be required to counter side effects.
Anticholinesterases rarely give complete symptomatic relief.

The balance between myasthenic and cholinergic (overdose) symptoms is very fine. The same patient may show myasthenic weakness and cholinergic weakness simultaneously in different muscle groups.

CHOLINERGIC OVERDOSAGE:
Muscle fasciculation
Increased secretions — sweating
                 — bronchorrhoea
Respiratory difficulty
Pupillary signs — miosis

All these warnings of overdosage may be masked if atropine is being taken

Ultimately cholinergic overdosage will result in generalised weakness — *cholinergic crisis*. Chronic high dosage may actually result in loss of postsynaptic acetylcholine receptors.

Steroids
Prednisolone may be used in patients who do not satisfactorily respond to anticholinesterase therapy. Thirty per cent remain in remission for up to 5 years following steroid treatment. Care should be taken as an exacerbation of symptoms is common 5–10 days after commencement. Alternate day dosage is used to reduce the incidence of drug induced complications.

Immunosuppressants other than steroids
Azothioprine. This drug appears useful in stabilising the disease and reducing the requirements for anticholinesterases. It is especially useful in patients who have proved refractory to steroids. Azothioprine therapy may take 6–12 months to produce a beneficial respone. The clincan must view the drug's advantages against complications of bone marrow suppression, hepatitis and/or other infection.

MYASTHENIA GRAVIS — TREATMENT *(contd)*

Thymectomy

When thymoma is not suspected, the benefits of thymectomy (20–30% remission, 50% improvement) must be weighed against the risk of sternotomy and postoperative respiratory difficulties in myasthenics.

Thymectomy seems to be of most benefit to young patients with generalised symptoms and a history of less than 5 years duration.

The transcervical operative approach is recommended by some; this procedure avoids splitting the sternum and has a lower operative morbidity, but this does not always achieve total thymectomy, thus reducing clinical benefit.

Plasmapheresis

In this procedure, the patient's plasma is 'exchanged' for albumin or another plasma expander. In this way IgG is removed and acetylcholine receptor antibody levels fall.

Several 'exchanges' are initially required and because of the 'rebound' of antibody levels after 2–3 weeks, either chronic intermittent exchange or simultaneous immunosuppressive therapy, e.g. steroids, azothioprine, is essential to maintain remission.

Plasmapheresis is probably most effective in producing short-term improvement and can be used in: 1. myasthenic crisis, 2. to improve clinical state before thymectomy, 3. to control exacerbation evoked by initiation of steroid therapy, 4. repeatedly in severely ill patients who might otherwise require prolonged hospitalisation.

SUMMARY OF TREATMENT

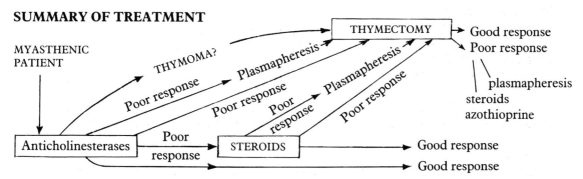

Anticholinesterases should not be required throughout the whole illness. When immunological control of the disease is obtained, these drugs may be stopped.

NEONATAL form of myasthenia gravis: this develops in a number of infants of myasthenic mothers.
— Suggested by poor crying/sucking and floppy limbs.
— Presents within 48 hours of birth and may persist until the end of 3rd month.
— Caused by passive transplacental passage of IgG (acetylcholine receptor antibodies).
— Treatment with anticholinesterases is required until spontaneous recovery occurs. Remission occurs following exchange transfusion.
This disorder may occur in infants even when their mother has been in remission for many years.

CONGENITAL form of myasthenia gravis.
This usually commences in infancy and persists through adult life. Receptor antibodies are not found and the disease may result from structural abnormalities of the receptors themselves. (A number of such disorders have been identified.)
Thymectomy is contraindicated in this disorder.

465

MULTIFOCAL NEUROLOGICAL DISEASE AND ITS MANAGEMENT

BACTERIAL INFECTIONS – MENINGITIS

ACUTE BACTERIAL MENINGITIS

Acute bacterial meningitis is an acute infection of the subarachnoid space and meninges characterised by polymorphonuclear cells in the cerebrospinal fluid. Bacteria may invade the subarachnoid space directly by spread from contiguous structures, e.g. sinuses, or more commonly, indirectly from the bloodstream.

Causative organisms

In neonates	— Gram -ve bacilli, e.g. *E. coli, Klebsiella.* *Haemophilus influenzae.*
In children	— *Haemophilus influenzae.* Pneumococcus (*Strep. pneumoniae*). Meningococcus. (*Neisseria meningitidis*).
In adults	— Pneumococcus. Meningococcus.

Other bacteria — *Listeria monocytogenes, Streptococcus pyogenes* and *Staphylococcus aureus* — are occasionally responsible.

Host factors (congenital or acquired immune deficiency, hyposplenism and alcoholism) predispose to infection.

Infections of mixed aetiology (two or more bacteria) may occur following head injury, mastoiditis or iatrogenically after lumbar puncture.

Pathology

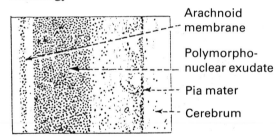

Arachnoid membrane

Polymorpho-nuclear exudate

Pia mater

Cerebrum

A purulent exudate most evident in the basal cisterns extends throughout the subarachnoid space.

The underlying brain, although not invaded by bacteria, becomes congested, oedematous and ischaemic.

The integrity of the pia mater protects against brain abscess formation.

The inflammatory exudate may affect vascular structures crossing the subarachnoid space producing an *arteritis* or *venous thrombophlebitis* with resultant *infarction*. Similarly, cranial nerves may suffer direct damage.

Hydrocephalus can result from obstruction to CSF flow in the ventricles and subarachnoid space.

Clinical

The classical clinical triad is fever, headache and neck stiffness.

Prodromal features (variable)
A respiratory infection
otitis media or pneumonia
associated with muscle pain
backache and lethargy.

Meningitic symptoms
Severe frontal/occipital headache
Stiff neck
Photophobia.

ACUTE BACTERIAL MENINGITIS

Clinical (*contd*)
Systemic signs:
– High fever. Transient erythematosus
  skin rash in meningococcal meningitis.

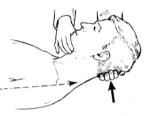

Meningitic signs:
Neck stiffness –
gentle flexion of
the neck is met
with boardlike
stiffness

Kernig's sign —
stretching the
lumbar roots
produces pain

Associated neurological signs
– Impaired conscious level (90%)
– Focal or generalised seizures are frequent.
– Cranial nerve signs occur in 15% of patients.
– Sensorineural deafness (not due to concurrent otitis media but to direct cochlear involvement) —
  20%
– Focal neurological signs — hemiparesis, dysphasia, hemianopia — occur in 10% of patients.

Non-neurological complications

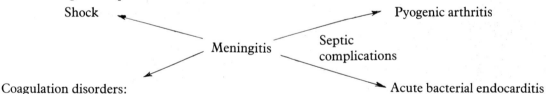

Shock

Pyogenic arthritis

Meningitis

Septic
complications

Coagulation disorders:
  Thrombocytopenia—disseminated intravascular coagulation.

Acute bacterial endocarditis

Features specific to causative bacteria

Haemophilus meningitis	*Meningococcal meningitis*	*Pneumococcal meningitis*
Generally occurs in small children. Preceding upper respiratory tract infection. Onset abrupt with a brief prodrome	Often occurs in epidemics where the organism is carried in the nasopharynx. Septicaemia can occur with arthralgia; purpuric skin rash. When overwhelming, confluent haemorrhages appear in the skin due to disseminated intravascular coagulation.	Predominantly an adult disorder. Usually associated with debilitation, e.g. alcoholism. May result from pneumonia middle ear sinus infection or follow splenectomy. Onset may be explosive, progressing to death within a few hours
Outcome Generally good Less than 5% mortality	Gradual onset — good prognosis Sudden onset with septicaemia — poor outcome Overall mortality — 10%	Mortality — 20%. Poor prognostic signs — coma, seizures, low cell count in CSF

469

ACUTE BACTERIAL MENINGITIS

Investigations

1. If patient is in coma or has papilloedema or focal neurological signs → exclude an intracranial mass with a *CT scan*. If the patient is deteriorating rapidly, take off blood cultures and commence antibiotics (see below) *prior* to scanning.
2. If above signs are absent or CT scan excludes a mass lesion → *confirm diagnosis with a lumbar puncture and identify the organism.*

CSF examination – moderate increase in pressure < 300 mmCSF.
    – Gram stain of spun-down sediment.

Gram +ve paired cocci = pneumococcus	Gram -ve bacilli = haemophilus	Gram -ve intra and extracellular cocci = meningococcus

– cell count is elevated, 100–10 000 cells/mm^3(80–90% polymorphonuclear leucocytes).
– glucose is depressed.
– enzyme lactic dehydrogenase is elevated.

Serological/immunological tests
    – countercurrent immunoelectrophoresis detects capsular antigen in CSF; leads to rapid diagnosis if CSF microscopy is unhelpful.

Blood cultures
    – *Haemophilus* isolated in 80% of cases of *Haemophilus meningitis*.
    – Pneumococcus and meningococcus in less than 50% of patients.
3. Check serum electrolytes.
    – important in view of the frequency of inappropriate antidiuretic hormone excretion in meningitis.
4. Detect the source of infection.
    Chest X-ray — pneumonia
    Sinus X-ray — sinusitis
    Skull X-ray — fracture
    Petrous views — mastoiditis

Treatment

Once meningitis is suspected, treatment must commence immediately, often before identification of the causative organism. Identification can be rapid if Gram stain is positive (70 – 80%), but this may depend on cultures or countercurrent immunoelectrophoresis.

Initial therapy (before organism identification)
    Neonates (above 1 month)   — ampicillin, 200 mg/kg/day i.v.
    Children (under 5 years)   — ampicillin, 200 mg/kg/day +
                                   chloramphenicol, 100 mg/kg/day i.v.
    Adults— penicillin G, 20 million units/day i.v.
            chloramphenicol, 2–4 g/day

ACUTE BACTERIAL MENINGITIS

Treatment (*contd*)
Therapy after organism identification

ORGANISM	ANTIBIOTIC	CHILD mg/kg/day	ADULT g/day	ALTERNATIVE THERAPY
Haemophilus	Chloramphenicol and/or	100	2–4	Ampicillin
	cefotaxime	200	6–12	Cefuroxime
Pneumococcus	Benzylpenicillin	180	20 million units	Chloramphenicol Cefotaxime Cefuroxime
Meningococcus	Benzylpenicillin	180	20 million units	Chloramphenicol Cetatamin
E. coli	Cefotaxime	200	6–12	Ampicillin Gentamicin
Listeria	Ampicillin ± gentamicin	200 5–7	8 (5–7 mg/kg/day)	Chloramphenicol Cotrimoxazole

Duration

Meningococcus ⎫
Haemophilus ⎬ continue for at least 1 week after afebrile.

Pneumococcus   — continue for 10–14 days after afebrile.

Remove any source of infection, e.g. mastoidectomy or sinus clearance.

In meningococcal meningitis the risk to household contacts is increased (500–800 x) and chemoprophylaxis should be offered — rifampicin 600 mg b.d. for 48 hours. Vaccines are also available.

Meningitis/CSF shunts

Meningitic infection may follow CSF drainage operations for hydrocephalus. This may occur in the immediate postoperative period or be delayed for weeks or months. Clinical features of raised intracranial pressure may coexist due to shunt blockage. Bacteraemia is inevitable and blood cultures identify the responsible organism — usually *Staphylococcus albus*. The infection seldom resolves with antibiotic therapy alone and shunt removal is usually required.

BACTERIAL INFECTIONS — CNS TUBERCULOSIS

Tuberculosis is an infection caused in man by one of two mycobacteria — *Mycobacterium tuberculosis* and *Mycobacterium bovis*. The disease involves the nervous system in less than 1% of patients.

MENINGITIS

This is the commonest manifestation of tuberculous infection of the nervous system. *In children,* it results from bacteraemia following the initial phase of primary pulmonary tuberculosis.

In adults, it may occur many years after the primary infection.

Following bacteraemia, metastatic foci of infection lodge in:
1. Meninges
2. Cerebral or spinal tissue
3. Choroid plexus

Rupture of these encapsulated foci

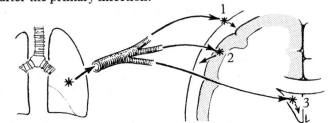

results in spread of infection into the subarachnoid space. In adults, reactivity of metastatic foci may occur spontaneously or result from impaired immunity (e.g. recent measles, alcohol abuse, administration of steroids).

The clinical features of tuberculous meningitis (TBM) result from:
— Infection.
— Exudation – which may obstruct the basal cisterns and result in hydrocephalus.
— Vasculitis – secondary to inflammation around vessels, resulting in infarction of brain and spinal cord.

The basal meninges are generally most severely affected.

Clinical features

The majority of patients are adults; childhood TBM is now rare.

Phase 1	Phase 2	Phase 3
Non-specific symptoms ➡	Confusion	➡ Coma
– Fever	Cranial nerve paresis	
– Lethargy	Meningism → Hemiparesis	
	Vasculitis Quadraparesis	
	Ataxia	
	Dysarthria	

Seizures may occur at the onset.

Atypically the illness may develop slowly over months presenting with dementia or rapidly like pyogenic (bacterial) meningitis. Occasionally cerebral features prevail rather than signs of meningitis.

Untreated, the illness may progress from phase 1 to death over a 3-week period.

Organisation of the inflammatory exudate may result in hydrocephalus/dementia/blindness.

TUBERCULOUS MENINGITIS

Investigations

General: Anaemia, leucocytosis. Hyponatraemia (if inappropriate ADH secretion is present).

Cerebrospinal fluid: A lymphocytic pleocytosis is usually present, though in acute cases polymorphonuclear cells may predominate — 500/mm^3.
   The protein is elevated — 100–400 mg/100 ml.
   The glucose level is usually less than two-thirds of simultaneously measured blood glucose.
   Microscopy (Ziehl Neelson stain) reveals acid-fast bacilli in 20% of patients.
   CSF culture (6 weeks in Lowenstein-Jensen medium) should confirm the diagnosis.

Chest X-ray: Reveals changes of old or recent tuberculosis in 50–70%.

PPD skin test (tuberculin): Positive to intermediate strength in 90%. Patients developing TBM while on steroids or with recently acquired primary tuberculosis may give a negative response.

Serum antibody tests: Lack specificity. Antigen agglutination tests look promising and are being evaluated.

CT scan: Shows meningeal enhancement on basal views, ventricular enlargement, associated infarction and tuberculomas in 10% (see page 346).

Diagnosis

Diagnosis is based on the clinical presentation with characteristic CSF findings. Even if Ziehl Neelsen staining is negative, in view of the progressive disease course do not await the results of cultures before starting treatment.

DIFFERENTIAL DIAGNOSIS of subacute/chronic meningitis (see pages 495, 496).

{
Viral meningoencephalitis (with *normal* CSF sugar).
Carcinomatous meningitis (with *high* CSF protein, *low* CSF sugar).
Partially treated bacterial meningitis.
Fungal meningitis. Sarcoidosis.
}

Treatment

If suspect, commence antituberculous treatment.
Recommended treatment programme:
Normal regime:

Isoniazid
Rifampicin   ——— 2 months ———>   Isoniazid   ———> 7 months
Pyrazinamide   Rifampicin

Drug resistance suspected due to previous antituberculous therapy, e.g.
   – Third World countries
   – History of previous infection.
→ Add a fourth drug — streptomycin or ethambutol.
   Isoniazid and pyrazinamide penetrate meninges well; other drugs penetrate less well especially when the inflammation begins to settle.

473

TUBERCULOUS MENINGITIS

Treatment *(contd)*

Side effects:
– Isoniazid may produce peripheral neuropathy — protect with pyridoxine 50 mg daily.
– Ethambutol may produce optic atrophy — check colour vision.
– Streptomycin may cause 8th cranial nerve damage.
– Nausea, vomiting, abnormal liver function and skin rashes may occur with all antituberculous drugs.

Intrathecal therapy: Since CSF penetration, especially with streptomycin, is poor, some recommend intrathecal treatment. Streptomycin 50 mg may be given daily or more frequently in seriously ill patients.

When an obstructive hydrocephalus occurs, combined intraventricular (through the shunt reservoir or drainage catheter) and lumbar intrathecal injections may be administered.

Steroid therapy: Many clinicians combine antituberculous therapy with steroids in the hope that these will minimise the risk of obliterative endarteritis and arachnoid adhesions. Although benefits are uncertain, steroids are recommended in patients with:
– deteriorating conscious level
– progressive neurological signs
– evidence of spinal block.

Hydrocephalus

Progressive dilatation of the ventricles impairing conscious level requires CSF drainage — either temporarily with a ventricular catheter (permitting intraventricular drug administration) or permanently with a ventriculoperitoneal/atrial shunt.

The course of treated tuberculous meningitis

Outcome is influenced by the patient's age, general state of health, timing of initiation of treatment and the development of arachnoiditis and vascular complications.

Treatment in early stages is associated with a 10% mortality, in later stages with a 50% mortality. Of those who survive, neurological sequelae persist in 30% — hemiplegia, hypothalamic/pituitary dysfunction, blindness, deafness, dementia and epilepsy.

With treatment, CSF sugar quickly returns to normal; the cellular reaction gradually diminishes over 3–4 months; the protein level may take a similar time to return to normal.

OTHER FORMS OF CNS TUBERCULOUS INFECTION

TUBERCULOMA
Tuberculomata may occur in cerebral hemispheres, cerebellum or brain stem with or without tuberculous meningitis, and may produce a space-occupying effect. Most resolve with antituberculous therapy. See page 473.

POTT'S DISEASE
Chronic epidural infection follows tuberculous osteomyelitis of the vertebral bodies. This arises in the lower thoracic region, can extend over several segments and may spread through the intervertebral foramen into pleura, peritoneum or psoas muscle (psoas abscess) — see page 388.

SPINAL ARACHNOIDITIS

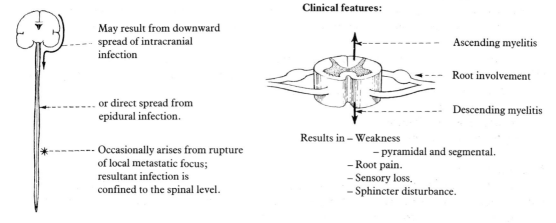

May result from downward spread of intracranial infection

or direct spread from epidural infection.

Occasionally arises from rupture of local metastatic focus; resultant infection is confined to the spinal level.

Clinical features:

Ascending myelitis

Root involvement

Descending myelitis

Results in – Weakness
          – pyramidal and segmental.
– Root pain.
– Sensory loss.
– Sphincter disturbance.

Diagnosis: Plain radiology, myelography and CSF examination.
Treatment: As for Pott's paraplegia
        – Surgical decompression if indicated and antituberculous treatment.

TUBERCULOUS ENCEPHALOPATHY
An autoimmune encephalopathy with features of acute allergic encephalomyelitis or haemorrhagic leukoencephalopathy (page 509) may complicate the course of tuberculous infection and contribute significantly to the neurological sequelae. Clinically, convulsions and deepening coma with extensor posturing characterise this complication.

TRANSVERSE MYELITIS
Transverse myelitis may occur during the successful treatment of tuberculosis and is not related to the usage of intrathecal therapy. It probably represents a delayed endarteritis.

SPIROCHAETAL INFECTIONS OF THE NERVOUS SYSTEM

SYPHILIS

This infectious disease is caused by the organism *Treponema pallidum*. Entry is by:
- inoculation through skin or mucous membrane (sexually transmitted) — acquired syphilis.
- transmission in utero — congenital syphilis.

The natural history of infection is divided into:

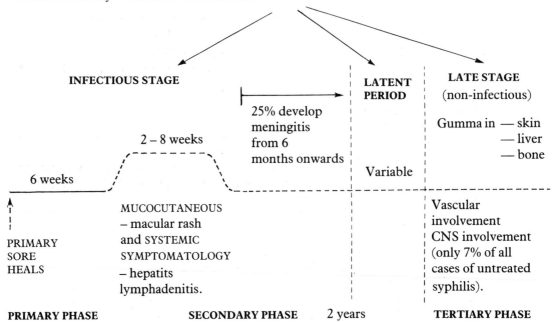

INFECTIOUS STAGE

6 weeks

2 – 8 weeks

25% develop
meningitis
from 6
months onwards

LATENT
PERIOD

Variable

LATE STAGE
(non-infectious)

Gumma in — skin
— liver
— bone

PRIMARY
SORE
HEALS

MUCOCUTANEOUS
– macular rash
and SYSTEMIC
SYMPTOMATOLOGY
– hepatits
lymphadenitis.

Vascular
involvement
CNS involvement
(only 7% of all
cases of untreated
syphilis).

PRIMARY PHASE   SECONDARY PHASE   2 years   TERTIARY PHASE

The *chancre* or *primary sore* on skin or mucous membrane represents the local tissue response to inoculation and is the first clinical event in acquired syphilis.

The organism, although present in all lesions, is more easily demonstrated in the primary and secondary phases.

In congenital syphilis fetal involvement can occur even though many years may elapse between conception and the mother's primary infection.

Widespread recognition and efficient treatment of the primary infection have greatly reduced the late or tertiary consequences.

Not all patients untreated in the secondary phase progress to the tertiary phase.

Investigations

Serological diagnosis depends on detection of antibodies.
1. Non-specific (Reagin) antibodies (IgG and IgM).
   Reagin tests involve complement fixation.
   The Venereal Disease Research Laboratory (VDRL) test is the commonest and when strongly positive indicates active disease.
2. Specific treponemal antibodies (do not differentiate between past and present infection).
   Fluorescent treponemal antibody absorption (FTA) test and
   Treponema immobilisation (TPI) test.

SPIROCHAETAL INFECTION — NEUROSYPHILIS

The initial event in neurosyphilis is meningitis. Of all untreated patients 25% develop an acute symptomatic syphilitic meningitis within 2 years of the primary infection.

ACUTE SYPHILITIC MENINGITIS: Three clinical forms are recognised:

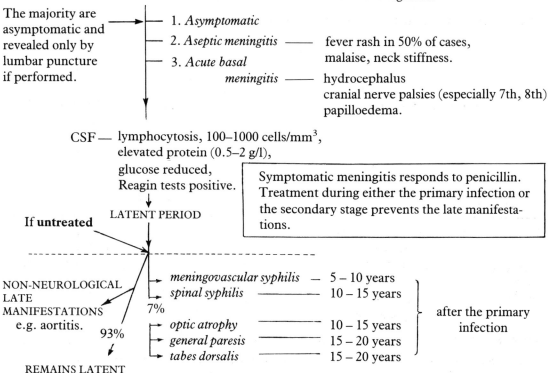

The majority are asymptomatic and revealed only by lumbar puncture if performed.

1. *Asymptomatic*
2. *Aseptic meningitis* —— fever rash in 50% of cases, malaise, neck stiffness.
3. *Acute basal meningitis* —— hydrocephalus cranial nerve palsies (especially 7th, 8th) papilloedema.

CSF — lymphocytosis, 100–1000 cells/mm^3, elevated protein (0.5–2 g/l), glucose reduced, Reagin tests positive.

LATENT PERIOD

If **untreated**

Symptomatic meningitis responds to penicillin. Treatment during either the primary infection or the secondary stage prevents the late manifestations.

NON-NEUROLOGICAL LATE MANIFESTATIONS e.g. aortitis. 93%

7%

REMAINS LATENT

meningovascular syphilis — 5 – 10 years
spinal syphilis —————— 10 – 15 years

optic atrophy —————— 10 – 15 years
general paresis —————— 15 – 20 years
tabes dorsalis —————— 15 – 20 years

after the primary infection

Late neurological complications occur in only 7% of **untreated** cases.

These forms are exceptionally rare and the clinical syndromes mentioned above seldom occur in a 'pure' form.

MENINGOVASCULAR SYPHILIS
'Early' late manifestation resulting in an obliterative endarteritis and periarteritis.

Presents as a 'stroke' in a young person — hemisphere, brain stem or spinal. Granulations around the base of the brain may produce cranial nerve palsies or even hydrocephalus.

CSF — lymphocytes 100/mm^3, protein ↑, gammaglobulin ↑, positive serology. Penicillin arrests progression.

SPINAL SYPHILIS
Chronic meningitis with subpial damage to the spinal cord.

Presents as a progressive paraplegia, occasionally with radicular pain and wasting in upper limbs — ERB's PARAPLEGIA. CSF — as meningovascular syphilis. Penicillin arrests progression.

OPTIC ATROPHY
Meningitis around optic nerve with subpial necrosis may be the only manifestation of late syphilis.
Presents as a constriction of the visual fields with a progressive pallor of the optic disc:
  – if both eyes are affected, the vision is rarely saved.
  – if only one eye is involved, treatment with penicillin will save the other.

SPIROCHAETAL INFECTION — NEUROSYPHILIS

GENERAL PARESIS

Characterised by dementia — with memory impairment, disordered judgement and disturbed affect — manic behaviour, delusions of grandeur (rare).

There are two phases:
1. Pre-paralytic — with progressive dementia.
2. Paralytic — when corticospinal and extrapyramidal symptoms and signs develop associated with involuntary movements (myoclonus).

Argyll Robertson pupils may be present (see page 133).

At autopsy, meningeal thickening, brain atrophy and perivascular infiltration with plasma cells and lymphocytes are evident; culture from the cortex may reveal an occasional treponema.

CSF — lymphocytes 50/mm^3, protein ↑ 0.5–2 g/l, gammaglobulin ↑.
Reagin tests in CSF positive in the majority.
Treatment in the preparalytic phase will halt progression in 40%.

TABES DORSALIS

Posterior spinal root and posterior column dysfunction – – – – – – – – – – – – →
account for symptoms.

Pupillary abnormality (Argyll Robertson) and optic atrophy occur. Peripheral reflexes are lost and joint position and vibration sensation is impaired. A positive Romberg's test (page 178) indicates a sensory ataxia.

Pain loss results in trophic lesions and occasionally a Charcot joint may develop. – – – – – – – – – – – – →
Urinary incontinence, impotence and constipation also occur. 'Lightning pains', visceral crises (abdominal pain/diarrhoea) and rectal crises (tenesmus) are frequent.

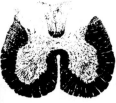

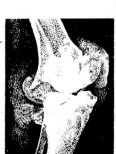

Repeated trauma to an insensitive joint results in 'painless' osteoarthritis and joint destruction.

The CSF is more normal than in general paresis. The Reagin test may be negative in 30 per cent. Treatment may produce some improvement; it will not reverse joint destruction.

SYPHILITIC GUMMA presenting as an intracranial mass is extremely rare.

SYPHILIS AND HIV INFECTION

In syphilis the role of cell-mediated immunity is uncertain. However, in AIDS, disturbed T-cell function results in accelerated drug-resistant forms of neurosyphilis.

Treatment of neurosyphilis

Penicillin G. ——— 2–4 megaunits i.v.
or   4-hourly for 10 days.
Procaine Penicillin — 600 000 units i.m.
                       daily for 15 days.
Benzathine Penicillin – 2–4 megaunits i.m. weekly x 3.

(When patient sensitive to penicillin
↓
erythromycin or
tetracycline may be given
orally over 30 days.)

The Jarisch-Herxheimer reaction — tachycardia/fever — occurs in one-third of patients within a few hours of commencing treatment; it is believed to be due to endotoxin release from killed organisms. Steroids should counter the reaction, especially in tertiary syphilis.
CSF follow up: CSF is checked initially and at 6 monthly intervals until normal.
Cell count and degree of positivity of VDRL are the best indicators of persistent infection.

SPIROCHAETAL INFECTIONS

LYME DISEASE

This is a disorder caused by the spirochaete *Borrelia Burgdorferi,* characterised by relapsing and remitting arthralgia associated with a characteristic skin rash *(erythema chronicum nigrans)* and neurological features. The organism, related to the treponemes, is prevalent throughout Europe and North America and is carried by ixodid ticks.

Clinical features

Only a minority of persons bitten by an infected tick develop the disease. Spirochaetocidal activity in normal serum and the immune response normally provide protection.

Stage 1: Spring/summer —

Tick bite → flu-like symptoms, arthralgia and skin rash (erythema chronicum nigrans).
Treatment with antibiotics is usually curative.

Untreated and small
number of treated patients.

Stage 2: Several weeks/months later —

Subacute lymphocytic meningitis — both illnesses are often mild, clear
Subacute encephalitis   spontaneously and occasionally are
     unrecognised.

Cranial nerve involvement — Facial nerve palsy with or without
     subacute lymphocytic meningitis.

Peripheral neuropathy — Subacute demyelinating and axonal sensory/motor
     neuropathy associated with severe root pain
     (radiculitis).

CSF examination in stage 2: Lymphocytosis   Elevated immunglobulins.
     Oligoclonal bands.   Elevated *anti*Burgdorferi antibodies.

An unknown proportion progress.

Stage 3: Several months/years later —

Arthritis

Diffuse CNS involvement — chronic/subacute encephalitis.
     — focal brain disease.

Diagnosis

     — *psychiatric* disease.

Antibody tests

– Immunofluorescence assay (IFA)
– Enzyme-linked immunoabsorbent assay (ELISA).

In endemic areas less than 5% of asymptomatic persons are positive, although with lower titres than symptomatic patients.

In patients from endemic areas:

with meningitis/CN palsy ⎤ diagnosis is definite, but
encephalitis/radiculitis ⎥ in stage 3 this is often
+CSF profile   ⎬ uncertain and blind trials
+positive serology   ⎦ of therapy are given.

Treatment

Stage 1 — Oral antibiotics: penicillin, erythromycin or tetracycline.
Stage 2 — I.v. penicillin G. 20 million units for 10 days (or cefotaxime).
Stage 3 — as stage 2.

If symptoms persist – wrong diagnosis with misleading titres, or
     – immune mediated damage.

SPIROCHAETAL INFECTIONS

LEPTOSPIROSIS

Leptospira interrogans is transmitted to man in the infected urine of wild and domestic animal carriers. Subclinical infection commonly occurs in high-risk occupations, e.g. sewer workers. Symptomatic illness is usually mild and only 10% of patients develop jaundice and haemorrhagic complications (Weil's disease).

Clinical features

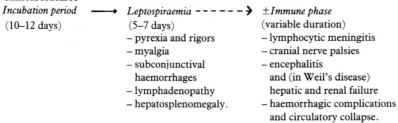

Incubation period ⟶ *Leptospiraemia* - - - - - → *±Immune phase*

(10–12 days)	(5–7 days)	(variable duration)
	– pyrexia and rigors	– lymphocytic meningitis
	– myalgia	– cranial nerve palsies
	– subconjunctival	– encephalitis
	haemorrhages	and (in Weil's disease)
	– lymphadenopathy	hepatic and renal failure
	– hepatosplenomegaly.	– haemorrhagic complications
		and circulatory collapse.

Diagnosis

Serological tests (complement fixation).

Treatment

The disease is usually self limiting and therapy unnecessary. In severe illness the role of antibiotics is unproven and support of renal/hepatic failure and management of haemorrhagic complications may be life saving.

PARASITIC INFECTIONS OF THE NERVOUS SYSTEM: PROTOZOA

TOXOPLASMOSIS
A world-wide parasitic infection affecting many species, including man.

Organism: An anaerobic intracellular protozoan, *Toxoplasma gondii*.
The majority of infections in man are asymptomatic (30% of the population have specific antibodies indicating previous exposure).

In the host

Organism - - - → 🦠 Multiplies and → 🦠 → Bloodstream → To involve organs
enters RE cell   cell ruptures   Lymphatics   e.g. liver, spleen, CNS, eye.

Transmission: Eating uncooked meat or contact with faeces of an infected dog or cat.

There are two forms of toxoplasmosis:

CONGENITAL — when a previously unaffected woman contracts infection during pregnancy (subclinical infection); transplacental spread results in fetal infection.

Premature delivery occurs in 25%.

Neurological complications:
 – hydrocephalus,
 – aqueduct stenosis,
 – microcephaly.
Non-neurological features:
 – skin rash, jaundice, hepatosplenomegaly, choroidoretinitis.
Skull X-ray shows:
 – curvilinear calcification (basal ganglion and periventricular regions).
 Varying degrees of organ involvement may occur.
The only manifestation may be choroidoretinitis in an otherwise healthy child.

ACQUIRED — symptomatic infection is uncommon and may be associated with underlying systemic disease or immunosuppression.

Fever and fatigue with muscle weakness and lymphadenopathy result. Abnormal lymphocytes in peripheral blood leads to confusion with *infectious mononucleosis*. The neurological features are those of a meningoencephalitis with focal signs and depressed conscious level. CT scan shows characteristic contrast ring enhancing lesions. Choroidoretinitis occasionally occurs.

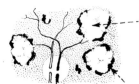

Areas of atrophic choroid, exposing the white sclera.

Retinal pigment epithelium becomes hyperplastic – densely pigmented areas result.

Diagnosis:
Organisms are seldom identified.
 Sabin Feldman Dye Test may demonstrate a rising titre.
 Complement fixation antibody test may provide a positive result.
N.B. Rubella, cytomegalovirus and herpes simplex can also spread transplacentally and cause jaundice and hepatosplenomegaly. Cytomegalovirus may also produce choroidoretinitis and intracranial calcification.

Treatment
Sulphadiazine and pyrimethamine (Dapaprim) for 3 weeks or longer in immunocompromised patients.
Give steroids when choroidoretinitis is present.

MALARIA
Plasmodium falciparum, the agent of malignant tertiary malaria, is responsible for *cerebral malaria*. Confusion, focal signs, convulsions and coma occur. Overall mortality is 10%. Complete recovery without sequelae is expected in survivors. Treatment is supportive.

481

VIRAL INFECTIONS

General principles

Invasion of the nervous system may occur as part of a generalised viral infection. Occasionally nervous system involvement is disproportionately severe and symptoms of generalised infection are slight.

Viruses enter the body through the: *respiratory tract,*
gastrointestinal tract,
genitourinary tract or by
inoculation through the skin.

Viral entry

— previous exposure ⟶ patient's IgA neutralises the virus

— no previous exposure ⟶ VIRAEMIA

Routes of spread to CNS

⟶ Massive viraemia ⟶ overcomes monocyte and reticuloendothelial defence systems ⟶ Invades CNS via capillaries and veins

⟶ Infection along peripheral nerves ⟶ Invades CNS

After CNS penetration, the clinical picture depends upon the particular virus and the cells of the nervous system which show a specific susceptibility.

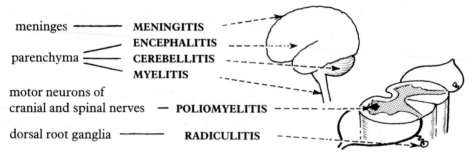

meninges — **MENINGITIS**

parenchyma — **ENCEPHALITIS**
CEREBELLITIS
MYELITIS

motor neurons of cranial and spinal nerves — **POLIOMYELITIS**

dorsal root ganglia — **RADICULITIS**

Some viruses cause a chronic, progressive infection, others remain dormant for many years within the nervous system before becoming symptomatic.

MENINGITIS

Meningitis is the commonest viral infection of the central nervous system. *Aseptic meningitis* includes viral meningitis as well as other forms of meningitis where routine culture reveals no other organisms.

Common causal viruses —
ENTEROVIRUSES
MUMPS VIRUS
HERPES SIMPLEX (subtype 2)
EPSTEIN-BARR VIRUS

Rare causal viruses —
LYMPHOCYTIC CHORIOMENINGITIS
HUMAN IMMUNODEFICIENCY VIRUS

VIRAL INFECTIONS — MENINGITIS

Clinical features of acute aseptic meningitis

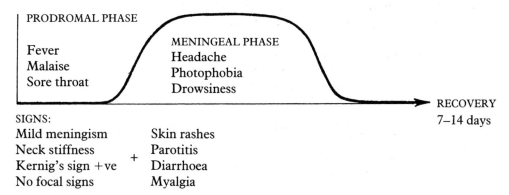

PRODROMAL PHASE

Fever
Malaise
Sore throat

MENINGEAL PHASE
Headache
Photophobia
Drowsiness

RECOVERY
7–14 days

SIGNS:

Mild meningism   Skin rashes
Neck stiffness   Parotitis
Kernig's sign +ve + Diarrhoea
No focal signs   Myalgia

Enterovirus infection — affects children/young adults and occurs seasonally in late summer.
    Spread is by the faecal/oral route.
    Accounts for 80% of cases in USA.
Mumps — affects children/young adults. Winter/spring incidence. Commonest world-wide cause.
Herpes simplex (type 2) — accounts for 5% of viral meningitis. Develops in 25% of patients
    with primary genital infection (suspect in sexually active adults).
Lymphocytic choriomeningitis — affects any age and is a consequence of airborne spread
    from rodent droppings.
Human Immunodeficiency Virus (HIV) — suspect in high risk groups (page 493) with meningitis.
    HIV antibodies are often absent and develop 1–3 months later during convalescence.

Investigations
CSF, obtained early, often contains recoverable virus. The CSF cell count is elevated
(lymphocytes or monocytes). Virus may be cultured from throat swabs or stool. Serological tests
on serum in acute and convalescent phases are especially valuable in detecting mumps and herpes
simplex (type 2).

Differential diagnosis
From other causes of an aseptic meningitis which are usually subacute or chronic in onset:
    – *Tuberculous* or *fungal* meningitis
    – *Leptospirosis*
    – *Sarcoidosis*
    – *Carcinomatous* meningitis
    – Partially treated *bacterial* meningitis
    – *Parameningeal* chronic infection which evokes a meningeal response, e.g. mastoiditis.
    The self-limiting and mild nature of viral meningitis should not lead to confusion with these
more serious disorders.

Prognosis is excellent and **treatment** symptomatic.
In severe herpes simplex meningitis, intravenous acyclovir may benefit.

VIRAL INFECTIONS — PARENCHYMAL

Viruses may act:

directly → acute viral encephalitis or meningoencephalitis,

after a latent period → 'slow' virus encephalitis,

or *indirectly via the immune system* → allergic or postinfectious encephalomyelitis,

postvaccinial encephalomyelitis.

Also, an encephalopathy may develop during the course of a viral illness in which inflammation is not a pathological feature — REYE'S SYNDROME.

ACUTE VIRAL ENCEPHALITIS

Viral infection causes neuronal and glial damage with associated inflammation and oedema. Viral encephalitis is a worldwide disorder with the highest incidence in the tropics.

Common causal viruses:

World-wide:

— Mumps

— Herpes simplex

— Varicella zoster

— Epstein-Barr

Specific areas:

Western equine — (vector) mosquito — USA

West Nile — (vector) mosquito — Africa/India

Russian spring summer — (vector) tick — eastern Europe

Encephalitis following childhood infections — measles, varicella, rubella — is presumed *postinfectious* and not due to direct viral invasion, though the measles virus has occasionally been isolated from the brain.

Clinical features:

Signs and symptoms:

General: pyrexia, myalgia, etc.

Specific to causative virus, e.g. features of infectious mononucleosis.

Meningeal involvement (slight) → neck stiffness, cellular response in CSF.

Signs and symptoms of parenchymal involvement – focal and/or diffuse.

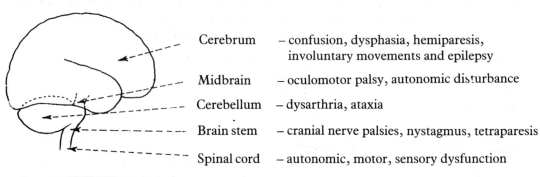

Cerebrum – confusion, dysphasia, hemiparesis, involuntary movements and epilepsy

Midbrain – oculomotor palsy, autonomic disturbance

Cerebellum – dysarthria, ataxia

Brain stem – cranial nerve palsies, nystagmus, tetraparesis

Spinal cord – autonomic, motor, sensory dysfunction

In general, the illness lasts for some weeks.

Prognosis is uncertain and depends on the causal virus,

e.g. herpes simplex — 20% mortality.

mumps — 2% mortality.

Neurological sequelae are likewise variable.

VIRAL INFECTIONS — PARENCHYMAL

HERPES SIMPLEX ENCEPHALITIS
Two subgroups of herpes simplex virus (HSV) are recognised:
1. Type I, responsible for oral and labial rashes as well as ENCEPHALITIS.
2. Type II, responsible for genital and neonatal infection as well as MENINGITIS.

   Most cases of encephalitis result from reactivation of the virus rather than from primary infection.

Clinical features
A world-wide disorder occurring during all seasons and affecting all ages.

   General symptoms at onset — headache, fever — with evolution over several days to seizures and impaired conscious level.

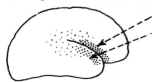

Inferior frontal and temporal lobes are selectively involved and signs and symptoms reflect this – olfactory or gustatory hallucinations, behavioural disturbance, complex partial seizures, dysphasia (dominant hemisphere) and hemiparesis.

Cerebral oedema may result in tentorial herniation.
In those who recover, a profound memory disturbance may be evident.

Investigations
CT scan shows low attenuation in the inferior frontal and temporal lobes – – → unless haemorrhage has occurred into necrotic regions. In early stages, the CT scan may be normal; in those patients an isotope brain scan may detect an area of increased uptake.

   CSF examination reveals 5–500 lymphocytes but the protein is only mildly elevated and the glucose is normal. CSF pressure may be raised.

   EEG examination shows generalised slowing with bursts of 'periodic' high voltage slow wave complexes over the involved temporal lobe.

N.B. In some patients only serial investigations may demonstrate the characteristic changes.

   Serological tests on acute and convalescent serum should eventually identify HSV infection. A fall in the *intrathecal herpes simplex immunoglobulin (IgM or IgG) antibody synthesis* results in a low CSF/serum ratio after 10–12 days, also providing late evidence of infection.

Differential diagnosis   Consider: — other forms of encephalitis
                                          — cerebral abscess
Diagnosis   — brain tumour.
Only biopsy can confirm the diagnosis in the acute phase.

This shows evidence of a necrotising encephalitis with intranuclear eosinophilic inclusion bodies

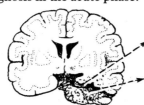

Demostrate herpes simplex antigen by immunofluorescence.

Isolate virus by culture (positive in 48 hours).

Treatment
Acyclovir (30 mg/kg/day) is given in divided dosage (to avoid renal toxicity) for at least 10 days.

   This treatment has reduced mortality from 70% to 20% with a similar reduction in neurological sequelae (memory disturbance, etc.).

   Since acyclovir is relatively non-toxic, many now advocate treatment with only CT or EEG evidence of HSV encephalitis.

485

VIRAL INFECTIONS

REYE'S SYNDROME
This rare encephalopathy, associated with fatty changes in the liver and other viscera, is almost exclusively confined to children. It occurs after viral or, rarely, bacterial infection and immunisation.

Incidence
1 per 100 000 children per year. Commoner in rural comunities.
Outbreaks described with certain virus infections — influenza A, B and varicella.

Pathology
Neurons and glial cells are swollen; the liver, heart and kidney show fatty infiltration.

Pathogenesis
Viral synergism with an environmental factor, e.g. salicylates, may be responsible.

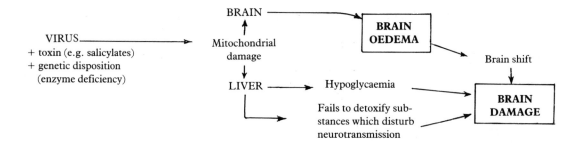

Clinical features

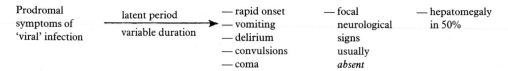

| Prodromal symptoms of 'viral' infection | latent period variable duration | — rapid onset — vomiting — delirium — convulsions — coma | — focal neurological signs usually *absent* | — hepatomegaly in 50% |

Death results from raised intracranial pressure.

Investigations
– Raised liver enzymes
– Elevated serum ammonia
– Hypoglycaemia (in infants)
– Prolonged prothrombin time
– Increase in serum fatty acids

Differential diagnosis
Consider other causes of raised intracranial pressure in childhood, especially
  – lead encephalopathy,
  – lateral sinus thrombosis, e.g. following mastoiditis.

Treatment
Treatment aims at lowering intracranial pressure with the aid of intracranial pressure monitoring (see page 50). In addition, blood glucose must be maintained and any associated coagulopathy treated.

Prognosis
Early diagnosis and supportive treatment has reduced the mortality from 80% to 30%.
   When raised intracranial pressure is present, mortality increases to 50% and a high proportion of survivors have cognitive disorders.

   A condition similar to Reye's syndrome occurs in some children with family history of 'sudden infant death'. A deficiency of medium chain acetyl-CoA dehydrogenase (an enzyme essential for fatty acid metabolism) is found. Carnitine deficiency results as a consequence of 'alternative pathway' fatty acid metabolism. *Siblings of children with Reye's syndrome should be screened for this disorder.*

VIRAL INFECTIONS — CHRONIC DISORDERS

In these disorders the virus infection results in a chronic progressive neurological condition.
The evidence of a
viral etiology is: *direct*   finding of inclusion bodies,
   and   demonstration of viral particles,
      isolation of virus,
   indirect   relationship of onset of symptoms to a preceding viral illness,
      transmission of illness from one host to the next.

Not all these features are present in any one illness.

SUBACUTE SCLEROSING PANENCEPHALITIS (SSPE)
Caused by measles-like *paramyxovirus* — isolated from brain biopsy.

Clinical features: A world-wide disorder. Incidence: 1 per million per year. Onset: between ages 7 – 10 years.

Stage 1	*Stage 2*	*Stage 3*
Behavioural problem	Chorioretinitis,	Lapses into rigid
Declining school performance	Myoclonic jerks	comatose state.
Progression → dementia.	Seizures, ataxia	
	Dystonia.	

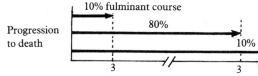

Progression to death

10% fulminant course
80%
10% – in this group, periods of stabilisation and even improvement may transiently occur.

3 months   3 years   4 – 10 years

The illness may occur after measles vaccination or following clinical infection at an early age (under 2 years).
Accompanying features of infection, i.e. pyrexia, leucocytosis, are *absent*.

Investigations

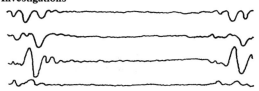

CSF examination shows elevated γ globulin with IgG oligoclonal bands; elevated measles antibodies (75% of total CSF IgG).

Blood examination shows elevated serum measles antibodies.

EEG – shows periodic high voltage slow wave complexes on a low voltage background trace.

Pathology
Changes involve both white and grey matter, especially in the posterior hemispheres. Brain stem, cerebellum and spinal cord are also affected.
    Oligodendrocytes contain eosinophilic inclusion bodies. Marked gliosis occurs with perivascular lymphocyte and plasma cell cuffing.

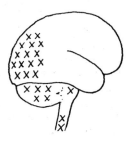

Treatment: There is no effective treatment. Since the introduction of measles vaccination there has been a marked reduction of SSPE.

Subacute measles encephalitis may follow measles infection in children on *immunosuppressive drug treatment* or with *hypogammaglobulinaemia*. The clinical course is different however from SSPE and EEG and CSF findings are less specific.

487

VIRAL INFECTIONS — CHRONIC PARENCHYMAL DISORDERS

PROGRESSIVE RUBELLA PANENCEPHALITIS
Similar to SSPE with a fatal outcome, caused by rubella virus.

Presents at a later age (10–15 years). .

Progressive dementia.

Ataxia. Spasticity. Myoclonus.

Treatment: No effective treatment

CSF shows high γ globulin.

EEG does *not* show periodic complexes of SSPE.

Antibodies elevated in serum and CSF to rubella.

Biopsy does *not* show inclusion bodies.

CREUTZFELDT-JAKOB DISEASE
Spongiform encephalopathic changes characterise this disorder, which presents as presenile dementia.

Incidence: 1 per million per year.   10 – 15% of cases are familial.   **Onset:** 5th to 6th decade.

Clinical course: Three phases are recognised.

1. *Prodromal*
   Vague onset
   Unsteadiness
   Memory disturbance
   Visual symptoms.

2. *Progressive*
   Progressing dementia
   Ataxia, corticospinal signs
   Visual loss (cortical)
   Myoclonus, chorea
   Muscle wasting (amyotrophy).

3. *Terminal*
   Mute, profoundly demented
   80% die within 12 months
   of onset.

Investigation
CSF — usually normal.

EEG — bilateral high voltage sharp waves on a
background of slow wave activity.

   The clinical picture and electroencephalogram suggest the
diagnosis only ultimately confirmed at postmortem.

Pathology
Moderate to severe atrophy occurs.
Frontal lobes are most affected
then parietal and occipital lobes
      then cerebellum
      and anterior horn
      cells in spinal cord.

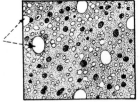

Vacuolation

Microscopically — Neuronal degeneration occurs with marked astrocytic proliferation.
Vacuolation of glial cells results in a characteristic spongiform appearance.

Aetiology
The realisation that other disorders characterised by spongiform changes were transmissible — KURU (a degenerative disorder found in New Guinea associated with cannibalism), BOVINE SPONGIFORM ENCEPHALOPATHY and SCRAPIE (a disorder in sheep) — led to the demonstration of transmission in Creutzfeldt-Jakob disease. Following primate inoculation, an illness characterised by confusion, ataxia and amyotrophy developed in 12–18 months.

   The mode of transmission in humans is unclear; it has been documented following corneal grafting and depth electrode implantation in neurosurgery, but does not appear communicable in that conjugal cases are unknown.

   Care should be taken in handling material from patients.

Treatment
There is no treatment.
Antiviral drugs are of no benefit.

POSTVIRAL OR ACUTE DISSEMINATED ENCEPHALOMYELITIS (see page 508)
PROGRESSIVE MULTIFOCAL LEUKOENCEPHALOPATHY (see page 509).

VIRAL INFECTIONS — MYELITIS AND POLIOMYELITIS

MYELITIS

Transverse myelitis is rare. It can occur in association with measles, mumps, Epstein-Barr, herpes zoster/simplex or enterovirus infections. Fever, back and limb pain precede paralysis, sensory loss and bladder disturbance. Initially paralised limbs are flaccid, but over 1–2 weeks spasticity and extensor plantar responses develop.

Investigations

Myelography when performed is normal. MRI may demonstrate focal cord signal changes. CSF shows elevated protein with a neutrophil or lymphocytic response. Serological tests will identify the causal virus.

Treatment

Supportive; the place of steroids remains unproven. About 30% recover fully; deficits of varying severity persist in the remainder.

It is not clear whether the pathological effects (perivenous demyelination) result from direct or delayed (immunological) reactions to the virus.

POLIOMYELITIS

An acute viral infection in which the anterior horn cells of the spinal cord and motor nuclei of the brain stem are selectively involved.

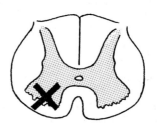

Causative viruses:

The poliovirus is an enterovirus (RNA virus).
  Three immunologically distinct strains have been isolated.
Immunity to one does *not* result in immunity to the other two.
  Coxsackie and echoviruses may produce a clinically identical disorder.

Pathology

Initially — inflammatory meningeal changes, followed by — inflammatory cell infiltration (polymorphs and lymphocytes) around the brain stem nuclei and anterior horn cells. Neurons may undergo necrosis or central chromatolysis.
Microglial proliferation follows.

Mode of spread

Spread by faecal/oral route. Once ingested the virus multiplies in the nasopharynx and gastrointestinal tract.

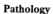

Penetration of GI tract results in viraemia but CNS involvement occurs in only a very small proportion. Most infected patients are asymptomatic. Virus excretion continues in the faeces for as long as three months after the initial infection — carrier state.

Epidemiology

A highly communicable disease which may result in epidemics.
Seasonal incidence — late summer/autumn.
World-wide distribution, although more frequent in northern temperate climates.
Prophylactic vaccination has produced a dramatic reduction in incidence in the last 25 years. In developing countries without a vaccination programme, the disease remains a problem.

Clinical features

Infection may result in:
  – Subclinical course + resultant immunity (majority)
  – Mild non-specific symptoms of viraemia + resultant immunity
  – Meningism without paralysis
    (PREPARALYTIC) + resultant immunity
  – Meningism followed by paralysis
    (PARALYTIC) + resultant immunity.

489

VIRAL INFECTIONS — POLIOMYELITIS

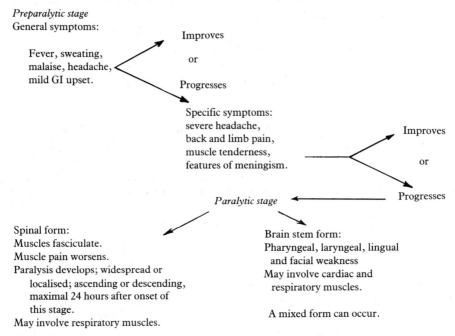

Preparalytic stage
General symptoms:

Fever, sweating,
malaise, headache,
mild GI upset.

Improves

or

Progresses

Specific symptoms:
severe headache,
back and limb pain,
muscle tenderness,
features of meningism.

Improves

or

Progresses

Paralytic stage

Spinal form:
Muscles fasciculate.
Muscle pain worsens.
Paralysis develops; widespread or
    localised; ascending or descending,
    maximal 24 hours after onset of
    this stage.
May involve respiratory muscles.

Brain stem form:
Pharyngeal, laryngeal, lingual
    and facial weakness
May involve cardiac and
    respiratory muscles.

A mixed form can occur.

Diagnosis
During the meningeal phase, consider other causes of acute meningitis.
    Once the paralytic phase ensues, distinguish from the Guillain-Barré syndrome and transverse myelitis.
    The clinical picture + CSF examination (polymorphs and lymphocytes increased; protein elevated with normal glucose) are sufficient to reach the diagnosis.
    Serological tests + virus isolation will confirm later.

Prognosis
In epidemics, a mortality of 25% results from respiratory paralysis. Improvement in muscle power usually commences one week after the onset of paralysis and continues for up to a year.
    Only a proportion of muscles remain permanently paralysed; in these, fasciculation may persist.
In affected limbs, bone growth becomes retarded with shortening as well as thinning.

Treatment
The patient is kept on bed rest and fluid balance carefully maintained.
    Respiratory failure may require ventilation.
    Avoid the development of deformities in affected limbs with physiotherapy and splinting.

Prophylaxis

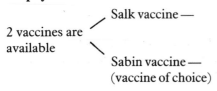

2 vaccines are
available

Salk vaccine — Formalin inactivated virus. 2 injections, 1 month apart, are followed by booster at 6 months; this prevents CNS invasion, but does not stop viraemia.

Sabin vaccine — Live attenuated virus given orally and will simulate
(vaccine of choice) subclinical infection. 3 doses 2 months apart.

VIRAL INFECTIONS — VARICELLA-ZOSTER INFECTION

Varicella (chickenpox) and herpes zoster (shingles) are different clinical manifestations of infection by the same virus — a DNA virus, VARICELLA ZOSTER.

Varicella may cause: — an acute encephalitis — postinfectious encephalomyelitis
                — viral meningitis   —postinfectious polyneuropathy
                                   (Guillain-Barré syndrome).

Herpes zoster is due to reactivation of the virus, dormant years after the primary infection (chickenpox).

Pathology: The virus involves the *dorsal root* (sensory) ganglion of the spinal cord or the *cranial nerve* sensory ganglion – trigeminal or geniculate. 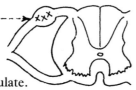 The inflammatory process may spread into the spinal cord and involve posterior and anterior horns. Similarly inflammatory changes may occur in the brain stem.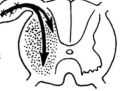

Haemorrhage occurs with neural loss and intense lymphocytic infiltration.

Clinical features

Most cases occur in patients over 50 years of age. Both sexes are affected equally. Recurrent attacks are rare.

Occurs more frequently in association with disorders in which immunity is disturbed, e.g. lymphoma. Also associated with spinal/nerve root trauma.

Initial feature: A vesicular skin rash associated with a burning, painful sensation. Vesicles contain clear fluid and conform to a *dermatome distribution*. After 1–3 weeks, the vesicles crust over and leave irregular skin depigmentation with scarring. The distribution of lesious reflects the particular nerve root involved.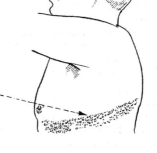

Motor weakness occurs in 20% due to spread of inflammation into the anterior horn cell territory. More widespread spinal (myelitis) or encephalic involvement can occur. In immunosuppressed patients extensive cutaneous lesions are common (disseminated zoster). Cranial nerve ganglia involvement:

– Trigeminal: usually ophthalmic division with vesicles above the eye and associated corneal ulceration — HERPES ZOSTER OPHTHALMICUS. Occasionally patients develop a contralateral hemiparesis due to a necrotising granulomatous angiitis involving the carotid artery and its branches.

– Geniculate: vesicles within the external auditory meatus and ear drum with a lower motor neuron VII nerve palsy — RAMSAY HUNT SYNDROME.

Diagnosis   Based on clinical features. CSF examination reveals a lymphocytic response.

Treatment

This depends on the severity and location of skin lesions. Mild disease requires symptomatic treatment only. Severe disease, involvement in immunodeficient patients, or ophthalmic vesicles require acyclovir (7.5 mg/kg slowly i.v. 3 times per day for 7 days).

POST HERPETIC NEURALGIA

This is a condition which occurs in 10% of all patients. The incidence rises with age. A chronic, uncomfortable, burning pain presents in the territory of the involved dermatome. Touching the skin may evoke severe, lancinating pains. The pathogenesis is unknown.

Treatment with antidepressants, anticonvulsants, e.g. carbamazepine, transcutaneous stimulation (TCS) or sympathetic ganglion block may help, but results are unpredictable.

OPPORTUNISTIC INFECTIONS

These infections occur in immunocompromised patients. Certain types of immunological deficiency tend to be associated with specific forms of infection.

	T cell/macrophage deficiency	*B cell immunoglobulin deficiency*	*Granulocyte deficiency*
Causal Diseases:	e.g. AIDS Lymphoreticular tumours Immunosuppressant drugs	Chronic lymphatic leukaemia Primary hypogammaglobulinaemia Splenectomy	Marrow infiltration Aplastic anaemia Chemotherapy/ radiotherapy
Organisms:			
Viruses –	Cytomegalovirus Herpes simplex/zoster JC virus	Measles enteroviruses	
Bacteria –	*Listeria* *Nocardia* *Mycobacterium*, etc.	*Streptococcus pneumoniae* *Haemophilus influenzae* *Pseudomonas aeruginosa*, etc.	Enterobacteria *Staphylococcus aureus* *Pseudomonas aeruginosa*, etc.
Fungi –	*Cryptococcus* *Aspergillus* *Candida* *Mucoraceae*		*Aspergillus* *Candida* *Mucoraceae*
Parasites –	*Toxoplasmosis*		

(Adapted from Singer 1980 Infections in the abnormal host. Yorke Medical Books.

CLINICAL SYNDROMES, DIAGNOSIS AND TREATMENT

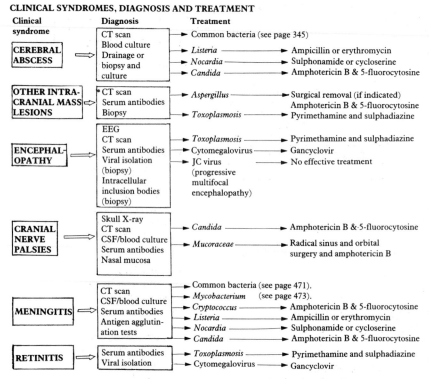

Clinical syndrome	Diagnosis	Treatment
CEREBRAL ABSCESS	CT scan Blood culture Drainage or biopsy and culture	Common bacteria (see page 345) *Listeria* → Ampicillin or erythromycin *Nocardia* → Sulphonamide or cycloserine *Candida* → Amphotericin B & 5-fluorocytosine
OTHER INTRA-CRANIAL MASS LESIONS	CT scan Serum antibodies Biopsy	*Aspergillus* → Surgical removal (if indicated) Amphotericin B & 5-fluorocytosine *Toxoplasmosis* → Pyrimethamine and sulphadiazine
ENCEPHAL-OPATHY	EEG CT scan Serum antibodies Viral isolation (biopsy) Intracellular inclusion bodies (biopsy)	*Toxoplasmosis* → Pyrimethamine and sulphadiazine Cytomegalovirus → Gancyclovir JC virus (progressive multifocal encephalopathy) → No effective treatment
CRANIAL NERVE PALSIES	Skull X-ray CT scan CSF/blood culture Serum antibodies Nasal mucosa	*Candida* → Amphotericin B & 5-fluorocytosine *Mucoraceae* → Radical sinus and orbital surgery and amphotericin B
MENINGITIS	CT scan CSF/blood culture Serum antibodies Antigen agglutination tests	Common bacteria (see page 471). *Mycobacterium* (see page 473). *Cryptococcus* → Amphotericin B & 5-fluorocytosine *Listeria* → Ampicillin or erythromycin *Nocardia* → Sulphonamide or cycloserine *Candida* → Amphotericin B & 5-fluorocytosine
RETINITIS	Serum antibodies Viral isolation	*Toxoplasmosis* → Pyrimethamine and sulphadiazine Cytomegalovirus → Gancyclovir

Other viral infections are dealt with in the appropriate section (pages 482-485).

ACQUIRED IMMUNODEFICIENCY SYNDROME (AIDS)

The retrovirus human immunodeficiency virus (HIV) has neurotropic and lymphotropic properties. It may invade the nervous system and also progressively destroy the immune system. AIDS is the end stage of chronic infection.

Prevalence of AIDS and HIV infection
Certain individuals are 'at risk' of infection:
– Homosexual males ⎫
– I.v. drug users ⎭ and heterosexual partners
– Babies born to infected individuals
– Recipients of blood products, e.g. haemophiliacs.
   The incidence of HIV infection in 'at risk' groups varies considerably.
Sexual education, supply of clean needles to addicts, active drug-dependence programmes and specific precautions in the preparation of blood products are necessary to control its spread.
   Current prevalence of HIV — USA 140/million (New York 991/million).
Patients with AIDS worldwide (1988) — over 82 000.

CLINICAL COURSE OF HIV INFECTION

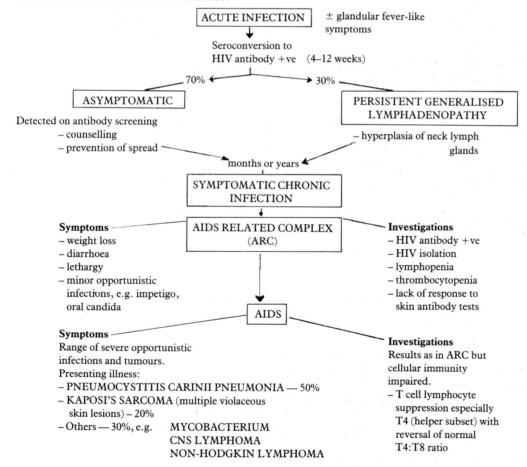

NEUROLOGICAL FEATURES OF HIV INFECTION

Neurological involvement develops in 80% of patients. It either occurs early, before or at seroconversion, due to a direct neurotropic effect, or later when AIDS is established.

HIV SYNDROMES AND INVESTIGATIONS

Cerebral tumours
Lymphoma ——— CT scan
Kaposi's sarcoma

Infections
Encephalitis
Cytomegalovirus
Herpes zoster/simplex ——— CT scan / Antibody tests / Biopsy
Toxoplasmosis
Progressive multifocal
    leukoencephalopathy
Cerebral abscess
E. coli
Aspergillus ——— CT scan / Aspiration/culture / Antibody tests
Candida
Nocardia
Meningitis
Aseptic (seroconversion)
Mycobacterium
Listeria ——— CSF exam and culture / Antibody tests
Aspergillus

Peripheral neuropathy
Herpes zoster radiculopathy
Cauda equina syndrome (cytomegalovirus)
Acute reversible demyelination (seroconversion)
Chronic demyelination ——— Nerve conduction studies / Antibody tests

AIDS dementia
Direct HIV infection with demyelination and perivascular inflammatory changes. Intellectual decline of subcortical type (page 125).

——— CT scan / Psychometry

Retinopathy
Cytomegalovirus
Toxoplasmosis

——— Fundal exam. / Antibody tests

Myelopathy
Acute reversible
    (seroconversion)
Ascending — cytomegalovirus
herpes zoster/
simplex ——— Myelography or Spinal CT/MRI / Antibody tests

Management

Opportunistic infection — treatment applies to the specific infection (see page 492). With known HIV+ve patients, invasive procedures such as biopsy are often avoided and trials of therapy are administered, e.g. cerebral toxoplasmosis — trial of pyrimethamine and sulphadiazine, monitored with CT scanning. If lesion does not resolve → biopsy (? lymphoma).

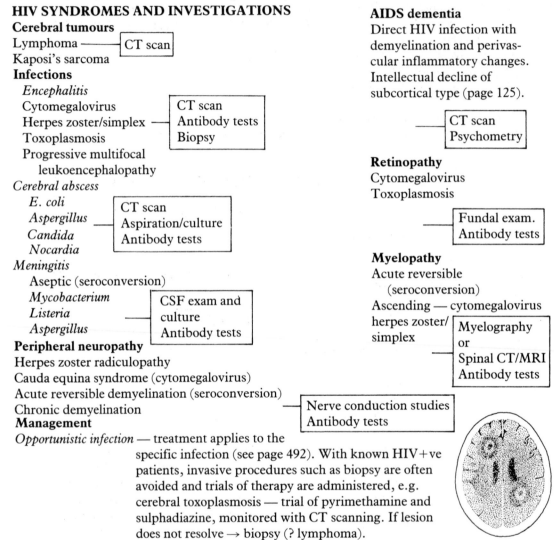

AIDS
Once AIDS is established, fatal infection or malignancy becomes inevitable. For this reason, treatments which boost the immune system or influence virus replication are currently under evaluation.

– Zidovudine (AZT), by interfering with nucleic acid synthesis, blocks HIV DNA formation and reduces virus replication. AZT is used at present in ARC and AIDS and prolongs survival. When given with Probenecid the dosage is reduced without loss of effectiveness.

Immune modulators, e.g. Interferon and Interleukin 2, stimulate the immune system and are of potential value.

SUBACUTE/CHRONIC MENINGITIS

This entity is characterised by symptoms and signs of meningeal irritation which persists and progresses over weeks without improvement. Unlike acute meningitis, the onset is insidious; cranial nerve signs and focal deficits such as hemiparesis, dementia and gradual deterioration of conscious level may predominate. The outcome depends upon aetiology and the instigation of appropriate treatment.

Chronic meningitis is associated with certain CSF findings.
– Lymphocytosis + low glucose
– Lymphocytosis + normal glucose.

Diagnosis depends upon CSF examination.

Lumbar puncture should be performed in suspicious cases as soon as CT scan has ruled out a mass lesion.

SUBACUTE/CHRONIC MENINGITIS WITH A MARKED REDUCTION IN CSF GLUCOSE

Causes	Diagnosis	Specific features	Treatment
M. tuberculosis	See page 473		
Fungi *Cryptococcus* *neoformans* *Nocardia* *Candida*	*CSF* Identification of organism with India ink stain. Antigen detected (latex agglutination). Culture *Serum* Anticryptococcal antibody tests	— Hydrocephalus may develop with progressive dementia	See page 492
Carcinomatous meningitis — lung/breast/ gastrointestinal tract Leukaemia/ lymphoma Glioma Medulloblastoma	Evidence of primary neoplasm. *CSF* Malignant cells seen in fresh centrifuged filtered sample. Tumour markers: – carcinoembryonic antigen (CEA) – ß-microglobulin	Back pain/ radicular involvement common. Hydrocephalus in 30%	Consider irradiation followed by intrathecal methotrexate or monoclonal targeting (see page 304). Leukaemia/lymph- oma requires specialist advice

SUBACUTE/CHRONIC MENINGITIS

SUBACUTE/CHRONIC MENINGITIS WITH SLIGHTLY REDUCED OR NORMAL CSF GLUCOSE

Causes	Diagnosis	Specific features	Treatment
Parameningeal infections Cerebral abscess Epidural abscess Sinusitis Mastoiditis	Evidence of primary infected source *X-rays* Sinuses, mastoids. *CT/MRI* scan — cerebral or cerebellar abscess *CSF* microscopy/ culture *Blood* cultures	Prodromal sinus or middle ear infection	Appropriate antibiotic therapy and, if indicated, surgical drainage of loculated parameningeal infection

Bacteria:
 Treponema
 Brucella
 Leptospira
 Listeria
 Borrelia
 Burgdorferi
	CSF
	 Isolate organism (if possible)
	 Serological tests
	 Serum
	 Serological tests
		Treponema — page 478
		   Sexual contact
		 Brucella ——————— Tetracycline
		   Contact with· Streptomycin
		   infected cattle
		 Leptospira page 480
		   Contact with
		   contaminated rat,
		   dog or cattle urine
		 Listeria
		   Contaminated — page 492
		   foods
		 Borrelia Burgdorferi — page 479
		   Tick bite	

Miscellaneous
 Parasites, e.g.
   toxoplasma — see page 481
 Sarcoidosis — see page 346
 Behçet's disease
 Systemic lupus
   erythematosus — see page 261			

Despite extensive investigation, a group of patients with chronic meningitis exists in whom no cause is found.

DEMYELINATING DISEASES — INTRODUCTION

Demyelinating disorders of the central nervous system affect *myelin* and/or *oligodendroglia* with relative sparing of *axons*.

The central nervous system is composed of *neurons* with *neuroectodermal* and *mesodermal* supporting cells.

The neuroectodermal cells comprise:
astrocytes
ependymal cells
oligodendrocytes.

The oligodendrocytes, like Schwann cells in the peripheral nervous system, are responsible for the formation of *myelin* around central nervous system *axons*.

One Schwann cell myelinates one axon but one oligodendrocyte may myelinate several contiguous axons, and the close proximity of cell to axon may not be obvious by light microscopy.

Oligodendrocytes are present in grey matter near neuronal cell bodies and in white matter near axons.

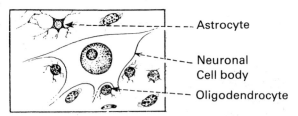

Myelin is composed of *protein* and *lipids*.
Protein accounts for 20% of total content.
The lipid fraction may divided into:
cholesterol
glycophosphatides
(lecithins)
sphingolipids
(sphingomyelins).

The laying down of myelin in the central nervous system commences at the fourth month of fetal life in the median longitudinal bundle, then in frontal and parietal lobes at birth. Most of the cerebrum is myelinated by the end of the 2nd year. Myelination continues until the 10th year of life.

Myelin disorders may be classified as diseases in which:
1. Myelin is inherently abnormal or was never properly formed — these disorders generally presenting in infancy and early childhood, e.g. *leukodystrophy*.
2. Myelin which was normal when formed breaks down as a consequence of inflammation, e.g. *multiple sclerosis*.

MULTIPLE SCLEROSIS

Multiple sclerosis (MS) is a common demyelinating disease, characterised by focal disturbance of function and a relapsing and remitting course.

The disease occurs most commonly in temperate climates and prevalence differs at various latitudes:

	Latitude (°N)	Rate/100 000
Orkneys and Shetlands	60	309
England (Cornwall)	51	63
Italy (Bari)	41	13

The disease usually occurs in young adults with a peak age incidence of 20 – 40 years. Slightly more females than males are affected. The risk of MS in relatives of patients increases 20 fold.

PATHOLOGY

Scattered lesions with a greyish colour, 1 mm to several cm in size, are present in the white matter of the brain and spinal cord and are referred to as *plaques*.

The lesions lie in close relationship to veins (postcapillary venules) — perivenous distribution.

RECENT LESIONS   ⟶   LATER   OLD LESIONS

Myelin destruction
Relative axon sparing
Perivenous infiltration
with mononuclear cells and
lymphocytes. Interstitial oedema is
evident in acute lesions
Breakdown of blood-brain barrier
occurs and may be essential for
myelin destruction.

Astrocyte proliferation

Relatively acellular and more
clearly demarcated. Within
these plaques bare axons are
surrounded by astrocytes

Thoracic spinal cord showing
established plaques of
demyelination

PATHOGENESIS

Immune deficiency has been suggested. This might explain the possible persistence of a latent virus and variations in immune status could be the basis of 'relapses and remissions'. Studies of humoral and cellular immunity both *in vivo* and *in vitro* are conflicting.

Hereditary/genetic factors appear significant. There is an increased familial incidence of multiple sclerosis. This has led to the study of *histocompatibility antigens* (HL-A). An association between A3, B7, B18 and DW2/DRW2 and multiple sclerosis has been demonstrated.

Viruses may be important in the development of multiple sclerosis, infection perhaps occurring in a genetically/immunologically susceptible host.
  Elevated serum and CSF antibody titres have been found to:
  – varicella zoster, measles, rubella and herpes simplex during relapse.
  It has been suggested that these antiviral antibodies are produced within the CSF.
  Oligoclonal bands present in M.S. in the CSF contain antibodies to several viruses.

Biochemical: No biochemical effect has been demonstrated — myelin appears normal before breakdown and the proposed excess of dietary fats or malabsorption of unsaturated fatty acids is unproven.

MULTIPLE SCLEROSIS

PATHOGENESIS (*contd*)
In summary — the causation is probably multifactorial.

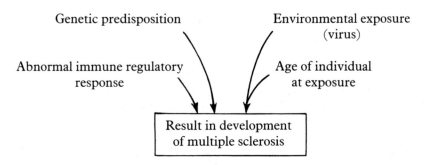

CLINICAL FEATURES

Peak age of onset	— 20–25 years
Childhood onset rare	— 2%
Patients presenting >50 years	— 5%
Patients presenting >60 years	— 1%

Initial symptoms may follow infection or injury, but usually there is no antecedent event.
Multiple sclerosis is usually characterised by:
1. Signs and symptoms of dissemination (widespread CNS involvement).
2. A relapsing and remitting course.

Symptoms at onset
1. *Vague symptoms:* lack of energy, headache, depression, aches in limbs — may result in diagnosis of psychoneurosis. These symptoms are eventually associated with:

2. *Precise symptoms:*
(initial symptom of
multiple sclerosis
expressed as a %)

Sensory disturbance	— 40%
Retrobulbar neuritis	— 17%
Limb weakness	— 12%
Diplopia	— 11%
Vertigo Ataxia 20% Sphincter disturbance	} 20%

Trigeminal neuralgia may be an early symptom of multiple sclerosis, and this should be considered in the young patient with paroxysmal facial pain.

499

MULTIPLE SCLEROSIS

Sensory symptoms

Numbness and paraesthesia are common and often so transient as to be forgotten. Paraesthesia is more often due to posterior column demyelination than to

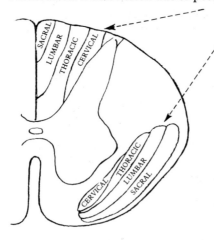

spinothalamic tract involvement.

Posterior column lesions result in impaired vibration sensation and joint position sensation.
In such cases a limb may be rendered 'useless' by the absence of positional awareness.

Lhermitte's sign: with cervical posterior column involvement sudden neck flexion will evoke a 'shock-like' sensation in the limbs.

Spinothalamic lesions result in dysaesthesia – an unpleasant feeling of burning, coldness or warmth, with associated sensory loss to pain and temperature contralateral to the lesion.

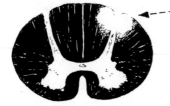

A plaque at the posterior root entry zone will result in loss of *all* sensory modalities in that particular root distribution.

Motor symptoms

Monoparesis and paraparesis are the most common motor symptoms. Hemiparesis and quadriparesis occur less commonly.

Paraparesis is the result of spinal demyelination, usually in the cervical region.

Signs: – Increased tone
– Hyperactive tendon reflexes, extensor plantar response and absent abdominal reflexes
– Pyramidal distribution weakness.

N.B. A plaque at the anterior root exit zone will result in lower motor neuron signs (reflex loss and segmental wasting)

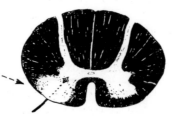

MULTIPLE SCLEROSIS

Disturbance of vision

Retrobulbar neuritis (RBN): Subacute visual loss associated with a central scotoma and recovery over some weeks. This disorder commonly occurs in young adults. The visual loss develops over several days and is often associated with pain on ocular movement (irritation of the dural membrane around the optic nerve). As colour vision (cones) is a function of the macular area, some disturbance in colour perception will occur.

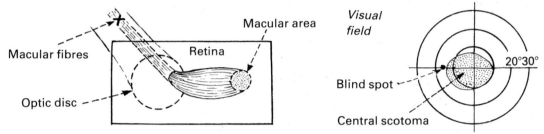

Usually only one eye is affected, although occasionally both eyes simultaneously or consecutively are involved.

On examination: Disturbance of visual function ranges from a small central scotoma to complete loss. Fundal examination reveals swelling — papillitis — in up to 50% of patients, depending upon the proximity of the plaque to the optic nerve head. 'Sheathing' from an inflammatory exudate around peripheral retinal venules is common. Reduced visual acuity distinguishes papillitis from papilloedema.

Investigation: Visual evoked responses (VERs) show delay. If recovery does not occur, high resolution CT or MRI of the optic nerve should exclude tumour.

Treatment: Steroids shorten the duration of visual loss and are used in bilateral disease. They also ease pain when present.

Outcome: 90% of patients recover most vision, although symptoms may transiently return following a hot bath or physical exercise — Uhthoff's phenomenon. Following recovery the optic disc develops an atrophic appearance with a pale 'punched out' temporal margin.

Subsequent course:
– No evidence of multiple sclerosis occurs in patient's lifetime.

or

– Bilateral RBN is followed by a transverse myelitis (Neuromyelitis optica, page 507).

or

– Symptoms and signs of demyelination elsewhere in the nervous system follow — multiple sclerosis.

Over a 15-year period from presentation, 40% of patients fall into the last group. Onset in winter and the presence of certain histocompatibility antigens, e.g. HLA DR2, increase the risk of subsequent MS.

It is important to appreciate that plaque formation in the optic nerve may be asymptomatic. Patients with symptoms and signs of nervous system dysfunction outwith the optic nerves may have fundal pallor and prolonged VERs.

501

MULTIPLE SCLEROISIS

Disturbance of ocular movement

Diplopia may result from demyelination affecting the intraparenchymal course of the III, IV or VI cranial nerves. Abnormality of eye movements with or without diplopia occurs when supranuclear or internuclear connections are involved. The latter results from a lesion in the medial longitudinal bundle (MLB) — *internuclear ophthalmoplegia* — and in young persons is pathognomonic of MS.

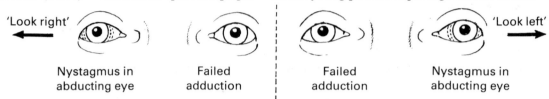

'Look right' — Nystagmus in abducting eye — Failed adduction — Failed adduction — Nystagmus in abducting eye — 'Look left'

Nystagmus may be an incidental finding on neurological examination. Its presence should be sought as evidence of a second lesion. It is unusual in multiple sclerosis when the eyes are in the primary position, and is commonly seen on lateral gaze.

Pupillary abnormalities may occur from:
– sympathetic involvement in the brain stem (Horner's syndrome)
– III nerve involvement, or
– II nerve involvement.

The swinging light test is a sensitive test of impaired afferent conduction in the II nerve. Alternating the light from one eye to the other results eventually in 'pupillary escape' — the pupil dilates despite the presence of direct light.

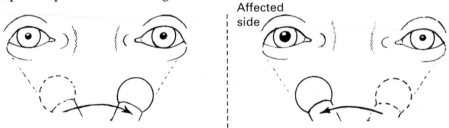

Affected side

OTHER FEATURES

Vestibular symptoms: Vertigo of central type may be a presenting problem or develop during the course of the illness. Hearing loss is rare.

Ataxia of gait and limb inco-ordination are frequently present. The gait ataxia may be cerebellar or sensory type (see Romberg's test). Limb inco-ordination, intention tremor and dysarthria indicate cerebellar involvement.

Sphincter disturbance with urgency or precipitancy of micturition and eventual incontinence occurs. Conversely urinary retention in a young person may be the first symptom of disease. On direct questioning, impotence is frequently found.

Mental changes: Mood change — euphoria or depression occur. Dementia develops in advanced cases. Generalised fatigue is common.

Emotional lability: Uncontrolled outbursts of crying or laughing, result from involvement of pseudobulbar pathways.

Paroxysmal (symptoms occurring momentarily throughout any stage of the disease): Paraesthesia, dysarthria, ataxia, pain, e.g. trigeminal neuralgia, photopsia (visual scintillations), epilepsy, Lhermitte's sign, Uhthoff's phenomenon.

MULTIPLE SCLEROSIS

CLINICAL COURSE

After the initial attack remission is usual and recovery complete. Thereafter relapses occur on average every two years and the likelihood of complete functional recovery lessens with each attack. The relapse rate is extremely variable from one patient to the next. The following clinical patterns may be recognised:

1. Acute MS:
Explosive onset
Death may occur in months
Dramatic recovery and prolonged remission may occur
Separation from acute disseminated encephalomyelitis (see page 508) is difficult.

2. Slowly progressive course with no relapse/remission. More common in older age group. Usually takes the form of a progressive myelopathy.

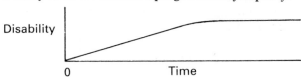

3. Relapsing course with accumulating disability.

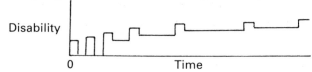

4. Benign form:
Abrupt onset — good remission —
long latent period.

Within this group could be
included those in whom plaques
appear as an incidental finding
at autopsy.

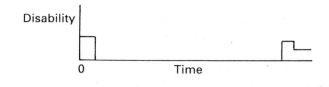

In such a variable disorder it is difficult to give a prognosis for an individual patient.
- After 15 years, 30% of patients are working and 40% walking.
- Progressive limb weakness in middle age — poor prognosis.
- Remitting visual and sensory onset in early adult life — good prognosis.

The best predictor of outcome is the degree of disability 5 years after the initial attack.

Classification can be made depending on pattern of CNS involvement.
The majority have a *generalised* form with optic nerve, cerebellum/brain stem and spinal lesions.
One-third develop an almost exclusively *spinal* form with spastic/ataxic gait and sphincter disturbance. Asymptomatic optic nerve involvement is frequent (abnormal VERs).
A *cerebellar* form occurs in a minority.

MULTIPLE SCLEROSIS

INVESTIGATIONS

There is no diagnostic test. Investigations only support the clinical suspicion.

Neurophysiological: Measurements of conduction within the central nervous system to detect a second asymptomatic lesion (see page 52).

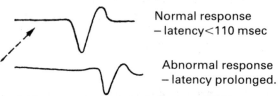

Normal response
– latency<110 msec

Abnormal response
– latency prolonged.

1. *Visual evoked potential (VEP).* In optic nerve involvement the latency of the large positive wave is delayed beyond 110 msec. The amplitude of the waves may also be reduced.

2. *Somatosensory evoked response (SSEP)* may detect central sensory pathway lesions.

3. *Brain stem auditory evoked potential (BAEP)* may detect brain stem lesions.

Cerebrospinal fluid examination by lumbar puncture

A mild pleocytosis (25 cells/mm^3), mainly lymphocytes, is occasionally found. The total protein may be elevated, although this rarely exceeds 100 mg/l. An increase in gammaglobulin occurs in 50–60% of cases. Electrophoresis of CSF using agar or acrylamide shows discrete bands which are not present in serum.

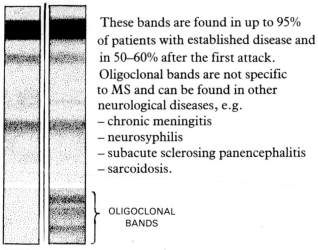

NORMAL

These bands are found in up to 95% of patients with established disease and in 50–60% after the first attack. Oligoclonal bands are not specific to MS and can be found in other neurological diseases, e.g.
– chronic meningitis
– neurosyphilis
– subacute sclerosing panencephalitis
– sarcoidosis.

OLIGOCLONAL BANDS

CT scanning/MRI

Delayed CT scanning following intravenous high-dose iodine-containing contrast shows multifocal enhancing white matter lesions in 25% of patients with clinically definite MS and recent symptoms.

MRI is more sensitive showing white matter disease in 90% of similar patients and is thus a valuable confirmatory investigation. Spin-echo (SE) sequences show hyperintense lesions on a T2 weighted image relative to surrounding brain.

Widespread MRI abnormalities are detected in 60% of patients presenting with first, often unifocal, symptoms and signs of disease. The MRI findings are not necessarily diagnostic; a similar distribution of white matter change occurs in vascular and granulomatous disorders.

Periventricular lesions, most evident at frontal and occipital horns. Abnormalities are also seen in the brain stem and cerebellum lesions of the optic nerves and spinal cord are more difficult to detect.

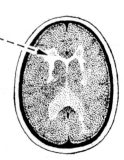

MULTIPLE SCLEROSIS

DIAGNOSIS

Diagnosis is based on demonstrating clinical, neurophysiological abnormalities or radiological lesions disseminated in time (relapses) and space (anatomical localisation).

In the established case with scattered signs and a history of relapse and remission a confident diagnosis can be made on clinical grounds alone. When this is not possible, neurophysiological, immunological and radiological investigations are indicated.

Difficulty arises:

1. With the first attack   2. With the nonremitting progressive form of disease

     3. In differentiating from other neurological disorders in which dissemination is a feature

Full investigation of that part of neuroaxis involved is mandatory,

e.g. With *spinal presentation* — myelography or MRI
     With *cerebellar presentation* — posterior fossa CT scan or MRI.

e.g. Collagen vascular disease
     Paraneoplastic syndromes
     Sarcoidosis.

Acute MS may be clinically inseparable from acute disseminated encephalomyelitis.

Solitary lesions strategically placed may give the impression of disseminated disease. This is especially so at the *foramen magnum* where a lesion may produce:

Cerebellar, brain stem and corticospinal signs — e.g. neurofibroma or
                                        Arnold-Chiari malformation.

Also in the *parasagittal region* where meningioma may produce symptoms and signs suggestive of progressive spinal cord disease.

Diagnostic criteria have been proposed (Poser Committee 1983). These were primarily conceived for research and clinical trials of therapy but are also of use to the clinician.

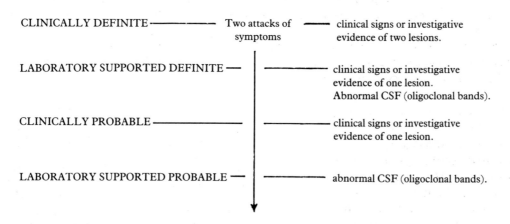

CLINICALLY DEFINITE ————— Two attacks of ——— clinical signs or investigative
                                       symptoms   evidence of two lesions.

LABORATORY SUPPORTED DEFINITE — ————— clinical signs or investigative
                                            evidence of one lesion.
                                            Abnormal CSF (oligoclonal bands).

CLINICALLY PROBABLE ———————— ————— clinical signs or investigative
                                            evidence of one lesion.

LABORATORY SUPPORTED PROBABLE — ————— abnormal CSF (oligoclonal bands).

(Modified from Poser 1983 Annals of Neurology 13:227–231.)

MULTIPLE SCLEROSIS — TREATMENT

SYMPTOMATIC/SUPPORTIVE

1. Spasticity. Spasms of flexor or extensor nature are painful and contractures will develop.

Drugs — antispastic, e.g. baclofen, dantrolene, diazepam.

Care must be taken not to make muscles too floppy and remove their 'splinting' effect. In severe contractures — tenotomy may help. When bladder/bowel function is lost — consider intrathecal baclofen, alcohol or phenol.

2. Urinary symptoms. Probanthene may be useful in the uninhibited bladder. The patient with precipitancy of micturition may need to pay close attention to his fluid load. Mandelamine and ascorbic acid will acidify urine and protect against infection.

Urinary infection, when it occurs, should be promptly treated.

3. Bowel symptoms. Stool softeners and high roughage diet should be recommended when constipation is a problem.

4. Paroxysmal pain of a burning dysaesthetic type may respond well to the anticonvulsants carbamazepine and phenytoin.

5. Seizures of a tonic/clonic or occasionally tonic nature will require anticonvulsants.

6. Pain and sphincter disturbance may be improved by dorsal column stimulation (DCS). The results of such electrical treatment are variable.

7. Cerebellar tremor may respond to clonazepam or isonizid with pyridoxine.

SPECIFIC AGAINST DISEASE PROCESS

1. Anti-inflammatory and immunosuppressive therapy

ACTH (adrenocorticotrophic hormone) may shorten the duration of relapses but will not influence the outcome.
Regime: i.m. 80 i.u. ACTH daily × 7 followed by i.m. 40 i.u. ACTH daily × 7.
Methylprednisolone (0.5g/day i.v. for 5 days) may be useful in acute relapses, but requires hospitalisation.

Immunosuppressive — cyclophosphamide, azothiaprine — no evidence of value and potentially dangerous; marrow toxicity, etc. Occasionally used in acute MS.

2. Enhancement of cell mediated immunity (depressed in MS?)
Transfer factor — disappointing.

Interferon (antiviral substance made by immunocompetent cells) has been suggested but not evaluated.

3. Physical treatment. Elevation of body temperature may aggravate symptoms — consequently body cooling has been applied in acute situations, also hyperbaric oxygen therapy, which appears to modify the animal model of MS (acute experimental allergic encephalomyelitis). This is of no proven short-term benefit.

4. Dietary measures, e.g. low gluten or polyunsaturated fat supplemented diets, again of no proven value.

IN SUMMARY — No available specific therapy of proven value.

OTHER DEMYELINATING DISEASES

NEUROMYELITIS OPTICA (Devic's disease)
A subacute disorder characterised by demyelination of the optic nerves and spinal cord. Initially considered a distinct entity, it is now regarded as a form of multiple sclerosis.

Clinical features
A history of upper respiratory infection may precede neurological symptoms.
Visual loss is rapid, bilateral and occasionally total.
Spinal cord symptoms follow — hours, days or occasionally weeks later.
Back pain and girdle pain. Paraesthesia in lower limbs.
Paralysis may ascend to involve respiratory muscles.
Urinary retention is common.
Recovery is complete in 60–70% of patients.

Examination

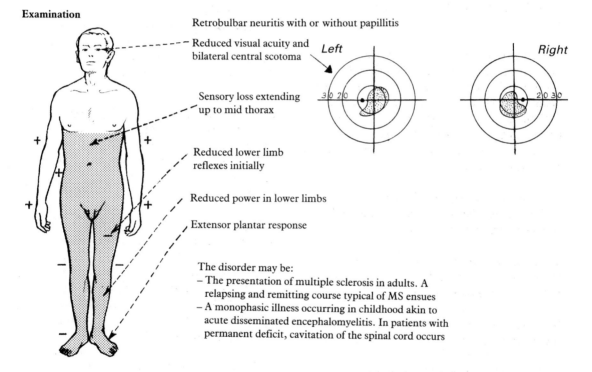

Retrobulbar neuritis with or without papillitis
Reduced visual acuity and bilateral central scotoma

Left   *Right*

Sensory loss extending up to mid thorax

Reduced lower limb reflexes initially

Reduced power in lower limbs

Extensor plantar response

The disorder may be:
– The presentation of multiple sclerosis in adults. A relapsing and remitting course typical of MS ensues
– A monophasic illness occurring in childhood akin to acute disseminated encephalomyelitis. In patients with permanent deficit, cavitation of the spinal cord occurs

Investigations
Visual evoked responses are prolonged. The CSF shows an elevated protein with a lymphocytosis occasionally as high as 1000 cells per mm³. Gammaglobulin may be elevated and oligoclonal bands present.

Treatment
Steroids are often given, but evidence of benefit anecdotal. Treatment is otherwise supportive.

DIFFUSE SCLEROSIS
A rare sporadic disorder of infancy or adolescence associated with widespread massive cerebral and spinal demyelination. The condition is unresponsive to treatment; diagnosis is made at autopsy.

507

OTHER DEMYELINATING DISEASES

POSTURAL OR ACUTE DISSEMINATED ENCEPHALOMYELITIS (ADEM)

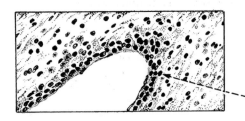

ADEM is an acute demyelinating disorder in which small foci of demyelination with a perivenous distribution are scattered throughout the brain and spinal cord. Lesions are 0.1–1.0 mm in diameter.

Microglial, plasma cell and lymphocyte exudate around the vein

This disorder may follow upper respiratory and gastrointestinal infections (viral), viral exanthems (measles, chickenpox, rubella, etc.) or immunisation with live or killed virus vaccines (influenza, rabies).

Measles is the commonest cause with 1 per 1000 primary infections; next Varicella zoster (chickenpox), 1 per 2000 primary infections.

The synonymous titles 'postinfectious' and 'postvaccinial' encephalomyelitis can also be applied to this condition.

Clinical features: Within days or weeks of resolution of the viral infection, fever, headache, nausea and vomiting develop. Meningeal symptoms (neck stiffness, photophobia) are then followed by drowsiness and multifocal neurological signs and symptoms — hemisphere brain stem/cerebellar/spinal cord and optic nerve involvement.

Predominantly *spinal*, *cerebral* or *cerebellar* forms occur, though usually the picture is mixed. Optic nerve involvement takes the form of retrobulbar neuritis. Rarely the peripheral nervous system is involved.

Outcome: 20% mortality.
Recovery may be complete. The cerebral form often results in permanent intellectual and behavioural deficits.

Diagnosis: No diagnostic test.
CSF — 20–200 mononuclear cells.
Total protein elevated with
γ globulin raised also.
Peripheral blood may be normal or show neutrophilia, lymphocytosis or lymphopenia.
The electroencephalogram (EEG) shows diffuse slow wave activity.

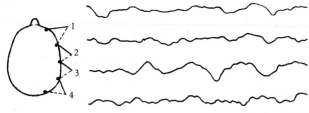

Generalised asynchronous delta activity

CT scan is normal. MRI shows small focal white matter changes.

Diagnosis is straightforward when there is an obvious preceding viral infection or immunisation. When viral infection *immediately* precedes, distinction from acute encephalitis is often impossible.

Separation from acute MS may be difficult. Fever, meningeal signs with elevated CSF protein above 100 mg/ml with cell count greater than 50 per mm³ suggest ADEM.

Pathologically, demyelination is limited to perivascular areas and lesions do not approach the same size as in MS.

Treatment: Steroids are used, although their efficacy is questionable. Large dosage is recommended during the acute phase.

OTHER DEMYELINATING DISEASES

ACUTE HAEMORRHAGIC LEUKOENCEPHALITIS
This is a rare demyelinating disease. It is regarded as a very acute form of postinfectious/acute disseminated encephalomyelitis.
Clinical picture: Antecedent viral infection, depression of conscious level and multifocal signs and symptoms. Focal features may suggest a mass lesion or even herpes simplex encephalitis.

The diagnosis is only really possible at biopsy or autopsy, but elevated CSF pressure, lymphocytosis and erythrocytes in CSF and xanthochromic appearance of fluid are all suggestive.
Pathology: Perivascular polymorph infiltration.
Microscopic and macroscopic haemorrhage.
Perivascular demyelination and necrotising
changes in vessels.
Treatment: Steroids in high dosage should be
used though evidence of value in this
rare condition is scant.

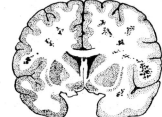

PROGRESSIVE MULTIFOCAL LEUKOENCEPHALOPATHY
This is a demyelinative disease occurring in association with systemic illness in which cell-mediated and occasionally humoral immunity is depressed, e.g. lymphoma, sarcoidosis, systemic lupus erythematosus. The disorder is due to reactivation of previous papavirus (JC strain) infection.
Clinical picture: Features of diffuse process — personality change, hemiparesis, cortical visual loss, seizures, etc. Duration of illness: 3–6 months. Non-remitting and fatal.
Pathology: Demyelination without inflammatory response.
Electron microscopy — papovavirus in oligodendroglia.
Diagnosis: CT scanning and MRI reveal widespread multifocal white matter damage. Definitive diagnosis is made from brain biopsy. Virus can be isolated by inoculation on to glial tissue culture.
Treatment: No effective treatment.

DYSMYELINATING DISEASES

Inborn errors of metabolism involving myelin formation may result in abnormal or arrested myelination. Several groups of disorders may express themselves in this way.
The *leukodystrophies* represent one such group and may be subdivided into:
1. Metachromatic leukodystrophy,   3. Adrenoleukodystrophy,
2. Globoid cell leukodystrophy,   4. Spongy sclerosis,
depending on pathological features.
Clinical features: Onset is in infancy or childhood. Metachromatic leukodystrophy may develop in early adult life.
The features are those of:
  – hypotonicity
  – progressive deterioration of conscious level with eventual flexion or extension to pain
  – seizures will occur throughout the illness.
Cerebellar ataxia and optic atrophy can occur.

Metachromatic leukodystrophy affects not only the central but also the peripheral nervous system. This disorder, when presenting in adult life may be mistaken for psychotic illness before the dementia becomes evident.

In adrenoleukodystrophy, features of Addison's disease coexist.

All show recessive Mendelian inheritance except adrenoleukodystrophy which is an X-linked recessive disorder.
Diagnosis: CSF examination may show protein elevation.
In metachromatic leukodystrophy, metachromatic bodies may be present in urine and diagnosis is confirmed by low urinary and leucocyte levels of arylsulpharase A and by sural nerve biopsy. Prenatal diagnosis can be made by amniocentesis.
Prognosis: These disorders are all progressive with death within months to 2–3 years.

509

NEUROLOGICAL COMPLICATIONS OF DRUGS AND TOXINS

Introduction

Drugs and toxins commonly involve the nervous system. They cause a wide spectrum of disorders of which most are potentially reversible on withdrawal of the causal agent.

Diagnosis is especially dependent upon history:
– Availability of drugs.
– Occupational/industrial exposure to toxins.

Drug toxicity may result from:
– The chronic abuse of drugs, e.g. barbiturates, opiates.
– The side effects of drug therapy, e.g. anticonvulsants, steroids.
– The wilfull overdosage of drugs, e.g. sedatives, antidepressants.

Toxin exposure may be:
– Accidental: industrial or household poisons, e.g. organophosphates, carbon monoxide, turpentine.
– Wilfull: solvent abuse.

History and examination

When drugs or toxins are suspected, the following clinical features are supportive.

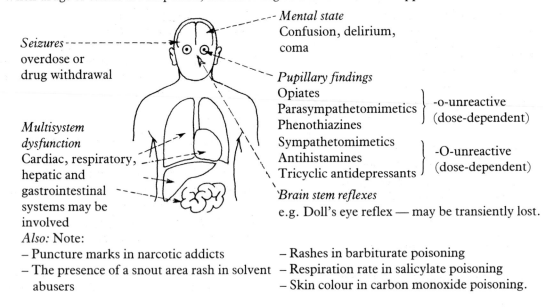

Seizures
overdose or
drug withdrawal

Mental state
Confusion, delirium,
coma

Pupillary findings
Opiates
Parasympathetomimetics } -o-unreactive
Phenothiazines   (dose-dependent)

Sympathetomimetics
Antihistamines } -O-unreactive
Tricyclic antidepressants   (dose-dependent)

Brain stem reflexes
e.g. Doll's eye reflex — may be transiently lost.

*Multisystem
dysfunction*
Cardiac, respiratory,
hepatic and
gastrointestinal
systems may be
involved
Also: Note:
– Puncture marks in narcotic addicts
– The presence of a snout area rash in solvent abusers

– Rashes in barbiturate poisoning
– Respiration rate in salicylate poisoning
– Skin colour in carbon monoxide poisoning.

Clinical features:

While the neurological picture is generally diffuse, certain pronounced symptoms occur with one drug or toxin and not with another. The following table should act as a guide to diagnosis and alert the clinician to the possible offending substance.

For treatment, the reader is advised to consult an appropriate pharmacology or general medical text.

DRUG-INDUCED NEUROLOGICAL SYNDROMES

This table is not all-inclusive but emphasises the more commonly prescribed drugs.

HEADACHE
Vasodilators: antihistamines, sympathomimetics, calcium channel blockers, bronchodilators, ergotamine
Dopamine agonists
Non-steroidal anti-inflammatories

SEIZURES
Antidepressants, antimicrobials: cycloserine, isoniazid, metronidazole, penicillin
Antineoplastics: vincristine, methotrexate, BCNU
Analgesics: pentazocine, fentanyl, opiates
Anaesthetics: ketamine, halothone, althesin
Bronchodilators. Sympathomimetics
Miscellaneous: amphetamine, baclofen, lithium, iodinated contrast media, insulin

CONFUSION/DELIRIUM
Anticholinergics. Anticonvulsants
Antimicrobials: isoniazid, rifampicin
Antineoplastics: vincristine
Dopamine agonists. Tranquillisers
Miscellaneous: cimetidine, ranitidine, lithium

PERIPHERAL NEUROPATHY
Antimicrobials: ethambutol, isoniazid, nitrofurantoin, metronidazole, dapsone
Antineoplastics: cytosine arabinoside, cisplatin, procarbazine, vincristine (and other vinca alkaloids)
Antirheumatics: colchicine, D-penicillamine, gold, indomethacin
Miscellaneous: cimetidine, phenytoin

VIII NERVE (VESTIBULAR & COCHLEAR) DAMAGE
Aminoglycoside antibiotics: gentamicin, kanamycin, neomycin, streptomycin
Miscellaneous: cisplatin, ethycrinic acid, quinine, salicylates

RETINOPATHY   *Antimalarials:*
↗   chloroquine, mepacrine
VISUAL DISTURBANCE   *Phenothiazines*
Miscellaneous: ethambutol, indomethacin, tamoxifen
↘

OPTIC NEURITIS   *Antimicrobials:* chloramphenicol dapsone, isoniazid, streptomycin
Miscellaneous: chlorpropamide

MOVEMENT DISORDERS
Antiemetics: metoclopramide
Butyrophenones: haloperidol, droperidol
Dopamine agonists. Phenothiazines: chlorpromazine, triflupromazine, thioridazine
Tricyclic antidepressants

ATAXIA
Anticonvulsants: carbamezepine, phenytoin, primidone
Antineoplastics: cytosine arabinoside. fluoracil
Phenothiazines: sedatives; barbiturates, chloral hydrate. *Tranquillisers:* diazepam

MUSCLE PAIN AND WEAKNESS
Antineoplastics: cytosine arabinoside, methotrexate, thiopeta
Miscellaneous: clofibrate D-penicillamine, diuretics, danazol, pindolol, nifedipine

Drug screen
Too often the clinician, when managing suspected drug or toxin overdosage, requests a 'drug screen'. The techniques used in detection, e.g. gas chromatography, thin-layer chromatography and immunological tests, are sophisticated and time-consuming and may require samples of serum, urine or both.

The clinician must 'narrow down the field' from the history and presenting symptoms/signs and discuss with the laboratory the class of drug or toxin he suspects. In this way detection will be more successful.

A knowledge of the blood level of some drugs, e.g. salicylates, barbiturates, is important in deciding the approach to treatment.

SPECIFIC SYNDROMES OF DRUGS AND TOXINS

NEUROLEPTIC MALIGNANT SYNDROME

A rare life-threatening disorder induced by initiation, increase or reintroduction of phenothiazine or butyrophenone drugs (e.g. chlorpromazine, haloperidol). The condition appears to result from acute dopamine receptor blockade and is characterised by *hyperpyrexia, bradykinesia, rigidity, autonomic disturbance* and *high serum muscle enzymes (creatine kinase)*. The causal drug should be withdrawn and the patient cooled. Give dopamine agonists with dantrolene sodium to control bradykinesia and rigidity respectively.

SOLVENT ABUSE

The abuse of volatile solvents is an increasing problem especially in children. The purpose of inhalation is to achieve a state of euphoria. Habituation develops. Commonly used substances are: aerosols, cleaning fluids, nail varnish remover, lighter fluids, 'model' glue. The 'active' components of these are simple carbon-based molecules, e.g. benzene, hexane and toluene.

Symptoms of acute intoxication:
- Euphoria
- Dysarthria, ataxia, diplopia
- Delusions and hallucinations occur, followed by
  seizures if exposure has been prolonged.
    Death may result:
- Aspiration/asphyxiation
- Cardiac arrhythmias
- Renal or hepatic damage.

Symptoms of chronic abuse:
- Behavioural disturbance.
- Chronic ataxia.
- Sensorimotor peripheral neuropathy.

Treatment of acute intoxication is symptomatic; there are no specific antidotes.

LEAD EXPOSURE

Lead has no biological function. It is present in normal diet as well as in the atmosphere from automobile fumes and in the water supply of old buildings containing lead tanks and piping. Occupation exposure occurs in plumbers, burners and smelters.

Lead excess interferes with *haem* synthesis. This results in the accumulation of 'blocked' metabolites such as aminolevulinic acid (ALA) in serum and urine.

Anaemia occurs with a characteristic finding in the blood film (basophilic stippling).

Both the peripheral and central nervous systems are affected.

ADULTS
A chronic motor neuropathy with minor sensory symptomatology. Axonal damage predominates.

rarely
Acute encephalopathy

CHILDREN
Peripheral neuropathy is rare.
Encephalopathy is characteristic.

Acute fulminating with confusion, impaired conscious level, coma, seizures, papilloedema.

Chronic with fatigue and irritability, headache, apathy.

In encephalopathy, diffuse neurological symptoms and signs may occur, e.g. vertigo, ataxia, paraparesis, hemiplegia.

Treatment

Chelating agents (e.g. calcium disodium edetate — EDTA — or D-penicillamine) and i.v. mannitol in acute encephalopathy with papilloedema.

In acute fulminating encephalopathy the mortality has been reduced to 5%, but neurological sequelae are common.

SPECIFIC SYNDROMES OF DRUGS AND TOXINS

COMPLICATIONS OF DRUG ABUSE

The increasing problem of 'recreational' drug abuse is associated with primary (direct) and secondary (infective/hypoxic) neurological disturbances.

	Cocaine	Metamphetamine	Heroin	Phencyclidine
Origin	Alkaloid from leaves of erythroxylon coca plant	Synthetic amphetamine	Alkaloid from poppy — papaver somiferin	Synthetic anaesthetic agent
Clinical use	Pain relief	Anorexia Narcolepsy Depression	Pain relief	Anaesthetic agent
Popular name(s)	'Coke', 'Snow', 'Crack' (potent pica base form)	'Speed' 'Uppers'		'Angel dust'
Method of taking	Oral Intranasal Intravenous	Oral Intravenous 'high speeding'	Oral Smoked Intravenous	Oral Smoked Intranasal
Mode of action	Blocks reuptake of dopamine and noradrenaline and augments neurotransmission (sympathetomimetic)	Increases release of dopamine and adrenaline and augments neurotransmission (sympathetomimetic)	Acts as opiate receptors located on the surface of neurons	Interference with multiple neurotransmitter function
Moderate dosage	Alertness ↑ Euphoria Blood pressure ↑	Alertness ↑ Euphoria Blood pressure ↑	Pupillary constriction Pleasurable abdominal sensation Facial flushing	Alertness ↑ Sweating Blood pressure ↑ Heart rate ↑
Excessive dosage	Blood pressure ↑ ↑ Temperature ↑ Respiration ↓ Cardiac dysrhythmia and sudden death	Blood pressure ↑ ↑ Temperature ↑ Respiration ↓ Cardiac dysrhythmia and sudden death	Pin-point pupils Respiration ↓ Coma	Dysarthria Psychosis Nystagmus Cardiac dysrhythmia Ataxia and sudden Vigilant but death unresponsive
Treatment	Haloperidol (blocks dopamine reuptake) Hypotensive agents Dysrhythmic agents Anticonvulsants	As for cocaine	Naloxone (opiate antagonist) Clonidine or Methadone (for withdrawal symptoms)	Haloperidol (for psychosis)
Neurological complications *Primary:*	Tremor Myoclonus Seizures	Chorea Intracranial haemorrhage (drug-induced vasculitis)	Myelitis Neuropathies and Plexopathies (immune mediated)	Dystonia Athetosis Seizures Rhabdomyalisis
Secondary:	*Infective, hypoxic and hypertensive complications* Intracranial haemorrhage Cerebral infarction Brain abscess Mycotic aneurysms	Intracranial haemorrhage	Postanoxic encephalopathy Brain abscess Mycotic aneurysms	Intracranial haemorrhage

All intravenous drug abusers are at risk of HIV infection and its complications (page 493)

METABOLIC ENCEPHALOPATHIES

In general terms, the clinical features of metabolic encephalopathy are relatively stereotyped.

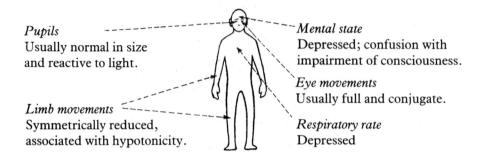

Pupils
Usually normal in size
and reactive to light.

Mental state
Depressed; confusion with
impairment of consciousness.

Eye movements
Usually full and conjugate.

Limb movements
Symmetrically reduced,
associated with hypotonicity.

Respiratory rate
Depressed

These features are characteristic but exceptions occur in specific encephalopathies —

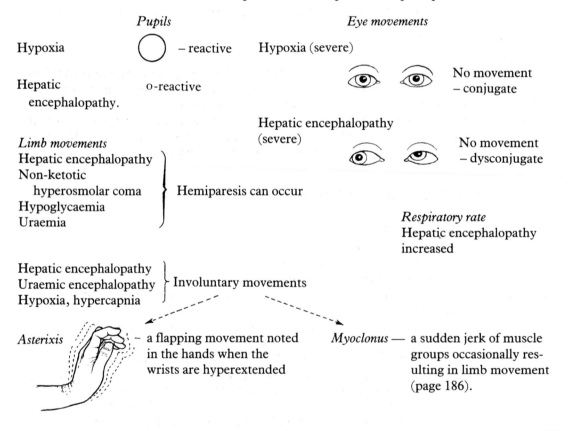

Pupils

Hypoxia   ◯ – reactive

Hepatic   o-reactive
  encephalopathy.

Eye movements

Hypoxia (severe)

No movement
– conjugate

Hepatic encephalopathy
(severe)

No movement
– dysconjugate

Limb movements
Hepatic encephalopathy
Non-ketotic
    hyperosmolar coma   } Hemiparesis can occur
Hypoglycaemia
Uraemia

Respiratory rate
Hepatic encephalopathy
increased

Hepatic encephalopathy
Uraemic encephalopathy } Involuntary movements
Hypoxia, hypercapnia

Asterixis – a flapping movement noted
in the hands when the
wrists are hyperextended

Myoclonus — a sudden jerk of muscle
groups occasionally res-
ulting in limb movement
(page 186).

Beware of the possibility of multiple pathology, e.g. an alcoholic patient with a chronic subdural haematoma may also have liver failure and thiamine deficiency.

CLASSIFICATION AND BIOCHEMICAL EVALUATION

Many metabolic disturbances cause an *acquired* encephalopathy in adults.
The most frequently encountered are:

– *Hypoxic*	Less commonly:
– *Hypercapnoeic*	– Hyponatraemia. Hypernatraemia.
– *Hypoglycaemic*	– Hypokalaemia. Hyperkalaemia.
– *Hyperglycaemic*	– Hypocalcaemia. Hypercalcaemia.
– *Hepatic*	– Hypothyroidism. Lactic acidosis.
– *Uraemic*	– Addison's disease.

Drugs and toxins producing encephalopathy are dealt with separately (page 510).

Laboratory assessment of suspected metabolic encephalopathy
All patients should have a basic biochemical screen:
– Serum urea and electrolytes.
– Liver function (albumin, globulin, bilirubin, alkaline phosphatase and enzymes) and random
    blood glucose.
– Blood gases (pH, PO_2 PCO_2).
– Serum ammonia.
– Electroencephalography — slow wave activity (theta or delta) supports the diagnosis of a diffuse
    dysfunction: hepatic encephalopathy shows a specific triphasic slow wave configuration.
– CT scan — if the above tests are normal or coexisting structural brain disease is suspected.
    Calculation of the *anion gap* may be helpful in the diagnosis of encephalopathies, especially *lactic
acidosis*. The sum of the anions (Cl^- and HCO_3^-) normally equals the sum of the cations (Na^+ and
K^+). An increase in the gap in the absence of ketones, salicylates and uraemia suggests lactic
acidosis.

SPECIFIC ENCEPHALOPATHIES

HYPOXIC ENCEPHALOPATHY
Impaired brain oxygenation results from:
– Reduced arterial oxygen pressure — lung disease.
– Reduced haemoglobin to carry oxygen — anaemia or blood loss.
– Reduced flow of blood containing oxygen (ischaemic hypoxia) — due to reduced cardiac output
    (with reduced cerebral blood flow).
– Biochemical block of cerebral utilisation of oxygen — rare (e.g. cyanide poisoning).
    When cerebral arterial PO_2 falls below 35 mmHg (4.5 kPa), anaerobic metabolism takes over;
this is not efficient and a further drop in PO_2 will result in neurological dysfunction. The extent of
hypoxic damage depends not only upon the duration of hypoxia but also on other factors, e.g. body
temperature — hypothermia protects against damage. The irreversibility of hypoxic damage is
explained by the 'no flow phenomenon' — after 3–5 minutes the endothelial lining of small vessels
swells — even with reversal of hypoxia, flow through these vessels is no longer possible.

SPECIFIC ENCEPHALOPATHIES

HYPOXIC ENCEPHALOPATHY (*contd*)
Pathology
As a consequence of high metabolic demand, some areas are more susceptible than others.

Vulnerability to hypoxia

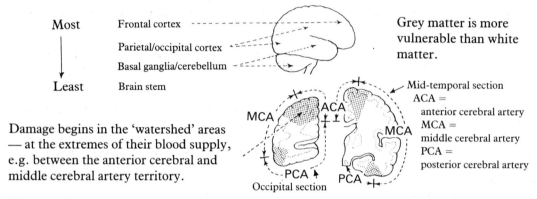

Most — Frontal cortex

Parietal/occipital cortex

Basal ganglia/cerebellum

Least — Brain stem

Grey matter is more vulnerable than white matter.

Damage begins in the 'watershed' areas — at the extremes of their blood supply, e.g. between the anterior cerebral and middle cerebral artery territory.

Mid-temporal section
ACA = anterior cerebral artery
MCA = middle cerebral artery
PCA = posterior cerebral artery

Occipital section

Microscopic changes depend upon the delay between the hypoxic event and death.

Immediate:	*At 48 hours:*	*At several days/weeks:*
Scattered petechial haemorrhages.	Cerebral oedema associated with petechial haemorrhage.	Necrosis in cortical grey matter and globus pallidus with associated astrocytic proliferation. The cerebellum and brain stem may also be affected.

Clinical features:
e.g. Severe hypoxia from circulatory arrest

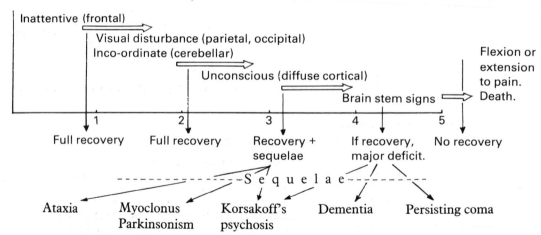

Inattentive (frontal)

Visual disturbance (parietal, occipital)
Inco-ordinate (cerebellar)

Unconscious (diffuse cortical)

Brain stem signs

Flexion or extension to pain. Death.

1 — Full recovery
2 — Full recovery
3 — Recovery + sequelae
4 — If recovery, major deficit.
5 — No recovery

- - - - - - - - - - - - Sequelae - - - - - - - -

Ataxia   Myoclonus   Korsakoff's   Dementia   Persisting coma
           Parkinsonism psychosis

Delayed hypoxic encephalopathy refers to the rare occurrence of a full clinical recovery followed after some weeks by a progressive picture → deterioration of conscious level → death. Widespread subcortical demyelination is found at autopsy.

SPECIFIC ENCEPHALOPATHIES

HYPERCAPNOEIC ENCEPHALOPATHY: the consequence of an elevated arterial carbon dioxide level.
Clinical features:
Headache, confusion, disorientation, involuntary movements.
Papilloedema, depressed limb reflexes, extensor plantar responses.

Diagnosis:
A $P\text{co}_2$ greater than 50 mmHg (6 kPa) with a reduced $P\text{o}_2$ is found on arterial blood sampling.
   The presence of headache, confusion and papilloedema may suggest intracranial tumour. If hypercapnia has not been diagnosed, such patients inevitably are referred for CT brain scan.

HYPOGLYCAEMIC ENCEPHALOPATHY: the consequence of insufficient glucose reaching the brain and may result
from: – overdosage of diabetic treatment
              – insulin secreting tumour — isulinoma
              – hepatic disease with reduction of liver glycogen.
Serum glucose levels of 1.5 mmol/1 are associated with the onset of encephalopathy. Levels of 0.5 mmol/1 are associated with coma.

Pathology:
Changes occur in the cerebral cortex — focal necrosis surrounded by neuronal degeneration. Subcortical grey matter (caudate nucleus) and cerebellum are vulnerable.

Clinical features:
These, as with hypoxia, depend upon the duration and severity of hypoglycaemia.

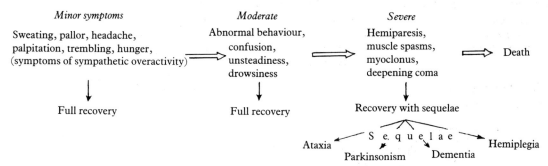

Repeated mild to moderate episodes may result in a chronic cerebellar ataxia.
   Repeated severe attacks may result in a mixed myelopathy/peripheral neuropathy which is distinguished from motor neuron disease by the presence of sensory signs.

HYPERGLYCAEMIC ENCEPHALOPATHY
Two types of encephalopathy develop as a consequence of hyperglycaemia:

Diabetic ketoacidotic coma
Accumulation of acetone and ketone bodies in blood results in acidosis. Hyperventilation ensues with a reduction in $P\text{co}_2$ and $H\text{co}_3^-$. Osmotic diuresis due to hyperglycaemia results in dehydration.
   The neurological presentation is that of confusion progressing to coma and, if untreated, death.

Diabetic hyperosmolar non-ketotic coma
This results from the hyperosmolar effect of severe hyperglycaemia. Reduction of the intracellular compartment results. Involuntary movements, seizures and hemiparesis may occur. Vascular thrombosis is not uncommon. Ketoacidosis is mild or does not occur.

517

SPECIFIC ENCEPHALOPATHIES

HEPATIC ENCEPHALOPATHY

Neurological signs and symptoms secondary to hepatic dysfunction may arise in:
- acute liver failure.
- chronic liver failure complicated by infection or gastrointestinal haemorrhage.
- chronic liver failure producing characteristic *hepatocerebral degeneration*.

Clinical features:

These may be divided into two groups:

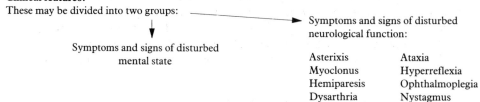

Symptoms and signs of disturbed
mental state

Symptoms and signs of disturbed
neurological function:

Asterixis	Ataxia
Myoclonus	Hyperreflexia
Hemiparesis	Ophthalmoplegia
Dysarthria	Nystagmus

The encephalopathy is progressive.

Pathology:

Neuronal loss with gliosis is noted in the cerebral cortex as well as basal ganglia, cerebellum and brain stem. Astrocytes with irregular and enlarged nuclei are characteristic.

Hepatocerebral degeneration produces varying symptoms and signs. Dementia is associated with dysarthria and ataxia. Primitive reflexes, choreoathetosis, myoclonus, tremor and pyramidal signs may also be present. Consciousness is *not* impaired.

URAEMIC ENCEPHALOPATHY

Clinical features:

These may be divided into two groups:

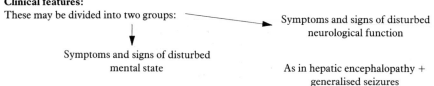

Symptoms and signs of disturbed
mental state

Symptoms and signs of disturbed
neurological function

As in hepatic encephalopathy +
generalised seizures

Pathology:

Uraemia may produce non-specific pathological findings in the nervous system. Peripheral nervous system involvement occurs in chronic renal failure (page 419).

Dialysis encephalopathy is encountered in persons on renal dialysis exposed to high aluminium levels in the dialysate. The features are those of dementia, behavioural changes, seizures and myoclonus. The condition progresses unless aluminium levels are controlled.

Specific investigations and treatment of individual metabolic encephalopathies do not come within the scope of this book.

NUTRITIONAL DISORDERS

INTRODUCTION

Nutritional deficiency presents a major problem in the developing world. In Western countries, alcoholism is the major cause of the neurological syndromes resulting from dietary deficiency with faddism and malabsorption disorders accounting for only a small number.

Vitamins appear important nutrients and certain disorders such as Wernicke Korsakoff syndrome (thiamine) or subacute combined degeneration (vit. B_{12}) are attributed to a single deficiency. Others such as polyneuropathy result from multiple deficiency.

Vitamin deficiency in itself does not always produce symptoms; a dietary excess of carbohydrate seems essential for the development of the neurological features of thiamine deficiency.

As a rule, nutritional disorders of the nervous system present clinically in a symmetrical manner.

WERNICKE KORSAKOFF SYNDROME

This syndrome is comprised of an acute and a chronic phase:

1. Wernick's disease (acute) and   **2. Korsakoff's psychosis** (chronic)

Ocular involvement   Ataxia   Confusion   Selective impairment of short-term (immediate) memory.

Cause:

Thiamine deficiency arising from poor nutrition.

Excessive alcohol intake
Hyperemesis gravidarum
Carcinoma
Renal dialysis.

N.B. Korsakoff's psychosis may also be caused by head injury, anoxia, epilepsy, encephalitis and vascular diseases.

WERNICKE'S DISEASE

Pathology:

Neuronal, axonal and myelin damage occur symmetrically in the mamillary bodies, the walls of the third ventricle, thalamus and periaqueductal grey matter. Secondary vascular proliferation and haemorrhages occur within these lesions.

WERNICKE KORSAKOFF SYNDROME

WERNICKE'S DISEASE (*contd*)

Clinical features: Develops acutely.

Ocular involvement:

Horizontal and vertical nystagmus is evident.

Unilateral or bilateral VI nerve paresis commonly occur.

Gaze palsies are less common.

Pupillary involvement and complete ophthalmoplegia are rare.

Retinal haemorrhages occasionally occur.

Confusion:

Disorientated.

Disinterested and inattentive. Coma is rare.

Withdrawal symptoms of alcohol:
– agitation, delusions and hallucinations develop following admission to hospital.

Ataxia — is often the presenting symptom.

Mild ataxia of gait or gross ataxia with inability to stand.

Lower limb (heel to shin) ataxia is modest. Upper limbs are spared.

Associated features:

Polyneuropathy is present in 80% of cases.

Vestibular disturbances will occur occasionally and accentuate the ataxia.

Autonomic disturbances, such as postural hypotension, may occur.

Investigation

Haematological and biological evidence of alcohol/nutritional deficiency, e.g. elevated MCV, abnormal LFTs, elevated Υ GT.

The blood *transketolase* (enzyme in hexose monophosphate shunt) is an index of thiamine levels, and should be measured immediately before being modified by hospital diet.

The blood *pyruvate* is less accurate.

Treatment

Beware, when giving i.v. dextrose infusions to confused patients, as this uses up the remaining thiamine and aggravates the condition.

50 mg thiamine i.v.
+
50 mg thiamine i.v.
} daily until normal diet is commenced, then supplement with oral thiamine.

Eyes improve — in days, though nystagmus may persist for months.

Ataxia improves — in weeks.

Overall mortality: 15% → coma → death.

KORSAKOFF'S PSYCHOSIS

Pathology

Lesions are identical in distribution to those of Wernicke's disease without haemorrhagic change.

Clinical features

There is a disturbance of memory in which new information cannot be stored. In addition the normal temporal sequence of established memories is disrupted, resulting in a semifictionalised account of the circumstances which the patient may find himself in — *confabulation*. This memory disturbance can only be tested for when the confusion of Wernicke's disease has cleared.

Treatment

Oral thiamine 100 t.d.s. should be continued for some months, although only a small proportion of patients show improved memory function.

SUBACUTE COMBINED DEGENERATION OF THE SPINAL CORD

Cause
B_{12} deficiency:
– Impaired absorption due to lack of intrinsic factor (idiopathic)
– Following total or partial gastrectomy or gastrojejunostomy
– Gastric malignancy
– Celiac disease
– Chronic pancreatic insufficiency

Pathology
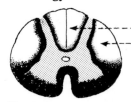
Spinal cord demyelination with eventual axon loss – affects:
posterior columns and
lateral columns (corticospinal and spinocerebellar tracts).
Corticospinal degeneration is most evident in the lower cord,
posterior column degeneration in the upper cord.
Peripheral nerve large myelinated fibre degeneration also occurs.

B_{12} deficiency resulting in neurological damage is usually associated with a *megaloblastic anaemia*, though a normal peripheral blood film may be found.

The exact role of B_{12} in tissue metabolism, especially within the nervous system, has not been defined.

Clinical features
Onset is subacute
Paraesthesia of extremities is the presenting symptom.
Numbness and distal weakness follow.
Walking becomes unsteady and spasticity is evident in the lower limbs with flexor or extensor spasms.

Examination
– Gait is ataxic (sensory ataxia).
– Motor power is diminished distally.
– Plantar responses are extensor.
– Sensory loss: loss of vibration and joint position sensation in the lower limbs. Stocking/glove sensory loss is found when peripheral nerves are involved.
– Reflex findings are variable and depend on the predominance of peripheral nerve or corticospinal tract involvement.

Associated features
Mental changes, due to anaemia or hemisphere demyelination, range from depression to progressive dementia.

Optic nerve involvement presents as visual loss with central or centrocaecal scotomas.

SUBACUTE COMBINED DEGENERATION OF THE SPINAL CORD

Diagnosis

Suspect in paraparesis with combined upper and lower motor neuron signs with 'stocking/glove' sensory loss.

Differentiate from other causes of acute myelopathy, e.g. cord compression, multiple sclerosis.

Investigation

Peripheral blood film.

Bone marrow — megaloblastic erythropoesis.

B_{12} (serum) low.

Investigation of underlying causes of B_{12} deficiency is essential:

– Radioactive B_{12} absorption tests.

– Endoscopy and biopsy.

– Barium meal and follow through.

– Investigation of small intestine function.

Treatment

When neurological dysfunction is present vit. B_{12} therapy must be started promptly — 1000 μg cyanocobalamin daily for several weeks and monthly thereafter.

Course and progression

Untreated, the disorder is progressive, the patient eventually becoming bed-bound.

If diagnosed and treated early (within 2 months of onset), complete recovery can be anticipated.

In established cases, only progression may be halted.

Caution:

When folic acid is prescribed for megaloblastic anaemia, it will improve the haematological picture of B_{12} deficiency with rapid and occasionally irreversible deterioration of the neurological symptoms and signs.

Calciferol (vit. D)

This vitamin is involved in muscle metabolism. Deficiency results in fatigue, muscle weakness and atrophy. These neurological features are associated with hypocalcaemia and osteomalacia.

Tocopherol (vit. E).

The role of this vitamin in the nervous system is unknown. Deficiency results from chronic fat malabsorption (e.g. celiac disease or cystic fibrosis) and results in widespread neurological disturbances — ataxia, ophthalmoplegia, seizures and corticospinal tract dysfunction. These are halted and often reversed by i.m. vit. E.

POLYNEUROPATHY

Deficiency of vitamin B complex — THIAMINE, PYRIDOXINE, PANTOTHENIC ACID — results in peripheral nerve damage.

The combination of polyneuropathy and cardiac involvement is referred to as **BERI-BERI**.

When oedema is also present it is termed wet beri-beri and, when absent, dry beri-beri.

Beri-beri occurs in rice eating countries.

In Western countries, alcoholism is the major cause of nutritional polyneuropathy with or without cardiac involvement.

Pathology

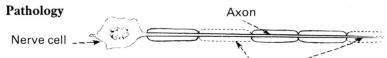

Axon

Nerve cell

Segmental demyelination and axonal degeneration occur simultaneously

The distal portions of nerves are initially affected.

Anterior horn cells and dorsal root ganglion cells undergo chromatolysis.

Vagus nerve and sympathetic trunk involvement occurs in severe cases.

Clinical features

Onset: subacute

Symptoms: Progressive distal weakness and sensory loss with painful tingling paraesthesia.

Signs:

1. Varing degrees of *areflexia* (only ankle reflexes are lost initially).
2. *Weakness* which is more marked distally than proximally and initially involves the lower limbs.
3. *Sensory loss* of a 'stocking/glove' type involving all modalities of sensation.
4. *Sympathetic* involvement results in sweating soles of feet and occasionally demonstrable orthostatic hypotension.
5. *Vagus nerve* involvement results in a hoarse voice and disturbance of swallowing.

Associated signs

Shiny skin on legs with poor distal hair growth. 'Hyperpathic' painful soles of feet.

Diagnosis

Suggested by nutritional/alcohol history.

Supported by investigations such as peripheral blood film (MCV), LETs and γGT.

Nerve conduction studies confirm the clinical picture and detect asymptomatic cases with minimal signs, e.g. reduced ankle reflexes, diminished peripheral vibration sensation.

Differential diagnosis

Consider other causes of subacute or chronic sensorimotor neuropathy (see page 418).

Treatment

Balanced diet with vitamin B group supplementation. Parental use of vitamins should be considered early in treatment.

Burning paraesthesia may respond to carbamazepine or to a lumbar sympathetic block.

Recovery may be very slow and incomplete but with the withdrawal of alcohol and adequate vitamin supplementation some improvement should occur.

TOXIC AND NUTRITIONAL AMBLYOPIA

A large number of toxic substances can produce impaired vision. Methyl alcohol causes sudden and permanent blindness. Chronic visual loss from optic neuritis develops in malnourished patients with a high tobacco consumption (Tobacco-alcohol amblyopia).

Pathology
Damage involves the papillomacular bundle within the optic nerves, chiasma and optic tracts. Retinal ganglion cells in the macular region are also affected.

Clinical features
– The condition slowly develops over weeks.
– Vision becomes hazy and blurred.
– Colour vision (red/green discrimination) is involved early.

Examination
– Bilateral involvement.
– Reduced visual acuity.
– Centrocaecal scotoma
  (a central field defect
  spreading from blind
  spot to macula and most easily detected with a red target).
– Fundal examination is normal, though optic atrophy will occur eventually.
– Coexistent Wernicke Korsakoff syndrome or polyneuropathy are common.

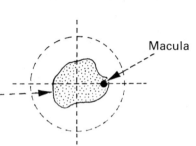

Macula

Treatment
Improvement in nutrition will halt progression and even result in gradual shrinkage of the scotoma.
Vitamin B supplementation, including B_{12}, should be administered.

SUBACUTE NECTROTISING ENCEPHALOMYELOPATHY (LEIGH'S DISEASE)
This rare autosomal recessive disorder presents in infancy and infrequently in adults. Weakness, hypotonia, dementia, ataxia and blindness culminate in death within months of onset. The pathological resemblance to Wernicke's disease suggests thiamine deficiency; temporary clinical benefit follows thiamine administration.

ALCOHOL RELATED DISORDERS

ALCOHOLIC MYOPATHY
Muscle damage (elevated creatine phosphokinase) is not uncommon in alcoholics following acute ingestion, but this is rarely symptomatic.

Acute necrotizing myopathy occurs after 'binge' drinking.
– Acute muscle necrosis ensues with pain/cramping and muscle tenderness/swelling.
– Myoglobin is excreted in the urine (myoglobinuria) after release
  from damaged muscles.
– Symptoms of alcohol withdrawal — delirium, etc. — coexist.
– Limb involvement may be markedly asymmetrical.
– Sometimes calf muscles are swollen and tender.
– Improvement occurs over weeks to months.
– Serum creatine phosphokinase (CPK) is
  elevated. Marked myoglobinuria when
  present may result in renal failure.
– Elevated serum K^+ may provoke cardiac arrhythmias.
– Aetiology appears due to the direct toxic effect of alcohol on muscle.
Chronic proximal weakness has been described, but is rare.

ALCOHOL RELATED DISORDERS

ALCOHOLIC DEMENTIA

Experimentally, chronic alcohol consumption results in neuronal loss. CT evidence of atrophy and neuropsychological impairment is common in alcoholics. However, whether or not these result from the direct toxic and dementing effect of alcohol remains uncertain.

ALCOHOLIC CEREBELLAR DEGENERATION

Alcoholic patients may develop a chronic cerebellar syndrome either as a sequel of Wernicke's disease or as a distinct clinical entity.

A long history of alcohol abuse is obtained.   Males are predominantly affected.

Onset is gradual and symptoms often stabilise.

Ataxia of gait with lower limb inco-ordination predominates. The upper limbs are spared.

Nystagmus is rarely present. Cerebellar dysarthria is usually mild.

Coexistent signs of neuropathy are often found.

Investigations: – Abnormal liver function tests. -Macrocytosis in peripheral blood film. -Elevated γGT.
     – CSF examination normal.
     – CT scanning may reveal cerebellar atrophy.

Progression → may evolve rapidly and reverse with improved nutrition and alcohol withdrawal.

↘ may evolve subacutely.

↘ may evolve chronically and slowly progress over many years.

Pathology: — Purkinje cell loss in cerebellar hemispheres and in superior cerebellar vermis.

Pathogenesis: — The disorder may be due to *nutritional deficiency,* especially thiamine, or else result from the direct toxic effect of alcohol or electrolyte disturbance on the cerebellum.

Differential diagnosis: — Distinguish from hereditary and other acquired ataxias, e.g. hypothyroidism, remote effects of carcinoma.

Treatment: — Alcohol withdrawal, a well balanced diet and adequate vitamin supplementation.

CENTRAL PONTINE MYELINOLYSIS

A history of alcohol abuse or debilitating disease such as carcinoma is obtained.

The lesion is one of demyelination with cavitation. Microscopically, myelin is lost, oligodendrocytes degenerate but neurons and axons are spared.

Clinically, an acute or subacute pontine lesion is suspected, evolving over a few days, with bulbar weakness and tetraparesis.

The limbs are flaccid with extensor plantar responses.

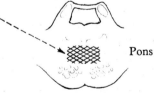

Pons

With progression of the lesion, eye signs become evident and conscious level becomes depressed → coma → death.

Investigations:

Electrolytic disturbances (low sodium, low phosphate) are found.

Liver function is normal. CSF examination is normal.

CT may demonstrate non-enhancing pontine low density. MRI appears more sensitive.

Recognition of this condition before death is important in view of its reversibility, though prior to CT/MRI availability it was diagnosed at autopsy. Vigorous supportive therapy with correction of metabolic abnormalities and vitamin supplementation is advised.

CORPUS CALLOSUM DEMYELINATION (syn: Marchiafava-Bignami disease)

This is a rare disorder occurring in malnourished alcoholics. It is rarely diagnosed in life.

The clinical picture is that of personality change with signs of frontal lobe disease.

The condition occurs most commonly in persons of Italian origin.

NON-METASTATIC MANIFESTATIONS OF MALIGNANT DISEASE

Disturbance of neurological function can occur in association with carcinoma without evidence of metastases. Brain, spinal cord, peripheral nerve and muscle may be affected, either separately or in combination. Other forms of malignancy such as the reticuloses may produce similar neurological syndromes.

Small cell carcinoma of the lung is the commonest malignancy to be associated with the non-metastatic syndromes. The mechanism of these syndromes is unclear, but neuronal damage may result from tumour peptide release or crossed antigenicity between tumour tissue and neurons.

The non-metastatic manifestations of malignancy are rare.

NON-METASTATIC NEUROLOGICAL SYNDROMES

The syndromes are not discreet, e.g. neuropathy and myopathy may coexist → carcinomatous neuromyopathy; encephalitis and myelopathy → carcinomatous encephalomyelitis.

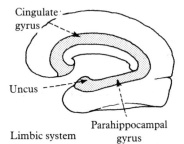

Encephalitis

Cerebellar degeneration

Myelopathy

Neuropathy

Myopathy

Neuromuscular junction disturbance
Myasthenic syndrome

ENCEPHALITIS

Cingulate gyrus

Uncus

Limbic system

Parahippocampal gyrus

Pathology
The encephalitic process selectively affects the limbic system — with neuronal loss, astrocytic proliferation and perivascular inflammatory changes.

Clinical features
Disturbance in behaviour precedes the development of complex partial (temporal lobe) seizures and memory impairment.
The course is progressive.

CEREBELLAR DEGENERATION

Usually associated with bronchial (small cell) or ovarian carcinoma.

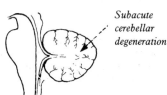

Subacute cerebellar degeneration

Pathology:
Purkinje cell loss with some involvement of the dentate nucleus. Brain stem changes also occur. Anti-Purkinje cell antibodies have occasionally been isolated.

Clinical features:
The patient presents with a rapidly developing ataxia.
Brain stem involvement results in nystagmus, opsiclonus and vertigo.
The course is one of rapid progression.

MYELITIS

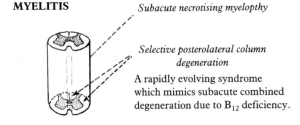

Subacute necrotising myelopthy

Selective posterolateral column degeneration

A rapidly evolving syndrome which mimics subacute combined degeneration due to B_{12} deficiency.

Pathology
Axonal and myelin destruction with microglial proliferation.

Clinical features:
Back pain with ascending paraesthesia, weakness and loss of sphincter control. Upper limb involvement is followed by respiratory paralysis and death.

NON-METASTATIC MANIFESTATIONS OF MALIGNANT DISEASE

NEUROPATHY (see page 425)

Sensory neuropathy: Destruction of the posterior root ganglion combined with axonal and demyelinative peripheral nerve damage causes progressive sensory symptoms. The neuropathy is subacute or chronic in evolution.

Sensorimotor neuropathy: A mixed neuropathy with weakness and sensory loss. The syndrome may predate the recognition of the underlying neoplasm.

Rarely, an acute neuropathy indistinguishable from postinfectious polyneuropathy may occur.

MYOPATHY

Establishing a causal relationship may be difficult.
– Muscle weakness can develop long before evidence of neoplasia.
– In patients with unexplained myopathy, malignancy may be detected only at autopsy.

Proximal myopathy: A slowly progressive syndrome with weakness of proximal limb muscles. In myopathy occurring in middle/late life, underlying neoplasm is a likely explanation.

Inflammatory myopathy (polymyositis/dermatomyositis) (see page 454):
The overall incidence of associated neoplasm in inflammatory myopathy is 15%. The typical patient is in middle age with a proximal weakness, elevated ESR and muscle enzymes with or without the skin features of dermatomyositis.

Myopathy with endocrine disturbance: Ectopic hormone production (by malignant cells) may induce a myopathy characterised by chronic progressive proximal weakness, e.g. ectopic ACTH production from oat cell carcinoma of lung.

Cachetic myopathy occurs in terminally ill, wasted patients.

THE MYASTHENIC SYNDROME (Eaton-Lambert syndrome)
A disorder of the neuromuscular junction.
Acetylcholine release following nerve stimulation is deficient.
This autoimmune disease is associated with malignancy (small cell carcinoma of the lung in 70% of sufferers).

Clinical features

The patient develops weakness of lower then upper limbs with a tendency to fatigue. Following brief exercise, power may paradoxically suddenly improve — second wind phenomenon. In contrast to myasthenia gravis ocular and bulbar muscles are rarely affected. Examination reveals a proximal pattern of wasting and weakness with diminished tendon reflexes. Up to 50% of patients experience symptoms of autonomic (cholinergic) dysfunction — impotence, dry mouth and visual disturbance.

Diagnosis

Confirmed electrophysiologically; the 'second wind phenomenon' is shown up as an incrementing response to repetitive nerve stimulation (as opposed to the decrementing response in myasthenia gravis, page 463).

Treatment

Guanidine hydrochloride and 4-aminopyridine enhance acetylcholine release by acting on calcium and potassium channels. These treatments are effective but toxic. 3, 4-diaminopyridine (less toxic), steroids and plasma exchange may also help.

These syndromes may respond to the removal of the underlying neoplasm. A totally resectible primary tumour is rarely encountered and the response to operation unpredictable.

The myasthenic syndrome may develop in the absence of neoplasia, especially in women.

527

DEGENERATIVE DISORDERS

Introduction

This heterogeneous group of neurological diseases is grouped together by the lack of known aetiology. As causes of such disease are identified (e.g. metabolic, viral) they have been reclassified in their appropriate category. Of the remaining conditions many are familial.

Characteristically these disorders:

– are gradually progressive
– are symmetrical (bilateral symptoms and signs)
– may affect one or several specific levels of the nervous system
– may demonstrate a specific pathology or just show neuronal atrophy and eventual loss without other features.

Classification

Degenerative disorders are classified according to the specific part or parts of the central/peripheral nervous system affected and according to the ensuing clinical manifestations.
The degenerative disorders may be alternatively termed the *system degenerations* because of their propensity to affect only part of the nervous system.

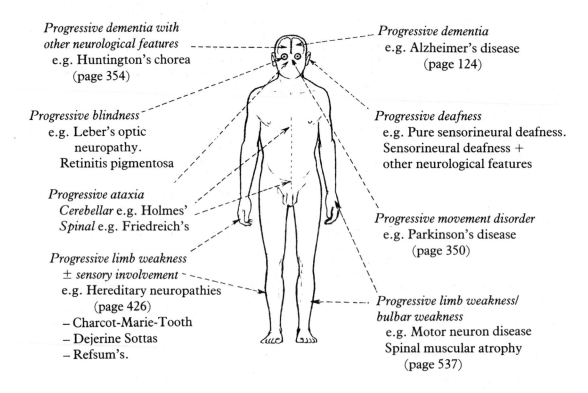

Progressive dementia with other neurological features
e.g. Huntington's chorea
(page 354)

Progressive blindness
e.g. Leber's optic neuropathy.
Retinitis pigmentosa

Progressive ataxia
Cerebellar e.g. Holmes'
Spinal e.g. Friedreich's

Progressive limb weakness
± *sensory involvement*
e.g. Hereditary neuropathies
(page 426)
– Charcot-Marie-Tooth
– Dejerine Sottas
– Refsum's.

Progressive dementia
e.g. Alzheimer's disease
(page 124)

Progressive deafness
e.g. Pure sensorineural deafness.
Sensorineural deafness +
other neurological features

Progressive movement disorder
e.g. Parkinson's disease
(page 350)

Progressive limb weakness/ bulbar weakness
e.g. Motor neuron disease
Spinal muscular atrophy
(page 537)

Most of these conditions are discussed in other chapters.

PROGRESSIVE BLINDNESS

LEBER'S OPTIC NEUROPATHY

Leber's optic neuropathy is a familial disorder of maternal inheritance with a tendency to affect males significantly more than females. The condition may result from defect of cyanide metabolism or of the enzyme thiosulphate transferase.

Pathology:

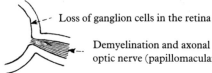

Loss of ganglion cells in the retina

Demyelination and axonal loss in the optic nerve (papillomacular bundle)

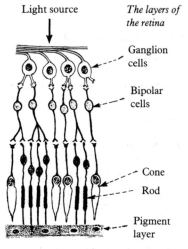

Light source

The layers of the retina

Ganglion cells

Bipolar cells

Cone

Rod

Pigment layer

Clinical features

Onset of visual loss in late teens/early twenties.
   – The first symptom is blurring of vision
   – Both eyes are simultaneously affected (rarely one eye months before the other).
   – Central vision is lost with large bilateral scotomata.
   Characteristically, blue/yellow colour discrimination is affected before red/green. The optic disc initially appears pink and swollen with an increase in small vessels, eventually becoming pale and atrophic.
   Visual impairment progresses with peripheral constriction of the fields. Complete visual loss seldom occurs. Occasionally vision can marginally improve.
   Associated symptoms and signs of a more generalised nervous system disorder occur in a proportion of cases — dementia, ataxia, progressive spastic paraplegia — and confusion with multiple sclerosis may arise.
   The diagnosis is made on the basis of a family history. Fluorescein angiography distinguishes this condition from acute bilateral optic neuritis. (Fluorescein 'leakage' does not occur in Leber's disease.)

Treatment: No treatment is effective.

RETINITIS PIGMENTOSA

A hereditary disorder of the retina which may be inherited as an autosomal dominant, recessive or X-linked disorder. All layers of the retina are affected.

Pathology:

Posterior pale cataracts and glaucoma are occasionally associated.

Loss of rods, degeneration of cones.
Bipolar and ganglion cells are also affected.
Pigment migrates to superficial layers.

The optic nerve may show some gliosis, but often is remarkably normal.

Clinical features

Onset of visual loss in childhood. Both eyes are simultaneously affected. Initially there is a failure of twilight vision. The child has difficulty in making his way as darkness falls (nyctalopia). The retina around the macular area is first affected resulting in a characteristic ring scotoma. This gradually spreads outwards; eventually only a small 'tunnel' of central vision is left. Finally, complete blindness occurs. The majority of patients are completely blind by 50 years of age.
   The fundal appearance is diagnostic as a result of the superficial migration of pigment.
   The electroretinogram — recording the electrical activity of the retina — is eventually lost.

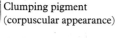

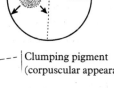

Clumping pigment (corpuscular appearance)

Pale optic disc

Attenuated vessels

Treatment

None. Vitamins and steroids have been tried unsuccessfully.

Associated conditions in retinitis pigmentosa

Several conditions are associated with retinitis pigmentosa:
– Hypogonadism/obesity/mental deficiency
– Spinocerebellar degeneration
– Polyneuropathy/sensorineural deafness
– Myopathy/ophthalmoplegia/heart block

– Laurence Moon syndrome
– Friedreich's ataxia
– Refsum's syndrome
– Kearns-Sayre syndrome } – Visual failure not progressive.

529

PROGRESSIVE ATAXIA

The degenerative disorders manifested by progressive ataxia are termed *spinocerebellar degenerations*. Further classification is difficult in view of the many descriptions of familial cases in the literature, often bearing the eponymous title of the original author. The clinical overlap in these various forms is such that a broad concept of the disorders is the only pragmatic approach to them.

Ataxias may be classified by age of onset, presence of associated features, mode of inheritance or site of dysfunction.

ATAXIA TELANGIECTASIA (Louis-Bar syndrome)

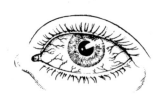

This multisystem disorder is characterised by progressive cerebellar ataxia, ocular and cutaneous telangiectasia and immunodeficiency. The disorder is of autosomal recessive inheritance affecting males and females equally.

Pathologically, widespread cerebellar neuronal loss occurs.

A progressive ataxia develops in infancy. Telangiectasia develops later, becoming more obvious after exposure to the sun.

Patients are eventually confined to a wheelchair and, because of associated low serum levels of IgE and IgM, are susceptible to repetitive infections.

Malignant neoplasms occur in 10% (lymphoma, glioma, thyroid adenoma).

Giving radiotherapy for these tumours has caused an increased incidence of chromosomal breakage and rearrangement, suggesting defective DNA repair mechanisms.

Treatment is symptomatic.

FRIEDREICH'S ATAXIA

Two forms of this disorder are recognised:

– early onset (8–20 years) autosomal recessive.
– late onset (over 20 years) autosomal dominant.

The recessive form more rapidly progresses.

Prevalence: 2 per 100 000 persons.

The underlying cause of this condition is probably metabolic.

Pathology:

Spinal: The spinal cord is shrunken, especially in the thoracic region.
There is degeneration and gliosis of:
1. — Posterior columns
2. — Corticospinal tracts
3. — Dorsal spinocerebellar tracts
4. — Ventral spinocerebellar tracts.
Dorsal roots and peripheral nerves are also shrunken when the condition is advanced.

Cerebellar: Changes in the cerebellum are less marked, there is Purkinje cell loss and atrophy of the dentate nucleus.

Peripheral nerves show loss of large myelinated axons and segmental demyelination.

The corticobulbar tract and cerebrum are relatively spared.

PROGRESSIVE ATAXIA

FRIEDREICH'S ATAXIA *(contd)*

Clinical features

Sexes are equally affected.

Disturbance of balance is the initial symptom, often associated with the development of scoliosis. A spastic, ataxic gait develops with inco-ordination of the limbs.

Corticospinal tract involvement results in limb weakness with absent abdominal reflexes and extensor plantar responses.

Posterior column involvement results in loss of vibration and joint position appreciation in the extremities.

Dorsal root and *peripheral nerve* involvement results in absent lower limb reflexes.

Involvement of myocardial muscle (cardiomyopathy) is common and results in cardiac failure or dysrhythmias.

Musculoskeletal abnormalities occur in 80% of cases.

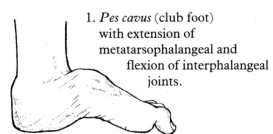

1. *Pes cavus* (club foot) with extension of metatarsophalangeal and flexion of interphalangeal joints.

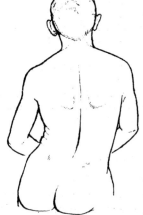

2. *Kyphoscoliosis* Excessive posterior and lateral curvature of the spine.

Optic atrophy, retinitis pigmentosa, nystagmus, distal wasting and convulsions may all be associated with Friedreich's ataxia.

The disease is progressive. Patients are usually unable to walk within 5 years of onset, and death from cardiac (cardiomyopathy) or pulmonary (kyphoscoliosis) complications occurs within 10–20 years. Arrested cases without progression do occur but are rare. Diabetes mellitus occurs in 10%.

Diagnosis

This is made on clinical grounds, usually with a known family history. It is considered when midline and limb ataxia develops in childhood. As the disease progresses the diagnosis becomes obvious, but initially exclusion of the many inborn errors of metabolism producing ataxia in childhood is necessary.

Nerve conduction velocities are prolonged.

Somatosensory evoked potential amplitudes are small and when optic nerve involvement is present visual evoked potentials are prolonged.

Aetiology

The biochemical basis of this disorder is unknown. Abnormalities of pyruvate dehydrogenase and mitochondrial enzymes have been suggested.

Treatment

Usually supportive. Choline and lecithin have been used for ataxia but without dramatic results. High-fat diet to bypass pyruvate dehydrogenase deficiency has had a limited success. Genetic counselling is advised. In the recessive form the risk of transmission to offspring is small.

531

PROGRESSIVE ATAXIA

ROUSSY-LEVY SYNDROME
A probable variant of Friedreich's ataxia, associated with features of hereditary motor sensory neuropathy.

MARIE'S SPASTIC ATAXIA
A further variant of Friedreich's ataxia, associated with features of a progressive spastic paraplegia (more marked than that found in pure Friedreich's ataxia).

CORTICAL CEREBELLAR DEGENERATION OF HOLMES
A mendelian dominant disorder.

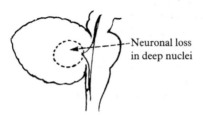

Neuronal loss in deep nuclei

Clinical features
Onset in middle age, with lower limb involvement, then dysarthria and upper limb spread.
    Seizures and myoclonus may ensue.
    The disorder is progressive over 12–15 years.
    Distinction should be made from acquired cerebellar degeneration, e.g.
– alcohol/nutritional,
– hypothyroidism,
– drugs, e.g. phenytoin

Progressive degeneration of the cerebellar cortex with Purkinje cell loss and reactive gliosis.

DYSSYNERGIA CEREBELLARIS MYOCLONICA
(Ramsay Hunt syndrome)

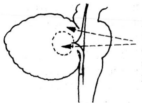

Myoclonus reflects the damage to the dentate nucleus and superior cerebellar peduncle

Characterised by the presence of myoclonus in an early onset cerebellar degeneration.
    Mendelian dominant disorder with onset in childhood. The disorder progresses with age. Myoclonic jerks of limbs and trunk are associated with nystagmus, dysarthria, ataxia of gait and stance and limb inco-ordination.
    Sodium valproate or clonazepam may suppress myoclonic jerks.

OLIVOPONTOCEREBELLAR DEGENERATION
A mendelian dominant disorder

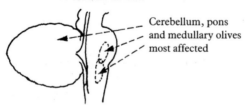

Cerebellum, pons and medullary olives most affected

Variable age of onset.
    Initial features are purely cerebellar then involvement of bulbar musculature and extrapyramidal features become evident.
    The patient becomes immobile and develops progressive speech and swallowing difficulties.
    Autonomic features may be associated.
    Survival ranges from 25–30 years from onset.

Diffuse cerebral atrophy and ventricular dilatation also occurs.

PROGRESSIVE SPASTICITY

HEREDITARY SPASTIC PARAPLEGIA
An autosomal dominant or recessive disorder with age of onset between 20 and 40 years.
    The patient presents with lower limb stiffness and difficulty in running. Weakness is mild, sphincter disturbance late and bulbar and upper limb function spared.

MOTOR NEURON DISEASE

Motor neuron disease (MND) consists of a group of disorders, all affecting in part the anterior horn cell. It is a progressive condition with no specific treatment.

Different terms are used to describe involvement at each level:
1. The motor cortex.
2. The corticobulbar pathway:
   PSEUDOBULBAR PALSY.
3. The cranial nerve nuclei:
   PROGRESSIVE BULBAR PALSY.
4. The corticospinal tract:
   PRIMARY LATERAL SCLEROSIS.
5. The anterior horn cell:
   PROGRESSIVE MUSCULAR ATROPHY.

When 4 and 5 predominate, the term AMYOTROPHIC LATERAL SCLEROSIS (ALS) is used.

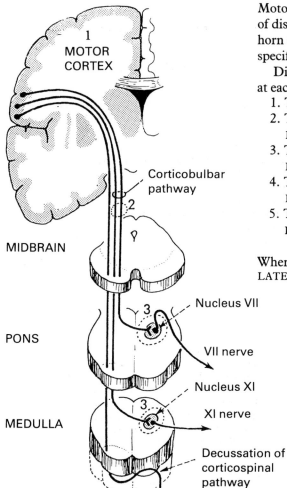

Epidemiology
Incidence: 1 per 100 000, except in endemic areas such as the Island of Guam. Clusters and conjugal cases have been reported.
Familial link in 5–10% of patients.
Sex ratio: male/female — 1–5/1
Mean age of onset — 55 years
               range — 16–77 years.
Mean survival — 3 years (50%),
               over 10 years (10%).

Pathology
Naked eye: Thinning of anterior roots of spinal cord.

Microscopic: Loss of neurons in motor cortex. Loss of neurons in cranial nerve nuclei and anterior horns. Section of brain stem: reduction of corticobulbar and corticospinal fibres.
No evidence of inflammatory response is seen in involved structures.

MOTOR NEURON DISEASE

AETIOLOGY

The cause of motor neuron disease is unknown. Several possibilities have been suggested:

– *Ageing:* Premature ageing in certain motor cells may result in increasing metabolic demand upon survivors. As a consequence the survivors also suffer premature loss. This process could be 'triggered' by genetic and environmental factors.

– *Viruses:* Slow virus infection has been suggested. Polio virus will acutely damage the anterior horn cell and 'slow' polio infection could theoretically produce motor neuron disease. Some claim that motor neuron disease follows acute poliomyelitis; however, when this occurs the clinical picture is not typical and may resemble more closely Spinal Muscular Atrophy (see later). Polio antibody titres remain normal. Virus-like particles have been reported in some patients with MND, but transmission to non-human primates has been unsuccessful.

– *Disordered carbohydrate metabolism:* Variable findings such as diabetic glucose tolerance curves, carbohydrate intolerance and insulin resistance, have been described in patients with motor neuron disease. No consistent abnormality has been found.

– *Toxins:* Certain metals, lead, selenium, mercury and manganese have been incriminated, but again evidence is inconclusive.

– *Minerals:* Clinical similarities between MND and neurological involvement in hyperparathyroidism and phosphate deficiency suggest a relationship with chronic calcium deficiency.

An increased incidence of *gastric surgery* in sufferers, the presence of *immune complexes* in small bowel biopsies and disordered *cellular immunity* have been noted but causative relationships are unclear.

CLINICAL FEATURES

At onset:

Combined upper and lower motor neuron features — 65%

Bulbar or pseudobulbar features — 25% (short survival)

Muscle weakness and atrophy — 10% (medium-long survival).

Pseudobulbar palsy

Features are due to degeneration of corticobulbar pathways to V, VII, X, XI and XII cranial nerve motor nuclei (with sparing of III, IV and VI).

There is an apparent weakness of the muscles of mastication and expression, the patient has difficulty in chewing and the face is expressionless. The jaw jerk (page 15) is exaggerated.

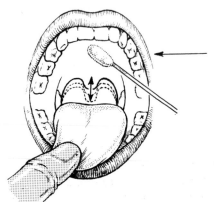

Food and fluid enter nasopharynx when swallowing – palatal weakness (X).

Gag reflex is brisk when soft palate is stimulated.

Speech is drawling and monotonous.

Swallowing is difficult (X).

Tongue is immobile, pointed and cannot protrude (XII).

The manifestations of emotions are increased producing *emotional lability* — unprovoked outbursts of laughing or crying result.

MOTOR NEURON DISEASE

Progressive bulbar palsy

The symptoms and signs are due to a disturbance of the motor cranial nuclei rather than corticobulbar tracts. The condition is distinguished from pseudobulbar palsy by the presence of lower motor neuron (nuclear) signs.

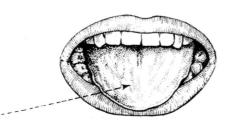

    Atrophy and *fasciculations* are present in cranial nerve innervated muscles.

    Fasciculations are visible muscle twitches which occur spontaneously and represent groups of discharging motor units.

    The tongue appears wasted and folded; fasciculations produce a writhing appearance. Jaw jerk and gag reflex are absent.

Primary lateral sclerosis

Signs of corticospinal tract disturbance with:
- – Increased tone.
- – Brisk reflexes.
- – Extensor plantar responses.
- – Distinctive distribution of weakness (extensors in upper limbs; flexors in lower limbs).

Spasticity is rarely severe (intact extrapyramidal inhibition).

Progressive muscular atrophy

Signs and symptoms are due to anterior horn cell involvement. Atrophy, weakness and fasciculations are the cardinal features.

The patient is often aware of fasciculation.

Muscle cramps are common.

Weakness is not as severe as the degree of wasting suggests.

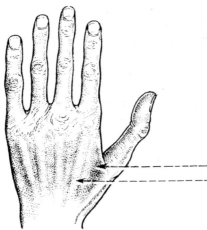

In the hand: wasting is evident. 1st dorsal interosseous muscle and tendons become prominent as hand muscles waste, giving 'guttered' appearance — SKELETON HAND.

As the disease progresses, these symptoms and signs spread to involve all skeletal muscles.

MOTOR NEURON DISEASE

Amyotrophic lateral sclerosis
Characterised by the unusual, almost diagnostic appearance of wasted, fasciculating muscles (anterior horn cell) with brisk reflexes (corticospinal tract). This is described as TONIC ATROPHY.

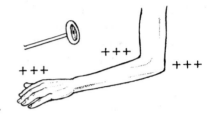

Relentless progression of symptoms and signs is inevitable.

DIAGNOSIS
The clinical findings are quite characteristic. These are supported by electromyography which reveals denervation with fibrillations widespread in different muscle groups (see EMG).

Differential diagnosis includes disorders which produce combined upper and lower motor neuron signs, e.g.
   Cervical spondylosis
   Spinal tumours.

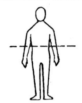

Segmental (LMN signs) weakness

Corticospinal muscle weakness

Hyperthyroidism and hyperparathyroidism produce muscle wasting and hyperreflexia.

Pseudobulbar palsy may result also from cerebrovascular disease or multiple sclerosis.

Progressive muscular atrophy may be confused with a spinal muscular atrophy, limb girdle dystrophy, diabetic amyotrophy or lead neuropathy.

N.B. *IN MOTOR NEURON DISEASE:*   *– Sensory signs do not occur*
                                     – Bladder is never involved
                                       – Ocular muscles are never affected.

TREATMENT
The diagnosis should be discussed fully with the patient and carers, and multidisciplinary support and counselling offered.

Symptomatic treatment:
Anarthria and dysarthria: —— Speech assessment and communication aids when indicated.
Dysphagia and aspiration:—— Cricopharyngeal myotomy. Feeding gastrostomy.
Nutrition: ——————— Estimate calorific content and supplement diet with vitamins.
Muscle weakness: ————Physiotherapy, walking aids. Splints, etc.
Respiratory failure: ——— Management poses problems. The value of assisted ventilation in a disorder that leads eventually to total paralysis is questionable.

Therapeutic trials
There is no proven treatment, nonetheless patients are only too keen to participate in clinical trials. These must always be properly designed and have scientific rationale.
Recent studies have evaluated:
    – Thyroid releasing hormone (THR)
    – L.theonine   – Testosterone
    – Cyclophosphamide   – Plasma exchange.

INHERITED MOTOR NEURON DISORDERS

SPINAL MUSCULAR ATROPHIES

These diseases have a hereditary basis and are characterised by degeneration of cranial nerve nuclei and anterior horn cells of the spinal cord. As with motor neuron disease these disorders solely affect the motor system. After Duchenne dystrophy they are the commonest cause of childhood neuromuscular disease.

Werdnig Hoffman disease

Acute infantile onset: 25% of patients.
This is an autosomal recessive disorder.

Reduced large fibres
in peripheral nerve

Grouped or 'neurogenic' atrophy of either type 1 or type 2 muscle fibres

Loss of anterior horn cells

Thinning of anterior root

Clinical features:
Reduced fetal movements in late pregnancy with weakness and hypotonia at birth.

The child lies with arms and legs abducted and externally rotated (hypotonic posture)

Contractures, wasting and fasciculation gradually become evident

} differentiate from other causes of 'floppy' infant.

May progress rapidly to death in 2–3 months.

In survivors, all motor milestones are delayed; 95% of all patients are dead by 18 months.

Kugelberg Welander disease

Late infantile or juvenile onset: 45% of patients.
Pathological features similar to Werdnig Hoffman disease. Both autosomal dominant and sex-linked recessive inheritances have been described.

Clinical features:
The disorder is characterised by wasting and weakness of proximal limb muscles. It is slowly progressive with great variability even within the same family. Survival into old age without serious disability can occur.

This disorder may easily be confused with limb girdle atrophy.

Adult onset: 8% of patients.
An autosomal dominant or recessive disorder. Motor function develops normally in childhood. Slowly progressive limb wasting and weakness appear in adult life. Cranial motor nerve weakness occurs in 50%. Corticospinal tract signs are rare. Life expectancy is normal. Confusion of spinal muscular atrophy with *acquired* motor neuron disease (MND) is common especially when the onset occurs asymmetrically. The presence of a family history and the slow rate of progression supports the former diagnosis.

Distal and scapuloperoneal forms

Differentiation from HMSN types I and II (page 426) and scapuloperoneal dystrophy (page 451) is clinically difficult and separation may only be possible on histological and neurophysiological grounds.

Juvenile bulbar palsy

An autosomal recessive disorder presenting in late childhood with drooling and dysarthria, progressing to aspiration pneumonia and respiratory failure. Limb involvement and pyramidal tract signs can occur. Few patients survive the second decade.

Management of spinal muscular atrophies

There is no specific treatment. Care is supportive.
Genetic counselling is essential to indicate the risks, e.g.
recessive form of adult onset: — risk to siblings 1 in 5   — risk to offspring 1 in 20.

NEUROCUTANEOUS SYNDROMES

These disorders are hereditary, characterised by multiorgan malformations and tumours. The literature includes many varieties of such conditions; most are extremely rare. Only the more major disorders are described below.

NEUROFIBROMATOSIS
Two distinct types occur:

Type 1
Characterised by café au lait spots and neurofibromas (Von Recklinghausen's disease).
Incidence: 1:4000
Inheritance: Autosomal dominant gene on chromosome 17.

Type 2
Characterised by tumours (schwannomas) of the eighth cranial nerve.

1: 50 000
Autosomal dominant gene on chromosome 22.

Pathology (type 1):
An embryological disorder in which localised overgrowth of *mesodermal* or *ectodermal* tissue produces tumours of:

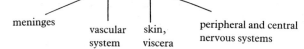

meninges | vascular system | skin, viscera | peripheral and central nervous systems

Clinical features (type 1):
Skin manifestations: —— Café au lait spots: light brown patches on the trunk with well demarcated edges.
Subcutaneous neurofibromata lying along peripheral nerves and enlarging with age.
Mollusca fibrosa: cutaneous fibromas – large, pedunculated and pink in colour
Plexiform neuroma: diffuse neurofibroma associated with skin and subcutaneous overgrowth and occasional underlying bony abnormality.
Skeletal manifestations: — 50% of patients exhibit scoliosis.
Subperiosteal neurofibromas may give rise to bone hypertrophy or rarification with pathological fractures.
Hypertension: — May result from intimal hyperplasia or coexistent phaeochromocytoma.
Neoplasia: — A high incidence of leukaemia, neuroblastoma, medullary thyroid carcinoma, and multiple endocrine neoplasia occurs.
Neurological manifestations: — Mental retardation and epilepsy occur in 10–15% of patients without intracranial neoplasm. Cerebrovascular accidents as a consequence of intimal hyperplasia are not uncommon. Three patterns of neurological neoplasia are recognised:

1. *Intracranial neoplasms:*
   Optic nerve glioma
   Acoustic nerve neuroma
   Multiple meningioma.

2. *Intraspinal neoplasms:*
   Meningioma
   Neurofibroma
   Glioma.

3. *Peripheral nerve neoplasms:*
   Neurofibroma — a proportion of which become sarcomatous.

Clinical features (type 2)
Skin and skeletal manifestations are absent.
Eighth nerve tumours often occur *bilaterally*.
Other intracranial and intraspinal neoplasms are common (as above).

NEUROCUTANEOUS SYNDROMES

NEUROFIBROMATOSIS *(continued)*

Diagnosis

A family history is obtained in over 50% of patients. In type 1, the cutaneous manifestations are characteristic, though they may be extremely mild with only café au lait spots (more than 6 in an individual is diagnostic). As a rule, the more florid the cutaneous manifestations the less likely is there nervous system involvement. CT scanning, MRI and myelography may be necessary when nervous system involvement is suspected.

Treatment

Plexiform neuromas may be removed for cosmetic reasons. The management of intracranial and intraspinal tumours has already been discussed.

TUBEROSE SCLEROSIS

Incidence: 1:30 000.

Autosomal dominant inheritance.

Characterised by skin lesions, epilepsy and occasionally mental retardation.

Pathology

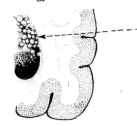

An embryological disorder.

Hard gliotic 'tubers' arise anywhere within the hemisphere but commonly around the ventricles. Projection into the ventricles produces a typical appearance like 'dripping candle wax'.

Tubers in the brain result from astrocytic overgrowth with large ⟶ vacuolated cells and loss of surrounding myelin.

Transition may occur from gliosis to a subependymal astrocytoma.

As well as skin lesions, primitive renal tumours and cystic lung hamartomas occur.

Clinical features

Skin manifestations

The cutaneous lesions are characteristic — adenoma sebaceum, a red raised papular-like rash over the nose, cheeks and skin, appears towards the end of the 1st year, though occasionally as late as the 5th year.

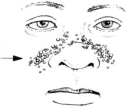

Depigmented areas on the trunk resembling vitiligo are common.

Fibromas and café au lait spots occur occasionally.

Neurological manifestations: — Mental retardation is present in 60% of patients, though the onset and its recognition may be delayed.

Seizures occur in almost all patients, often as early as the 1st week of life. Attacks are initially focal motor and eventually become generalised. The response to anticonvulsants is variable.

Intracranial neoplasms — astrocytomas — arise from tubers usually close to the ventricles and may result in an obstructive hydrocephalus.

Neoplasia: — Renal carcinoma occurs in 50% of patients. Retinal tumours (hamartomas) and muscle tumours (rhabdomyomas) are common, the latter often involving the heart.

Diagnosis:

The presence of epilepsy and adenoma sebaceum is diagnostic.

CT scan may show subependymal areas of calcium deposition. MRI shows uncalcified subependymal tubers. Other developmental abnormalities may be evident, e.g. microgyria.

Treatment:

Anticonvulsant therapy for epilepsy. Surgical removal of symptomatic lesions.

NEUROCUTANEOUS SYNDROMES

STURGE-WEBER SYNDROME

This disorder is characterised by a facial angioma associated with a leptomeningeal venous angioma. There is no clear pattern of inheritance.

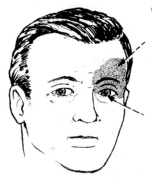

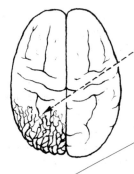

CAPILLARY NAEVUS
or 'port wine stain' usually involving forehead and eyelid conforming to the 1st or 1st and 2nd divisions of the trigeminal nerve.

EYE DISORDERS
are common -buphthalmos (congenital glaucoma), choroidal angioma.

Thickened leptomeninges, commonly ipsilateral to the facial naevus and full of abnormal vessels, overly an **ATROPHIC HEMISPHERE** with degenerative changes and vascular calcification usually most marked in the parieto-occipital vessels.

↓

EPILEPSY occurs in 90%, usually presenting in infancy.

HEMIPARESIS, HOMONYMOUS HEMIANOPIA, occur in 30%.
BEHAVIOURAL DISORDER AND MENTAL RETARDATION occur in 50%.

Skull X-ray shows parallel linear calcification (tram-line sign) and CT scan, in addition, shows the associated atrophic change. Angiography demonstrates dilated deep cerebral veins with decreased cortical drainage. Arteriovenous and dural venous sinus malformations are present in 30%.

Treatment

Intractable epilepsy may require lobectomy, or even hemispherectomy. Some recommend early excision of the surface lesion, but the rarity of the condition prevents thorough treatment evaluation.

VON HIPPEL-LINDAU DISEASE

An autosomal dominant disorder in which haemangioblastomas are found in the cerebellum, spinal canal and retina, and are associated with a number of visceral pathologies:
– Renal angioma
– Renal cell carcinoma
– Phaeochromocytoma
– Pancreatic adenoma/cyst
– Erythrocytosis.

Any of the above may produce signs and symptoms.
Retinal haemangioblastoma is seen on fundoscopy — — — — — — — — — — →
and may produce sudden blindness. These often produce the earliest clinical manifestation of disease. Confirm with fluorescin angiography and treat with cryotherapy or photocoagulation.

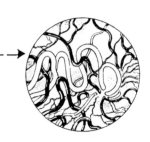

Cerebellar haemangioblastoma presents with progressive ataxia. Compression of the fourth ventricle may cause hydrocephalus with a subsequent rise in intracranial pressure.

Spinal canal haemangioblastoma — intradural or intramedullary lesion presenting with signs and symptoms of cord or root compression.
Supratentorial haemangioblastomas are exceedingly rare.
In long-term survivors, renal carcinoma and phaeochromocytoma are the principal causes of death.
Treatment: depends on symptomatology.

540 **ATAXIA TELANGIECTASIA** — see page 530.

FURTHER READING

ADAMS, J.H., CORSELLIS, J.A.N. and DUCHEN, L.W. (1984) Greenfield's Neuropathology. 4th Edition, Edward Arnold, London.

AMINOFF, M.J. (ed) (1989) Neurology and General Medicine. Churchill Livingstone, Edinburgh.

ASBURY, A.K., McKHANN, G.M. and McDONALD, W.I. (eds) (1986) Diseases of the Nervous System (2 vols). W.B. Saunders & Co. Philadelphia.

BARNETT, H.J.M., STEIN, B.M., MOHR, J.P. and YATSU, F.M. (eds) (1986) Stroke (2 vols). Churchill Livingstone, Edinburgh.

BRODAL, A. (1981) Neurological Anatomy. 3rd Edition, Oxford University Press.

JENNETT, W.B. and TEASDALE, G.M. (1981) Management of Head Injuries. Davis, Philadelphia.

ROWLAND, L.P. (ed) (1989) Merritt's Textbook of Neurology. 8th Edition, Lea & Febiger, Philadelphia, London.

RUSSELL, D.S. and RUBINSTEIN, L.J. (1977) Pathology of Tumours of the Nervous System. 4th Edition, Edward Arnold, London.

MILLER, J.D. (ed) (1987) Northfield's Surgery of the Central Nervous System. 2nd Edition, Blackwell, Oxford.

WILKINS, R.H. and RENGACHARY, S.S. (eds) (1985) Neurosurgery (3 vols). McGraw-Hill, New York.

INDEX